COMMUNICATION YEARBOOK 12

COMMUNICATION YEARBOOK 12

Edited by
JAMES A. ANDERSON

Routledge
Taylor & Francis Group
NEW YORK AND LONDON

First published in 1989

This edition first published in 2012
by Routledge
711 Third Avenue, New York, NY 10017

Simultaneously published in the UK
by Routledge
2 Park Square, Milton Park, Abingdon, Oxon, OX14 4RN

Routledge is an imprint of the Taylor & Francis Group, an informa business

British Library Cataloguing in Publication Data
A catalogue record for this book is available from the British Library

ISBN 13: 978-0-415-88009-1 (Set)
eISBN 13: 978-0-203-80297-7 (Set)
ISBN 13: 978-0-415-87320-8 (Volume 12)
eISBN 13: 978-0-203-85676-5 (Volume 12)

Publisher's Note
The publisher has gone to great lengths to ensure the quality of this reprint but points out that some imperfections in the original copies may be apparent.

Communication Yearbook/12

edited by
JAMES A. ANDERSON

Published Annually for the
International Communication
Association

SAGE PUBLICATIONS
The Publishers of Professional Social Science
Newbury Park London New Delhi

For information address:

SAGE Publications, Inc.
2111 West Hillcrest Drive
Newbury Park, California 91320

SAGE Publications Ltd.
28 Banner Street
London EC1Y 8QE
England

SAGE Publications India Pvt. Ltd.
M-32 Market
Greater Kailash I
New Delhi 110 048 India

Printed in the United States of America

Library of Congress: 76-45943
ISBN 0-8039-3348-7

FIRST PRINTING 1989

CONTENTS

Preface 11

SECTION 1: DISCOURSE AND RELATIONSHIPS

1. **Structures of Discourse and Structures of Power**
Teun A. van Dijk 18

Commentaries

Power, Discourse, and Ideology:
The Micropractices of Common Sense
Leonard C. Hawes 60

The Irrationality of Power
Ruth Wodak 76

2. **Coherence: A Meaningful Adhesive for Discourse**
Kathy Kellermann and Carra Sleight 95

Commentaries

On Coherence Judgments and Their Multiple Causes:
A View from the Message-Variable Paradigm
James J. Bradac 130

About Coherence
Sally Jackson and Scott Jacobs 146

3. **A Dialectical Analysis of the Tensions, Functions and Strategic Challenges of Communication in Young Adult Friendships**
William K. Rawlins 157

Commentaries

Further Dialectics: Strangers, Friends,
and Historical Transformations
David R. Maines 190

What Is Friendship? A Hermeneutical Quibble
Allen Scult 203

4. **Second-Guessing Theory: Review and Extension**
Dean E. Hewes and Maudie L. Graham 213

Commentaries

On Second-Guessing the Theory of Second-Guessing:
A Comment
Michael E. Roloff 249

Second-Guessing Second-Guessing: Yet Another Comment
Gerald R. Miller 266

SECTION 2: INTERCULTURAL RELATIONSHIPS AND CULTURAL IDENTITY

5. **Intercultural Communication Revisited: Conceptualization, Paradigm Building, and Methodological Approaches**
Fred L. Casmir and Nobleza C. Asuncion-Lande 278

Commentary

Ceteris Paribus in the Global Village: A Research Agenda for Intercultural Communication Theory Building
William J. Starosta 310

6. **Culture and the Development of Interpersonal Relationships**
William B. Gudykunst 315

Commentaries

Uncertainty in Interpersonal Relationships: A Predicted Outcome Value Interpretation of Gudykunst's Research Program
Michael Sunnafrank 355

Culture and Interpersonal Relationship Development: Some Conceptual Issues
Stella Ting-Toomey 371

7. **Cultural Identity and Modes of Communication**
Jan Servaes 383

Commentaries

The Relationship Between Cultural Identity and Modes of Communication
Cees J. Hamelink 417

Poststructuralist Concepts in Culture and Communication
Syed A. Rahim 427

SECTION 3: TECHNOLOGY AND COMMUNICATION SYSTEMS

8. **Issues and Concepts in Research on Computer-Mediated Communication Systems**
Ronald E. Rice 436

Commentaries

Classifying Mediated Communication Systems
Carrie Heeter 477

Commentary on Issues and Concepts in Research on Computer-Mediated Communication Systems
Jerome Johnston 490

9. **Designing Communication Systems for Human Systems: Values and Assumptions of "Socially Open Architecture"**
Stephen R. Acker 498

Commentaries

Interactive Communication Systems, Values, and the Requirement of Self-Reflection
Eric S. Fredin 533

Toward an Open Architecture and User-Centered Approach to Media Design
Diana Gagnon 547

SECTION 4: MEDIA CULTURAL STUDIES

10. **The Return of the "Critical" and the Challenge of Radical Dissent: Critical Theory, Cultural Studies, and American Mass Communication Research**
Hanno Hardt 558

Commentaries

Cultural Studies: From Old World to New World
Farrell Corcoran 601

Critical Theory and Empirical Critique in Mass Communication Research: Some Methodological Considerations
Slavko Splichal 618

SECTION 5: ORGANIZATIONS AND GIFTS

11. **One-Way Communication Transfers in Loosely Coupled Systems**
Larry Davis Browning and Sheila C. Henderson 638

Commentaries

Social Indicators of One-Way Transfers in Organizations
Kenneth E. Boulding 670

One-Way Transfers and Organizational Cohesion
Karl E. Weick and J. Douglas Orton 675

Index 688

About the Editor 695

About the Authors 696

THE INTERNATIONAL COMMUNICATION ASSOCIATION

The *Communication Yearbook* series is sponsored by the International Communication Association, one of several major scholarly organizations in the communication field. It is composed of 2,500 communication scholars, teachers, and practitioners.

Throughout its 40-year history, the Association has been particularly important to those in the field of communication who have sought a forum where the behavioral science perspective was predominant. The International Communication Association has also been attractive to a number of individuals from a variety of disciplines who hold communication to be central to work within their primary fields of endeavor. The Association has been an important stimulant to the infusion of behavioral concepts in communication study and teaching, and has played a significant role in defining a broadened set of boundaries of the discipline as a whole.

The International Communication Association is a pluralist organization composed of ten subdivisions: Information Systems, Interpersonal Communication, Mass Communication, Organizational Communication, Intercultural and Development Communication, Political Communication, Instructional and Developmental Communication, Health Communication, Philosophy of Communication, and Human Communication Technology.

In addition to *Communication Yearbook*, the Association publishes *Human Communication Research, Communication Theory,* the *ICA Newsletter*, and *ICA Directory*. Several divisions also publish newsletters and occasional papers.

PREFACE

This volume of *Communication Yearbook* was developed with separate emphases on interpersonal and intercultural studies. Mediated, organizational, and technology interests are also represented. This preface is charged with the responsibility of illuminating the central themes of the chapters contained herein. In this volume, our authors pursue issues in relationships, the interpretation of texts, the construct of culture and that of technology, and the course of development in scholarship. My comments follow this list.

RELATIONSHIPS

Four authors (van Dijk, Rawlins, Gudykunst, and Browning) and their commentators (Hawes, Wodak, Maines, Scult, Sunnafrank, Ting-Toomey, Weick, Boulding, and Orton) address the nature of the relationship in varying ways. van Dijk investigates the relationship from the perspective of power and its instantiation in discourse and text production. Power is given a clear empirical trace. Wodak, in her following commentary, shows how family and other social practices develop power as a relational resource in which individuals can order themselves vis-à-vis one another (see also Servaes's discussion of power in Chapter 10). She demonstrates the naturalized and irrational character of this resource in her analysis of the realization of anti-Semitism in Austrian newspapers and Viennese conversations. Hawes, for his part, works the articulation between societal macropractices and the micropractices of conversation as together they create the possibility and expression of power.

Rawlins and his commentators, Maines and Scult, use the peculiar nature of friendship to investigate the relationship construct as a moment-by-moment construction, albeit with a history and ideological inertia, but still in constant danger of collapse. The construction is maintained in an effortful management of strategies and tactics on a dialectical field of change. When that management fails, as Maines points out, friendship can become a ready site of violence. Maines goes on to show that friendship is a rather recent relational practice depending on the presence of strangers for its full expression. The stranger, as a continuous presence, is a phenomenon of the city rather than the community. Further, modern privatization and post-modern fragmentation have loaded current friendships with the dilemma of intimacy and distance. Scult pursues friendship as a necessary condition for the practice of good judgment, as such judgment requires the human consciousness to come to and realize an understanding of the other. Scult seeks to extract Rawlins's moral vision of friendship that Scult claims underlies the analysis.

Using the theories of social penetration and uncertainty reduction, Gudykunst posits the essence of a relationship as knowledge about the other. A relationship gains in power and intimacy as the breadth and depth of knowledge, reciprocal or not, is increased. Having claimed knowledge as the center, the course of a relationship can be traced according to the influences that would facilitate or impede circulation of information. For Gudykunst, the variations of culture are part of those influences. Knowledge, of course, invokes prediction and control, which places the relationship in the most primitive of survival needs. This theme is picked up and made explicit in Sunnafrank's alternative formulation within predicted-outcomes-value theory which adds the proviso that the work of uncertainty reduction needs to be seen as worth the effort. Ting-Toomey, however, seems to doubt that increasing certainty is an adequate explanation. She offers a reciprocal management of demands for certainty *and* uncertainty, among many other pairings, as the manner in which we know a relationship exists and flourishes.

Finally, in this four-chapter tour of the relationship, Browning and Henderson call into question both reward and reciprocity as the limiting characteristics of relationships by examining, in the special arena of information (rather than goods), the genuineness of gifts (or one-way transfers). The clarity of the vision of a relationship as an economic exchange (or a psychological demand for reward) is significantly blurred in their reported episodes of risk-taking without personal gain—the altruistic gift. Browning and Henderson argue that the giving of gifts can be, but is not necessarily, an exchange. In some ways, then, a relationship can be characterized by the practice of gifting. Weick and Orton point out, however, that it is a highlighted characteristic in what is otherwise an overdetermined practice of exchange. Nevertheless, gifts confound, obligate, and bind individuals in ways that exchange cannot. For Boulding, gifting is a sign of an integrative social system in which there is a mutual recognition of obligation, the performance of which may well be asynchronous.

The 12 articles that I have collected in this section address the relationship within the contexts of widely separated issues. Nonetheless, their juxtaposition demonstrates that the assumptive or explicit formulation of the relational construct is an important empowering move. How could social penetration, uncertainty reduction, or predicted-outcomes-value theory deal with an altruistic gift of information? What sustains the dialectical field of friendship? Where is the naturalized resource of power in the practices of gift? One fascination with these articles, even beyond their separate identities and worth, has to be in the differential consequences of this empowering move. The authors represent a range of argument that itself is impressive.

TEXTS

Two sets of authors, Kellermann and Sleight and Hewes and Graham, continue what is a discipline-wide attempt to unravel the relationship between the text (used in the most generic sense) and the auditor (a text receiver/interpreter of any sort). Both right what Miller sees as a long-standing fault in our research by placing the emphasis on the auditor. Kellermann and Sleight engage the relationship within the context of textual coherence and, I think, show the internal conflicts that the analyst faces as the field moves from the notion of the text as a meaning-delivery system to that of the text as an interpretive resource. Kellermann and Sleight are considerably closer to the latter as they conclude that coherence is a judgment by the auditor that can be made, even if the text is incomprehensible (e.g., in an unknown language). They also conclude that this judgment is dependent on the consonance between text and interpretive schemata and that the proper interpretive schemata can be cued by textual qualities. This argument appears to use a recalcitrant computer metaphor (one that will probably respond to its instructions) to solve the problem of how much interpretive freedom to grant to the auditor. Jackson and Jacobs, in their commentary on this issue, point out that neither Kellermann and Sleight, nor themselves, in their modeling alternative, nor the field in general has dealt with the ontology of interpretation; although nearly everyone claims it. In his commentary, Bradac concludes that by granting triggering cues to the text, Kellermann and Sleight remain "squarely in the message-variable paradigm" (p. 421). Bradac, interestingly, also questions the ecological validity of coherence judgments, puzzling if they might occur only in the expert mind.

Hewes and Graham, along with their commentators, Miller and Roloff, also struggle with the issue of the boundaries of text and interpretation. Hewes and Graham look at an interpretive process they call "second-guessing," which they attribute to the auditor, but they wonder (à la Kellermann and Sleight) what textual cues invoke this interpretive process. They simplify their problem by holding second-guessing to be a learned skill, sociologically located in human experience, and motivated by the "basic human need to reduce uncertainty" (p. 223). Hewes and Graham, therefore, have made, at least, an initial move at the ontology of this interpretive process. Their move comes in for some criticism by Miller who wonders if the result does represent some ideological commitment to an academic style of reasoning—a question that aligns with Bradac's foregoing comment. Roloff indicates, however, that Hewes and Graham are describing a strategic, rather than merely active, auditor.

As we refocus on the auditor after decades of research which privileged the text, I sense an uncertainty as to how much the analyst can let go of the security of the message-driven position in the exploration of the more chaotic interpretation one. Kellermann and Sleight don't go very far according to their commentators. Hewes and Graham are more daring, but quite forthrightly point out the precautions they have taken to not lose their way back. As an example of this concern, Kellermann and Sleight's use of schemata can be seen as an attempt to locate a cognitive text amenable to all the traditional forms of analysis between the external text and the auditor. The understanding of the interpretive process, then, is simplified in a traditional analysis of the content of these cognitive texts. Hewes and Graham move us more closely to the cognizing auditor but restrict interpretation to socially normative outcomes—what a text really says. Our collective struggle with interpretation is well-reflected in these two works.

CULTURE

The authors also struggle with the nature of culture. For Casmir and Asuncion-Lande, culture is a relational process that (ultimately) promotes survival. Gudykunst sees culture as a set of characteristics that affects behavioral performances. A given culture is defined in the particular collection. Servaes sees culture as the "normative context" that "mediates all human perceptions." Our commentators, too, take strongly different positions: Hamelink, commenting on Servaes, argues a very liberal position of each culture having multiple expressions among which individuals may move. Hawes, developing his position on power, takes the Althusserian ideological apparatus stance that accepts Hamelink's differences but fixes them in a hegemonic relationship and restricts individual movement.

The differences in definition are, of course, required by the different claims these authors wish to make. One cannot get to Gudykunst's analysis from Servaes's definition or make an easy claim to a cultural identity from a collection of traits. The utilitarian nature of these different definitions is more adequately shown in the commentary by Rahim (of Servaes) and by Starosta (of Casmir and Asuncion-Lande).

TECHNOLOGY

If we consider technology as the devices, practices, and codes that define and regulate these devices and practices, and the knowledge we claim about all three, then the authors present an enlightened view from the usual fixation on the devices alone. Rice's analysis of the research opportunities and requirements in computer-mediated communication systems clearly lays out the broad scope required. His commentators, Heeter and Johnson, with their emphasis on separate elements, show the value of working figures against the background of the larger picture. Acker, in his analysis of socially open architecture, takes on the interaction of these multiple elements in a specific concern for design. Equally important, Acker and commentators, Gagnon and Fredin, re-present the user/consumer as not only an active participant but also the point of actualization at which technology comes into view. These three authors are not of one thought on this cognizing and creating user, just as the authors are not of one mind on the cognizing auditor, but they all represent the same movement in the field.

SCHOLARSHIP

While all authors practice it, Hardt, Corcoran, Splichal, and Casmir/Asuncion-Lande directly address scholarship in communication. A connecting theme in all four of these articles is that we must have a good grasp of the past to understand where we presently stand. A singular interest in only the current fails to see the continuing idea in the dazzle of that idea's latest conceptualization. While there is some value in the ingenuous excitement that can result, the real loss is in the failure to see the value of the work that went before.

Hardt and his commentators, Corcoran and Splichal, in their combined analysis of the precedences and current advances of cultural studies in the United States, provide a useful critique of the epistemic, ideological, economic, and professional instrumentalities of scholarly camps. Certainly the epistemic innovation that can be sustained by a line of thought is not the sole reason for, and it may not even be central to, its ascendancy in the intellectual community.

ACKNOWLEDGMENTS

My first thanks must go to the authors and commentators who produced these original works in a painfully short time. While they draw on their extended history of study, their commitment to the intensity of effort required calls for our recognition. My thanks to the many reviewers who provided advice and counsel, especially Dennis Alexander, Douglas Birkhead, Yuro Dissanayake, David Eason, Susan Tyler Eastman, Richard Rieke, and Mary Strine. Alexis Olds has been the perfect editorial associate, and the University of Utah's Department of Communication continues its unflagging support.

SECTION 1

DISCOURSE AND RELATIONSHIPS

1 Structures of Discourse and Structures of Power

TEUN A. VAN DIJK
University of Amsterdam

This chapter examines some of the relationships between discourse and social power. After a brief theoretical analysis of these relationships, we review some of the recent work in this new area of research. Although we draw upon studies of power in several disciplines, our major perspective is found in the ways power is enacted, expressed, described, concealed, or legitimated by text and talk in the social context. We pay special attention to the role of ideology, but unlike most studies in sociology and political science, we formulate this ideological link in terms of a theory of social cognition. This formulation enables us to build the indispensable theoretical bridge between societal power of classes, groups, or institutions at the macro level of analysis and the enactment of power in interaction and discourse at the social micro level. Thus our review of other work in this field focuses on the impact of specific power structures on various discourse genres and their characteristic structures.

THE discourse analytical theory that forms the background of this study presupposes, but also extends, my earlier work on discourse (e.g., van Dijk, 1977, 1980, 1981; van Dijk & Kintsch, 1983), as well as other approaches of current discourse analysis (see the contributions in van Dijk, 1985a). That is, continuing my recent work on news discourse, and on racism in discourse, which will briefly be reviewed here, this chapter shows a more social approach to discourse, and bears witness to a more general development toward a critical study of text and talk in the social context.

Our discourse analytical framework and the obvious space limitations of a single chapter impose a number of restrictions. First, we presuppose but do

AUTHOR'S NOTE: For critical remarks and suggestions on the first version of this chapter, I am indebted to James Anderson, Charles Berger, Norman Fairclough, Cheris Kramarae, and Ruth Wodak.

Correspondence and requests for reprints: Teun A. van Dijk, University of Amsterdam, Department of General Literary Studies, Section of Discourse Studies, 210 Spuistraat, 1012 VT Amsterdam, The Netherlands.

Communication Yearbook 12, pp. 18-59

not discuss or review current work on the more general relationships between power and language, which has been the focus of several recent studies (Kramarae, Shulz, & O'Barr, 1984; Mey, 1985). Our discussion focuses on discourse as a specific "textual" form of language use in the social context and only some of the sociolinguistic work that deals with the role of dominance or power in language variation and style (Scherer & Giles, 1979). Second, we must ignore much of the related field of the study of power in interpersonal communication, a field that has been aptly reviewed already by Berger (1985) (see also Seibold, Cantrill, & Meyers, 1985) as we are interested in social or societal power rather than in personal power. Third, we must regrettably limit ourselves to the role of power in "Western" cultures. Therefore, we neglect the insights into the role of power in other cultures obtained in some work in the ethnography of speaking (Bauman & Scherzer, 1974; Saville-Troike, 1982), or in the current work on intercultural communication. Fourth, feminist studies on male dominance and power in language have already been discussed (see the extensive bibliography of Kramarae, Thorne, & Henley, 1983), therefore, we limit ourselves to a brief review of research focusing on gender power and discourse. To further constrain the size of our review, few references will be made to the many interesting studies on the relationships between language, discourse, power, and ideology in several European and Latin American countries.

THE ANALYSIS OF POWER

The analysis of power in several disciplines has created an extensive literature. Some recent work includes studies by Dahl (1957, 1961), Debnam (1984), Galbraith (1985), Lukes (1974, 1986), Milliband (1983), Mills (1956), Therborn (1980), White (1976), and Wrong (1979), among many others. Most of this work is carried out within the boundaries of sociology and political science. It cannot be our task in this chapter to review or summarize this rich tradition. Therefore, we select a number of major properties of social power and reconstruct those within our own theoretical framework. It should be understood, however, that in our opinion the complex notion of power cannot simply be accounted for in a single definition. A full-fledged, interdisciplinary theory is necessary to capture its most important implications and applications. The properties of power that are relevant for our discussion may be summarized as follows:

(1) Social power is a property of the relationship between groups, classes, or other social formations, or between persons as social members. Although we may speak of personal forms of power, this individual power is less relevant for our systematic account of the role of power in discourse as social interaction.

(2) At an elementary but fundamental level of analysis, social power relationships are characteristically manifested in interaction. Thus we say that group A (or its members) has power over group B (or its members) when the real or potential actions of A exercise social control over B. Since the notion of action itself involves the notion of (cognitive) control by agents, the social control over B by the actions of A induces a limitation of the self-control of B. In other words, the exercise of power by A results in the limitation of B's social freedom of action.

(3) Except in the case of bodily force, power of A over B's actual or possible actions presupposes that A must have control over the cognitive conditions of actions of B, such as desires, wishes, plans, and beliefs. For whatever reasons, B may accept or agree to do as A wishes, or to follow the law, rules, or consensus to act in agreement with (the interests of) A. In other words, social power is usually indirect and operates through the "minds" of people, for instance by managing the necessary information or opinions they need to plan and execute their actions. Most forms of social power in our society imply this kind of "mental control," typically exercised through persuasion or other forms of discursive communication, or resulting from fear of sanctions by A in case of noncompliance by B with A's wishes. It is at this point that our analysis of the role of discourse in the exercise, maintenance, or legitimation of power becomes relevant. Note, however, that this "mental mediation" of power also leaves room for variable degrees of freedom and resistance of those who are subjected to the exercise of power.

(4) A's power needs a basis, that is, resources that socially enable the exercise of power, or the application of sanctions in case of noncompliance. These resources usually consist of socially valued, but unequally distributed attributes or possessions, such as wealth, position, rank, status, authority, knowledge, expertise, or privileges, or even mere membership in a dominant or majority group. Power is a form of social control if its basis consists of socially relevant resources. Generally, power is intentionally or unwittingly exercised by A in order to maintain or enlarge this power basis of A, or to prevent B from acquiring it. In other words, the exercise of power by A is usually in A's interest.

(5) Crucial in the exercise or the maintenance of power is the fact that for A to exert mental control over B, B must know about A's wishes, wants, preferences, or intentions. Apart from direct communication, for instance in speech acts such as commands, request, or threats, this knowledge may be inferred from cultural beliefs, norms, or values; through a shared (or contested) consensus within an ideological framework; or from the observation and interpretation of A's social actions.

(6) Total social control in contemporary Western societies is further limited by the field and the scope of power of power agents. That is, power agents may be powerful in only one social domain—politics, the economy, or education—or in specific social situations as in the classroom or in court. Similarly, the

scope of their actions may be limited to a few people or extend to a whole class or group of people or to specific actions. And finally, the powerful may be assigned special responsibilities in their exercise of power. Besides this form of power distribution, which also involves various forms of power sharing, there is the important dimension of resistance: Dominated groups and their members are seldom completely powerless. Under specific socioeconomic, historical, or cultural conditions, such groups may engage in various forms of resistance, that is, in the enactment of counterpower, which in turn may make the powerful less powerful, or even vulnerable, typically so in revolutions. Therefore, the enactment of power is not simply a form of a action, but a form of social interaction.

(7) The exercise and maintenance of social power presupposes an ideological framework. This framework, which consists of socially shared, interest-related fundamental cognitions of a group and its members, is mainly acquired, confirmed, or changed through communication and discourse.

(8) It should be repeated that power must be analyzed in relation to various forms of counterpower or resistance by dominated groups (or by action groups that represent such groups), which also is a condition for the analysis of social and historical challenge and change.

DISCOURSE CONTROL AND THE MODES OF DISCURSIVE REPRODUCTION

One important condition for the exercise of social control through discourse is the control of discourse and discourse production itself. Therefore, the central questions are: Who can say or write what to whom in what situations? Who has access to the various forms or genres of discourse or to the means of its reproduction? The less powerful people are, the less they have access to various forms of text or talk. Ultimately, the powerless have literally "nothing to say," nobody to talk to, or must remain silent when more powerful people are speaking, as is the case for children, prisoners, defendants, and (in some cultures, including sometimes our own) women. In everyday life, most people have active access as speakers only to conversation with family members, friends, or colleagues on the job. Occasionally, in more formal dialogues, they may speak to institutional representatives, or with job superiors, but in that case they have a more passive and reactive role. At the police station, in the courtroom, at the welfare agency, in the classroom, or in other institutions of the social bureaucracy, they are expected to speak, or to give information, only when requested or ordered to do so. For most formal, public, or printed discourse types (including those of the mass media) the less powerful are usually only recipients.

More powerful groups and their members control or have access to an increasingly wide and varied range of discourse roles, genres, occasions, and styles. They control formal dialogues with subordinates, chair meetings, issue commands or laws, write (or have written) many types of reports, books, instructions, stories, or various mass media discourses. They are not only active speakers in most situations, but they may take the initiative in verbal encounters or public discourses, set the "tone" or style of text or talk, determine its topics, and decide who will be participant or recipient of their discourses. It is important to stress that power not only shows "in" or "through" discourse, but is relevant as a societal force "behind" discourse. At this point, the relation between discourse and power is close, and a rather direct manifestation of the power of class, group, or institution, and of the relative position or status of their members (Bernstein, 1971-1975; Mueller, 1973; Schatzman & Strauss, 1972).

Power is directly exercised and expressed through differential access to various genres, contents, and styles of discourse. This control may be analyzed more systematically in terms of the forms of (re)production of discourse, namely, those of material production, articulation, distribution, and influence. Thus mass media organizations and their (often international) corporate owners control both the financial and the technological production conditions of discourse, for instance those of the newspaper, television, printing business, as well as the telecommunication and computer industries (Becker, Hedebro, & Paldán, 1986; Mattelart, 1979; Schiller, 1973). Through selective investments, budget control, hiring (and firing), and sometimes through direct editorial influence or directives, they may also partly control the contents or at least the latitude of consensus and dissent of most forms of public discourse. For the privately operated media that depend on advertising, this indirect control may also be exercised by large corporate clients and even by prominent (mostly institutional) news actors that regularly supply information on which the media depend. These same power groups also control the various modes of distribution, especially of mass media discourse, and therefore also partly control the modes of influence of public text and talk.

The production mode of articulation is controlled by what may be called the "symbolic elites," such as journalists, writers, artists, directors, academics, and other groups that exercise power on the basis of "symbolic capital" (Bourdieu, 1977, 1984; Bourdieu & Passeron, 1977). They have relative freedom, and hence relative power, in deciding about the discourse genres within their domain of power and determine topics, style, or presentation of discourse. This symbolic power is not limited to articulation per se, but also extends to the mode of influence: They may set the agendas of public discussion, influence topical relevance, manage the amount and type of information, especially who is being publicly portrayed and in what way. They are the manufacturers of public knowledge, beliefs, attitudes, norms, values, morals, and ideologies. Hence their symbolic power is also a form of ideological power. Despite the problems with the notion of "elite" (Domhoff & Ballard, 1968), we maintain this term to denote an extended concept (contrasted with Mills, 1956, for example) involving exclusive social control by a small group. That is, we claim that besides the political, military, and economic elites, the symbolic elites play an essential role in the ideological supporting framework for the exercise or maintenance of power in our modern, information and communication societies.

Because, however, most of these elites are managed by the state or private corporations, they too have constraints on their freedom of articulation that emerge in various properties of their discourse. The voice of the elite is often the voice of the corporate or institutional master. The interests and ideologies of the elites are usually not fundamentally different from those who pay or support them. Only a few groups (e.g., novelists and some academics) have the possibility to exercise counterpower, which still must be expressed within the constraints of publication. The dependence of the elite is typically ideologically concealed by various professional norms, values, or codes, for instance, by the widespread belief in "freedom of expression" in the mass media (Altheide, 1985; Boyd-Barrett & Braham, 1987; Davis & Walton, 1983; Downing, 1980; Fishman, 1980; Gans, 1979; Golding & Murdock, 1979; Hall, Hobson, Lowe, & Willis, 1980).

STRATEGIES OF COGNITIVE CONTROL AND IDEOLOGICAL REPRODUCTION

If most forms of discursive power in our society are of the persuasive type as claimed earlier, then, despite the essential and often ultimate control of the modes of production and distribution (especially for mass mediated discourse) the decisive influence on the "minds" of the people is symbolically rather than economically controlled. Similarly, recognizing the control expressed over the less powerful in the socioeconomic domain (money, jobs, welfare), a major component in the exercise and maintenance of power is ideological, and is based on various types of acceptance, negotiation, and challenge, and consensus. It is, therefore, crucial to analyze the strategic role of discourse and its agents (speakers, writers, editors, and so on) in the reproduction of this form of sociocultural hegemony. Given that the symbolic elites have major control over this mode of influence through the genres, topics, argumentation, style, rhetoric, or presentation of public text and talk, their symbolic power is considerable, albeit exercised within a set of constraints.

A New Approach to Ideology

Because the notion of ideology is crucial for our argument about the role of discourse in the enactment or legitimation of power, it deserves a few remarks, although it is impossible even to summarize the classical proposals and the current discussions on the subject (see Abercrombie, Hill, & Turner, 1980; Barrett, Corrigan, Kuhn, & Wolf, 1979; Brown, 1973; Centre for Contemporary Cultural Studies [CCCS], 1978; Donald & Hall, 1986; Kinloch, 1981; Manning, 1980). Despite the variety of approaches to the concept of ideology, it is generally assumed that the term refers to group or class "consciousness," whether or not explicitly elaborated in an ideological system, which underlies the socioeconomic, political, and cultural practices of group members in such a way that their (group or class) interests are (in principle, optimally) realized. Both the ideology itself and the ideological practices derived from it are often acquired, enacted, or organized through various institutions, such as the state, the media, education, or the church, as well as in informal institutions such as the family. Classical Marxist analyses suggest, more specifically, that the dominant ideology in a given period is usually the ideology of those who control the means of ideological reproduction, namely, the ruling class. This may imply that certain dominated groups or classes may develop biased conceptions of their socioeconomic position ("false consciousness"), which in turn may lead them to act against their own basic interests. Conversely, the dominant groups or classes tend to conceal their ideology (and hence their interests), and will aim to get their ideology generally accepted as a "general" or "natural" system of values, norms, and goals. In that case, ideological reproduction assumes the nature of consensus formation, and the power derived from it takes on a hegemonic form.

Ignoring many details and complexities, our analysis of ideology takes a somewhat different and more specific direction than traditionally crafted (see also van Dijk, 1987f). Although there are undeniably social practices and institutions that play an important role in the expression, enactment, or reproduction of ideology, we first assume that ideology "itself" is not the same as these practices and institutions. Rather, we assume that ideology is a form of social cognition, shared by the members of a group, class, or other social formation (see, for example, Fiske & Taylor, 1984, for a more general introduction to the study of social cognition). This assumption does not mean that ideology is simply a set of beliefs of attitudes. Their sociocognitive nature is more elemental. An ideology according to this analysis is a complex cognitive framework that controls the formation, transformation, and application of other social cognitions, such as knowledge, opinions, and attitudes, and social representations, including social prejudices. This ideological framework itself consists of socially relevant norms, values, goals, and principles, which are selected, combined, and applied in such a way that they favor perception, interpretation, and action in social practices that are in the overall interest of the group. In this way, an ideology assigns coherence among social attitudes, which in turn codetermine social practices. It should be stressed that ideological social cognitions are not systems of individual beliefs or opinions, but essentially those of members of social formations or institutions. Similarly, according to this analysis, we do not use terms such as "false" in order to denote specific "biased" ideologies. All ideologies (including scientific ones) embody an interest-dependent (re)construction of social reality. (One appropriate criterion for the evaluation of such a construction would be its relevance or effectiveness for the social practices of social formations and their members in the realization of their goals or interests.)

The acquisition of an ideology, however, is not just guided by the "objective interests" of each group or class; although on many occasions, and historically, these interests may eventually override other conditions of ideological (re)production. Therefore, discourse and communication, we suggested, play a central role in the (trans)formation of ideology. In that perspective, it is indeed crucial to examine who, and by what processes, controls the means or institutions of ideological (re)production, such as the media or education. Although the formation of the fundamental sociocognitive framework of ideology is a very complex process, it at least needs a basis of (true or false) beliefs. This chapter tries to show that discourse, and in particular discourse of powerful institutions and groups, is the essential social practice that mediates and manages these beliefs (Roloff & Berger, 1982). Contrary to most approaches to ideology in the social and political sciences, we aim at a more systematic sociocognitive analysis of ideological frameworks, and of the processes involved in their (trans)formation and application. This goal means that ideologies need to be spelled out in detail, and that it should be shown how such group cognitions influence social constructions of reality, social practices, and hence, the (trans)formation of societal structures. Similarly, we need an explicit analysis of the structures, strategies, and processes of discourse and its specific role in the reproduction of ideologies. In other words, much classical work on ideology derives from typical macroanalyses of society to the neglect of the actual structures and processes at the micro level of the operation of ideology. This global and superficial approach also prevents the establishment of the link between societal or group ideologies (and the power structures they determine, conceal, or legitimate) with concrete social practices of intra- or intergroup interaction, including the precise role of discourse in ideological (trans)formations.

Discourse and Ideological Reproduction

To form and change their minds, people make use of a multitude of discourses, including interpersonal ones, and of the information derived from them. Note, however, that the complexity of text processing and of attitude formation, of course, does not allow immediate transformations of public beliefs and opinions, let alone of highly organized attitudes and ideologies (Petty & Cacioppo, 1981; Roloff & Miller, 1980; van Dijk & Kintsch, 1983). And yet, it is the symbolic elite and its discourses that control the types of discourses, the topics, the types and the amount of information, the selection or censoring of arguments, and the nature of rhetorical operations. These conditions essentially determine the contents and the organization of public knowledge, the hierarchies of beliefs, and the pervasiveness of the consensus, which in turn are potent factors in the formation and the reproduction of opinions, attitudes, and ideologies (Burton & Carlen, 1979).

In the news media, this strategic control of knowledge is exercised through restricted topic selection, and more generally by specific reconstructions of social and political realities (Hall et al., 1980; Tuchman, 1978; van Dijk, 1987b, 1987c). This process is itself governed by a system of news values and professional ideologies about news and newsworthiness, which happen to favor attention for and the interests of various elite actors, persons, groups, classes, institutions, nations, or world regions (Galtung & Ruge, 1965). Preferential access and coverage (whether positive or negative) of news actors is one factor in the mass mediated reproduction of social power (Brown, Bybee, Wearden, & Murdock, 1982). The same is true in education, where the curriculum, textbooks, educational materials, and lessons are also governed by educational objectives, subjects, topics, and learning strategies that mostly happen to be consistent with the values or interests of the various power elite groups (Apple, 1979; Lorimer, 1984; Young, 1971). Therefore, we see that the symbolic elites that control the style and content of media and educational discourse are also those who have partial control of the mode of influence, and hence of ideological reproduction in society.

The symbolic elites, we suggested, are not independent of other, mostly economic and political, power groups (Bagdikian, 1983). There may be conflict and contradiction between the interests and, therefore, the ideologies of these respective power groups. These other power groups not only have direct or indirect means to control symbolic production, they have their own strategies for the manufacture of opinion. For the media, these strategies consist in the institutional or organizational supply of (favorable) information in press releases, press conferences, interviews, leaks, or other forms of preferred access to newsmakers. Journalistic routines are such that these preformulations are more likely to be reproduced than other forms of source discourse (Collins, Curran, Garnham, Scannell, Schlesinger, & Sparks, 1986; Gans, 1979; Tuchman, 1978; van Dijk, 1987b).

In education, the overall constraint of avoiding "controversial" issues censors most radical social and political views that are inconsistent with dominant sociopolitical ideologies. More concretely, state organizations or corporations may supply free educational materials, advertise in educational journals, and have other ways to influence teachers and textbook content (Domhoff, 1983).

Similarly, the power elites also have the access to measures to control dissent and resistance, for example, through selective hiring and funding, by subtle or more overt censorship, through defamation campaigns, and by other means to silence "radicals" and their media (Domhoff, 1983; Downing, 1984; Gamble, 1986). Thus in many western countries it is sufficient to be branded as a "communist," or as an opponent of our type of "freedom," or of similar dominant values, in order to be disqualified as a serious formulator of counterideologies. This is a potent strategy to keep the symbolic elite itself under control, both internally and externally. In other words, there is a broad array of economic, cultural, and symbolic strategies through which the various power groups may concurrently, though sometimes not without mutual conflict and contradiction, manage knowledge and information, convey dominant goals and values, and thereby provide the building blocks of dominant ideologies. The consensus-shaping power of these ideologies provides the conditions that make a "conspiracy" of these power groups unnecessary.

THE ANALYSIS OF POWER AND DISCOURSE

Within this very general framework of social power and the control of discourse, we may now focus more specifically on the many ways discourse is related to this form of social control.

Discourse Genres and Power

We begin our analysis with a typology of the ways power is enacted by discourse as a form of social interaction:

(1) Direct control of action is achieved through discourses that have directive pragmatic function (elocutionary force), such as commands, threats, laws, regulations, instructions, and more indirectly by recommendations and advice. Speakers often have an institutional role, and their discourses are often backed by institutional power. Compliance in this case is often obtained by legal or other institutional sanctions.

(2) Persuasive discourse types, such as advertisements and propaganda, also aim at influencing future actions of recipients. Their power is based on economic, financial, or, in general, corporate or institutional resources, and exercised through access to the mass media and onto widespread public attention. Compliance in this case is manufactured by rhetorical means, for example, by repetition and argumentation, but of course backed up by the usual mechanisms of market control.

(3) Beyond these prescriptive discourse forms, future actions may also be influenced by descriptions of future or possible events, actions, or situations; for instance, in predictions, plans, scenarios, programs, and warnings, sometimes combined with different forms of advice. The power groups involved here are usually professionals ("experts"), and their power basis often the control of knowledge and technology (Pettigrew, 1972). The rhetorical means often consist of argumentation and the description of undesired alternative courses of action. More implicitly, scholarly reports about social or economic developments may thus influence future action.

(4) Various types of sometimes widespread and, hence, possibly influential narrative, such as novels or movies, may describe the (un)desirability of future

actions, and may have recourse to a rhetoric of dramatic or emotional appeals, or to various forms of topical or stylistic originality. The power groups involved here form what we called the symbolic elites. A specific case of this class of discourses is news reports in the media, which not only describe current events and their possible consequences, but which essentially portray the actions, and represent the opinions of the political, economic, military, and social power elites. It is mainly in this way that the consensual basis of power is manufactured, and how the general public gets to know who has power and what the powerful want. This is a crucial condition for the development of the supporting ideological framework of power, but also for various forms of resistance ("know thine enemies").

This first typology shows that the discursive enactment of power is mostly persuasive. Powerful groups or institutions only rarely have to prescribe what the less powerful should do, although ultimately such directives may be decisive in controlling others, as is especially the case in state control. Rather, they argue by providing economic, political, social, or moral reasons, and by managing the control of relevant information. In this way, communication may be biased through selective release of information that is favorable to the power elites, or by constraining information that is unfavorable to them. The realization of these goals may be facilitated by various rhetorical or artistic means.

Levels of Discourse and Power

A second dimension goes beyond this simple typology of discourse genres and their contributions to social control. It features the various levels of discourse that may specifically enact, manifest, express, describe, signal, conceal, or legitimate power relations between discourse participants or the groups they belong to.

Thus as we have seen earlier, power may first be enacted at the pragmatic level through limited access, or by the control of speech acts, such as commands, formal accusations, indictments, acquittals, or other institutional speech acts. Second, in conversational interaction, one partner may control or dominate turn allocation, self-presentation strategies, and the control of any other level of spontaneous talk or formal dialogue. Third, selection of discourse type or genre may be controlled by more powerful speakers, for instance in the classroom, courtroom, or within the corporation: Sometimes stories of personal experiences are allowed, but more often than not, they tend to be censored in favor of the controlled discourse genres of the business at hand, for instance interrogations. Fourth, outside of everyday conversation, topics are mostly controlled by the rules of the communicative situation, but their initiation, change, or variation are usually controlled or evaluated by the more powerful speaker. The same is true for style and rhetoric.

Dimensions of Power

The analysis of power structures allows us to list other relevant categories, namely, those dimensions of power that may have an impact on discourse and its structures: The various institutions of power, the internal power structures of these institutions, power relations between different social groups, and the scope or domain of the exercise of power by (members of) these institutions or groups. Without a further analysis of these structures and dimensions of social power, we simply argue here that they are also manifested in the various structures of "powerful" text and talk.

In this list we first find the major power institutions, such as the government, parliament, state agencies, the judiciary, the military, big corporations, the political parties, the media, the unions, the churches, and the institutions of education. Each of these institutions may be associated with its specific discourse genres, communicative events, topics, styles, and rhetorics. Second, there is the usual hierarchy of position, rank, or status within these institutions and these imply different speech acts, genres, or styles, for example, those signaling authority and command.

Third, parallel and sometimes combined with the institutions, we have, group power relations, such as those between the rich and the poor, men and women, adults and children, white and black, nationals and foreigners, the highly educated and those who have little education, heterosexuals and homosexuals, believers and nonbelievers, the moderates and the radicals, the healthy and the sick, the famous and the unknown, and generally those between *Us* and *Them*. Both within institutional and in everyday, informal interaction, these power relations may be structurally enacted by the members of the respective dominant groups. As is the case for institutional members, members of dominant groups may derive their individually exercised power from the overall power of the group they belong to. The effect on discourse in these cases will be especially obvious in the unbalanced control of dialogue, turn taking, speech acts, topic choice, and style.

Fourth, the enactment of power may be analyzed as to its domain of action or scope and type of influence. Some institutions or their leading members may accomplish discursive acts that affect whole nations, states, cities, or large organizations, or they may affect life and death, health, personal freedom, employment, education, or the private lives of other people, whereas other institutions or their members have a less broad and a less serious impact on other people.

Finally, we may distinguish between the various kinds of legitimacy for these forms of social control, which may vary between total control imposed or maintained by force (as in a dictatorship, and in some domains also in a democratic system of government), on the one hand, and partial control sanctioned by an elite, by a majority, or on the other hand, by a more or less general consensus. These (gradual) differences reflect the possible sanctions of the powerful, as well as the acceptance or resistance of those subjected to the enactment of power.

These differences in the modes of legitimation are also manifest in different genres, topics, and styles of discourse. Discussion, argumentation, and debate, for example, are not characteristic of dictatorial discourse. Hence the importance of the amount and nature of discursive legitimation in these different sorts of power systems. It may be expected that each political system, viewed as an institutionalization of power, for instance by the state, is associated with its own characteristic orders or modes of discourse. Since the principles (norms, rules, values, goals) of legitimacy are embedded in an ideology, the processes of legitimation will also appear as discursive processes.

Different Approaches

With these various dimensions of power in mind, we should be able to make the next step and establish systematic links between these dimensions and the various structural dimensions of discourse. However, this may be done in different ways and from different, complementary perspectives. Thus the social scientist may start with an analysis of the dimensions of social power just mentioned and then examine through what discourses or discursive properties these power structures are expressed, enacted, or legitimated. This (macro) approach favors a more general and integrated analysis of various discourse genres and properties related to a class, institution, or group (for instance, the discourse of the legal system, or the patriarchal power of men over women). On the other hand, the sociolinguist will usually start with an analysis of specific properties of language use or discourse, and try to show how these may vary, or depend on, different social positions, relations, or dimensions, for example, those of class, gender, ethnic group, or situation. This perspective will usually pay more detailed attention to linguistic properties of text and talk, and take a more general view of the various social "circumstances" of such properties.

We opt for an approach that combines the advantages of these two alternatives, namely the analysis of discursive (sub)genres and communicative events in social situations (Brown & Fraser, 1979). Such a "situation analysis" requires an integration of both discourse analysis and social analysis. Through an interdisciplinary study of everyday conversations, classroom dialogues, job interviews, service encounters, doctors' consultations, court trials, boardroom meetings, parliamentary debates, news reporting, advertising, or lawmaking, among many other communicative events, we are able to assess both the relevant discourse structures and the relevant structures of dominance and control in the social context. That is, understanding these communicative genres requires an analysis of participant representation, interactional strategies, turn allocation, topic and code selection, stylistic registers, rhetorical operations, and also an analysis of the roles, relations, rules, norms, or other social constraints that govern the interaction of participants as social group members. In this way, we capture both the properties and processes of text and talk, and the micromechanisms of social interaction and societal structure. Also, this level and scope of analysis allows a sociocognitive assessment of knowledge, opinions, attitudes, ideologies, and other social representations that exercise the cognitive control of acting agents in such situations. Finally, these social microstructures (e.g., the lesson) may in turn be related (e.g., by comparison or generalization) to relevant social macrostructures, such as institutions (e.g., the school, the education system, and their ideologies) and overall social relations (e.g., the dominance of whites over blacks) (Knorr-Cetina & Cicourel, 1981).

POWER IN DISCOURSE: A REVIEW

In the previous sections, I have given a brief theoretical analysis of the notion of power and its links with discourse and communication. We have witnessed how the powerful have recourse to many strategies that allow them to control the material and symbolic production of text and talk, and, therefore, part of the cognitive processes that underlie the cognitive management and the manufacturing of consent from the less powerful. On several occasions, this discussion has mentioned some properties of discourse that are specifically affected by this process of (re)productive control, for instance, conversational turn taking, topics, and style. In the remainder of this chapter, we analyze in more detail how power is actually expressed, signaled, reproduced, or legitimated in various structures of text and talk. Whereas the previous sections focused on various social strategies of discourse and communication control, we will now systematically examine the discursive strategies that implement such (inter)actions, and briefly review empirical studies that show power "at work" in text and talk. We will organize our discussion around a few selected discourse types, namely, subgenres or communicative events, that also embody typical social relations, including specific power relations. In this discussion, a reinterpretation of research will sometimes be necessary, for instance, when the notion of power is not used as such. We begin with various sorts of spoken, dialogical discourse, and then discuss written types of text. We will focus on social power and disregard types of individual power, influence, or status in interpersonal communication (see, Berger, 1985 for a review of this work, and Brooke & Ng, 1986, and Falbo & Peplau, 1980, for empirical studies on interpersonal influence).

Conversation

Although the analysis of conversation generally presupposes that speakers have equal social roles (Sacks, Schegloff, & Jefferson, 1974; Atkinson & Heritage, 1984; McLaughlin, 1984), it is obvious that group and institutional membership of speakers, and in general social inequality, introduce differences in control over the ongoing dialogue. These differences appear, for instance, in talk between men and women, adults and children, whites and blacks, the rich and the poor, or between the more or less educated. It is assumed that such control by the more powerful speaker may extend to turn allocation or appropriation, speech act choice, topic selection and change, and style. The enactment of this control, however, need not be static, but may be dynamically negotiated or challenged by the less powerful speakers. In other words, talk is continuously contextualized by signaling various conditions or constraints of the social situation in general, and by the social relationships between the speech participants, in particular. And although it makes sense to make a distinction between everyday, personal, or informal talk, on the one hand, and, on the other hand, formal, institutional discourse, it should be stressed that informal or private discourse may be imbued with formal and institutional constraints. Conversely, institutional discourse also may be informal and an everyday accomplishment among other social practices.

Conversation Between Parents and Children

One of the more obvious power differences in many cultures is that between parents and children. Although there is important cultural variation (Snow & Furgeson, 1977), and differences between fathers and mothers (Gleason & Geif, 1986), parental control is generally enacted in parent-child talk in many ways: "The low status of children in stratified societies can keep them silent, forbid them to initiate or discuss certain topics, prevent them from interrupting, or require them to use a special deferential variety of speech" (Ervin-Tripp & Strage, 1985, p. 68).

As these and other authors show in detail, parents may also control child behavior more directly, for example, through scolding, threatening, directing, or correcting children in talk. More indirect forms of action control in parent-child talk may take the form of advice, requests, or inducement through promises. These differences in parental control in talk have often been related to class differences (Cook-Gumperz, 1973). Relevant to our discussion of social power, social representations of power are acquired and displayed rather early, as through different forms of discursive politeness and deference, or through verbal power play and ritual (Bavelas, Rogers, & Millar, 1985; Ervin-Tripp, O'Connor, & Rosenberg, 1984; Labov, 1972; Lein & Brenneis, 1978).

Conversation Between Women and Men

The power differences between women and men and their manifestation in language have received extensive attention, especially during the last decade, and by feminist researchers (Eakins & Eakins, 1978; Kramarae, 1980, 1983; Spender, 1980; Thorne & Henley, 1975; and Thorne, Kramarae, & Henley,

1983, who provide an extensive bibliography). Therefore, we mention only a few general conclusions of this important work, which in many respects has become paradigmatic for the analysis of power in language and communication, and focus on the more recent studies of gender power in discourse (for a brief review, see West & Zimmerman, 1985).

Although differences may sometimes be subtle and dependent on situation (Leet-Pellegrini, 1980), and on social position (Werner, 1983), it has been found that women generally "do more work" than men do in conversation, by giving more topical support, by showing more interest, or by withdrawing in situations of conflict (Falbo & Peplau, 1980; Fishman, 1983). Several studies document that men tend to interrupt women more often, especially at irregular turn transition places (Eakins & Eakins, 1978; Natale, Entin, & Jaffe, 1979; West & Zimmerman, 1983).

Some of the studies collected by Trömel-Plötz (1984) show that male dominance is not restricted to informal situations, such as the home, but also appears in public contexts, such as television talk shows, which are moderated mostly by men (see also Owsley & Scotton, 1984). For instance, women tend to get the floor less often than men do, and men talk longer, more often, and use long, complicated sentences and various types of pseudostructuring of conversational contributions.

Gender differences in talk may also be studied in a more general perspective as instances of "powerful" and "powerless" speech, which may be found in other social situations (Bradac & Street, 1986; Erickson, Lind, Johnson, & O'Barr, 1978), to which we turn next.

Racist Talk

What is true for the subordination of women in talk, also holds for discourse addressed to, or about blacks and other minority groups in many Western countries (Smitherman-Donaldson & van Dijk, 1987). White group power may also be exercised through verbal abuse and derogation of minority group members (Allport, 1954). Although there are many historical and literary sources that document the pervasiveness of racial slurs, there are few systematic studies of their usage and functions. Kennedy (1959) provides a brief list of "etiquette rules" for the ways blacks and whites should address each other in the period of Jim Crow racism in the United States. One of these rules was that blacks should never be addressed as "Mr.," "Mrs.," "Sir," or "Ma'am," but by first names only, whereas whites always must be addressed in the polite form. Although the last decades have seen much of this verbally expressed racism mitigated because of changing official norms and laws, racial slurs still exist in everyday white talk. Verbal derogation of blacks, as well as of Chinese, Italian, Mexican, or Puerto Rican Americans is common in the United States, and of Turkish, Moroccan, South Asians, Caribbean, and other minorities or immigrants in Western Europe (Helmreich, 1984).

Ethnic conflict may also be manifested in different speech styles that lead to misunderstanding and stereotyping (Kochman, 1981). Within a German project on language acquisition by immigrant workers, attention was paid to the ways these "Gastarbeiter" were addressed in terms of a perceived, simplified "foreigner German" (Dittmar & Stutterheim, 1985; Klein & Dittmar, 1979). Often, such talk by itself may signal superiority of the speakers and their group. This is an interesting specific case of the functions of linguistic accommodation and conflict in interethnic communication (Giles & Powesland, 1975; Giles & Smith, 1979; Gumperz, 1982a, 1982b).

Much recent research on prejudice and racism suggests that even if racist opinions, talk, and action have become more indirect and subtle in certain contexts, basic attitudes may not have changed very much (Barker, 1981; Dovidio & Gaertner, 1986; Essed, 1984). Greenberg, Kirkland, and Pyszczynski (1987) show that the use of racial slurs by experimental confederates against black subjects may activate such basic attitudes among white subjects and result in more negative evaluations of these black subjects. Among the conservative elites, racist discourse has taken a more "cultural" orientation during the last decade. Such discourse emphasize assumed cultural differences between in-groups and out-groups, and sometimes subtly advocates nationalist cultural autonomy of the dominant white group (Seidel, 1987a, 1987b).

In my own work on the expression of ethnic opinions and prejudice in everyday talk, such explicit racial slurs appear to be rare, both in the Netherlands and in California (van Dijk, 1984a, 1987a). However, the informal interviews on which my research is based are typically examples of talk with relative strangers (university students), and, therefore, such talk is likely to be heavily monitored by official norms of nondiscrimination. In fact, white people routinely express their knowledge of such norms, and elaborately affirm that whatever they may say about "foreigners" they do not mean to be racists.

Therefore, the overall strategy of talk about minorities is twofold. On the one hand, many white people express negative experiences and opinions about ethnic minority groups. On the other hand, however, this negative "other-presentation" is systematically balanced by positive self-presentation, namely, as tolerant, nonracist, understanding citizens. This overall strategy is implemented by many local strategies and tactics, such as apparent denials and concessions ("I have nothing against them, but . . ." "There are also good ones among them, but . . ." and so on), contrasts that emphasize group differences, competition, generally the us/them opposition ("We work hard, and they don't have to do anything"), and transfer ("I don't mind, but other people in the country, city, street, or department do"). Besides such semantic and rhetorical strategies of positive self-presentation, negative other-presentation is mainly implemented by argumentation and concrete storytelling. Stories are based one's own personal experiences, and, therefore, "true" and good "evidence" for negative conclusions. Most of these stories feature events and actions of minority groups that are perceived to violate dominant (white) norms, values, goals, and interests, but which also happen to substantiate current stereotypes and prejudices. Often, the news media are used to legitimate such stories and opinions, for instance by referring to minority crime "about which you read in the paper everyday." More subtly, conversational properties such as hesitations, repairs, and corrections provide insight into the underlying cognitive processes and monitoring in such talk. Lexical choice and the use of identifying pronouns and demonstratives also suggest social distance: "them," "those people," "those Turks (Mexicans, and so on)." In this way, everyday talk among white majority group members reproduces such prejudices within the ingroup, while at the same time verbally confirming group membership, and group goals and norms, which in turn are relevant in the maintenance of white group power.

Institutional Dialogue

Dialogues with and within institutions or organizations are forms of institutional interaction, and, therefore, also enact, display, signal, or legitimate a multitude of power relations (Pettigrew, 1973; Pfeffer, 1981). Participants in such interactions may follow context dependent rules and norms of interaction, but may also negotiate different roles or positions, including those of status, hierarchy, or expertise. Another difference with everyday, informal conversation is that institutional members are mostly professionals, experts "at work" (see also Coleman, 1984, 1985b). Let us examine some of the more prominent subgenres of institutional dialogue.

Job Interviews

Ragan (1983) showed that in job interviews power differences manifest themselves in what she calls "aligning actions," such as accounts, metatalk, side sequences, digressions, or qualifiers. Interviewers more often had recourse to strategies that control conversational pace and progress, such as formulations, metatalk, and metacommunicative digressions. Applicants, on the contrary, are more often engaged in justifying or explaining their behavior, for instance through accounts, qualifiers, and "you knows," even when these were unnecessary. This study complements earlier social psychological work on the (power) effect of language attitudes in job interviews, which shows that otherwise identical applicants may be discriminated against because of their foreign accent, for instance, by getting lower evaluations for higher-level jobs and higher evaluations for lower-level jobs (Kalin & Rayko, 1980).

In a series of experimental studies, Bradac and associates examined the role of powerful and powerless styles in job interviews (Bradac & Mulac, 1984). As in early studies of women's language, hesitations, and tag questions were found to characterize the powerless style (see also Bradac & Street, 1986). We shall see that similar results have been found in styles of courtroom talk.

Doctor-Patient Discourse

Doctor-patient discourse is just one specific example of medical discourse in general (Fisher & Todd, 1983, 1986; Freeman & Heller, 1987), which has often been criticized for a variety of reasons, including the abuse of power by medical practitioners. Edelman (1974), in a critical article, shows how the language of people in the helping professions, typically in psychiatry, in many ways conceals the real nature of their intentions and actions, which are geared toward the control of patients. In this way, direct power may be masked by the discourse of "helping," in which patients who have good reasons to be angry may be categorized as "aggressive." Such patients will be put in what is euphemistically called a "quiet room" instead of "solitary confinement." Similarly, the use of such terms as "predelinquent" may mean that professionals get carte blanche in the "treatment" of (mostly powerless, e.g., young, poor) people who have shown no sign of deviance. Professional power here combines with the power of class and age. Indeed, as we shall see next, power seldom comes alone: Institutional power is frequently enacted at the same time as group power derived from gender, class, race, age, subculture, or nationality (see also Sabsay & Platt, 1985).

West (1984) shows that the inherent social asymmetry in doctor-patient relationships is also displayed in their conversations, and that gender and race play a role here: Male doctors interrupt patients (especially black patients) much more often than the reverse, without any medical function or relevance; on the contrary, these interruptions make them miss important information. Female doctors, however, are interrupted more often by their (male) patients. Generally, in doctor-patient talk there is an imbalance in information exchange: Doctors initiate most questions and patients stutter when asking their few questions, with the exception of a specific type of conditional query. West concludes that, "Quantitative and qualitative evidence suggests that physicians stand in nearly godlike relation to their patients—as entities 'not to be questioned'" (West, 1984, p. 51). Formal expressions are used to address the doctor, whereas doctors tend to use the first names of patients, especially when the patients are black. Fisher and Todd (1983) also find an interaction between medical and gender power. They showed that female patients are subject to "friendly persuasion" by (male) practitioners to use birth control pills, while being kept uninformed about the pills' possible negative effects or about alternative forms of birth control.

In a critical analysis of clinical interviews, Mishler (1984) found discursive evidence for the domination of what he calls the "biomedical voice" of doctors, and concludes: "Typically, the voice of the lifeworld was suppressed and patients' efforts to provide accounts of their problems within the context of their lifeworld situations were disrupted and fragmented" (p. 190). Treichler, Frankel, Kramarae, Zoppi, and Beckman (1984) argue that the physician's focus on biomedical aspects hinders the full expression of the patient's concerns. Thus concerns readily expressed to a medical student were not included in the physician's medical records. Doctors are found to use irony in showing dismissal of the patient's complaints. Finally, just as for job interviews, social psychological work on language attitudes shows that doctors may evaluate their patients differently depending upon whether or not they have a dialect or sociolect accent (Fielding & Evered, 1980).

What has been found for general practitioners may be expected to be true for other medical professionals. Coleman and Burton (1985) studied control in dentist-patient consultations in Great Britain, and found that dentists control both verbal and nonverbal activity: Dentists talk 71% and patients 26% of the time, (assistants 3%). Dentists have more turns, and longer turns (4.6 versus 2.1 seconds). Obviously, control in this case takes a very literal form: Patients usually have their mouths open, but are still prevented from speaking in such a situation, and, therefore, have little to say in the first place. Compliance with dentists' power may also depend on fear of pain. Thus the authors found that dentists regularly respond to patients' reports by making no acknowledgment, by minimizing them as irrelevant, or by dismissing them as incorrect. As is the case for most professional forms of power, the major resource of dentist dominance is expertise (see also Candlin, Burton, & Coleman, 1980).

As noted earlier, power may derive from institutional organization and routinization. Medical power is a characteristic example. The results of the studies just reviewed should also be interpreted in that perspective. Thus Strong (1979) specifies some other factors that limit the freedom of patients in consultation discourse: Doctors use technical language (see also Coleman, 1985a); there are few doctors and many patients; doctors are organized and patients are usually not; doctors have high status; in some countries, there are no or few (affordable) alternatives for the public health service provided by doctors, and, therefore, little medical competition and reduced possibilities for second opinions. We see that the local enactment and organization of power in doctor-patient talk is intricately interwoven with more general social and institutional forms of control.

These findings are also relevant in counseling or admission interviews, in which professionals act as gatekeepers of institutions and may exert relevant group power on the differential conversational treatment of minority clients or candidates (Erickson & Shultz, 1982; Mehan, 1986). Similarly, in classroom talk, teachers may be expected to exercise control over students through a series of strategies: They decide about discourse type, they initiate and evaluate topics and question-answer sequences, they monitor student speech style, and generally control both the written and spoken discourses of the students. Unfortunately, although there is much work on classroom dialogues (Sinclair & Brazil, 1982; Stoll, 1983; Wilkinson, 1982), little specific attention is paid to these routine enactments of institutional power.

Discourse in Court

More than in most other institutional contexts, the enactment of power in court is systematically governed by explicitly formulated rules and procedures of dialogical interaction between the judge, the prosecution, defense counsel, and the defendant. Much work has been done on courtroom dialogues in the tradition of conversational analysis, but again, little attention has been paid to such social dimensions as power, control, or dominance (Atkinson & Drew, 1979). The stylistic power of highly technical jargon shared by the participating legal representatives may be internally balanced among these professionals, but ultimately further subordinates the defendant. The combined powers of indictment by the prosecution, judicial courtroom control, and final judgment may be expected to show in what court officials say and imply dominance toward the defendant, toward witnesses, and even toward the defense counsel. Conversely, whatever defendants, in their inherent position of subordination, may say, it "may be used against them," which places a special burden on their talk.

In court, the distribution of speaking turns and speech acts is strictly regulated. Unlike most other situations of dialogical interaction, defendants have the obligation to talk when requested to do so, and to answer questions with specific statements, such as simply "Yes" or "No" (Walker, 1982). Refusal to talk or to answer questions may be sanctioned as contempt of court. Harris (1984) examined how questions in court are used to control defendants or witnesses and found that question syntax appeared to be important for what will count as an appropriate response. He also found that information control is exercised by questioning sequences, rather than by long accounts, which also firmly establish the control of the questioner. Most questions are for yes/no questions that restrict possible answers because they contain already completed propositions. Thus questioning rules and strategies, as well as legal power, together regulate the choice of a restricted set of speech acts: Most questions ask for information or make accusations (see also Mead, 1985; Shuy, 1986). Obviously, these discursive methods of control in the courtroom may vary according to the procedures of direct or cross-examination (see also Adelswärd, Aronsson, Jönsson, & Linell, 1987).

Besides turn taking, sequencing, speech acts, and topic control, style may be an important feature of self-presentation and persuasion of defendants and witnesses, although these may not always be preserved in courtroom transcripts (Walker, 1986; see also Parkinson, Geisler, & Pelias, 1983). These strategies of interaction and impression formation in court were examined by Erickson, Lind, Johnson, & O'Barr (1978) in their influential study of powerful and powerless styles. These authors found that powerless style can be characterized by the frequent use of intensifiers, hedges, hesitation forms, and questioning intonation, whereas powerful style is marked by less frequent use of these features. Experiments suggest that powerful style results in greater attraction to the witness, independent of sex of witness or subject, but that powerful style leads to enhanced perceived credibility only when witness and subject are of the same sex (see also Bradac, Hemphill, & Tardy, 1981). In a later experimental study, these authors show that the evaluation of the defendants or witnesses may also depend on whether the defense counsel relinquishes control by letting them tell their own stories (Lind & O'Barr, 1979).

As in all cases already discussed, factors of class, gender, and race play a role, and may possibly reinforce or mitigate the subordination of the defendant. Thus Wodak (1984, 1985) shows that middle-class defendants are better able to build a positive image in court proceedings. They know the strategies of courtroom interactions, tell coherent stories, and mention plausible facts. Working-class defendants, however, appear to perform less successfully on these crucial tasks. Such class differences also appear in the way the judge addresses the defendant, for instance through forms of politeness, patience, understanding, and showing interest in the occupation of professional, middle-class defendants. On the other hand, Maynard (1985), in a study of plea bargaining, suggests that the discursive characterization of defendants in terms of specific categories (old, woman, minority) may sometimes be taken as arguments to dismiss a case. That is, unlike cases of discrimination, age, class, or race may sometimes be used to reduce the responsibility of the defendant. Maynard claims that knowledge of the social interaction (of justice) is needed to make conclusions about discrimination, and that general assumptions about unfair treatment of the less powerful in court may not always be warranted.

Whereas the enactment and reproduction of legal power surfaces most concretely in courtroom interaction, it also characterizes other types of legal and bureaucratic discourse, such as laws, contracts, regulations, and many other texts. Besides the power embodied in their pragmatic functions of legal directives, such texts also indirectly manifest power by their exclusive "legalese." This archaic lexical, syntactic, and rhetorical style not only symbolizes and reproduces a legal tradition, thus facilitating communication among legal professionals, but obviously excludes lay persons from effective understanding, communication, and, hence, resistance (Charrow, 1982; Di Pietro, 1982; Danet, 1980, 1984; Radtke, 1981).

Organizational Discourse

Discourse in business organizations has, unfortunately, led to fewer studies of details of dialogical interaction. Especially in "vertical" communication between bosses and their subordinates, such talk is obviously an enactment and expression of hierarchical power (McPhee & Tompkins, 1985). In their review of organizational communication, Blair, Roberts, & McKechnie (1985) found that managers spend 78% of their time with verbal communication; when leaders dominate leader-subordinate communications, subordinates react by deferring; and there is more self-disclosure upward than downward in the organization. Focusing more on the content of such talk Riley (1983) found in an analysis of interviews that power in organizations is expressed through signification, legitimation, and domination. Verbal symbols, such as (military) metaphors, myths, jokes, and legends, dominate the discussions, whereas game metaphors provide legitimation by expressing possible sanctions.

Power differentials in business may be expected to show in different forms of politeness, deference, and, hence, in forms of address (Brown & Levinson, 1978). Slobin, Miller, and Porter (1972) studied forms of address in business corporations and found that the first name is used primarily when subordinates are addressed by their superiors. Conversely, title and last name are used when talking to higher management, who communicate among themselves mostly on a first-name basis. These different forms of address appear to be more or less independent of age differences. The authors not only found, expectedly, more self-disclosure among fellow workers, but found nonreciprocal self-disclosure to immediate superiors (even when no first names are used). These results confirm the rules established by Brown and his associates (Brown & Gilman, 1960; Brown & Ford, 1972): The greater the status difference, the greater the tendency toward nonreciprocal address. However, unlike the findings by Brown et al., subordinates show more self-disclosure to bosses than the reverse. That is, the use of first names in business contexts is not always associated with greater familiarity, and vice versa.

Whereas organizational hierarchy and power may be directly enacted in commands, orders, instructions, or other directives, power may also be expressed by representation. Members in the organization may be expected to talk about daily events, and thus try to make sense of their lives. Such experiences are typically expressed in narrative. In one of the few studies of its kind, Kelly (1985) analyzed scripts and schemata of stories told by people at different levels of "high-tech" organizations. He found that many of these stories focused on the boss, and whether positive or negative, they emphasized the power structure and at the same time legitimated it.

Political Discourse

Since the rhetorical treatises of classical Greece and Rome, political discourse—and its persuasive power—have received much attention as a special object of study (Chaffee, 1975; Nimmo & Sanders, 1981; Seidel, 1985). Unlike most other discourse forms, political discourse may be relevant for all citizens. Its power derives both from this scope and from its various degrees of legitimacy. Few forms of oral discourse are as well known, routinely quoted, or distributed as widely through the mass media as that of top politicians, such as the president or prime minister. Especially in the United States, speeches and media performances of the president are both a prominent social or political event, and a preferred object of study (Hart, 1984; Lindegren-Lerman, 1983). This dominant presence in, and preferential access to, the media may be interpreted as a manifestation of political power.

In light of what we just assumed, we may expect many studies to deal with political discourse. This is indeed the case, but many of these studies focus on what is commonly called "political language," which mostly means specific lexical style (see Bergsdorf, 1983; Edelman, 1964; Guespin, 1976; Hudson, 1978; Shapiro, 1984). Thus ideologies have been studied through analysis of preferential use of specific words or concepts, typically so for extremist politicians of the left or the right (fascist or communist language). It is interesting, however, to go beyond the study of single words, and look into other discourse structures, of which some are even less in the control of the speaker, and therefore often more revealing of attitudes and ideologies (see also Guespin, 1976; Pecheux, 1975). Although only indirectly interested in the analysis of power, Atkinson (1984) investigated various properties of political oratory, such as the management of applause by political speakers, and the careful preparation of such performance by experts (for instance by taking speech lessons). Against the background of my remarks on gender and especially racial power, it is interesting to note that Atkinson found that applause is particularly likely after passages in which different outgroups are negatively discussed.

Institutional Texts

Whatever the power of directors, top politicians, corporate boards, professors, judges, or doctors in face-to-face discourse, their real power seems to have formal consequences only when somehow "fixed" in writing or print. Therefore, many types of formal dialogues, such as meetings, interviews, or debates, have a written counterpart in the form of minutes, protocols, or other official transcripts that define the "record" of the encounter, and are often the institutional or legal basis for any further action or decision making.

Institutional dialogues are often accompanied by various types of text, which function as guidelines or reference for the accomplishment of the spoken discourse. Thus most formal meetings involve a written agenda as well as various kinds of documents. Courtroom dialogue is related to many written texts, such as law texts, a formal indictment, written statements, witness reports, and a final judgment. Even in oral consultation, doctors may sometimes have recourse to medical handbooks and make notes, and the encounter is often closed after writing out a prescription or a referral to a specialist. Records in medical organizations play a vital role. School or university lessons are unthinkable without textbooks or a host of other written (or to be written) materials. In other words, most formal business, even when accomplished orally, requires written texts as its basis or its consequence. Thus texts are literally the consolidation of communicative power in most institutional contexts.

Written discourse is, for the most part, explicitly programmed or planned and, therefore, better controlled. In complex ways, this property has implications for the exercise of power. Whereas less monitored, face-to-face encounters allow the exercise of illegitimate dominance, for instance against women or ethnic minorities in service encounters, job interviews or counseling discourse, written discourse is, in principle, often public, and therefore its writers may be held accountable. This publicness may imply that in texts, power may need to be enacted and formulated in more indirect, veiled, formalized ways, especially when such power is not legally or organizationally established. Another factor that makes the exercise of power through written communication less direct is that often authors of institutional texts are not identical with the public speakers, senders, or sources of such discourse. Public discourse, therefore, is often a form of collective, institutional discourse, as is the power it enacts.

Media Discourse: News Reports and News Production

There can be little doubt that of all forms of printed text, those of the mass media are most pervasive, if not most influential, when judged by the power criteria of recipient scope. Besides the spoken and visual discourses of television, newspaper texts play a vital role in public communication. Contrary to popular and scholarly beliefs, news in the press is usually better recalled than is television news (Robinson & Levy, 1986), and perceived to be qualitatively superior (Bruhn Jensen, 1986), which may enhance its persuasive influence, and therefore its power.

We have seen that many power holders (as well as their talk) get routine coverage by the news media, and thus their power may be further confirmed and legitimated. Even when the power of the media is a form of mediating power, it has is own autonomous role in the production and reproduction of social power structures. Through selective source use, news beat routines, and story topic selection, the news media decide which news actors are being publicly represented, what is being said about them, and, especially, how it is said. Much recent work on news production has shown that these processes are not arbitrary, and not simply determined by intuitive, journalistic notions of interestingness. Journalists learn how to portray the power of others, and at the same time learn how to contribute to the power of their own organization, for example, by making it independent of other organizations (Turow, 1983). Newsworthiness is based on ideological and professional criteria that grant preferential media access to elite persons, organizations, and nations, thereby recognizing and legitimating their power (Galtung & Ruge, 1965; Gans, 1979). Similarly, the routine organization of news production favors news gathering in the institutional contexts that guarantee a constant source of news stories, such as the major political bodies of the state, the police, the courts, and the big corporations (Fishman, 1980; Tuchman, 1978). In sum, the corporate embedding of most Western media, especially newspapers, as well as the routine organization of news production, the reliance on readily available and credible sources, and the general professional and ideological aspects of newsworthiness, all concur in social cognitions and text production that favor stories about the most powerful people, groups, or institutions in society (van Dijk, 1987b). In this way, instead of simply being a mouthpiece of the elite, the media also show that they are an inherent part of the societal power structure, of which they manage the symbolic dimension.

Such power is, of course, locally embodied and exercised by media professionals. The question then arises: How do journalists reproduce or challenge the ideologies they are confronted with? Critical media scholars have emphasized that because of their socialization and class membership, journalists tend to reproduce the dominant ideologies of the elite (Hall et al., 1980). It has also been argued, however, that journalists are critical of dominant politics and business, and do not always share the ideologies of these elites (see a review of this position in Altheide, 1985). Despite these contradictions, we may assume with the critical theorists that media practices usually remain within the boundaries of a flexible, but dominant consensus, even when there is room for occasional dissent and criticism. Fundamental norms, values, and power arrangements are seldom explicitly challenged in the dominant news media. In fact, this latitude of dissent is itself organized and controlled. Opposition, also by the media, is limited by the boundaries set by the powerful institutions, and may thus also become routinized.

One important aspect of the process of power (re)production is how journalists acquire the professional and ideological frameworks that guide their daily practice. Turow (1983) examined the processes whereby journalists learn how to portray institutional power. He argues that the media, just like other organizations, want to reduce their dependence on other organizations. They cope with environmental risks through routines. Journalists, writers, and directors must produce creative products, but these must be successful. This happens, for example, through formulas, both in fiction (plots, characters, and settings), and in news reports. This analysis from an organizational point of view partly agrees with the microsociological analysis of news production routines studied by Tuchman (1978).

In a series of discourse analytical case studies of news in the press, I examined how subordinate social groups are represented in news reports (van Dijk, 1987c; see also van Dijk, 1985b). Minorities, refugees, squatters, and Third World countries and peoples appear to be represented in ways that are often rather similar, that is, in contrast with the portrayal of powerful groups and nations. The general conclusion of these studies is that these and other outgroups (a) tend to have less access to the dominant mass media, (b) are used less as credible and routine sources, (c) are described stereotypically if not negatively, primarily as a "problem," if not as a burden or even as a threat to our valued resources, (d) are assumed to be "deficient" or "backward" in many ways, as compared to our norms, goals, expertise, or culture, and, therefore, (e) need our (altruistic) help, understanding, or support, assuming they adapt to our social and political norms and ideology. These general implications may be inferred from the analysis of news production routines, amount, size, and prominence of presentation, dominant topics, as well as style of news reporting (see also Cohen & Young, 1981, for studies with similar conclusions).

Within the framework of the New International Information Order debate, I examined the international coverage of a characteristic media event—the assassination of President-Elect Bechir Gemayel of Lebanon in September 1982 (van Dijk, 1984b, 1987c). In addition to the usual content analytical study of this coverage in newspapers (from some hundred countries), I performed a more qualitative analysis of news discourse. It may be expected that political, ideological, cultural, or regional differences influence the perception, interpretation, and description of this event, which was taking place in the confused and controversial Middle East conflict. I found that although there may have been differences of size, and especially of editorial commentary, the news reports themselves were surprisingly similar as to their schematic, conventional format, and as to their topical contents. An unexpected, major difference was found between first world and Third World newspapers as to their use of their own correspondents: Most Third World newspapers relied on the Western news agencies. My interpretation of these findings was that on the one hand, there may be historical and professional conditions that impose an internationally pervasive news schema for the press reproduction of news events, but that, on the other hand, Western dominance and power, in many complex ways, was an explanation of the pervasiveness of "Western" formats in reporting. Time constraints, lack of money and correspondents, Western-influenced professional socialization, and other factors will favor more or less the same type of stories in Western and non-Western countries. Stories from and about Third World countries are most likely to be either written by Western journalists or adapted to international (i.e., Western) agency formats in order to reach and be used by these agencies and their (rich) Western clients.

These conclusions partly confirm some of the critiques leveled by many Third World countries against the information hegemony of European and U.S. media organizations (UNESCO, 1980; Mankekar, 1978; see also the discussions in Richstad & Anderson, 1981, and in Atwood, Bullion & Murphy, 1982). As may be expected, Western news media and politicians have forcefully rejected these allegations, and usually ignore results from scholarly research that support them (Fascell, 1979). For my study of power and discourse, it is interesting to witness that such rejections are typically framed in terms of "attack on the freedom of the press." My analysis of power suggests that in such cases the notion of "freedom" may often simply be translated as (our) "power" or "control."

Knowledge acquisition and opinion formation about most events in the world appears to be largely based on news discourse in the press and on television, which is shared daily by millions of others. Probably no other discourse type is so pervasive and so shared and read by so many people at more or less the same time. Its power potential, therefore, is enormous, and close scrutiny of the schemata, topics, and style of news reports is therefore crucial to our understanding of the exercise of political, economic, social, and cultural power, and of the communication and acquisition of the ideologies that support it.

This potential does not mean that media power can simply be understood in terms of simplistic, direct "effects." Depending on socioeconomic and sociocultural differences, people obviously interpret, represent, and evaluate news reports and news events quite differently, and, hence, form different opinions, attitudes, and ideologies. Although in some specific cases, direct forms of influence indeed do exist, especially when there are no other information sources and when no counterinformation is available or relevant, we should see the power of news media discourse in more structural terms. Structural influence implies the development of a socially shared, selective knowledge basis, goals, norms, values, and the interpretation frameworks based on them. Media power thus implies the exclusion of alternative sources, alternative information, and other relevancies in the description of world events. Governments and/or media corporations may effectively control the publication or broadcasting of such alternative "voices," and therefore limit the information freedom of citizens, for instance by prohibiting, harassing, or marginalizing the "radical" media (Downing, 1984).

Another feature that has often been found to characterize Western news discourse is the ethnocentric, stereotypical portrayal of Third World nations and peoples. Although not all news about the Third World is of the "coups and earthquakes" brand (Rosenblum, 1981; Schramm & Atwood, 1981), it certainly focuses on only a few types of events and actors, which are generally stereotypical if not negative: poverty, lack of (our type of) democracy, dictatorship, violence and civil war, and technological and cultural "backwardness" (see Said, 1981, for the currently highly relevant coverage of Islam). Downing (1980) found that Third World leaders are often portrayed in a condescending way, and seldom are allowed to speak for themselves.

The same is true for ethnic and racial minorities and their representation in Western countries and their media. Hartmann and Husband (1974), in their classic study of racism and the press, concluded from a content analysis of the British press that (Third World) immigrants tend to be portrayed primarily as "problem people," as people who threaten our valued resources (space, housing, work, education), if not simply as welfare cheats or criminals. I found similar evidence in our qualitative studies of the Dutch press (van Dijk, 1983, 1987c). Ethnic minority groups in the Netherlands (immigrant workers from Mediterranean countries, and people from former colonies, such as Indonesia and Surinam) do not have routine access to news beats or the newspaper columns, and are seldom employed by the media. If they are portrayed at all, the topics tend to be stereotypical or negative, focusing on immigration difficulties and illegality, emphasizing perceived cultural differences and the problems entailed by them, language and educational problems, their competition for housing and employment, and their illegal or criminal activities, centered around dominant notions such as aggression, violence, and drug abuse (see also Hall, Cretcher, Jefferson, Clanks, & Roberts, 1978). These ethnocentric, if not prejudiced and racist, portrayals can be found at all levels of textual organization, including headlining, the relevance hierarchy of news reports, and in style and rhetoric. Note that these expressions of group power may be very subtle and indirect in the quality press and on television. Overt racial abuse is exceptional. Rather, "ethnic" properties and situations are described in a manner that may be used by readers as components or arguments in the development of ethnic prejudice. These results show agreement with the general conclusions found in most other studies of racism in the media in other Western countries (Ebel & Fiala, 1983; Hartmann & Husband, 1974; Merten, 1986; Troyna, 1981; Wilson & Gutiérrez, 1985; see also the papers in Smitherman-Donaldson & van Dijk, 1987).

A characteristic feature of the syntactic style of reporting about outgroups of various kinds appears in several studies of the expression of semantic and social roles. Fowler, Hodge, Kress, and Trew (1979) studied the news coverage in the British press of racial disturbances in London. They found that the ideology of newspapers showed in the ways the participants of varying power were represented in sentential syntax, namely, as active agents, placed in first subject position, or in later positions in passive sentences, or as implied, but absent actors. They found that when the authorities are associated with negative acts, they tend to be placed in later positions, or simply left out of the sentence. Conversely, minorities, who are usually in later, dependent syntactic positions, typically occupy first subject positions as soon as they are negative actors (see also Fowler, 1985; Kress, 1985; Kress & Hodge, 1979). In this way, the negative characteristics of ingroups or elites may be downgraded and those of outgroups emphasized. This action is in agreement with current social psychological theories of prejudice and intergroup perception (Hamilton, 1981; Tajfel, 1981; van Dijk, 1987a).

I reached the same conclusions in an analysis of the headlines in news reports about ethnic groups in the Dutch press (van Dijk, 1987e), as well as in my study of refugee immigration to the Netherlands (van Dijk, 1987c). Ingroup perspective, ethnocentrism, and group power, consequently also influence the syntactic formulation of underlying semantic representations. Further, Downing (1980) shows that such biased representations hold for minorities in Western countries and for peoples in Third World countries alike. Sykes (1985, 1987) arrives at similar conclusions in her study of official British (welfare) discourse about ethnic minorities: Syntactic structures of sentences suggest the passiveness and dependence of black youth and downgrades their own active initiative.

The importance of these various studies of racism in the mass media is that they show an interesting interaction between group power and organizational power. White journalists (also mostly male) write both as professional representatives of media institutions and, at the same time, as members of the dominant, white, Western group. This position shapes their social cognitions and, therefore, their processing of information about outgroups. Social position and social cognition allows them to exercise their power by writing, and continuing to write despite many protests and studies, in a stereotypical or even negative way about relatively powerless ethnic or racial minority groups. Typically, they may do so unwittingly and will mostly forcefully reject the conclusion, made by ethnic groups and black or white researchers, that such reporting is ethnocentric, if not racist.

The effectiveness of media power also shows in the sources people use for their knowledge and attitude formation about ethnic groups (Hartmann & Husband, 1974). In the interviews we collected in Amsterdam about white people's experiences with and opinions about their "foreign" neighbors, it appears that they often refer to the newspaper to warrant prejudices about ethnic groups (van Dijk, 1987a). Stereotypical media topics also appear to be dominant topics in everyday talk. Even when the media are ambiguous in their various discourses, the information they communicate may, nevertheless, be used to develop and confirm extant racist attitudes. The same is more generally true of racist discourse by other powerful groups or elites, for instance in the polity (Reeves, 1983).

Similar conclusions hold for the representation in the media of the working class, of women (especially feminists), of youth, demonstrators, squatters, punks, and all social groups that tend to be discriminated against, marginalized, subordinated, or stereotyped but that also engage in various forms of resistance that may be seen as a bid for counterpower (see Cohen & Young, 1981; Halloran, Elliott, & Murdock, 1970; Tuchman, Daniels, & Benet, 1978; van Dijk, 1987c).

In a series of studies of television news about industrial conflicts in Great Britain, the Glasgow University Media Group (1976, 1980, 1982) concludes that the presentation of the major participants in these conflicts tends to be subtly in favor of employers and, therefore, negative for strikers. This bias is manufactured through time and type of interviews: Employers tend to be interviewed in quiet contexts and in dominant positions, for instance in their offices, whereas strikers—if interviewed at all—are asked questions in the disturbing noise of the picket line. Camera angles and position, and the topical association by citizens of strikes with trouble, also reveal the antistrike perspective of the media. Lexical choice represents strikers as demanding, whereas government or employers are represented more positively as making offers or otherwise as being in control. Workers are not said to "offer" their labor under specified conditions. These and many other features of news production, source contact, interviewing, presentation, quotation, dominant topics, associations, and style, subtly convey the social and ideological positions involved, including those of the media themselves.

What holds for news also holds for other media discourse, such as advertising. Here, corporations and advertising agencies combine powers in the production of persuasive discourse for public consumption. Unlike corporate representations in news reports, their public display in advertising, and hence, their possible influence, is bought. The power of resistance by the public may be reduced by many tactical means (Percy & Rossiter, 1980). Like news reports, however, advertisements tend to reproduce social power structures and stereotypes, for instance of women or blacks (Culley & Bennett, 1976; Dyer, 1982; Greenberg & Mazingo, 1976; Goffman, 1979; King & Stott, 1977; Manstead & Cullogh, 1981; Tuchman, Daniels, & Bent, 1978; Wilson & Gutiérrez, 1985). In this framework, Goffman (1979) speaks of the "ritualization of subordination." Advertisements attract public attention while at the same time controlling exposure and opinion and concealing corporate power through complex strategies of incompleteness, novelty, ambiguity, repetition, and positive self-presentation (Davis & Walton, 1983; Packard, 1957; Tolmach Lakoff, 1981).

Textbooks

Like the mass media, educational discourse derives its power from its enormous scope. Unlike most other types of texts, textbooks are obligatory reading for many people, which is a second major condition of their power. Together with instructional dialogues, textbooks are used extensively by all citizens during their formal education. The knowledge and attitudes expressed and conveyed by such learning materials, again, reflect a dominant consensus, if not the interests of the most powerful groups and institutions of societies. Because textbooks and the educational programs they are intended to realize should, in principle, serve public interests, they are seldom allowed to be "controversial." In other words, alternative, critical, radical voices are usually censored or mitigated (McHoul, 1986).

Many studies have shown that most textbooks reproduce a nationalistic, ethnocentric, or racist view of the world—of other peoples as well as of ethnic minority groups (Ferro, 1981; Klein, 1986; Milner, 1983; Preiswerk, 1980; van Dijk, 1987d). The observations are familiar from our news media analysis: underrepresentation, voicelessness, and stereotyping. Minority groups and their history and culture tend to be ignored, and a few stereotypical cultural differences are emphasized and often negatively contrasted with properties of the "own" group, nation, or culture. Although cultural differentiation and pride may be a feature of all or most groups, cultures, or countries, Western or white dominance is shown through special attention to "our" superior technology, culture, and political system. Third World countries and (black) minorities may thus be portrayed as "backward" compared to "our" position and development, if not as "primitive," "lazy," and "stupid." At the same time, the dominant white group or the Western world has its "burden" to "help these people," through aid, welfare, or technological advice. Although there are variations among textbooks (and in some countries these properties of books for children seem to change slowly), these messages dominate the history, geography, social science, or language textbooks in many countries of the Western world (and Japan). Again, opposition, for example, by teachers, requires extensive knowledge of, and access to other sources of information, and the (usually restricted) freedom to deviate from established curricula and traditions. Thus, together with the media, textbooks and other educational materials form the core of both symbolic power and the textual reproduction and legitimation of power in society (Bourdieu, 1984; Bourdieu & Passeron, 1977).

CONCLUSIONS

In this chapter, we have examined some of the relationships between social power and discourse. We started from a general analysis of social power in terms of group-based or institutional control over actions and cognitions of other people and groups, usually in the interest of the powerful. Generally, an increase in power diminishes freedom for those who are subjected to this power. This interaction may be restricted to a specific social domain, and also affect the power holder. At the same time, the exercise of power may lead to resistence and the exercise of counterpower. Social power was further analyzed in terms of its institutional or group basis, its domain, scope, and legitimation. Personal power, which is not analyzed in this chapter, may sometimes emphasize, but also counter, these forms of social power. Indeed, some women may dominate their husbands, some students their teachers, and some children their parents; and conversely, not all doctors or men are medical or male chauvinists. Despite these personal differences, we focused on more general, structural properties of power relations and discourse in society.

Text and talk appear to play a crucial role in the exercise of power. Thus discourse may directly and coercively enact power, through directive speech acts, and through text types such as laws, regulations, or instructions. Power may also be manifested more indirectly in discourse, as representation in the form of an expression, description, or legitimation of powerful actors or their actions and ideologies. Discursive power is often directly or indirectly persuasive, and, therefore, features reasons, arguments, promises, examples, or other rhetorical means that enhance the probability that recipients build the desired mental representations. One crucial strategy in the concealment of power is to persuade the powerless that wanted actions are in their own interest.

Discursive power also involves the control over discourse itself: Who is speaking in what contexts; who has access to various types and means of communication; and which recipients can be reached? We found that there is a direct correlation between the scope of discourse and the scope of power: The powerless generally may have control only in everyday conversation, and are merely passive recipients of official and media discourse. The powerful have recourse to a large variety of dialogical, and especially printed, formal forms of text and talk, and, in principle, can reach large groups of people. Thus the powerful control discourse through control of its material production, its formulation, and its distribution. Crucial in the exercise of power, then, is the control of the formation of social cognitions through the subtle management of knowledge and beliefs, the preformulation of beliefs, or the censorship of counterideologies. These representations form the essential cognitive link between social power itself and the production and understanding of discourse and its social functions in the enactment of power.

Against this more general background of the analysis of the links between power and discourse, our more concrete discourse analysis focused on the central micro-units of power and discourse, namely, communicative events, such as everyday conversations, courtroom trials, or classroom talk. In a review of some recent work, we thus examined how power is expressed, described, displayed, or legitimated in various genres of text and talk, and at various levels of analysis, such as speech acts, turn taking, topic selection, style, and rhetoric. Special attention was paid to the various ways institutional power is enacted by professionals and experts over their clients, and to the ways women and minority groups are subjected to power strategies, both in institutional dialogue and in media texts, such as news reports, textbooks, and advertising. It was found that in this way, communicative events may be structured by several dimensions of power at the same time, not only those of the institution, but those of gender, race, and class.

Our theoretical analysis and our review show that whether in its direct or in its indirect forms, power is both enacted and reproduced in and by discourse. Without communication—text and talk—power in society can hardly be exercised and legitimated. Power presupposes knowledge, beliefs, and ideologies to sustain and reproduce it. Discourse structurally shows and communicates these crucial conditions of reproduction for all societal levels, dimensions, and contexts. This chapter has presented an outline of these processes. Much further theoretical and empirical work will be necessary to fill in the many details of this discursive enactment and reproduction of power.

REFERENCES

Abercrombie, N., Hill, S., & Turner, B. S. (1980). *The dominant ideology thesis.* London: George, Allen & Unwin.

Adelswärd, V., Aronsson, K., Jönsson, L., & Linell, P. (1987). The unequal distribution of interactional space: Dominance and control in courtroom interaction. *Text, 7,* 313-346.

Allport, G. W. (1954). *The nature of prejudice.* Garden City, NY: Doubleday, Anchor.
Altheide, D. (1985). *Media power.* Beverly Hills, CA: Sage.
Apple, M. W. (1979). *Ideology and curriculum.* London: Routledge & Kegan Paul.
Atkinson, J. M. (1984). *Our masters' voices. The language and body language of politics.* London: Methuen.
Atkinson, J. M., & Drew, P. (1979). *Order in court. The organisation of verbal interaction in judicial settings.* London: Methuen.
Atkinson, J. M., & Heritage, J. (Eds.). (1984). *Structures of social action. Studies in conversational analysis.* Cambridge: Cambridge University Press.
Atwood, L. E., Bullion, S. J., & Murphy, S. M. (1982). *International perspectives on news.* Carbondale: Southern Illinois University Press.
Bagdikian, B. H. (1983). *The media monopoly.* Boston: Beacon Press.
Barker, M. (1981). *The new racism.* London: Junction.
Barrett, M., Corrigan, P., Kuhn, A., & Wolff, J. (Eds.). (1979). *Ideology and cultural production.* London: Croom Helm.
Bauman, R., & Scherzer, J. (Eds.). (1974). *Explorations in the ethnography of speaking.* Cambridge: Cambridge University Press.
Bavelas, J. B., Rogers, L. E., & Millar, F. E. (1985). Interpersonal conflict. In T. A. van Dijk (Ed.), *Handbook of discourse analysis: Vol. 4. Discourse analysis in society* (pp. 9-26). London: Academic Press.
Becker, J., Hedebro, G., & Paldán (Eds.). (1986). *Communication and domination: Essays to honor Herbert I. Schiller.* Norwood, NJ: Ablex.
Berger, C. R. (1985). Social power and interpersonal communication. In M. L. Knapp & G. R. Miller (Eds.), *Handbook of interpersonal communication* (pp. 439-496). Beverly Hills, CA: Sage.
Bergsdorf, W. (1983). *Herrschaft und Sprache. Studie zur politischen Termonilogie der Bundesrespublik Deutschland.* Pfullingen: Neske Verlag.
Bernstein, B. (1971-1975). *Class, codes, control* (3 vols.). London: Routledge & Kegan Paul.
Blair, R., Roberts, K. H., & McKechnie, P. (1985). Vertical and network communication in organizations. In R. D. McPhee & P. K. Tompkins (Eds.), *Organizational communication: Traditional themes and new directions* (pp. 55-77). Beverly Hills, CA: Sage.
Bourdieu, P. (1977). *Outline of a theory of practice.* Cambridge: Cambridge University Press.
Bourdieu, P. (1984). *Home academicus.* Paris: Minuit.
Bourdieu, P., & Passeron, J.-C. (1977). *Reproduction in education, society and culture.* Beverly Hills, CA: Sage.
Boyd-Barrett, O., & Braham, P. (Eds.). (1987). *Media, knowledge and power.* London: Croom Helm.
Bradac, J. J., & Mulac, A. (1984). A molecular view of powerful and powerless speech styles. *Communication Monographs, 51,* 307-319.
Bradac, J. J., & Street, R. (1986). *Powerful and powerless styles revisited: A theoretical analysis.* Paper presented at the annual meeting of the Speech Communication Association, Chicago.
Bradac, J. J., Hemphill, M. R., & Tardy, C. H. (1981). Language style on trial: Effects of "powerful" and "powerless" speech upon judgments of victims and villains. *Western Journal of Speech Communication, 45,* 327-341.
Brooke, M. E., & Ng, S. H. (1986). Language and social influence in small conversational groups. *Journal of Language and Social Psychology, 5,* 201-210.
Brown, J. D., Bybee, C. R., Wearden, S. T., & Murdock, D. (1982). *Invisible power: News sources and the limits of diversity.* Paper presented at the annual meeting of the Association for Education in Journalism, Athens, OH.
Brown, L. B. (1973). *Ideology.* Harmondsworth: Penguin.
Brown, R., & Ford, M. (1972). Address in American English. In S. Moscovici (Ed.), *The psychosociology of language* (pp. 243-262). Chicago: Markham.
Brown, P., & Fraser, C. (1979). Speech as a marker of situation. In K. R. Scherer & H. Giles

(Eds.), *Social markers in speech* (pp.33-62.). Cambridge: Cambridge University Press.
Brown, R., & Gilman, A. (1960). The pronouns of power and solidarity. In T. A. Sebeok (Ed.), *Style in language* (pp. 253-277). Cambridge: MIT Press.
Brown, P., & Levinson, S. C. (1978). Universals in language use: Politeness phenomena. In E. N. Goody (Ed.), *Questions and politeness* (pp. 56-289). Cambridge: Cambridge University Press.
Bruhn Jensen, K. (1986). *Making sense of the news*. Aarhus, Denmark: Aarhus University Press.
Burton, F., & Carlen, P. (1979). *Official discourse. On discourse analysis, government publications, ideology and the state*. London: Routledge & Kegan Paul.
Candlin, C., Burton, J., & Coleman, H. (1980). *Dentist-patient communication: A report to the general dental council*. Lancaster, England: University of Lancaster, Department of Linguistics and Modern English Language.
Centre for Contemporary Cultural Studies (1978). *On ideology*. London: Hutchinson.
Chaffee, S. H. (Ed.). (1975). *Political communication*. Beverly Hills, CA: Sage.
Charrow, V. R. (1982). Language in the bureaucracy. In R. J. Di Pietro (Ed.), *Linguistics and the professions* (pp. 173-188). Norwood, NJ: Ablex.
Cicourel, Aaron V. (1973). *Cognitive sociology*. Harmondsworth: Penguin.
Cohen, S., & Young, J. (Eds.). (1981). *The manufacture of news. Deviance, social problems and the mass media*. London: Constable,
Coleman, H. (Ed.). (1984). Language and work 1: Law, industry, education. *International Journal of the Sociology of Language, 49* (special issue).
Coleman, H. (1985a). Talking shop: An overview of language and work. *International Journal of the Sociology of Language, 51*, 105-129.
Coleman, H. (Ed.). (1985b). Language at work 2. The health professions. *International Journal of the Sociology of Language, 51*. (special issue).
Coleman, H., & Burton, J. (1985). Aspects of control in the dentist-patient relationship. *International Journal of the Sociology of Language, 51*, 75-104.
Collins, R., Curran, J., Garnham, N., Scannell, P., Schlesinger, P., & Sparks, C. (Eds.). (1986). *Media, culture and society*. London: Sage.
Cook-Gumperz, J. (1973). *Social control and socialization*. London: Routledge & Kegan Paul.
Culley, J. D., & Bennett, R. (1976). Selling women, selling blacks. *Journal of Communication, 26*, 160-174.
Dahl, R. A. (1957). The concept of power. *Behavioural Science, 2*, 201-215.
Dahl, R. A. (1961). *Who governs? Democracy and power in an American city*. New Haven, CT: Yale University Press.
Danet, B. (1980). Language in the legal process. *Law and Society Review, 14*, 445-565.
Danet, B. (Ed.). (1984). Legal discourse. *Text, 4*(1/3) (special issue).
Davis, H., & Walton, P. (Eds.). (1983). *Language, image, media*. Oxford: Blackwell.
Debnam, G. (1984). *The analysis of power*. London: Macmillan.
Di Pietro, R. J. (1982). *Linguistics and the professions*. Norwood, NJ: Ablex.
Dittmar, N., & von Stutterheim, C. (1985). On the discourse of immigrant workers. In T. A. van Dijk (Ed.), *Handbook of Discourse Analysis: Vol. 4. Discourse analysis in society* (pp. 125-152). London: Academic Press.
Domhoff, G. W. (1978). *The powers that be: Processes of ruling class domination in America*. New York: Random House.
Domhoff, G. W., & Ballard, H. B. (Eds.). (1968). *C. Wright Mills and the power elite*. Boston: Beacon Press.
Donald, J., & Hall, S. (Eds.). (1986). *Politics and ideology*. Milton Keynes: Open University Press.
Dovidio, J. F., & Gaertner, S. L. (Eds.). (1986). *Prejudice, discrimination and racism*. New York: Academic Press.
Downes, W. (1984). *Language and society*. London: Fontana.
Downing, J. (1980). *The media machine*. London: Pluto.
Downing, J. (1984). *Radical media*. Boston: Southend.

Dyer, G. (1982). *Advertising as communication.* London: Methuen.
Eakins, B. W., & Eakins, R. G. (1978). *Sex differences in human communication.* Boston: Houghton Mifflin.
Ebel, M., & Fiala, P. (1983). *Sous le consensus, la xénophobie.* Lausanne: Institut de Science Politique.
Edelman, M. (1964). *The symbolic uses of politics.* Urbana: University of Illinois Press.
Edelman, M. (1974). The political language of the helping professions. *Politics and Society, 4,* 295-310.
Erickson, B., Lind, A. A., Johnson, B. C., & O'Barr W. M. (1978). Speech style and impression formation in a court setting: The effects of "powerful" and "powerless" speech. *Journal of Experimental Social Psychology, 14,* 266-279.
Erickson, F., & Shultz, J. (1982). *The counselor as gatekeeper: Social interaction in interviews.* New York: Academic Press.
Ervin-Tripp, S., O'Connor, M. C., & Rosenberg, J. (1984). Language and power in the family. In C. Kramarae, M. Schulz, & W. M. O'Barr (Eds.), *Language and power* (pp. 116-135). Beverly Hills, CA: Sage.
Ervin-Tripp, S., & Strage, A. (1985). Parent-Child discourse. In T. A. van Dijk (Ed.), *Handbook of discourse analysis: Vol. 3. Discourse and dialogue* (pp. 67-78). London: Academic Press.
Essed, P.J.M. (1984). *Alledaags racisme* (Everyday racism). Amsterdam: Sara. (To be published in English by Hunter House, Claremont, CA).
Falbo, T., & Peplau, L. A. (1980). Power strategies in intimate relationships. *Journal of Personality and Social Psychology, 38,* 618-628.
Farr, R. M., & Moscovici, S. (Eds.). (1984). *Social representations.* Cambridge: Cambridge University Press.
Fascell, D. B. (Ed.). (1979). *International news: Freedom under attack.* Beverly Hills, CA: Sage.
Ferro, M. (1981). *Comment on raconte l'Histoire aux enfants à travers le monde entier.* Paris: Payot.
Fielding, G., & Evered, C. (1980). The influence of patients' speech upon doctors: The diagnostic interview. In R. N. St. Clair & H. Giles (Eds.), *The social and psychological contexts of language* (pp. 51-72). Hillsdale, NJ: Lawrence Erlbaum.
Fisher, S., & Todd, A. D. (1983). *The social organization of doctor-patient communication.* Washington, DC: Center for Applied Linguistics.
Fisher, S., & Todd, A. D. (Eds.). (1986). *Discourse and institutional authority: Medicine, education and law.* Norwood, NJ: Ablex.
Fishman, M. (1980). *Manufacturing the news.* Austin: University of Texas Press.
Fishman, P. (1983). Interaction: The work women do. In B. Thorne, C. Kramarae, & N. Henley (Eds.), *Language, gender and society* (pp. 89-101). New York: Pergamon.
Fiske, S. T., & Taylor, S. E. (1984). *Social cognition.* Reading, MA: Addison-Wesley.
Fowler, R. (1985). Power. In T. A. van Dijk (Ed.), *Handbook of discourse analysis: Vol. 4. Discourse analysis in society* (pp. 61-82). London: Academic Press.
Fowler, R., Hodge, B., Kress, G., & Trew, T. (1979). *Language and control.* London: Routledge & Kegan Paul.
Freeman, S. H., & Heller, M. S. (1987). Medical discourse. *Text, 7* (special issue).
Galbraith, J. K. (1985). *The anatomy of power.* London: Corgi.
Galtung, J., & Ruge, M. H. (1965). The structure of foreign news. *Journal of Peace Research, 2,* 64-91.
Gamble, A. (1986). The political economy of freedom. In R. Levitas (Ed.), *The ideology of the new right* (pp. 25-54). Cambridge, MA: Polity.
Gans, H. (1979). *Deciding what's news.* New York: Pantheon.
Giles, H., & Powesland, P. F. (1975). *Speech style and social evaluation.* London: Academic Press.
Giles, H., & Smith, P. M. (1979). Accommodation theory: Optimal levels of convergence. In H. Giles, & R. N. St. Clair (Eds.), *Language and social psychology* (pp. 45-65). Oxford: Basil

Blackwell.
Glasgow University Media Group. (1976). *Bad news.* London: Routledge & Kegan Paul.
Glasgow University Media Group. (1980). *More bad news.* London: Routledge & Kegan Paul.
Glasgow University Media Group. (1982). *Really bad news.* London: Writers and Readers.
Gleason, Y. B., & Geif, E. B. (1986). Men's speech to young children. In B. Thorne, C. Kramarae, & N. Henley (Eds.), *Language, gender and society* (pp. 140-150). Rowley, MA: Newbury House.
Goffman, E. (1967). *Interaction ritual: Essays on face-to-face behavior.* Garden City, NY: Doubleday.
Goffman, E. (1979). *Gender advertisements.* New York: Harper & Row.
Golding, P., & Murdock, G. (1979). Ideology and the mass media: The question of determination. In M. Barrett, P. Corrigan, A. Kuhn, & J. Wolff (Eds.), *Ideology and cultural production* (pp. 198-224). London: Croom Helm.
Graber, Doris A. (1984). *Processing the news.* New York: Longman.
Greenberg, B. S., & Mazingo, S. L. (1976). Racial issues in mass media institutions. In P. A. Katz (Ed.), *Towards the elimination of racism* (pp. 309-340). New York: Pergamon.
Greenberg, J., Kirkland, S., & Pyszczynski, (1987). Some theoretical notions and preliminary research concerning derogatory labels. In G. Smitherman-Donaldson & T. A. van Dijk (Eds.), *Discourse and communication.* Detroit, MI: Wayne State University Press.
Guespin L. (Ed.). (1976). Typologie du discours politique. *Langages, 41.*
Gumperz, J. (1982). *Discourse strategies.* Cambridge: Cambridge University Press.
Gumperz, J. (Ed.). (1982). *Language and social identity.* Cambridge: Cambridge University Press.
Hall, S., Critcher, C., Jefferson, T., Clarke, J., & Roberts, B. (1978). *Policing the crisis: Mugging, the State and law and order.* London: Methuen.
Hall, S., Hobson, D., Lowe, A., & Willis, P. (Eds.). (1980). *Culture, media, language.* London: Hutchinson.
Halloran, J. D., Elliott, P. & Murdock, G. (1970). *Demonstrations and communication: A case study.* Harmondsworth: Penguin.
Hamilton, D. (Ed.). (1981). *Cognitive processes in stereotyping and intergroup behavior.* Hillsdale, NJ: Lawrence Erlbaum.
Harris, S. (1984). Questions as a mode of control in magistrates' court. *International Journal of the Sociology of Language, 49,* 5-27.
Hart, R. P. (1984). *Verbal style and the presidency.* Orlando, FL: Academic Press.
Hartmann, P., & Husband, C. (1974). *Racism and the mass media.* London: Davis-Poynter.
Helmreich, W. B. (1984). *The things they say behind your back. Stereotypes and the myths behind them.* New Brunswick, NJ: Transaction Books.
Hudson, K. (1978). *The language of modern politics.* London: Methuen.
Kalin, R., & Rayko, D. (1980). The social significance of speech in the job interview. In R. N. St. Clair & H. Giles (Eds.), *The social and psychological contexts of language* (pp. 39-50). Hillsdale, NJ: Lawrence Erlbaum.
Kelly, J. W. (1985). *Storytelling in high tech organizations: A medium for sharing culture.* Paper presented at the annual meeting of the Western Speech Communication Association, Fresno, CA.
Kennedy, S. (1959). *Jim Crow guide to the U.S.A.* London: Lawrence and Wishart.
King, J., & Stott, M. (Eds.). (1977). *Is this your life? Images of women in the media.* London: Virago.
Kinloch, G. C. (1981). *Ideology and contemporary sociological theory.* Englewood Cliffs, NJ: Prentice-Hall.
Klein, G. (1986). *Reading into racism.* London: Routledge & Kegan Paul.
Klein, W., & Dittmar, N. (1979). *Developing grammars: The acquisition of German by foreign workers.* Heidelberg & New York: Springer Verlag.
Knorr-Cetina, K., & Cicourel, A. V. (Eds.). (1981). *Advances in social theory and methodology.*

Towards an integration of micro- and macrosociologies. London: Routledge & Kegan Paul.
Kochman, T. (1981). *Black and white styles in conflict*. Chicago: University of Chicago Press.
Kramarae, C. (1980). *Voices and words of women and men*. Oxford & New York: Pergamon.
Kramarae, C. (1983). *Women and men speaking*. Rowley, MA: Newbury House.
Kramarae, C., Schulz, M., & O'Barr, W. M. (1984). Towards an understanding of language and power. In C. Kramarae, M. Schulz, & W. M. O'Barr (Eds.), *Language and power* (pp. 9-22). Beverly Hills, CA: Sage.
Kramarae, C., Thorne, B., & Henley, N. (1983). Sex similarities and differences in language, speech, and nonverbal communication: An annotated bibliography. In B. Thorne, C. Kramarae, & N. Henley (Eds.), *Language, gender and society*, (pp. 151-331). Rowley, MA: Newbury House.
Kress, G. (1985). Ideological structures in discourse. In T. A. van Dijk (Ed.), *Handbook of discourse analysis: Vol. 4. Discourse analysis in society* (pp. 27-42). London: Academic Press.
Kress, G., & Hodge, B. (1979). *Language and ideology*. London: Routledge & Kegan Paul.
Labov, W. (1972). Rules for ritual insults. In D. Sudnow (Ed.), *Studies in social interaction* (pp. 120-169). New York: Free Press.
Leet-Pellegrini, H. M, (1980). Conversational dominance as a function of gender and expertise. In H. Giles, W. P. Robinson, & P. M. Smith (Eds.), *Language: Social psychological perspectives* (pp. 97-104). New York: Pergamon.
Lein, L., & Brenneis, D. (1978). Children's disputes in three speech communities. *Language in Society, 7*, 299-323.
Lind, E. A., & O'Barr, W. M. (1979). The social significance of speech in the courtroom. In H. Giles & R. N. St. Clair (Eds.), *Language and social psychology* (pp. 66-87). Oxford: Basil Blackwell.
Lindegren-Lerman, C. (1983). Dominant discourse: The institutional voice and the control of topic. In H. Davis & P. Walton (Eds.), *Language, image, media* (pp. 75-103). Oxford: Basil Blackwell.
Lorimer, R. (1984). *Defining the curriculum: The role of the publisher*. Paper presented at the annual meeting of the American Educational Research Association, New Orleans.
Lukes, S. (1974). *Power: A radical view*. London: Macmillan.
Lukes, S. (Ed.). (1986). *Power*. Oxford: Basil Blackwell.
Mankekar, D. R. (1978). *One-way flow: Neo-colonialism via news media*. New Delhi: Clarion.
Manning, D. J. (Ed.). (1980). *The form of ideology*. London: George, Allen & Unwin.
Manstead, T., & McCullogh, C. (1981). Sex role stereotyping in British television ads. *British Journal of Social Psychology, 20*, 171-180.
Mattelart, A. (1979). *The multinational corporations and the control of culture: The ideological apparatus of imperialism*. Atlantic Highlands, NJ: Harvester.
Maynard, D. W. (1985). The analysis of plea bargaining discourse. In T. A. van Dijk (Ed.), *Handbook of discourse analysis: Vol. 4. Discourse analysis in society* (pp. 153-179). London: Academic Press.
McHoul, A. W. (1986). Writing, sexism, and schooling: A discourse-analytic investigation of some recent documents on sexism and education in Queensland. In S. Fisher & A. D. Todd (Eds.), *Discourse and institutional authority: Medicine, education and law* (pp. 187-202). Norwood, NJ: Ablex.
McLaughlin, M. L. (1984). *Conversation: How talk is organized*. Beverly Hills, CA: Sage.
McPhee, R. D., & Tompkins, P. K. (Eds.). (1985). *Organizational communication: Traditional themes and new directions*. Beverly Hills, CA: Sage.
Mead, R. (1985). Courtroom discourse. *English Language Research, Discourse Analysis Monographs, 9* (University of Birmingham).
Mehan, H. (1979). *Learning lessons*. Cambridge, MA: Harvard University Press.
Mehan, H. (1986). The role of language and the language of role in institutional decision making. In S. Fisher & A. D. Todd (Eds.), *Discourse and institutional authority: Medicine, education, and law* (pp. 140-163). Norwood, NJ: Ablex.

Merten, K. (1986). *Das Bild der Ausländer in der deutschen Presse.* Frankfurt: Gagyeli Verlag.
Mey, J. (1985). Whose language: A study in linguistic pragmatics. Amsterdam: Benjamins.
Milliband, R. (1983). *Class power and state power.* London: Verso.
Mills, C. W. (1956). *The power elite.* New York: Oxford University Press.
Milner, D. (1983). *Children and race. Ten years on.* London: Ward Lock Educational.
Mishler, E. G. (1984). *The discourse of medicine: Dialectics in medical interviews.* Norwood, NJ: Ablex.
Mueller, C. (1973). *The politics of communication: A study of the political sociology of language, socialization, and legitimation.* New York: Oxford University Press.
Natale, M., Entin, E., & Jaffe, J. (1979). Vocal interruptions in dyadic communication as a function of speech and social anxiety. *Journal of Personality and Social Psychology, 37,* 865-878.
Nimmo, D. D., & Sanders, K. R. (Eds.). (1981). *Handbook of political communication.* Beverly Hills, CA: Sage.
Owsley, H. H., & Scotton, C. M. (1984). The conversational expression of power by television interviewers. *Journal of Social Psychology, 123,* 696-735.
Packard, V. (1957). *The hidden persuaders.* New York: Pocket Books.
Parkinson, M. G., Geisler, D., & Pelias, M. H. (1983). The effects of verbal skills on trial success. *Journal of the American Forensic Association, 20,* 16-22.
Pecheux, M. (1975). Analyse du discourse. Langue et ideologies. *Langages, 37.*
Percy, L., & Rossiter, J. R. (1980). *Advertising strategy: A communication theory approach.* New York: Praeger.
Pettigrew, A. M. (1972). Information control as a power resource. *Sociology, 6,* 187-204.
Pettigrew, A. M. (1973). *The politics of organizational decision making.* London: Tavistock.
Petty, R. E., & Cacioppo, J. T. (1981). *Attitudes and persuasion: Classic and contemporary approaches.* Dubuque, IA: Wm. C. Brown.
Pfeffer, J. (1981). *Power in organizations.* Marshfield, MA: Pitman.
Preiswerk, R. (Ed.). (1980). *The slant of the pen. Racism in children's books.* Geneva: World Council of Churches.
Radtke, I. (Ed.). (1981). *Die Sprache des Rechts und der Verwaltung. Volume II of Deutsche Akademie für Sprache und Dichtung, Die öffentliche Sprachgebrauch.* Stuttgart: Klett-Cotta.
Ragan, S. L. (1983). Alignment and conversational coherence. In R. T. Craig & K. Tracy (Eds.), *Conversational coherence* (pp. 157-171). Beverly Hills, CA: Sage.
Reeves, F. (1983). *British racial discourse.* Cambridge: Cambridge University Press.
Richstad, J., & Anderson, M. H. (Eds.). (1981). *Crisis in international news.* New York: Columbia University Press.
Riley, P. (1983). A structurationist account of political culture. *Administrative Science Quarterly, 28,* 414-437.
Robinson, J. P., & Levy, M. R. (1986). *The main source. Learning from television news.* Beverly Hills, CA: Sage.
Roloff, M. E., & Berger, C. R. (Eds.). (1982). *Social cognition and communication.* Beverly Hills, CA: Sage.
Roloff, M. E., & Miller, G. R. (Eds.). (1980). *Persuasion: New directions in theory and research.* Beverly Hills, CA: Sage.
Rosenblum, M. (1981). *Coups and earthquakes: Reporting the world to America.* New York: Harper & Row.
Sabsay, S., & Platt, M. (1985). *Social setting, stigma and communicative competence.* Amsterdam: Benjamins.
Sacks, H., Schegloff, E. A., & Jefferson, G. A. (1974). A simplest systematics for the organization of turn taking for conversation. *Language, 50,* 696-735.
Said, E. W. (1981). *Covering Islam.* Henley, Oxfordshire: Routledge & Kegan Paul.
Saville-Troike, M. (1982). *The ethnography of communication.* Oxford: Basil Blackwell.
Schatzman, L., & Strauss, A. (1972). Social class and modes of communication. In S. Moscovici

(Ed.), *The psychosociology of language* (pp. 206-221). Chicago: Markham.
Scherer, K. R., & Giles, H. (1979). *Social markers in speech.* Cambridge: Cambridge University Press.
Schiller, H. I. (1973). *The mind managers.* Boston: Beacon Press.
Schramm, W., & Atwood, E. (1981). *Circulation of news in the Third World: A study of Asia.* Hong Kong: Chinese University Press.
Seibold, D. R., Cantrill, J. G., & Meyers, R. A. (1985). Communication and interpersonal influence. In M. L. Knapp & G. R. Miller (Eds.), *Handbook of interpersonal communication* (pp. 551-611). Beverly Hills, CA: Sage.
Seidel, G. (1985). Political discourse analysis. In T. A. van Dijk (Ed.), *Handbook of discourse analysis: Vol. 4. Discourse analysis in society* (pp. 43-60). London: Academic Press.
Seidel, G. (1987a). The white discursive order: The British New Rights's discourse on cultural racism, with particular reference to the *Salisbury Review.* In I. Zavala, T. A. van Dijk, & M. Diaz-Diocaretz (Eds.), *Literature, discourse, psychiatry.* Amsterdam: Benjamins.
Seidel, G. (1987b). The British New Right's "enemy within": The anti-racists. In G. Smitherman-Donaldson & T. A. van Dijk (Eds.), *Discourse and discrimination.* Detroit: Wayne State University Press.
Shapiro, M. (Ed.). (1984). *Language and politics.* Oxford: Basil Blackwell.
Shuy, R. W. (1986). Some linguistic contributions to a criminal court case. In S. Fisher & A. D. Todd (Eds.), *Discourse and institutional authority: Medicine, education and law* (pp. 234-249). Norwood, NJ: Ablex.
Sinclair, J. McH., & Brazil, D. (1982). *Teacher talk.* Oxford: Oxford University Press.
Slobin, D. I., Miller, S. H., & Porter, L. W. (1972). Forms of address and social relations in a business organization. In S. Moscovici (Ed.), *The psychosociology of language* (pp. 263-272).
Smitherman-Donaldson, G., & van Dijk, T. A. (Eds.). (1987). *Discourse and discrimination.* Detroit: Wayne State University Press.
Snow, C., & Furgeson, C. (Eds.). (1977). *Talking to children.* New York: Cambridge University Press.
Spender, D. (1980). *Man made language.* London: Routledge & Kegan Paul.
Stoll, E. A. (1983). *A naturalistic study of talk in the classroom.* Unpublished doctoral dissertation, University of Utah.
Strong, P. M. (1979). *The ceremonial order of the clinic: Parents, doctors and medical bureaucracies.* London: Routledge & Kegan Paul.
Sykes, M. (1985). Discrimination in discourse. In T. A. van Dijk (Ed.), *Handbook of discourse analysis: Vol. 4. Discourse analysis in society* (pp. 83-101). London: Academic Press.
Sykes, M. (1987). From "rights" to "needs": Official discourse and the "welfarisation" of race. In G. Smitherman-Donaldson & T. A. van Dijk (Eds.), *Discourse and discrimination.* Detroit: Wayne State University Press.
Tajfel, H. (1981). *Human groups and social categories.* Cambridge: Cambridge University Press.
Therborn, G. (1980). *The ideology of power and the power of ideology.* London: Verso.
Thorne, B., & Henly, N. (Eds.). (1975). *Language and sex: Difference and dominance.* Rowley, MA: Newbury House.
Thorne, B., Kramarae, C., & Henley, N. (Eds.). (1983). *Language, gender and society.* Rowley, MA: Newbury House.
Tolmach Lakoff, R. (1981). Persuasive discourse and ordinary conversation: With examples from advertising. In D. Tannen (Ed.), *Analyzing discourse: Text and talk* (pp. 25-42). Washington, DC: Georgetown University Press.
Treichler, P., Frankel, R. M., Kramarae, C., Zoppi, C., & Beckman, H. B. (1984). Problems and *prob*lems: Power relationships in a medical interview. In C. Kramarae, M. Schultz, & W. M. O'Barr (Eds.), *Language and power* (pp. 43-61). Beverly Hills, CA: Sage.
Trömel-Plötz, S. (Ed.). (1984). *Gewalt durch Sprache. De Vergewaltigung von Frauen in Gesprachen.* Frankfurt: Fischer.
Troyna, B. (1981). *Public awareness and the media: A study of reporting on race.* London:

Commission for Racial Equality.
Tuchman, G. (1978). *Making news.* New York: Free Press.
Tuchman, G., Daniels, A. K., & Benet, J. (Eds.). (1978). *Hearth and home: Images of women in the mass media.* New York: Oxford University Press.
Turow, J. (1983). Learning to portray institutional power: The socialization of creators of mass media organization. In R. D. McPhee & P. K. Tompkins (Eds.), *Organizational communication: Traditional themes and new directions* (pp. 211-234). Beverly Hills, CA: Sage.
UNESCO. (1980). *Many voices, one world.* Report by the International Commission for the Study of Communication Problems (chaired by Sean MacBride). Paris: UNESCO, London: Kogan Page.
van Dijk, T. A. (1977). *Text and context.* London: Longman.
van Dijk, T. A. (1980). *Macrostructures.* Hillsdale, NJ: Lawrence Erlbaum.
van Dijk, T. A. (1981). *Studies in the pragmatics of discourse.* The Hague & Berlin: Mouton/de Gruyter.
van Dijk, T. A. (1983). *Minderheden in the media* (Minorities in the media). Amsterdam: Socialistische Uitgeverij Amsterdam.
van Dijk, T. A. (1984a). *Prejudice and discourse. An analysis of ethnic prejudice in cognition and conversation.* Amsterdam: Benjamins.
van Dijk, T. A. (1984b). *Structures of international news. A case study of the world's press.* Unpublished manuscript. University of Amsterdam, Department of General Literary Studies, Section of Discourse Studies.
van Dijk, T. A. (1987a). *Communicating racism: Ethnic prejudice in thought and talk.* Beverly Hills, CA: Sage.
van Dijk, T. A. (1987b). *News as discourse.* Hillsdale, NJ: Lawrence Erlbaum.
van Dijk, T. A. (1987c). *News analysis: Case studies of national and international news: Lebanon, ethnic minorities, refugees, squatters.* Hillsdale, NJ: Lawrence Erlbaum.
van Dijk, T. A. (1987d). *Schoolvoorbeelden van racism* (Textbook examples of racism). Amsterdam: Socialistische Uitgeverij Amsterdam.
van Dijk, T. A. (1987e). How "they" hit the headlines: Ethnic minorities in the press. In G. Smitherman-Donaldson & T. A. van Dijk (Eds.), *Discourse and discrimination.* Detroit: Wayne State University Press.
van Dijk, T. A. (1987f). *Social cognition, social power and social discourse.* Paper presented at the International Conference on Social Psychology and Language, Bristol.
van Dijk, T. A. (Ed.). (1985a). *Handbook of discourse analysis* (4 vols.). London: Academic Press.
van Dijk, T. A. (Ed.). (1985b). *Discourse and communication. New approaches to the analysis of mass media discourse and communication.* Berlin: de Gruyter.
van Dijk, T. A., & Kintsch, W. (1983). *Strategies of discourse comprehension.* New York: Academic Press.
Walker, A. G. (1982). Patterns and implications of co-speech in a legal setting. In R. J. Di Pietro (Ed.), *Linguistics and the professions* (pp. 101-112). Norwood, NJ: Ablex.
Walker, A. G. (1986). The verbatim record: The myth and the reality. In S. Fisher & A. D. Todd (Eds.), *Discourse and institutional authority: Medicine, education and law* (pp. 205-222). Norwood, NJ: Lawrence Erlbaum.
Werner, F. (1983). *Gesprächsverhalten von Frauen and Männer.* Frankfurt: Lang.
West, C. (1984). *Routine complications: Troubles with talk between doctors and patients.* Bloomington: Indiana University Press.
West, C., & Zimmerman, D. H. (1983). Small insults: A study of interruptions in cross-sex conversations between unacquainted persons. In B. Thorne, C. Kramarae, & N. Henley (Eds.), *Language, gender and society* (pp. 102-117). Rowley, MA: Newbury House.
West, C., & Zimmerman, D. H. (1985). Gender, language and discourse. In T. A van Dijk (Ed.), *Handbook of discourse analysis: Vol. 4. Discourse analysis in society* (pp. 103-14). London: Academic Press.

White, D. M. (1976). *The concept of power*. Morristown, NJ: General Learning Press.
Wilkinson, L. C. (Ed.). (1982). *Communicating in the classroom*. New York: Academic Press.
Wilson, C., & Gutiérrez, F. (1985). *Minorities and media*. Beverly Hills, CA: Sage.
Wodak, R. (1984). Determination of guilt: Discourse in the courtroom. In C. Kramarae, M. Schulz, & W. M. O'Barr (Eds.), *Language and power* (pp. 89-100). Beverly Hills, CA: Sage.
Wodak, R. (1985). The interaction between judge and defendant. In T. A. van Dijk (Ed.), *Handbook of discourse analysis: Vol. 4. Discourse analysis in society* (pp. 181-191). London: Academic Press.
Wrong, D. H. (1979). *Power: Its forms, bases and uses*. Oxford: Basil Blackwell.
Young, M. (Ed.). (1971). *Knowledge and control. New directions for the sociology of education*. London: Collier-Macmillan.
Zumbühl, U. (1984). "Ich darf noch ganz kurz. . . ": Die männliche Gesschwätzigkeit am Beispiel von zwei TV-Diskussionssendungen. In S. Trömel-Plötz (Ed.), *Gewalt durch Sprache. Die Vergewaltigung von Frauen in Gesprächen* (pp. 233-245). Frankfurt: Fischer.

Power, Discourse, and Ideology: The Micropractices of Common Sense

LEONARD C. HAWES
University of Utah

Common sense is the deposit of prejudice laid down in the mind before the age of eighteen.

—Albert Einstein

In his essay on discourse structures and power structures, van Dijk sets for himself the task of theorizing a bridge between, on the macroscopic side of the chasm, the embodiment of power in classes, groups, and institutions, and on the microscopic side, the enactment of power in face-to-face, social interaction. I, too, am at work on such a project, but I am beginning from a rather different assumptive site, and consequently I make use of quite different conceptual equipment. The aim of my commentary is to mark points along the two lines of work that constitute significant differences. It is with the implications of these differences that this commentary stakes its claim to value.

Power, discourse, and *ideology* stand together as the foundation for van Dijk's essay; they are the founding constructs for my commentary as well. The crucial differences are in the ways these constructs get defined and come to be used. More specifically, van Dijk and I share an interest in studying "the ways power is enacted, expressed, described, concealed, or legitimated by text and talk in the social context. We pay special attention to the role of ideology" (van Dijk, p. 18). I focus much more directly on discourse as discursive practices than I do on its textuality, and textual practices; van Dijk, at times,

Correspondence and requests for reprints: Leonard C. Hawes, Department of Communication, University of Utah, Salt Lake City, UT 84112.

Communication Yearbook 12, pp. 60-75

appears to use "discourse" and "text" interchangeably. For me, "discourse" is performance and enactment whereas "text" is recorded, or otherwise inscribed, discourse. van Dijk chooses not to review work on the general relationship between "power" and "language," in order to focus on discourse as a "textual" form of language-use in the social context. I admit to not understanding what this qualification means. What is language besides its discursive performances and its textual productions and reproductions? On the matter of levels of conceptualization, van Dijk is interested in "social or societal power" rather than in "personal power" (van Dijk, p. 19). I choose not to make a distinction between the two "levels"; or rather, I don't know where to draw the line that separates the "personal level" from the "social level" of analysis. For me, the micropractices of conversation and the macropractices of institutions anchor two ends of a continuum. Power is, for my purposes, relational, and is expressed in and through embodied discursive practices; for van Dijk, power appears to be a property or attribute of persons and/or social formations.

Working in the European, critical Marxist tradition, I explicate the overdetermined and structurally causal relations of *power, discourse,* and *ideology*. This point of view draws its life from two, not always harmonious, intellectual traditions: first, from structuralism, as it is manifested in Saussure's (1960) linguistics, Lévi-Strauss's (1963; 1967; 1969) structural anthropology, Barthes's (1964; 1972) semiotics, Lacan's (1968; 1977; 1978) structuralist reading of Freud, and Althusser's (1971; 1977) structuralist reading of Marx; and second, from culturalism, as it is manifested in Hoggart's (1957) study of literacy, Thompson's (1963) study of the English working class, Williams's studies of television (1975), literature (1977), and the sociology of culture (1981), and Hall, Critcher, Jefferson, Clarke and Roberts's (1978) study of the social production of news.

I theorize *power, discourse,* and *ideology* as three facets of a multifaceted phenomenon; they become independent constructs only for purposes of analytic convenience. The task is to think of them as a totality. Toward that end, *discourse* becomes a constellation of communicative practices; *practices* are characteristic ways of communicating—of speaking and listening, of writing and reading. *Ideology* is discursively inscribed and deployed; it is evidenced in practice's characteristic, conventional, common, typical, ordinary styles. *Style* comprises these practices, whose effects are, among other functions, ideological. The *power* of ideological practices, then, is its seemingly transparent nature; insofar as ideology's practices are seemingly *both* transparent *and* minuscule, seemingly *both* conventional *and* innocent, seemingly *both* mundane *and* inconsequential, they are *both* overlooked *and* taken-for-granted.

The extent to which power is (wrongly) assumed to be only of macroscopic proportions, to be exercised by monolithic, reified agents, such as corporations and institutions, is the extent to which its capillarylike infrastructure of interactional micropractices is overlooked. This is *not* to argue that macroscopic social formations do not exercise power. It is, rather, to argue that power works at all levels of experience, and to be confused on this point is to invite the conclusion that the individual is powerless when pitted against the State. The error is a mismatch of scale, a confusion at the level of theory (Laclau, 1983; LeFort, 1983). Power is *both* enabling *and* constraining, *both* productive *and* repressive, *both* microscopic *and* macroscopic, when adequately theorized (Foucault, 1980). Taking on such a theoretical project, however, is not possible in the limited space of this commentary, so I shall merely sketch out such an undertaking, but in sufficient detail to provide the grounds for an alternative reading of the discourse analytic and sociolinguistic material van Dijk reviews.

Section I of this commentary theorizes *ideology* from a structuralist-Marxist point of view; specifically, I develop *ideology* on a foundation of Althusser (1977), Hall (1985), Bakhtin (1984), and Volosinov (1973; 1976). Section II theorizes *discourse,* not as textuality, but as conversational practice, as the spatio-temporal practices of making time take place. The works of Bourdieu (1977), Bakhtin (1981), Certeau (1984), and Baudrillard (1981) are most pertinent to this theoretical discussion. In Section III, *power* is developed not at the macroscopic, societal level, but at the microscopic, mundane level; what Foucault would call the microphysics of power. The work of Certeau (1984) on the *narrative of tact* is pivotal to such a discussion of power.

IDEOLOGY

van Dijk formulates ideology in terms of a theory of social cognition; his rationale for this move is that a theory of social cognition provides a theoretical bridge between macro level and micro level analyses. Rather than moving "up and in"—"up" to a social level and "in" to a cognitive domain—I move "down and out"—"down" to a conversational level and "out" to the domain of practice. These two distinct approaches, I find, complement one another in some very heuristic ways.

The work of ideology is to maintain the conditions that ensure the production and reproduction of the relations of power and control in the contexts of everyday living (Barth, 1976; Larrain, 1983). On this view, *language* is a system of signed differences with no positive terms; it comprises the category system of codes that pass as reality. To theorize *language* as an avenue to ideology and consciousness requires, in turn, an explication of semiotic theory and its relations to a theory of discourse (Coward & Ellis, 1977; Fowler Hodge, Kress, & Trew, 1979; Kress & Hodge; 1979). The hallmark of critical theory is its positioning of language in the rethinking of consciousness and ideology. For Marx (1973), consciousness originates in social relations, in the existing relations of production. Consciousness must express itself in concrete, material forms to be accessible to other subjects. One family of such concrete structurational formats comprises conversational practices (Giddens, 1979). *Conversation* is a term designating a large but finite set of material practices. The question is: How are conversational micro-practices and societal macropractices articulated?

Leaving aside, for the purposes of this discussion, the configuration of issues in the debate on the relations between the economic base and the cultural superstructure, and at the same time accepting the proposition that social formations are born of dominant modes of production, it follows that in order to continue to be productive, social formations must perpetually reproduce the conditions of their production. To maintain themselves, social institutions and cultural formations reproduce both the productive forces of production and the social relations that empower such production and reproduction. Althusser (1977) theorizes ideology as being essential to the production and reproduction of subjects capable of reproducing the relations of production, thereby underwriting State power. The power of the State is ensured by means of the Repressive State Apparatus—the police, the penal system, the army—and the Ideological State Apparatuses—education, religion, family, law, politics, trade unions, communications, culture.

The end-point of all ideology is the interpellation of people as subjects; the elementary ideological effect is that the practices that produce subjects are, themselves, transparent. The dominant ideological State apparatus, having replaced the church, is the school. Schools not only inculcate particular knowledges and skills, but inscribe the rules of good conduct and responsible citizenship (Apple, 1979; Burton & Carlen, 1979). For Althusser (1977), ideology represents the imaginary relationship of individuals to their real conditions of existence (p. 162); reflected in the imaginary representation of the world found in an ideology are the conditions of the existence of people, that is, their real world (p. 164). Hall (1985) paraphrases Althusser's formulation of ideology as, "systems of representation—composed of concepts, ideas, myths, or images—in which men and women live their imaginary relations to the real conditions of existence" (p. 103). Systems of representation are the codes of intelligibility, the formats for experiencing the material conditions of everyday life. These systems represent and mediate the immediate conditions of existence. It is impossible to experience real conditions immediately, thus all practices of representation are ideological, which does not imply that all representational practices are *nothing but* ideology. Conversational practices are formats that mediate our experience of the real conditions of existence, and mediated experience stands in an imaginary relation to the real. Such mediating practices deploy systems of representation, and they are, in that sense and to that extent, ideological.

The concepts of *cognition* and *cognitive/mental mediation* become unnecessary in the critical-theoretical formulation of ideology, consciousness, and the subject. For Althusser (1977), our *ideas materialize in actions, which, in turn, are inserted into practices governed by rituals, which are themselves defined by ideological apparatuses* (p. 169). In short, ideas are material practices rather than idealist concepts, and the effectivity of such material practices is the production and reproduction of the category of the subject and its relations to its ideas and to those of other subjects. By way of extending Althusser, Coward and Ellis (1977) define ideology as representational practices that close off meanings and produce subjects as their supports. It is meaning, as closure, that delimits and fixes the individual as a subject of and for discourse. The work of ideology is the production of the continuity of the unitary ego as such a subject; by closing off the inherent openness of discourse and its contradictions, ideology produces the experience of meaning and of the singularity of the subject.

The subject as a sign, however, is in process: ideology works to punctuate this process of becoming, which produces the momentary appearance of a monadic subject speaking with a singular voice originating from within a corporeal body. Bakhtin (1984) maintains, in his study of Dostoevsky's poetics, that the subject/heroes that Dostoevsky creates speak themselves into conscious being in the very process of speaking. Rather than creating a finished and completed subject speaking monologically, Dostoevsky writes subjects who speak themselves into their own autonomous consciousness in a world inhabited by other polyphonic subjects in the process of becoming conscious in the ongoing stream of speech. Subjects speak utterances structured by their material circumstances that then form up and flesh out their experience.

Speaking dialogically is speaking *with* a multiplicity of other voices, rather than speaking *for* others and their experience. Dialogical discourse is speech that opens onto the threshold of crisis and possibility at every moment. Its speaker is not a finalized subject, but a subject in process, a subject always coming to consciousness by means of speaking the truth of his or her experience. From such a theoretical perspective, speaking dialogically clarifies events and experiences for a subject such that the truth at which a speaker is arriving is the truth of its own consciousness; it is speech that is conscious of itself, speech productive of a self-conscious subject (Bakhtin, 1984, pp. 259-422).

As dialogical speech, conversational practices surround corporeal bodies; these bodies are the material embodiments of language. Speaking dialogically is both a matter *of* the body—the body as a surface for, as well as a field of, inscribed signifiers—and a matter *other than* the body. The body is not a causal mechanism driven by cognitive machinery, but is a materially embodied configuration of signifiers that speaks its material consciousness, and, in so doing, speaks its material context. Consciousness cannot be located *inside* a monadic subject, any more than reality can exist *on* a single plane (Schaefer, 1981). Reality is not an *external* backdrop against which *internally* driven subjects interact.

Volosinov (1973) maintains that the notion of a qualitative difference between the *inner* and the *outer* is illusory (pp. 25-26). The structure of experience is as social as is the structure of ideology, and as the structure of ideological experience, an *utterance* is a Janus-faced act; it is directed simultaneously toward the addresser and toward the addressee. The two faces constitute the two poles of a continuum along which experience congeals ideologically. The "I experience," at its extreme, loses its ideological structuration, and with it its sociological apprehendability. It approaches the physiological reaction of animality in losing its verbal delineation. At the other extreme is the "we experience," characterized by a high degree of differentiation, which is characterized as the mark of the growth of consciousness (pp. 38-40). The more differentiated the collective in which a subject orients itself, the more vivid and complex its conscious experience.

Consciousness, then, is inherently ideological; it is constituted in the polyphony of subjects conversing the truth of their experience of material reality. Outside the embodiment of material signs, consciousness is an illusion; embodied utterances, as gesture and speech, configure experience by tying life together and sharpening its differentiations. Volosinov uses the term *behavioral ideology* to delineate the unsystematized speech that endows every act, and therefore every conscious state, with meaning (pp. 83, 91-93). To characterize speech as ideological is to grant it ontological status. As discourse, conversed speech is thought actualized as social practice. When speech is distributed conversationally, which is to say, when it is dialogical and polyphonic, it calls for a response. An utterance stands as a challenge to a precedent; it summons a riposte from an other subject bodying forth to consciousness. Such consciousness of self as subject rests on a semiotic foundation of division, difference, opposition, contradiction, claim and counterclaim, challenge and riposte: It rests on conversation.

Bourdieu (1977) concerns himself with the logic of exchange systems, whose underlying structure is challenge/riposte. A synchronic system of gift-exchange, temporally inflated into a diachronic model, is a political economy whose currency is gifts and whose logic is dialectical. The rights and obligations of differentially distributed power materialize at the same time they are hidden from themselves in temporality: hidden in the irreversible process of giving gifts. Giving a gift is taking a turn, it is presenting a challenge to reply, it is reciprocating in kind but not in identity. Escalation is the most apparent way to engage in the regulated improvisation of such an autopoetic exchange system. In the very same moment that a challenge becomes a riposte, the power claimed by the turn hides itself in its appearance as a gift, a seemingly cooperative gesture. In this way, a conversational turn is a doubled structure; two transformations are produced in a single stroke: challenge becomes riposte and cooperation becomes contestation.

This dialectic of challenge/riposte articulates the exchange systems of Foucault's (1977) microphysics of power insofar as such power is not a determinate effect of the dialectic, but is the structural ambivalence of the domain of practice. It is the region of socioideology, the slip space between individual style and sociocultural tempo. The generative principles for the movement of this dialectic of exchange are not located in abstracted and disembodied rules. Rather, practical consciousness is inscribed on and embodied in the infant from its earliest moments of life. An infant becomes the material sign, signifier, and signified configured as codes in sociocultural circuitries of exchange. The infant's body is the material of socioideological formations.

DISCOURSE

When an infant is born, it is deposited into the symbolic realm of language; it enters a speech community comprising discursive practices that have locative positions for individuals to occupy as subjects. For their subject, the discursive practices make sense; they make meaning. As a subject *of* and *to* these practices, an individual is both *per-formed* and *pro-noun-ced* as a speaking/listening subject articulated to an interpersonal circuitry of social relations and formations. Making meaning in and through subjects is hardly an innocent activity: It is a material struggle, a struggle over the interpretation of events, and a struggle over the power of subjects. Conversational practices presuppose underlying, unstated codes of reality, performing them rather than saying them. Ideology, then, takes its material form in and through the effect of discursive practices that make sense when the underlying codes are presupposed.

For Bourdieu (1977), these configured codes, these socioideological formations, these *dispositions,* are learned—without being explicitly modeled, taught, or instructed—in and through daily participation in the practices of everyday life. *Dispositions,* then, are conversed subjects; they are the material embodiments of everyday practices (p. 72). As discursive practices, conversed language shapes the experiences of its subject's consciousness with the enclosed meanings to sociohistorical conditions. It is the articulation of meaning to experience, the closing off of both meaning and experience, that constitutes the ideological nature of conversational practices. Such practices sustain productive relations and structure in dominance; they laminate meaning to experience, producing conscious subjects; they produce historical continuity in the very process of reproducing sociocultural formations. In this fashion, conversational practices mediate consciousness and ideology simultaneously.

Located at the axis of speech/language, conversational formats interpellate subjects who, in turn, interanimate the production and reproduction of everyday life. The verb *to converse* consists of two Latin root terms: *con* and *vertere*, which means *to turn together in a continuing process of reversal.*

Conversational formats are discursive practices whose movement is doubled, whose turning and reversing interpellate authorial positions as both fixed pronouncements and as unfinished subjects-in-process. Insofar as language is that which all its collusional members assume they know—what goes without saying—language is a practical consciousness, a *common* sense. Speech, however, is a discursive consciousness, an *individuated* sense, insofar as it is that which must be said precisely because it cannot go without saying. So, speech can be thought as the discursive appropriation of practical consciousness, what Bakhtin (Clark & Holquist, 1984), in "The Architectonics of Answerability," calls the *utterance* (pp. 63-94).

It would be a mistake to theorize conversation as a totality, as a coherent and unitary phenomenon. The critical task is to deconstruct the construct of conversation, to describe the micropractices that interpellate an individual into discursive formations as a conversed subject, to explode that totalized gloss into the ideological practices that are the small change of everyday life. The hailing of an individual into the realm of language as a speaking subject is, in large measure, the inscription of identity and difference, of presence and absence, of sound and silence, of self and other. In the realm of language, an individual is alternately subject and object. Subjectivization, then, is division and oscillation coded in conversational formats and performed by means of exchanging.

The giving and taking of turns inscribes a world of subjects, objects, and their interpenetrated relations. Inasmuch as turns are valued, sought, avoided, given, and taken, the way in which conversation is distributed among its members can be thought in politico-economic terms. As with any political economy, the organization of distributional rights and obligations reproduces the very material conditions it organizes. Conversational practices are the structures of sharing and community insofar as turns are distributive; by that, I mean conversational practices are turn-taking systems. Much of social existence is structured in and around the taking of turns. Ideologies are conventionally transparent arrangements for assessing who has what rights and obligations in the scheme of things.

To illustrate: common goods is a fundamentally different mode of distribution than is individual portioning. The analogy is to buffet dining as opposed to à la carte dining. For a buffet, the choices are all present and available. For a la carte, someone presupposes the right to determine for you how much you get and how often. The more fascist the dining, the more the regime presumes the right to serve the portions. The rights of distribution come to be centrally controlled rather than locally administered. The analogy is apposite for conversation; in a family system, for instance, turns are distributed somewhere along the buffet/à la carte continuum. The variety of a subject's tactics for taking turns is either maximized or minimized, either liberated or constrained. Control, to the extreme of passivity, is the objective of fascism; freedom, to the exteme of chaos, is the objective of anarchism. Somewhere along that continuum, a system formulates a communal ideology in the material forms of rights and obligations.

Structures and codes of turn distribution become conventionalized as familiarity and common sense (see van Dijk's discussion of sexism in "Conversation Between Women and Men," and racism in "Racist Talk"). A subject's identity, then, is a conventional collection of discursive micro-practices: Tactics for giving and taking turns. A turn is an opening, a possibility to *be* and to *do*. But what is done with turns is integrally related to how and when turns materialize and how turns are fleshed out with particular content (see van Dijk's discussion of "Job Interviews," "Doctor-Patient Interviews," and "Discourse in Court"). Coming to language as a conversed subject is coming to pragmatic, ethical, aesthetic, political, and spiritual consciousness. There is, in the very production and consumption of conversational practices, a morality whose ideology glosses the appropriation of time, and informs the necessary relations of production and consumption (see Foucault, 1985, pp. 25-32). The ideological effectivity of conversational practices is the production and consumption of an ordinary everyday life of common sense and common places.

The property of conversational practices most responsible for the production and reproduction of this ordinariness and mundaneity are their transparent methods of *cutting out* and *turning over,* of animating social action. In his critique of Foucault's (1977) microphysics of power, and Bourdieu's (1977) notion of *habitus,* Certeau (1984) argues that each theoretical discourse *cuts out* a particular phenomenon from its naturally occuring context and then inverts it, or *turns it over.* In Foucault's case, the "it" is the microphysical practices of surveillance and discipline, and in Bourdieu's case, the "it" is the domestic practices of *habitus.* The discourse cuts one of its features out of its context and turns it into the principle that explains everything.

My argument here is that conversational discourse operates in much the same fashion; conversational practices privilege the position of the speaker, and, in so doing, turn the speaker into an *authority.* Conversational practices cut out individuated subjects from the social collectivity and invest those subjects with the authority produced by its logic of valued differences, its logic of status. Baudrillard (1981) stipulated four different sociologics: (1) a *functional logic* of use value, which is a logic of practical operations or a logic of utility, the object of which is the *instrument*; (2) an *economic logic* of exchange value, which is a logic of equivalence or a logic of the market whose object is the *commodity*; (3) a *logic of symbolic exchange,* which is a logic of ambivalence, a logic of the gift whose object is the *symbol*; and (4) a *logic of sign value,* which is a logic of difference, a logic of status whose object is the *sign* (pp. 66, 67). Conversational practices predicated on a *logic of exchange value* produce objects as commodities. The logic of equivalence, which is a logic of the market, cuts out subjects from the social collectivity and turns them over into commodified objects whose values are determined by this market logic of equivalence.

Practices predicated on a *logic of symbolic exchange* operate on a logic of ambivalence as opposed to equivalence, and produce symbols rather than commodities: The paradigmatic symbol is the gift (Mauss, 1970). The conversational practices of symbolic exchange produce symbols, here broadly defined to include everything from glances, smiles, frowns, and gestures of all sorts, to teasing, joking, and tokens of familiarity whose value is their meaning and worth on a relationship market. On a relationship market, symbols are differentially valued and exchanged, much like commodities on an economic market. However, the symbol, exchanged as a gift, is not intended to be appropriated by an individual subject and accumulated as part of one's economic worth, but to affirm and reaffirm the relationship that its exchange reconstitutes. The gift is not *kept*; in fact, it dissolves in its being given: What remains is its memoric and historical traces. What comes into sharper relief is the circuitry of exchange, the political economy of relationship.

Conversational practices predicated on a *logic of sign value,* which is a logic of difference and status, produce signs as markers of differences. For Baudrillard, this logic of sign value is the logic of the production of commodity consumption as signs of status difference. Or perhaps more succinctly, consumption is its own form of production, and what is produced in consumption is the network of signs marking out status differentiations. In terms of conversational practices, conversing is an act not of accumulation but of consumption. Conversational practices produce the differences among codes at the same time they consume the temporary alliances among them. So vertical contradictions are transformed into horizontal differences. The differences have the status of signs in the political economy of sign value systems, which is to say that contradictory meanings are appropriated by conversational practices and made over into the surfaces of different significations.

POWER

Why would a body break into the silence of anonymity with the sounds of identity? In large measure, because conversational practices are the media of everyday life. They are a way of living as well as a way of knowing; they are ontological as well as epistemological. They are practical from beginning to end insofar as they are ways of doing: Subjective identity becomes a conversation's traces. Conversational practices, then, are ways of taking and giving turns, ways of appropriating and surrendering places in time as a speaker among speakers, an authority among authorities. They are ways of uttering speech to articulate the collaboration and collusion of language. They are ways of marking, locating, and positioning conversed subjects in relation to one another.

Corporeal bodies are inscribed as mobile repositories of memory and consciousness, and it is in this discursivized sense that conversational practices organize ways of knowing into forms of doing, of putting practical knowledge into discursive practice. It is the immediacy of the contradiction of collective living that conversational practices mediate by informing and formatting them as experience, as more or less coherent structures of feeling and thinking. This mediatization produces the identities and commonplaces required for the production and consumption of the common sense of everday life.

Conversational practices mediate the immediate vertical circumstances by turning and inverting them into horizontal differences, thereby transforming meaning into signification. In undercutting and dispersing problematic contradictories, in horizontalizing vertical dilemmas, in laying to rest inscrutible paradoxes, conversational practices are ideological through and through. Their per-forming mediates the immediate, re-presents the present, and empirically evidences the way things are, at least for the time being. Turns produce their speakers as interlocutors, as bricoleurs, as interpellated subjects taking what they find, mediating it, thereby refashioning it. The ways a turn takes what it finds—and what it finds are the material conditions of the imaginary relations to the real conditions of existence—and produces an utterance, necessarily rearranges, reforms, and reproduces the material conditions which are its raw materials.

Once the analogic relations of practical knowledge are digitalized via their transformation into the discursive practices of conversation, gaps and absences are produced; the continuity of practical knowledge becomes the discontinuity of discursive practice. The turning and reversing of conversing break up analogic experience into digital, circumstantial experience, the formats of which are the performative structures of conversed speech. It is this digitalizing of the analogic that produces the gaps and absences that, in the same stroke, define and separate the codes of our material circumstances. It is these gaps and lacunae that are the spaces for *occasions*—the places for time to appear as the experience, memory, and practical intelligence that momentarily bridge the gap by filling it in with what's missing, thereby producing the temporality of meaning. But in so doing, of course, it also produces, as a consequence of having rearranged those circumstances in the production of meaning, the spatiality of significance by producing other gaps and spaces between the codes of material circumstances. What must be said and done to fill in the gaps and ruptures between codes of changing circumstances, thereby stitching together the seams of temporary coherence, changes with each utterance, which summons another turning reversal to address and redress the newly produced gaps—the spaces for the possibility of new occasions. *Utterance,* here, is the name for the ways and means of the turning, of the practices for making time take place in the conjunctures of everyday life circumstances.

Bourdieu's (1977) concern with the individual operations of exchange locates the practicing subject within the moment of the practice's production, rather than outside of practice and time. He aims at a science of the dialectical relations between theoretical and practical knowledge that includes scientific as well as everyday practices. Instead of positioning it outside of everyday temporality, and off to one side of the dialectical relation—the better to reconstruct its possibility conditions and operating rules—he locates the practicing subject as close to the seam of space/time as possible.

The operation of the practices of everyday life presupposes that subjects do not recognize, are not conscious of, the rules and mechanisms of the exchange system that an analyst's model exposes by temporally collapsing it, rendering diachronic practice as synchronic structure. As a temporally deflated structure of layered relations, practices now appear to be reversibly granularized rather than irreversibly temporalized. Inflating the structuralist model with the time of the subject's practices produces a dialectic of two opposing truths: The reversible sign value system of relations of power is as true as, even if overshadowed by, the irreversible symbolic exchange system.

Temporalizing the structural relations of power doesn't invalidate the political economic model, but instead produces a symbolic exchange model, and each system generates the possibility of the other. Time is the medium through which the spatio-structural contradictions are worked out, and concern shifts to the practices of and for *making time take place*. For Bourdieu, such practices are *strategies*; for Certeau, they are *tactics*. Both refer to temporal practices that materialize in space but are not inscribed "once and for all." Intervals between durations of actions constitute the temporal embodiments and amplifications of contradictions that are resolved, more or less adequately, by *tempo*. Variable intervals of time between actions accommodate the acceptable array of contradictions to be taken account of practically, to be appropriated and worked on in time, and that materialize in practice.

Conversation is a gloss for this broadly deployed set of practices of selection and realization for producing and reproducing the substantive tempo of everyday life, a tempo whose structure resolves appropriatable contradictions and suppresses the materialization of others. As a multi-mediated set of practices, *conversation* is the play of a spontaneous semiology that orchestrates the regulated improvisation of practices whose region of production lies somewhere between the seemingly open set of mundane practices of everyday life, and the more constrained practices of custom, ceremony, and ritual (Turner, 1982); between individual style and social custom. Conversation consists of those practices for being carried along, without being carried away or carried beyond practical knowledge, which is the ground of the very possibility of conversing.

In the format of utterances, conversational practices break into the silent stasis of practical consciousness by taking place momentarily, and, in so doing, putting into practice (i.e., discursivizing) whatever is done at that moment. The taking of turns is possible to the extent that subjects presuppose a covenant: A subject grants a speaking turn to Other, and, in so doing, produces an implicit promise or a subsequent turn and continued access to the turn-taking economy. Much as a plastic overlay organizes without obscuring that which it covers, the turn-taking formats of speaking and listening organize that which appears to be transparent common sense. The ideological labor of conversational micropractices is to appear to be neutral and labor-free. Their purpose is to conceal themselves, making room for the content that takes its place. Formats of micropractices constitute the seemingly transparent contexts in and through which the content of common sense is routinely inscribed.

Utterances, thereby, articulate subjects to spatio-temporal contexts, and may be formulated in a variety of grammatical tenses, but the structures of experience being encoded can, and do, come from times and places other than the tense in which the turn is currently being produced. Furthermore, a *here* of a speaker is separated from a *there* of a listener; a *now* of speaking and listening is articulated to a *then*, of memory and imagination. In this perpetual articulation and disarticulation, *utterances make time* (now/then), *take place* (here/there). Memory and history are the products of the ideological labor of reproducing forms of communal life and structures of experience produced in other times and places. Structures of experience, initially inscribed in infancy and early childhood, are reproduced throughout a subject's lifetime. In fact, an individual comes to be recognized as a subject having an identity, as being the selfsame subject over time, to the extent that he or she reproduces identical and near-identical formats of speech and structures of experience. Space/time, then, is a doubled structure, produced by means of conversational practices; there is the spatio-temporal positioning of the speaking subject's corporeal body, and there is the grammatico-historical positioning of the language being spoken.

The pivotal concern in all of this is how the practical consciousness of existence gets discursively distributed as the coded formats of communal life. How do the dialectical relations get deployed in the material and spiritual structures of everyday experience? Conversational practices are mimetically valid and ideologically productive; their self-imitation remains transparent. The beginning of a turn announces a possible future moment in which speaking will have ceased and an other subject will have been articulated to a turn. As attention and orientation are managed in and through conversational turn-taking, possibilities come into view, collapse, dissolve, and fold back the imaginable. In this mimetic fashion, conversational practices format and distribute the experiential world by means of structuring turns of speaking and listening. Turns are taken and given in *particular ways,* and it is the *style* of the taking and giving, the tactical flair, that captures attention or fails to capture attention. It is through the seeming transparency of conversational codes that the traces of intentionality are evidenced. Agreement, disagreement, deference, partronage, status, control, knowledge, racism, sexism, integrity, trust, honor, hatred, desire, are only a handful of such structures coded in the micropractices of conversation (in addition to van Dijk's extensive bibliography, see Benthall & Polhemus, 1975; Coulthard & Montgomery, 1981; Craig & Tracy, 1983; Goodwin, 1981; Halliday, 1978; Heritage, 1984; Sandywell, Silverman, Roche, Filmer, & Phillipson, 1975; Spacks, 1985; Stubbs, 1983).

Taking a turn by producing an utterance is, at one and the same moment, a radical assertion of individuality and difference, and a repressive insistence on punctuating reality in the narrative formats of tradition and convention. The conversational practices of making time take place are simultaneously fascistic and revolutionary: Fascistic insofar as individuals are obligated to be subjects of conventional turns as evidence of membership and good faith; and revolutionary insofar as a turn can be taken that violates convention and tradition, and foundationally reorganizes both practical and discursive knowledge along with their attendant power relations. Ways of inscribing spaces of time are, then, by their very nature, both an assertion and a repression; as such, turns are moves in the relations of power and signification.

Power relations are evident in the most microscopic of social practices, evident because the nature of collective living marks differences that become, upon their materialization, signs of values—commodities marking status difference—and power relations. To live in the everyday world of postmodern capitalism is to live in a world of constantly shifting alliances with signs. Conversational practices are ways of modifying one's positionality among signs of power, means of shifting alliances, methods of accommodating individuated benefits, and techniques for taking care of one's practical affairs. This lateralization of contradictories is a narrative movement; the formats informing experience are narrative, and these narratives are the structures of feeling of our imaginary relationships to our real conditions of existence (Jameson, 1981).

Insofar as theory encodes practices, and practice informs time, conversation is a discourse that is both memory and practice: the *narrative of tact*. Certeau (1984) characterizes an "art" as a practice for which there is no enuciation; it is practical knowledge that has yet to be discursivized; it is use value without the commodifying algorithm to produce exchange value. For Certeau, speaking is such an art, an art of doing and of thinking, constituting theory and practice simultaneously. In short, it is the art of story telling (p. 33). As an art of speaking, story telling produces effects, not objects; narration, not description. As the narrative of tact, conversation is the style of the tactics for taking turns that enact memory and produce experience.

The circuitry of interpersonal relations, the domain of time-bound experience, is a temporary one at best; it comprises temporary islands of interpersonal alliances in spatial seas of ever-accelerating changes. The question is not so much one of taking over the centralized, repressive State apparatus, but is more a matter of how to live everyday life at the margins, within the workings of the ideological State apparatuses, with subjects whose tactics for producing and consuming experience form up the dialectics of conversational practices for the enactment of transient communities and relations. And the narratives of legitimation change as macroscopic technological innovations extend the spatial boundaries of reality. It falls to the time binding micropractices of conversation to produce and reproduce narratives whose legitimacy is decreasingly grounded in the spatial and increasingly grounded in the temporary.

REFERENCES

Althusser, L. (1971). Ideology and ideological state apparatuses. In *Lenin and philosophy and other essays*. London: New Left.

Althusser, L. (1977). *For Marx*. London: New Left.

Apple, M. W. (1979). *Ideology and curriculum*. London: Routledge & Kegan Paul.

Bakhtin, M. (1981). *The dialogic imagination: Four essays*. Austin: University of Texas Press.

Bakhtin, M. (1984). *Problems of Dostoevsky's poetics*. Minneapolis: University of Minnesota Press.

Barth, H. (1976). *Truth and ideology*. Berkeley: University of California Press.

Barthes, R. (1964). *Elements of semiology*. New York: Hill & Wang.

Barthes, R. (1972). *Mythologies*. London: Jonathan Cape.

Baudrillard, J. (1981). *For a critique of the political economy of the sign*. St. Louis: Telos.

Benthall, J., & Polhemus, T. (1975). *The body as a medium of expression*. New York: E. P. Dutton.

Bourdieu, P. (1977). *Outline of a theory of practice*. Cambridge: Cambridge University Press.

Burton, F., & Carlen, P. (1979). *Official discourse: The English used by teachers and pupils*. London: Routledge & Kegan Paul.

Certeau, M. de. (1984). *The practice of everyday life*. Berkeley: University of California Press.

Clark, K., & Holquist, M. (1984). *Mikhail Bakhtin*. Cambridge: Belknap/Harvard.

Coulthard, M., & Montgomery, M. (1981). *Studies in discourse analysis*. London: Routledge & Kegan Paul.

Coward, R., & Ellis, J. (1977). *Language and materialism*. London: Routledge & Kegan Paul.

Craig, R. T., & Tracy, K. (Eds.). (1983). *Conversational coherence: Form, structure, and strategy*. Beverly Hills: Sage.

Foucault, M. (1977). *Discipline and punish*. New York: Vintage.

Foucault, M. (1980). *Power/knowledge: Selected interviews and other writings*. New York: Pantheon.

Foucault, M. (1985). *The use of pleasure: The history of sexuality* (Vol. 2). New York: Pantheon.

Fowler, R., Hodge, B., Kress, G., & Trew, T. (1979). *Language and control*. London: Routledge & Kegan Paul

Giddens, A. (1979). *Central problems in social theory: Action, structure and contradiction in social analysis*. Berkeley: University of California Press.

Goodwin, C. (1981). *Conversational organization: Interaction between speakers and hearers.* New York: Academic Press.
Hall, S. (1982). The rediscovery of "ideology": return of the repressed in media studies. In M. Gurevitch, T. Bennett, J. Curran, & J. Woollacot (Eds.) *Culture, society and the media* (pp. 56-90). London: Methuen.
Hall, S. (1985). Signification, representation, ideology: Althusser and the post-structuralist debates. *Critical Studies in Mass Communication, 2,* 91-114.
Hall, S. Critcher, C., Jefferson, T., Clarke, J., & Roberts. B. (1978). *Policing the crisis.* London: Macmillan.
Halliday, M.A.K. (1978). *Language as social semiotic.* Baltimore: University Park Press.
Heritage, J. (1984). *Garfinkel and ethnomethedology.* Cambridge: Polity Press.
Hoggart, R. (1957). *The uses of literacy.* London: Chatto & Windus.
Jameson, F. (1981). *The political unconscious: Narrative as a socially symbolic act.* Ithaca, NY: Cornell University Press.
Kress, G., & Hodge, R. (1979). *Language as ideology.* London: Routledge & Kegan Paul.
Lacan, J. (1968). *The language of the self: The function of language in psychoanalysis.* New York: Delta.
Lacan, J. (1977). *Ecrits: A selection.* New York: Norton.
Lacan, J. (1978). *The four fundamental concepts of psychoanalysis.* New York: Norton.
Laclau, E. (1983). The impossibility of society. *Canadian Journal of Political and Social Theory, 7,* 21-24.
Larrain, J. (1983). *Marxism and ideology.* London: Macmillan.
Lefort, C. (1983). On the genesis of ideology in modern societies. *Canadian Journal of Political and Social Theory, 7,* 43-83.
Levi-Strauss, C. (1963). *Structural anthropology.* New York: Basic.
Levi-Strauss, C. (1967). *The scope of anthropology.* London: Jonathan Cape.
Levi-Strauss, C. (1969). *The elementary structures of kinship.* London: Eyre & Spottiswoode.
Marx, K. (1973). *Grundrisse.* New York: Vintage.
Marx, K., & Engels, F. (1970). *The German ideology.* New York: International Publishers.
Mauss, M (1970). *The gift.* London: Routledge.
Sandywell, B., Silverman, E., Roche, M., Filmer, P., & Phillipson, M. (1975). *Problems of reflexivity and dialectics in sociological inquiry: Language theorizing difference.* London: Routledge & Kegan Paul.
Saussure, F. de (1960). *Course in general linguistics.* London: P. Owen.
Schaefer, R. (1981). Narration in psychoanalytic dialogue. In W.J.T. Mitchell (Ed.), *On narrative.* Chicago: University of Chicago Press.
Spacks, P. M. (1985). *Gossip.* Chicago: University of Chicago Press.
Stubbs, M. (1983). *Discourse analysis.* Chicago: University of Chicago Press.
Thompson, E. P. (1963). *The making of the English working class.* London: Gollancz.
Turner, V. (1982). *From ritual to theatre: The human seriousness of play.* New York: Performing Arts Journal Publications.
Volosinov, V. N. (1973). *Marxism and the Philosophy of Language.* New York: Seminar Press.
Volosinov, V. N. (1976). *Freudianism: A Marxist critique.* New York: Academic Press.
Williams, R. (1975). *Television: Technology and cultural form.* New York: Schocken.
Williams, R. (1981). *The sociology of culture.* New York: Schocken.
Williams. R. (1977). *Marxism and literature.* Oxford: Oxford University Press.

The Irrationality of Power

RUTH WODAK
University of Vienna

> No matter how one looks at it, the command in its self-contained, complete form—that is, the form in which we find it today after a long period of development—has become the single most dangerous element in the social life of man. One must have the courage to resist it and undermine its power. Ways and means must be found to keep the majority of mankind free from it. One dare not allow it to do any more than just scratch the skin. Its barbs must become no more than harmless leeches, which can easily be brushed off.
>
> Canetti (1980, p. 371)

As a complex, interdisciplinary phenomenon, power requires an interdisciplinary approach that includes sociology, social psychology, sociolinguistics, history, economics, psychoanalysis, and discourse analysis. Whereas van Dijk concentrates on sociopsychological, economic, and cognitive concepts, I would like to base my investigation on psychoanalytical, sociological and sociolinguistic aspects. Only an analysis of all the aspects can do justice to the problem of who is powerful or powerless, where, why, and how.

Therefore, I would like to proceed from the *internal perspective* and from the *irrationality of power,* from the level of feelings, from the *interaction* between the powerful and the powerless, and from their motives. I am chiefly interested in the *dialectic* between the *internal and the external perspectives,* between the masses and the individual, between collective and private discourse. Ideologies and power can be productive only if they can be related to everyday experience and prevailing sentiment. Thus newspapers can print only what their readers understand and expect, though these expectations can also be titillated and reinforced.

van Dijk, on the other hand, takes as his starting point the power of the elite over the masses, which is especially exemplified by the power the former exercises over the media. (However, he ignores Bourdieu's [1982] innovative and very useful concept of "symbolic power" [see Wodak, in press-b]).

Correspondence and requests for reprints: Ruth Wodak, Department of Linguistics, University of Vienna, Leichtensteinstrasse 46a, Vienna, A 1090, Austria.

Communication Yearbook 12, pp. 76-94

Ideologies, viewed chiefly as collections of cognitive and sociocognitive concepts, are centrally regulated and imparted "from the top," manipulating attitudes and public opinion. The effect is assumed to be unidirectional.

In what follows, I give my approach to the dominant aspects of "power and discourse." To save space, I have briefly outlined the main points we will engage.

The *relational character of power*: Of prime importance here is power viewed as the interaction between the powerful and the powerless. Power and powerlessness, and the powerful and the powerless, must be specifically defined for each situation and setting. One must also distinguish between the different forms in which power is exercised; these may be subtle or very obvious (through "feelings of guilt," brute force, or even extermination).

The *effect of power* on those subjected to it: Whether it be exercised through fear, threats, force, punishment, feelings of guilt, and so on, power, as a psychological phenomenon, requires irrational and emotional levels in order to sustain itself (see Strotzka, 1984). In *Massenpsychologie und Ich-Analyse,* Freud described—and almost seemed to predict—the dialectic interplay between the *Führerkult* (cult of the leader) and the dutiful masses. Through identification and projection, people regress at times, give up their "superegos," and are trustingly obedient. Understanding, reflection, and cognitive awareness are thus almost inoperative.

From the viewpoint of microanalysis and *verstehende* description, the *manner in which power is affected* is multileveled, multidimensional, often dysfunctional, subtle, affective, systematic, and unique to each situation. The unidimensionality of van Dijk's static categories and his empirical quantitative methods are not adequate for a detailed treatment of such interactions. Participatory observation, case studies, and qualitative methods are necessary. It is only by employing both methods (quantitative as well as qualitative, verstehend and descriptive, external and internal) that social language behavior as the manifestation of the exercising of power can be subtly differentiated and explained.

Finally (and critically), the *theoretical concepts of the non-English-speaking world are ignored,* as is the long tradition of sociolinguistics, which has, since its beginnings, been concerned with the phenomenon of power (see Bernstein, 1981; Dittmar, 1985a, 1985b; Ehlich & Rehbein, 1986; Wodak, 1981, 1984, 1986, in press-a, in press-b; Bourdieu, 1982; Soeffner, 1979; Lutz & Wodak, 1987; Pfeiffer, Strouhal, & Wodak, 1987). Because of the limited space available to me, I will restrict myself in the following to Arendt's and Habermas's concept (see next) and dispense with a critical survey of the literature. Similarly, I will limit myself to van Dijk's description of supplemental perspectives rather than overburden the reader with a comprehensive review of the research in the area (see Ammon, Dittmar, & Mattheier, 1988).

van Dijk does consider both the relational character and the significance of interaction in his framework. Concepts such as domination, authority, ideology, control, and manipulation are defined with regard to the sociocognitive concept he uses as his basis, while historical, sociolinguistic, and social-psychological considerations are incomplete. His concept, however, remains too deterministic, monocausal, and restrictive; mediating agencies and social dialectics are missing. In the end, he limits himself to an external perspective and to an analysis of control over the means of production (as well as of texts) as the basis of power. Paying particular attention to historical and social consideration, I would like to expand on the subtle and irrational forms of power by examining each individual situation without bringing the materialistic argumentation into question.

AN APPROACH TO UNDERSTANDING POWER: HABERMAS'S COMMUNICATIVE CONCEPT

Weber (1968) defines power as the possibility of imposing one's own will on others, even in the face of resistance. Hannah Arendt (1986) regards power as a political institution, "as manifestation and materialization of power" (p. 64). Parsons (1986) prefers to view power in the sense of the institutionalization of authority and, therefore, as "the rights of collective agents to mobilize performances and define them as binding obligation" (p. 97). Finally, Foucault (1977) presents interesting relationships between power structure and the structures of discourse, especially the limitations they impose in institutions by means of the principles of division, exclusion, and brevity (p. 47). These "procedures" (Foucault, 1977, p. 7) of discourse control, selection, and organization in institutions must be investigated, with particular reference to samples of texts. They are indeed a question of power: Who is in the position to control, select, organize, and channel it? Which of these procedures are legitimate in an institution (e.g., in a hospital) and which are not? Where does one draw the line? (see Lalouschek, Menz, & Wodak, 1987).[1]

Nevertheless, Habermas's definition appears to be the more practical, because it does not limit power to institutions and hierarchies, but considers behavior in a wide range of situations. I would like to use this broader view as a departure point, dealing above all with communicative models. My concept of language behavior, therefore, involves the inclusion of both cognitive and emotional factors, as follows:

> Power arises from the human ability to act (or to do something) as well as to come together with others and get along with them. The fundamental phenomenon of power is the instrumentation of an alien will in communication that is directed towards understanding. (Habermas, 1982, p. 104)

We therefore constantly ask ourselves: Who exercises power over whom, how, where, and with what means; who accepts it, and how; who resists it, and how; who refuses to comply with it, and how; who goes along with it; who does not? To explore these questions from the internal perspective—the psychoanalytical point of view—I would like to investigate the dialectic of collective and individual discourse in the dissemination of ideologies and power using examples from research on prejudice.

INTERNAL AND EXTERNAL PERSPECTIVES: DISCOURSE AND POWER AS TOPIC AND CHALLENGE

As mentioned, power must be defined in relation to a particular situation and to particular discourse. This stance points to the discrepancy between two strategies of research, that is, between systems research and *Lebenswelt* research. In order to be able to describe "power and language" and "power and discourse," both a macrosociological and a sociolinguistic description of the system (the institution) and a multilevel analysis of various and unique interactions (language behavior) with a microlinguistic basis will be necessary. In the end, what we want to understand is the why, when, where, and how of who is powerful, how power develops, and what its effect is, and finally, what role language plays in it (Wodak, 1988).

It is Dittmar's (1985a) view that theory construction is possible only if one can succeed in "building a constructive interdisciplinary bridge between the *language system and language use,* and the culture-specific "Lebenswelt and the institutionalized social system." Dittmar thereby takes up the question posed by Habermas (1981), who describes the discrepancy between two types of research. On the one hand, one observes an individual's behavior from the *internal pespective* and attempts to understand it; on the other hand, one looks at the social institutions from an *observer perspective* and abstracts from the subjects' behavior. This difference corresponds to the conflict between qualitatively oriented research and quantifying methods (see also Ehn, 1986; Auwärter, 1983). Habermas (1981) suggests a resolution, as follows:

> A connection between the two is possible, however, namely through the *semanticization of the interactions* and by means of the *shared language.* With every shared definition of a situation, they, the participants, determine the boundaries between external nature, society, and internal nature, while at the same time renewing the delimitation between themselves as interpreters on the one hand, and the outside world and their perspective inner worlds on the other hand. (p. 186)

Communicative behavior is based, therefore, on a cooperative process of interpretation, in which the interactors always refer simultaneously to something in the objective, in the social, and in the subjective world, even if sometimes (or usually) only one component in an utterance is explicitly focused on.

Habermas's approach appears to me to be especially pertinent here. For if language and culture are constituents of the Lebenswelt (p. 190) and if "culture" at the same time represents a "developmental process for particular institutions and relationships involving domination" and if language and culture are created, maintained, and orally passed on by participating subjects, then such a dichotomy is not necessary but can be integrated by means of a theory of communicative behavior and by means of a theory of socialization and culture.

> The entities that should be subsumed under the external perspective of an observer's systems-theoretical concepts must be identified in advance as the "Lebenswelten" of social groups and be understood in terms of their symbolic structures. (Habermas, 1981, p. 227)

This statement refers to the interaction and the dialectic between external and internal perspective. It claims that identification and understanding can be achieved only through language. A sociolinguistic theory of power that seeks to link microanalysis and macroanalysis must, therefore, attempt to combine both perspectives, not only in the formation of hypotheses, but in the method used.

The *ethnopsychoanalytical approach* (Erdheim, 1984) could certainly be taken as a model. Without explicitly carrying out a linguistic analysis, this school is able to conclusively demonstrate both the theoretically and empirically founded connection between the individual, the Lebenswelt, identity, and personality structure on the one hand, and social processes, domination, power relationships, and culture on the other. Erdheim considers two relevant points: (1) socialization within the family, and (2) the tensions between the individual, the family, and culture. These points bring us to the cornerstones of the language barrier theory, that is, to "social inequality and power" and "socialization, planning strategies, and codes" (see also, Bernstein, 1981). As I have discussed socialization in a more detailed manner elsewhere (see Wodak, in press-a), here I will limit myself to the issue of "power and language."

In his work on mass psychology, Freud (1976) shows that *institutions function like individuals,* though the price that must be paid for this is high: "institutions function like individuals, but only by robbing their members of their characteristic qualities" (Erdheim, 1984, p. 190).

Because, however, institutions are based on individuals, or participating subjects, they can also be understood from the internal perspective. While institutionally "robbed" of his or her characteristics, the individual feels comfortable in the security of the institution and initially does not question it because the institution possesses his or her characteristics. Of relevance to the issue of the development of a sociolinguistic theory of power is that the individual and the Lebenswelt, as well as society, the institution, and culture do not stand at opposite poles and are not different "entities," but that they are related to and can be understood through each other. Society, collective consciousness and subconsciousness, rituals, ceremonies, myths, and ideologies can also be explained by taboos and the suppression of wishes and drives typical to the individual (see Wodak, Menz, Lutz, & Gruber, 1985).

What specific significance does this have both for a sociolinguistic theory of "discourse and power" and for empirical research (see Wodak, 1986, in press-d)? (a) The incompatibility of internal and external perspectives must be rejected. (b) Thus a theory must combine the linguistic manifestations of the family, of socialization, and of power and society. (c) It must operate with a *multimethod approach,* proceed qualitatively and quantitatively, and combine static and dynamic categories (see Dittmar, 1985a, p. 2). (d) *Several levels* must likewise be involved in the *interpretation,* whereby it is expedient to include as much information as possible from a wide range of sources on the topic under investigation (see Wodak, in press-b). (e) *Microanalyses* should not neglect the social framework, and *macroanalyses* should be supplemented by verstehende, qualitative microresearch. (f) The *interdisciplinary nature* should be emphasized. Language analysis must include a sociopsychological communication theory and a historical and social context as well as a social theory. (g) Because power is never only rational and functional, the *cognitive* dimension should not be overemphasized. The linguistic behavior of both the powerful and the powerless is the result of conscious and unconscious processes, as well as automatic and spontaneous ones. It is imperative that the *affective* and *emotional* levels not be ignored.

THE IRRATIONALITY OF POWER: THE PSYCHOANALYTIC AND PSYCHOLINGUISTIC APPROACH

Affective and irrational factors as well as the mechanisms of mass psychology, which in turn require concepts from individual psychology, are not often considered in the analysis of power, even in the literature of sociology and social psychology. How is power exercised and by whom? Why is it accepted, tolerated, and even acceded to?

Obviously power does not have only a negative effect; one is sometimes ready to identify with the powerful and put one's own values and identities last. And even if power is not affected by means of total control as in Orwell's *1984* (as it is not in a pluralistic society), fear or a self-indulging helplessness can still be the result. Let me take the "family" as an example: It is not necessary to beat children, shout at them, and bring them up in a completely repressive environment in order for them to be obedient and to recognize guilt and fear. More subtle mechanisms are at work (see Wodak, 1984; Wodak & Schulz, 1986).

In my view, the psychoanalytic approach is well suited to arriving at an answer to the questions just posed. By extending psychoanalytic concepts through ethnopsychoanalysis (Erdheim, 1984), the individual-psychological level can be socially integrated (see the foregoing comments and Wodak, 1988).

> The psychoanalytic approach to the problems of power lies on the one hand . . . in ideas of grandeur as well as in the impoverished relationship of narcissism; and on the other hand, it lies in the desire to dominate and to be dominated, as well as in the causes of suffering and in sadomasochistic suffering. (Strotzka, 1984, p. 69)

Certain character structures and personality types (see Adorno, 1973) predestine many people with a desire to exercise power. This determination is connected with fantasies of grandeur, an unstable identity, and uncontrollable aggression, whereby certain psychodynamic processes are held responsible in the development of the individual. The impaired self-esteem of such people is strengthened by the powerlessness of others. Their detachment makes the suppression of others possible without arousing guilt in themselves. Furthermore, such people know how to exploit their feelings of omnipotence in order to captivate others (charismatic personalities) (see Freud, 1976). But it is not only the powerful who have power—the powerless do as well.

> The indirect power that the ill and the handicapped exercise over their surroundings is often considerable.
>
> One might take the case of the elderly mother who does not release her child from the symbiotic relationship for the child's entire life thereby making it impossible for the child to have an independent existence; or consider the hysterical woman who tyrannizes her husband and children with her fits and threats to commit suicide; or the class at school or the group at work, which not only can drive their teacher or supervisor crazy merely by passive resistance, but can also reduce production to a minimum, regardless of what it consists of. Children's power over their parents and patients' power over their doctors are likewise often denied. (Strotzka, 1984, p. 51)

Powerlessness can be identified within the aspect of "sadomasochism," which Strotzka (1984, p. 69ff.) does not interpret as a sexual perversion. Just as there are typical powerful individuals, there are also typical powerless ones: They offer themselves as objects of suppression to the powerful, who need these masochistic types in order to develop (Strotzka, p. 71). Anticipation of punishment, therefore, means pleasure. This explains why, if it is in any way possible, there is not more resistance to violence, power, domination, and authority. Power plays, viewed by the outsider as awful, be they in the nuclear family, in partnerships, or institutions, and so on, are experienced subjectively and differently by the participants as pleasurable suffering.

Fromm (1980) distinguished between sadistic and destructive personalities. The latter attempt to destroy the object, whereas the former need it in order to dominate it and fear its loss. The desire for power is, therefore, the most important manifestation of sadism (see also Strotzka, 1984, p. 72ff.).

Subtle discourse analytic studies of political language and domination can also reveal these psychological, historical, and social components in their complexity. I refer the reader to Sauer (1987), Maas (1985), Wodak and Feistritzer (in press), and Gruber and Wodak (1987). Without this psychological-affective level it would not be possible—as Strotzka (1984, p. 208ff.) shows—to fully explain phenomena such as National Socialism (the particular role that illusion and myth play in the legitimization of domination will be examined next, especially the function of prejudice in the setting up of a scapegoat).

LANGUAGE AND PREJUDICE: LANGUAGE AND POWER

"If the Arguments Are Lacking, One Must Fall Back on the Jew."

Sociolinguistics can make an important contribution in explaining the phenomenon of the transmission of power through prejudice. Ideologies use language in varied ways and constitute themselves through them. Forms of the shaping of prejudice and of its effect on language use in the public sphere can be demonstrated through language analysis.

I would, at this point, like to make some general remarks about the dialectic interplay between language, ideology, and prejudice (see in detail Wodak, 1988; in press-a, in press-b; Wodak et al., 1985).

Ideology manifests itself linguistically, has its effect through language and on it, and is only made possible and established through it. Therefore, linguistic behavior has a direct impact on social practice.

Ideological language has a dual character: It is both an expression and a transmitter of ideological thought. It manipulates and is at the same time manipulated.

There are special "languages of ideology": Each is a complete, closed system with a claim to truth, and with its own values and meanings. Language is able to allow, thanks to its distorted mythical functionings, that which serves power to appear as "positive." This appearance occurs, for instance, in party platforms, manifestos, and in the "fundamental works" on ideology (see Wodak, in press-d; Wodak & Feistritzer, in press). This isolation does not, of course, exist in everyday language use.

Ideologies, as structures of myths, establish a secondary reality and thus also a social practice; they make the previous reality taboo and supersede it. A new dimension of meanings and values is produced that expresses itself in new concepts and connotations.

The elimination of reflection is achieved by means of stereotypes and clichés, which possess a systematic linguistic realization: Certain areas thereby become taboo, others are "automated," many are freed from history (or history is paraphrased or rewritten).

Such a closed, ideological structure for anti-Semitism existed only to a certain degree in the Third Reich. Clearly, present-day anti-Semitism is no longer effective as such a total pseudoscientific, ideological system. However, it can very easily fall back on relics of Nazi anti-Semitism; one encounters linguistics borrowings from it everywhere.

In a linguistic analysis of anti-Semitic prejudices, it is not enough to investigate all the levels of linguistic utterances (vocabulary, sentence structure, the text level and linguistic strategies, and semiotic elements in posters or caricatures). Contributing factors in the production and reception of texts must also be considered. There is a dynamic interrelation between the individual who produces an utterance, the text, and the addressee of the utterance. Sociolinguistic factors (age, social status, sex, political socialization, and so on) must be taken into consideration, both in the production of texts (in the broadest sense) and in their reception. The participants' knowledge of the world, which influences their expectations, attitudes, and prejudices is "understood," that is, interpreted, as a linguistic utterance (see Lutz & Wodak, 1987; van Dijk, 1984).

The analysis of current forms of anti-Semitism requires asking: In the presence of what foreknowledge and in which social classes do forms of anti-Semitic discourse appear? This analysis can explain why we need only to operate with allusions to voice anti-Semitic prejudices in present-day political discourse, for example, when we speak of "certain groups" or dishonorable persons. It is enough to quote or allude to the expressions of the old anti-Semitism in order to achieve an anti-Semitic effect. Sociolinguistics can contribute to an understanding of subtle forms of utterances of prejudices and to making their functionings and power transparent. It can also make a contribution in cases in which prejudices are allegedly only quoted and the quoter wants to leave the anti-Semitisms to the interpretations of the hearer, with the comment "*honni soit qui mal y pense.*" Moreover, whatever power anti-Semitism has, it no longer needs to be broken down into separate classes after the holocaust.

The Function of Anti-Semitic Prejudices

Anti-Semitism reveals itself to be too complex and multileveled a phenomenon for one explanatory approach to be adequate. Social psychology and prejudice research can certainly verify empirically that all people want to and must reduce the "complexity of the world" by means of certain stereotypes, experiences, and automations. But, why the Jews offer themselves as a target of aggression, as a scapegoat, as the enemy without, and as a projection surface, requires further explanation. In addition, we are struck by the apparent contradiction that anti-Semitism is at its strongest in Austria, in those places where there are hardly any or no Jews (anti-Semitism without Jews). And, certain linguistic patterns (quotes, allusions) allow taboos and the shifting of responsibility (anti-Semitism without anti-Semites).

What purpose then does anti-Semitism serve—sui bono? According to Adorno (1973):

> The "irrational" Jewish cliché seems to fulfill similar functions [reduction of complexity]. For the extremely prejudiced person, they are stereotyped to the limit and, at the same time, are personalized in a stronger way than any other bogey. This is because they are not defined on the basis of profession or social role, but rather on the basis of their existence as such. . . . The foreignness of Jews seems to be the most convenient formula to deal with the alienation of society. Blaming the Jews for all existing evil lights up the darkness of reality like a headlight, which affords one a rapid and extensive orientation. The less anti-Jewish fantasies correspond to actual experience and the more they are kept "clean," so to speak, from the defilement of society, the less they are exposed to disturbances from the dialectic of experience, which is prevented by the rigidity of the stereotypes. Anti-Semitism is the panacea that ensures intellectual equilibrium, counter "kathexis," and a channeling of the desires for "change." (p. 123ff.)

Thus anti-Semitic clichés create an image of "the Jew" as the enemy in a stereotypical and rigid way as the continued presence of prejudice in history demonstrates. This usually has little to do with experience—one need not know any Jews in order to believe and use these concepts of the enemy. In fact, just the opposite is true: The less personal experience one has with Jews, the wider the door seems to be open to anti-Semitic projection. Although I cannot make a detailed analysis of this discourse within the scope of this article (see Maas, 1985; Wodak, 1988), I would like to point out at least three current typical groups of patterns of prejudice or anti-Jewish language use. For the present, I view these distinctions as purely heuristic:

(1) *Relics of the Nazi period:* These are either neologisms from the ideological structure of the Third Reich or older concepts that were redefined ("*Volk,*" "gassing," "mixed marriage").

(2) *Direct and hostile injunctions* mainly appear in graffiti or implicitly in headlines ("kill the Jews," "dirty Jews").

(3) *Argumentation and generalizations* are embedded in typical patterns of prejudice and, from a historical point of view, concern themselves with typical topics. I would like to present a taxonomy of five recurring topics that also have some bearing on our examples (the linguistic forms and the extent of their manifestation will be discussed with concrete examples in the following section): (a) *Conspiracy theory:* World Jewry owns and dominates the press, the banks, and so on; the Jews are a people without a country and are plotting a Zionist/communist/capitalist world conspiracy. (b) *Dishonesty:* Jews are usurers, sharks, liars, slippery, dishonest, and so on. (c) *Jewish intelligence:* Jews dominate art, science, and culture; they are revolutionary, subversive, self-destructive, domestic, fanatical, and threaten traditional values. (d) *Murderers of Christ:* The Jews killed Christ and are therefore the enemies of Christians. (e) *Being different:* Jews are foreign; they look different: hair, lips,

skin color, nose, hunchback; they are parasites on those who "serve" them; they are sexually perverse; and so on.

The range of these anti-Semitic topics proves Adorno to be right: much of what is too difficult and incomprehensible in modern society is blamed on the Jews. The Jew is the scapegoat, and remains so despite so many terrible historical events and, as the most recent Austrian history shows, ultimately prove themselves to the prejudiced as "worthy" of their prejudice (for a detailed analysis and categories, see Wodak, in press-b; DeCillia, Mitten, & Wodak, 1987).

The following case studies (the contrast between prejudice discourse in the media and spontaneous oral arguments) should demonstrate the multilevel nature, the complexity, and the power of prejudices. The effect of these clichés, stereotypes, argumentation, and *Feindbilder* (concepts of the enemy) would not be explainable if one did not assume a connection between collective and individual discourse. This connection also makes the unconscious adoption of collective experience and organization of the world apparent. The effect and the successful implementation of anti-Semitism in present-day Austria would not be conceivable without the historical dimension up to the last century and the family tradition of the time.

Some Examples from *Die Kronenzeitung* and *Die Presse*

In the following, I want to examine some passages in regard to the presentation strategy used and also in regard to the extent to which anti-Semitic language use manifests itself. It is especially interesting to see if both newspapers employ similar strategies or if their anti-Semitic language use is reader-dependent (i.e., oriented toward a target group). The analysis is qualitative and, for the present purposes, disregards further indicators inherent in the text (along the parameters of text linguistics) (see Wodak, 1984). A quantification is also not included (see Wodak, DeCillia, Blüml, & Andraschko, 1987). The prejudices, stereotypes, and clichés that are to be found in the passages are representative examples of the public discourse allowed in Austria and thus, are representative, in part, of the collective norm. The examples are presented under headings describing the strategy employed. (Items emphasized by the author indicate especially pertinent sections.)

Both newspapers from which these examples are taken claim to be nonpartisan. During the 1986 election campaign, they were both strongly pro-Waldheim, although this position manifested itself in different ways. *Die Neue Kronenzeitung* (*NKZ*) circulation during the week is about 1,020,000 and on Sunday over 1,400,000. It is the most widely read newspaper in Austria. It characterizes itself as "independent" and is a daily tabloid; it is conservative, but it cannot be categorized as party-bound.

Die Presse belongs to the Austrian *Wirtschaftsbund* (Business Federation). Its weekly circulation is about 55,000 and on Saturday over 70,000. It follows a middle-class, right-wing-liberal line and is not a party organ, although its sympathies lie with the conservative Austrian People's Party (*Volkspartei*).

Turning the Persecuted into the Persecutor[2]

Items: The Jews are the Persecutor, Waldheim as the Persecuted

The World Jewish Congress and the media that it *influences persecuted* Waldheim and *threatened* Austria, which brought forth an *act of defiance* on the part of the Austrians . . .(*NKZ,* May 4, 1986, p. 2).

No, the *deliberate attack* on Waldheim was totally merciless. (*Presse,* April 3, 1986, p. 1)

Items: Jews Create Anti-Semitism

The man who wants to make a *Nazi-monster* out of Waldheim and in doing so evokes at most *abominable anti-Semitic reactions.* (*NKZ,* April 3, 1986, p. 3).

In regard to the discussion about a possible wave of anti-Semitism in Austria due to the activities of the World Jewish Congress . . . (*Presse,* March 26, 1986, p. 4)

Group Solidarity as a Product of the Creation of "Feindbilder"

Items: Identification with Waldheim

Any *decent* person who still retains the ability to judge must be *deeply* shocked by the humiliating events in New York and Israel. (*NKZ,* June 19, 1986, p. 8)

The patriotism which expressed itself in the election results was of a different kind: it was sparked off by the *horrible and total defamations* that this country was subjected to. The motto was not "*Now more than ever*" ["*Jetzt erst recht*"] but obviously, "*Just to spite you*" ["*Justament*"]. For the first time in a long time, the Austrians have again demonstrated something like national pride. (*Presse,* June 9, 1986, p. 1)

Items: "Interference" Will Not Be Tolerated

Severe measures must be taken to quell the continuing *insistent* interference from abroad. (*NKZ,* letter to the editor, May 1, 1986, p. 20)

No matter what Kurt Waldheim has done—is it the World Jewish Congress' business to pass judgement, or that of the Austrian people? (*Presse,* March 25, 1986, p. 1)

Scapegoat Strategy (Against the World Jewish Congress)

Items: Producing a Demon (Jewish Trick)

The World Jewish Congress, which, because of its connections, has access to the Reagan administration, has been named as the *manipulator* of all the "intriguing." That's where Waldheim was bad-mouthed. (*NKZ,* April 26, 1986, p. 2)

The *"propaganda machinery of the World Jewish Congress"* (*Presse,* March, 29/30/31, 1986, p. 1)

Items: Degradation—Qualification

But, *my young ladies and gentlemen* of the World Jewish Congress, that is not how the situation was then! (*NKZ,* April 20, 1986, p. 6)

And that Waldheim, the insignificant first lieutenant and clerk on the staff of the "*Wehrmacht,*" is supposed to be a "Nazi" is so *outrageous* that one should *not really* concern himself further with it *at all.* (*NKZ,* June 1, 1986, p. 6)

"Christ" (= Waldheim) Murderers

It is not difficult to understand that Israel too has joined the *World Jewish Congress' slaughtering of Waldheim.* (*NKZ,* May 25, 1986)

Title: "Politics on Good Friday"

There they are, those who wash their hands in innocence, in the same way today as then, the crowds, who called out to a *cowardly judge: "Crucify him!"* (*Presse,* March 28, 1986, p. 1)

Analysis and Interpretation

The gross, blatant anti-Semitism, and the exploitation of these prejudices for deliberate political maneuvering is shocking. Especially striking are the affective adjectives ("abominable," "insistent") in the passages, as are the degrading address (for example, to the World Jewish Congress—"my young ladies and gentlemen"), the pairs of opposites, and the deliberate use of colloquial words ("bad-mouthed"). From the point of view of argumentation, *Die Presse* is certainly subtler, although the choice of words has the characteristics of slogans, and emotionally loaded concepts dominate. One does not even stop at blatant abuse. Not "Justament"! That the name of the World Jewish Congress naturally lends itself to an association with "world conspiracy" is fully exploited.

What differences can we find between the two newspapers (about the anti-Semitic tendencies, there is no doubt)? Differences were apparent even at first glance; I have selected a few, as follows.

Die Presse

The anti-Semitic utterances in *Die Presse* are subtler and tend to be built into the argumentation rather than being expressed in blatant stereotypes. Although Jewish persons and communities are referred to, they are seldom explicitly named. Insinuations are employed, but in such a way as to make the newspaper less open to attack. Therefore, a macro- and a microlinguistic analysis are especially necessary to identify the pseudo-logical argumentation in *Die Presse* columns. Even in the case of the item "Crucify him," the World Congress is not explicitly named. Allusions make a hypocritical "retreat" possible.

Die Kronenzeitung

The use of anti-Semitic language is blatant here. The vocabulary, the adjectives, the repetitions, the trivializing, and colloquial usages in very simple syntax are easy for everyone to understand and are openly defamatory. The writers certainly do not mince words; allusions and quotations do not seem to be at all necessary (this method indeed differs from Reimann's "famous" series, 1973; see Marin, 1983; DeCillia, Mitten & Wodak, 1987). It is both surprising and alarming that the most widely read Austrian daily paper dares to be so openly anti-Semitic. And we should not be astonished that the "new" anti-Semitism could assume such forms given the possible effect of this media propaganda.

Both newspapers are directed at their respective readership (on the one hand, at business and at the intellectual, and on the other hand, at the average citizen). The danger inherent in the more subtle argumentation is certainly greater, since it has the appearance of being more factual and objective. In contrast, the striking anti-Semitism makes an impression more easily with its sloganizing.

Anti-Semetic Language in Spontaneous Speech: The Memorial Vigil

In June 1987, a memorial vigil took place on St. Stephen's Square in Vienna, directly in the center of the city. It had been organized by the "Republican Club," a left-liberal organization that had been formed mainly to counteract the anti-Semitism that surfaced during the 1986 presidential election campaign but that continues to concern itself with similar issues. The vigil commemorated Austrian war victims, especially those who had been killed in concentration camps.

The memorial vigil caused quite a sensation. Clusters of people formed spontaneously. Many seemed to consider the mere presence of those maintaining the vigil a provocation that invited, if not demanded, a response. In point of fact, many did feel provoked and began—out of the blue—to express opinions and attitudes, to vent aggression, tell stories, and so on. We recorded these discussions on a daily basis, since we had never had the opportunity to obtain material of this sort. There were discussions and arguments about a myriad of topics, for example, social benefits and pensions, the election campaign, Austria's past, and the Jews.

Since a detailed discourse analysis of these discussions would exceed the scope of this article, I shall concentrate on the content of one text and the lines of argument it contains. This is done in order to suggest the symmetry, if not in fact the symbiotic indispensability, between the stereotypes, clichės, allusions, and so on, employed therein (as examples of anti-Semitic language use) and the discourse found in the mass print media.

A Brief Summary of the Content

In the passage chosen (for a complete analysis, see Wodak, in press-d), there is an argument about who is responsible for resurrecting the discussions about Austria's past. One speaker is clear that the Jews are to blame. Another participant attempts to refute this contrarational discourse, but does so by introducing as an argument the cliché about how much the Jews have done for Austrian culture.

Later in the discussion the initial speaker relates a "prejudice story," in which a specific (presumably apocryphal) anecdote is used to illustrate a general prejudice, namely, that of the cutthroat Jewish businessman and usurer. This story is, in turn, followed by a second prejudiced discourse, different from the first in that the generalized statements it contains (Jews take work away from others, all psychiatrists and lawyers are Jews, and so on) are not accompanied by corresponding illustrative examples.

The exchange ends with a summary admonition: Let things be; there are more important things to discuss.

The Line(s) of Argument

The examples from this one discussion reveal several of the stereotypes and many of the argumentation strategies currently in the public discourse in contemporary Austria.

The first speaker feels that he is being attacked as an Austrian and aligns himself with Waldheim against the "bad outside interference." This particular attitude reached a peak during the 1986 election campaign with the Waldheim campaign slogan "We Austrians will elect whom *we* choose"—"Now more than ever" (see Wodak, 1988). The German expression "*das Ausland*" (the foreigner) is a singular usage that imputes a unity or oneness of things non-Austrian, and as such is more potentially emotive and threatening than the plural "foreign countries," its closest English equivalent. The language is to a certain extent coded, for when speakers referred to das Ausland they normally meant the United States. This was clear from the initial speaker's further line of argument: After excoriating the pernicious interference from abroad, he turned to the United States where, he claimed, Reagan and Meese (Meese's name was known in Austria principally as a consequence of the "watch list" decision) were themselves mere marionettes of the Jews. Thus even when the ostensible target is das Ausland the images of the Jews as the genuine enemy, and the conspiratorial theme that suggests that the world at large acts at their behest, are never far from the surface.

A second speaker argues in a matter-of-fact way and attempts to refute the generalizations and correct what he considers the distorted picture of the past. In this effort, he receives support from others gathered in the group.

A third speaker then offers the "let the past be" argument. Those who were guilty, she maintains, have been punished anyway, while the rest are, in an innovative turn of phrase, "innocent perpetrators."

At this point, yet another speaker enters the discussion by introducing what I would like to call the *Iudaeus ex machina,* the Jew as scapegoat for all occasions. The anecdote refers to a Jew who had entered into a business arrangement with a farmer, but who had cheated the farmer by respecting his part of the bargain, that is, for acting like a businessman. The spectre of the village Jew thus enters the discussion. That this anecdote should illustrate "the other side" of anti-Semitism—that there is something to it, as the speaker concludes—is, however, possible only by means of a straightforward double standard of rights and duties. It also suggests the speaker's readiness to convert the persecuted into the persecutor.

Other participants in the discussion do not sense, or at least do not react to, the convoluted logic and inapplicability of the chosen story for the intended messages; the form seems to appeal to familiar patterns of experience. The arguments his opponents use to counter this anecdote are predictable enough: *One* story is not sufficient, one says, but this concedes the legitimacy of the anecdote as an argument.

This storyteller then brings up all the others who died in the war (those who "did their duty"), asks why the Jews are a "chosen people," and why the Jews are deserving of any special sympathy. One previous speaker then contributes the ambiguous remarks, "I don't see any dirty Jews." From the context it becomes clear that she is referring to Jews who do manual work, but such slips are certainly not accidental. The collocation, "dirty Jew" can also refer in general to East European Jews, when it is not intended as a blanket attributive adjective. That this might indeed be the case is suggested by the string of generalizations she then introduces, encouraged by the story about the farmer: Jews are lazy; they do not do manual work; they are psychiatrists (i.e., they have power over people—a possible latent allusion to Freud); the Jews are to blame for the recent anti-Semitism; they arouse feelings of anti-Semitism in others by stirring up trouble and threatening jobs; and so on.

Having found common ground, the storyteller and the woman together make a general appeal to sympathy—one should feel concern for all victims—and to tolerance—one should let things be. In the end, however, the Jews are guilty, because they (presumably) exhibit neither quality. The conditional nature of these appeals is obscured by the superficial universality of the formulations. Those who do not share these assumptions make themselves *eo ipso* guilty.

We have already encountered all these lines of argument (as strategies) in the newspaper analysis. The mechanisms of repression and of shifting the blame; where and in what ways a quasi-logical argument lapses into incoherence, only to be rescued by the Jews, who suddenly appear as perpetrators, manipulators, troublemakers, usurers, lazy intellectuals, and so on, are all typical of the scapegoat syndrome. The three principal mottos could be: "Let us be;" "The Jews are guilty;" "We are innocent perpetrators."

Collective and Individual Anti-Semitic Discourse

I would now like to compare the strategies and clichés in the newspapers with those in the spontaneous discussion: Conspiracy theory, turning the persecuted into the persecutor, having a scapegoat and a Manichean portrayal of events, all appear in both. Only religious motifs are missing. Political anti-Semitism dominates the discussion. The counterarguments adhere to the official line: the Jews are a people just like any other; Waldheim is not Austria, and the Jews have contributed a lot to Austria's culture. The individual discourse reflects the political climate: Prejudices have assumed a public character; the media influence the languages employed and link up exactly with the individual experience schemata and the prejudiced utterances that were previously tabooed or at most were permissible among a closed circle of friends. However, in contrast to the newspaper, insults and negative judgments appear more in the argumentation, in the general statements and in the stories, not blatantly in the choice of words, as in *Die Kronenzeitung*. Whether this can be attributed to the fact that it was a public discussion (who knows what else the storyteller and the woman might have had to say to each other) or whether it is still indeed taboo cannot be determined on the basis of these examples.

Our case study suggests that power and manipulation work in at least two ways: Certainly the power of the elites, even in pluralistic societies, controls the mass media, the information dissemination, and also which information is transmitted in what qualitative way. However, to see this process of manipulation as unidirectional would be far too simplistic. The qualitative analysis of our spontaneous speech data confirms our claim that previous experience, knowledge, attitudes, and prejudices must be collectively shared. Otherwise the mass media would not be successful.

Thus the purely sociocognitive, quantitative, and unidirectional approach to power—demonstrated by van Dijk both in his analysis of print media and in his microanalysis of prejudice stories—is too narrow. In place of this we propose a more differentiated approach, the use of qualitative data and a multilevel analysis. For only such a conception can adequately comprehend irrational forms of power and of powerful persons.

NOTES

1. In our participatory study in a clinic in a large Viennese hospital, it could be seen just how complex the structure of power is, and in what a contradictory way latent functions and official hierarchies often operate. Certain myths also play a role in the exercising of power in a hospital: for example, omniscience, time, curability, and efficiency. Both doctors and patients believe in these myths and cooperate as they interact with one another. If this were not the case, it would be difficult to explain why a conversation "works" and is accepted despite a minimum of eight interruptions, three new beginnings, and a great deal of misunderstanding. Power expresses itself in manifest and subtle ways: In a manifest way, when the patient is addressed with "Who is she?" in a subtle way when "there's just enough time [to deal with a patient]"; referencing time as money (see Lalouschek, Menz, & Wodak, 1987).

2. The opposition *persecuted/persecutor* represents the least undesirable rendering of the German *Opfer/Tater*. The German *Tater* implies a more neutral form of agency than the more obviously normative *persecutor*. Elsewhere the word *Tater* is rendered, although also unsatisfactory, as *perpetrator*.

REFERENCES

Adorno, T. (1973). *Der autoritäre Charakter*. Frankfurt: Suhrkamp.

Ammon, U., Dittmar, N., & Mattheier, K. (Eds.). (1988). *Handbook of sociolinguistics*. Amsterdam: de Gruyter.

Arendt, H. (1986). *Communicative power*. In S. Lukes (Ed.), *Power* (pp. 59-74). Oxford: Basil Blackwell.

Auwärter, M. (1983). Sprachgebrauch in Abhängigkeit von Merkmalen der Sprecher und der Sprechsituation. *Max Planck Institut für Bildungsforschung, Studien und Berichte, 42*. Berlin West.

Bernstein, B. (1981). Codes, modalities, and the process of cultural reproduction: A model. *Language and Society, 10*, 327-363.

Bourdieu, P. (1982). *Die feinen Unterschiede: Zur Kritik der gesellschaftlichen Urteilskraft*. Frankfurt: Suhrkamp.

Canetti, E. (1980). *Masse und Macht*. Frankfurt: Fischer.

DeCillia, R., Mitten, R., & Wodak, R. (1987). Von der Kunst, antisemitisch zu sein. In K. Weinberger & F. Jelinek (Eds.), *Judentum in Wien* (pp. 94-107). Vienna: Historisches Museum der Stadt Wien.

Dittmar, N. (1985a). *Bausteine zu einer übergreifenden theoretischen Perspektive der Soziolinguistik*. Unpublished manuscript.

Dittmar, N. (1985b). *Sprache und soziale Ungleichheit*. Unpublished manuscript.

Ehn, M. (1986). *Sozial Deviante erzählen ihre Lebensgeschichte*. Unpublished master's thesis, University of Vienna.

Ehlich, K., & Rehbein, J. (1986). *Muster und Institution*. Tübingen: Niemeyer.

Erdheim, M. (1984). *Die gesellschaftliche Produktion von Unbewusstheit*. Frankfurt: Suhrkamp.

Foucault, M. (1977). *Die Ordnung des Diskurses*. München: Fink.

Freud, S. (1976). *Massenpsychologie und Ich-Analyse*. (Vol. XIII, pp. 73-161). Frankfurt: Fischer.

Fromm, E. (1980). *Anatomie der menschlichen Destruktivität*. Stuttgart: Klett.

Gruber, H., & Wodak, R. (Eds.). (1987). "Jetzt erst recht?!" Sozio- und textlinguistische Untersuchungen zur Medienberichterstattung im Bundespräsidentschaftswahlkampf. *Wiener Linguistische Gazette*, 38-39.

Habermas, J. (1981). *Theorie des kommunikativen Handelns* (Vol. II). Frankfurt: Suhrkamp.

Habermas, J. (1982). *Politik, Kunst, Religion.* Ditzingen: Reclam.

Lalouschek, J., Menz, F., & Wodak, R. (1987). *Das Leben in der Ambulanz: Ambulanzgespräche.* Projectreport.

Lutz, B., & Wodak, R. (1987). *Information für Informierte: Linguistische Studien in zur Verstandlichkeit und Verstehen von Hörfunknachrichten.* Vienna: Akademie der Wissenschaften.

Mass, U. (1985). *Als der Geist der Gemeinschaft eine Sprache fand: Sprache im Nationalsozialismus.* Opladen: Deutsche Verlagsanstalt.

Marin, B. (1983). Ein historisch neuartiger "Antisemitismus ohne Antisemiten." In J. Bunzl & B. Marin (Eds.), *Antisemitismus in Österreich* (pp. 171-192). Innsbruck: Inn-Verlag.

Parsons, T. (1986). Power and the social system. In S. Lukes (Ed.), *Power* (pp. 94-103), Oxford: Basil Blackwell.

Pfeiffer, O., Strouhal, E., & Wodak, R. (1987). *Recht auf Sprache.* Vienna: Orac.

Reimann, V. (1973). Die Juden in Österreich. Series. *Kronenzeitung.*

Sauer, C. (1987). Stil, NS-Propaganda und Besatzungspresse. In R. Wodak (Ed.), *Language, Power, and Ideology.*

Soeffner, H. (Ed.). (1979). *Interpretative Verfahren in den Sozial- und Textwissenschaften.* Stuttgart: Metzler.

Strotzka, H. (1984). *Macht: Ein psychoanalytische Essay.* Vienna: Zsolnay.

van Dijk, T. A. (1984). *Prejudice in discourse.* Amsterdam: Benjamins.

Wodak, R. (1981). *Des Wort in der Gruppe.* Vienna: Akademie der Wissenschaften.

Wodak, R. (1984). *Hilflose Nähe—Mutter und Töchter erzählen.* Vienna: Bundesverlag.

Wodak, R. (1986). *Language behavior in therapy groups.* Los Angeles: University of California Press.

Wodak, R. (1987). Antisemitismus 1986/87: Vorüberlegungen zu einer sozio- und textlinguistischen Studie öffentlichen Sprachgebrauchs in den Medien in Österreich. *Akzente, 9/10,* 17-18.

Wodak, R. (1988). Wie über Juden geredet wird: Textlinguistische Analyse öffentlichen Sprachgebrauchs in den Medien im Österreich des Jahres 1986. *Journal für Sozialforschung, 28,* 7-137.

Wodak, R. (in press-a). Internal perspective—external perspective: Remarks on the development of sociolinguistic theory.

Wodak, R. (in press-b). The reality of political jargon in 1968 and the presentation in the media. In R. Wodak, (Ed.), *Language, Power, and Ideology.*

Wodak, R. (in press-c). *Die sprachliche Inszenierung des Nationalsozialiosmus: Einige soziolinguistische überlegungen.* Wein.

Wodak, R. (in press-d). *Opfer der Opfer.* Stuttgart: Deutsche Verlag.

Wodak, R., Menz, F., Lutz, B., & Gruber, H. (1985). *Die Sprache der Mächtigen—die Sprache der Ohnmachtigen: Der Fall Hainburg.* Vienna: Bohlau.

Wodak, R., & Schulz, M. (1986). *The language of love and guilt.* Amsterdam: Benjamins.

Wodak, R., & Feistritzer, G. (in press). *Sprache und Ideologie: Zur Analyse von Parteiprogrammen.*

Wodak, R., DeCillia, R., Bluml, K., & Andraschko, E. (1987). *Sprache und Macht—Sprache und Politik.* Vienna: Bundesverlag.

2 Coherence: A Meaningful Adhesive for Discourse

KATHY KELLERMANN
CARRA SLEIGHT
Michigan State University

Rejecting relevance, topicality, cohesive devices, syntactic structure, and comprehension as synonymous with and as necessary and/or sufficient for coherence, this chapter develops coherence as a cognitive judgment on the meaningful state of a text. This judgment of meaningfulness is determined by the relationship between the inferential demands of a text and the knowledge structures (schemata) available to the individual to accommodate those demands. Text therefore can be brought into the domain of coherence by varying knowledge structures.

THE varying uses of the term *coherence* make it difficult to understand the concept. A sampling of definitions of coherence find it described as a well-structured text (Badzinski, 1985), what makes a set of sentences form a text (Frederiksen, 1977), how one utterance follows another in a rational, rule-governed manner (Dascal & Katriel, 1979), the requirement that each succeeding sentence connect with what has already been introduced (e.g., Kieras, 1978), successful topic management (Tracy, 1985), the presence of a knowledge-based relation (van Dijk, 1977a), the cognitive correlate of cohesion (Moe & Irwin, 1986), the rational relation an utterance bears to some goal (Jacobs & Jackson, 1983), and a property assigned to another's continuous action (Sorensen, 1981).

To add to the confusion, these definitions vary in terms of their level of analysis, identification with cohesion, presumptions of connectedness, and concern with relevance. In terms of level of analysis, some scholars (e.g., Langleben, 1983) talk about the coherence of a sentence; others reject the applicability of coherence to such a small fragment of discourse (e.g., Garnham, Oakhill, & Johnson-Laird, 1982; Hobbs, 1982, 1983). The question argued here is whether coherence resides at some micro or macro level of the text. Cohesion is often viewed as being nested inside coherence, with cohesion being the local or micro level of *textual* (macro, global) coherence. Other scholars, however, use the words *cohesion* and *coherence* interchangeably.

Correspondence and requests for reprints: Kathy Kellermann, Department of Communication, Michigan State University, East Lansing, MI 48824.

Communication Yearbook 12, pp. 95-129

Connectedness is another area of dispute. Connectedness at the local level has been argued to be (1) a necessary condition (e.g., van Dijk, 1977b), (2) a sufficient condition (e.g., Labov, 1972), and (3) an irrelevant condition for global coherence (e.g., Keenan, Baillet, & Brown, 1984). Moreover, connectedness has often been translated to mean *relevance,* another term that has been both differentiated from (Jackson, Jacobs, & Rossi, 1986) and used interchangeably with (e.g., Tracy, 1985) coherence.

A final confusion is the problem of the *locus* of coherence. Does coherence reside in the discourse itself or is it imposed by the receiver of the discourse? While Halliday and Hasan (1976) devote their energies to identifying coherent *textual* structures, Levy (1979) argues explicitly that coherence is a mental phenomenon rather than a textual one.

This chapter seeks to clarify the concept of coherence by identifying what coherence is as well as what coherence is not. Prior to exploring the nature of coherence, however, we would like to make explicit a number of our working assumptions. First, our interest is in conversational behavior, so we focus our analysis on conversational coherence rather than on the coherence of written texts. Although we will draw from the textual literature in our analysis, we will limit our claims to conversational coherence.

Second, we believe that a conversation involves more than just the words that are uttered. Interlocutors bring their knowledge, emotions, and experiences with them to conversational encounters; their goals, plans, and understandings influence what is said as well as how what is said is interpreted. In other words, textual analyses without consideration of the beliefs, expectations, knowledge, and so on of producers and recipients of the discourse is limited in its ability to produce valid results.

Third, we believe that people communicate with a "coherence expectation"; that is, people are motivated to want to produce coherent discourse and expect that others are producing coherent discourse. We are not saying that people *always* produce or perceive discourse to be coherent; rather, we believe people *expect* themselves and others to be coherent. Even when a person produces intentionally obscure or unusual discourse, it is a general assumption of conversational interaction that it is to be interpreted as coherent (Bellert, 1970; Charolles, 1983). People will undertake effort so as to perceive conversation as coherent (Brown & Yule, 1983; Grice, 1975, 1978; Levinson, 1983). Indeed, this expectation of coherence can lead to effort that will overcome structural problems of the text (de Beaugrande, 1980; Hopper, 1981; Sanders, 1983).

Fourth, we believe that an understanding and application of cognitive principles are *necessary* to the exploration of coherence in conversations. As conversation is symbolic behavior, the ability to manipulate those symbols and supply meaning to those symbols requires the use of cognitive processes. However, the processing and production of symbolic behavior occurs within the capacities and limitations of people as information processors. A common cognitive principle is that human beings are limited-capacity processors. We cannot attend to all stimuli that impinge on our senses, and we are limited in our abilities to process information. Consequently, information must be "sorted," so that we admit some for further processing and disregard the rest. Given information is admitted for further processing; it enters the short-term memory store, which also has a limited-capacity in terms of both the quantity of information that can be held there and the time available for processing the information. These limited processing capabilities lead individuals to parse or chunk incoming information (such as conversations) so as to extract critical information before it is "lost."

Parsing is designed to permit more efficient use of our limited capacities. Information is parsed according to two interrelated processes. Top-down processing implies that the conversation is being directed and interpreted by knowledge structures rather than responding to cues from the environment, the conversational partner, and the like. By contrast, bottom-up processing occurs when actual conversational behaviors are attended and processed for meaning.

Most conversational interaction probably occurs in response to both top-down and bottom-up processing. Indeed, it is the *relative mix* of top-down and bottom-up processing that is critical. To the extent preplanned tactics or preexistent knowledge structures are employed to direct or interpret a conversation, the degree of active, on-line processing will vary. Thus it is possible that persons can interact relatively mindlessly or quite mindfully (Langer, 1978). For example, the more top-down processing occurring, the less attentive individuals need to be to the actual conversation. In such situations, verbal slips or other actions slips are likely to occur and not necessarily be noticed (Norman, 1981).

We believe that, by preference, processing of conversational discourse is heavily weighted toward top-down processing. Human beings are seen as cognitive misers, hoarding their cognitive energy (Fiske & Taylor, 1984; Taylor, 1980). One means of reducing cognitive load and hoarding energy is through top-down processing. In conversational interactions, "top-down" sets of generalized and situationally specific routines can be deployed as information enters in a "bottom-up" fashion. We believe that missing information in memory obstructs the flow of conversation, in terms of both processing and production. An interlocutor can attempt to obtain the information through memory search and inferential procedures or conversational repair attempts. Memory search and inferential procedures generally require extra processing energy to resolve the difficulty, whereas repair attempts require conversational processing energy. The memory search and inferential procedures serve as a top-down procedure while conversational repair serves as a bottom-up procedure to "failed" top-down processing.

Since conversations do not exist in a vacuum, devoid of the knowledge, goals, plans, beliefs, attitudes, and inferences of interlocutors, an understanding of conversational coherence necessitates the employment of cognitive principles. We will argue throughout this chapter that coherence is a *judgment* about discourse, a product of the cognitive processing of conversations. The act of using language (or nonverbal symbols) for communication engages cognitive processes. The determination of coherence is an output of the cognitive processing of discourse. In essence, we will argue that coherence is a judgment of *meaningfulness* of discourse (not to be confused with identification of meaning or comprehension). We will begin, however, by arguing "what coherence is *not*." In this way, the current definitions and claims in the literature concerning relevance, topicality, cohesive devices, and discourse structure can be reviewed, compared, and clarified in preparation for a reframing of the construct.

WHAT COHERENCE IS NOT

In the literature on coherence, relevance, topicality, cohesive devices, and syntactic structure are all used at times as synonyms for coherence and/or for each other. At other times, they are viewed as distinct determinants of coherence. These approaches generally presume that coherence is a feature of the *text*. We will argue that each of these approaches is inadequate for defining coherence in that such textual features do not provide adequate grounds for understanding how *judgments* of coherence are determined, and that relevance, topical relevance, cohesive devices, and syntactic structure are neither necessary nor sufficient conditions for coherence.

Coherence Is Not Relevance

The construct of relevance gained prominence with the publication of Grice's theory of conversational implicature in 1975. Grice's maxims of quantity, quality, relation, and manner are the means by which conversationalists are to interact (cooperate) with one another to attain the goal of meaningful (coherent) conversation to the ultimate end of understanding and being understood. Subsequent researchers have tended to focus on the ill-defined maxim of relation, "Be relevant," which has supplanted the notion of where relevance might lead. Relevant talk has thus become equivalent to coherent talk. In this perspective, relevance is usually defined as local relatedness, while coherence is considered to be global relatedness (Clark & Haviland, 1977; Hobbs, 1979; Jackson, Jacobs, & Rossi, 1986; McLaughlin, 1984; Tracy, 1982, 1984a). Wilson and Sperber (1981) even argue that the cooperative principle should be subsumed by the maxim of relation. This claim serves only as more evidence that the subgoal of cooperation has been misunderstood. Although it is possible that all four maxims may be unified under the idea of relation/relevance, the reason talkers are relevant is in order to cooperate so that their talk might be coherent and potentially understood.

Relevance is not the ultimate goal in spite of what Wilson and Sperber's claim implies.

In this perspective of relevance, if utterances are sequentially ordered such that each utterance is conditionally relevant to a preceding one, the conversation as a whole is claimed to be coherent (Dascal & Katriel, 1979). Labov (1972) has argued that if no such relevance relation holds between each and every utterance of a conversation, then that conversation is incoherent. van Dijk (1977a) tempers the claim by suggesting that relevance is a necessary though not sufficient condition for coherence. All of these works presume that both relevance and coherence are assessments of the germaneness of an utterance or set of utterances to prior utterances or to some overarching topic. In other words, the *level* of *analysis* (global/local) may vary, but the nature of the assessment is the same.

We agree with Grice, who did not claim that relevance was isomorphic with coherence. Coherence is different from relevance; the presence or absence of one does not signal the presence or absence of the other. Though both coherence and relevance are judgments persons make about the *relation* of text, the *types* of relation being assessed are quite different. Coherence references meaningfulness, while relevance references pertinence or centrality. In other words, relevance is concerned with the degree to which utterances are germane to some matter at hand (such as a topic), while coherence is concerned with the potential interpretative implications of an utterance. Presuming isomorphic meanings for these two constructs confuses two *different* types to judgments of relatedness.

We would argue that local relevance—that is, "a relevant remark is one that chains to something in the last sentence or two of a speaker's message" (Tracy, 1984b, p. 447)—is neither a necessary nor sufficient basis for coherence. If coherence and relevance are isomorphic in meaning, then it would be impossible to find instances of either (a) coherent but irrelevant utterances or (b) incoherent but relevant utterances. In fact, it is easy to find both of these outcomes. First, incoherence does not imply irrelevance. Recently, a colleague was relating a story about the presentation of a convention paper. The author of the paper was described was being "incoherent" because the "sense" of his or her remarks was not apparent. However, the author's presentation was *not* described as irrelevant; indeed, there seemed to be a presumption of relevance of the presentation to the nature of the paper. In other words, the utterances were judged to be relevant though incoherent.

Second, coherence does not imply relevance. A person who is a "boring" storyteller often "clutters" up the story with unnecessary, trivial details. These details do not affect the *coherence* of the discourse, rather they affect perceptions of the relevance of parts of the discourse.

Typically, relevance has been investigated by looking only at the local relations among sequential utterances. A unit of analysis, however, should not be the sole determinant of a construct. For instance, a two (or more) sentence (or word) interchange could be both irrelevant (one sentence may be unrelated to the other) and coherent (taken together they are meaningful to the talkers). Such a process is how an indirect response to a question can count as a direct answer (Brockway, 1981; Nofsinger, 1976). In some circumstances, we may even be obligated to be irrelevant to attain the goal of a coherent interchange (Tracy, 1984a). In conversations, digressions do occur that may impinge on a judgment of relevance, though few would judge such digressions as incoherent (Dascal & Katriel, 1979). Relevance and coherence should *not* be treated as synonyms. Coherence is a judgment that a discourse of any length has been judged to be meaningful. Relevance is a judgment of pertinence between two pieces of discourse, regardless of their length. While relevance may facilitate coherence, it is not isomorphic with it *and* the presence or absence of one does not guarantee the presence or absence of another.

Topical Relevance Is Not Coherence

Topical relevance is concerned with whether utterances are pertinent to some predefined topic in the conversation. Topical relevance suggests that coherence is dependent on talk being "on the topic."

Topical relevance is not necessary for coherence. If relevance is a judgment of relatedness, then talkers within a context will determine what is or is not pertinent to the discourse. Because an irrelevant comment may be seen as coherent, coherence does not rely on "relatedness factors," such as topicality. In fact, topics might change from one utterance to the next and still elicit a judgment that the conversation is coherent. Topic *changes* (as distinct from transition-based shifts) are points at which what is being uttered is *unrelated* to what has gone before. Yet, conversations with topic changes are not perceived as *incoherent* (Maynard, 1980).

Topics are generally defined to be "what discourse is about" (Fletcher, 1984), although there is considerable disagreement over what this "aboutness" references. Local notions of topic focus on topic as a serial characteristic of sentences: Each sentence becomes the topic for the one that follows it (Chafe, 1976; Crow, 1983; Schank, 1977). Global notions maintain that topic refers to the main point or theme of a message (Reichman, 1978; Schank, 1977; Schwarz & Flammer, 1981; van Dijk, 1977a). The topic is identified as being in the top position in an information hierarchy that will vary from interchange to interchange (Tracy, 1985).

The ability to identify either the local or the "top" topic suggests a cognitive process performed by talkers as conversations proceed. Talkers "topicalize" discourse as it proceeds and are not dependent on a topic at any level in order to find discourse meaningful (Coulthard, 1977; Dascal & Katriel, 1979). Recent work, however, indicates that persons can topicalize discourse (to some degree) when instructed to do so, though natural processing of conversations is *not* done with meaningful units of topics (Palmer & Badzinski, 1985). If topics are not meaningful units, then the idea of topical relevance loses much of its force. If people do not process conversations topically, then it is difficult to argue that a *judgment* resulting from that cognitive processing is dependent on a nonexistent processing strategy.

The lack of topical relevance will not necessarily bring about judgments of incoherence, as can be witnessed in the rather rapid topic changes (without seeming transition) that occur in initial interactions. Similarly, conversational digressions represent two successive topic shifts (to the digression, away from the digression) that, while perhaps lacking in relevance, do not disrupt the *coherence* of the conversation (Dascal & Katriel, 1979). Finally, utterances that regulate the flow of talk or otherwise manage the interaction are often not topical, though their presence does not generally lead to judgments of incoherence. The lack of topic continuity may elicit judgments of irrelevance but, as we have argued, relevance is distinct from coherence.

Topical relevance is not sufficient for coherence. Even if persons producing discourse remain on the same topic (by whatever definition), the utterances need not be seen as coherent. A topic, whether local or global, is generally viewed to be a measure of semantic content (Jackson, Jacobs, & Rossi, 1986); that is, a topic isolates the "important" elements of the content of discourse (Brown & Yule, 1983). However, the relatedness of the semantic content of one utterance to that of the next does not ensure judgments of coherence. Jackson, Jacobs, and Rossi (1986) report that across three experiments, responses linked propositionally or referentially to initiating remarks were rated low in relevance. Other conditions and/or variables are sometimes needed for such judgments to be made. First, utterances related to a specific topic might need to occur in a given order to be found meaningful (Irwin, 1986; Jackson, Jacobs, & Rossi, 1986), as in a recipe. Second, the goals of interactants need to be considered in determining coherence. The degree of topical relevance from utterance may vary depending on the goal the speaker has in mind (Tracy, 1985; Tracy & Moran, 1982, 1983). Finally, world knowledge of a perfectly topically linked discourse may be needed before a judgment of coherence can be made (van Dijk, 1977a). Therefore, comments that demonstrate topical relevance alone will be insufficient to garner judgments of coherence; other factors must be brought to bear.

In sum, topical relevance is neither necessary nor sufficient for conversational coherence. Bransford and Johnson (1972) make precisely this point when they argue that the topic of a written passage does not determine optimal comprehension of the passage. Similarly, Kieras (1978) argues that the topic or theme of a set of sentences is unrelated to their degree of coherence. A conversation may be perceived as coherent even when utterances are *not* topically relevant just as the presence of topical relevance does not guarantee coherence.

Cohesion Is Not Coherence

Cohesion is generally analyzed at the local level of text through the identification of linguistic devices that link together phrases, utterances, or sentences. Though attempts to be judged as producing coherent discourse may well lead persons to employ cohesive devices, the presence of cohesive devices implies nothing about the ultimate coherence of a discourse. In other words, we argue that the causal relationship between cohesive devices and coherence is *not* that cohesive devices cause coherence but that the attempt to be perceived as coherent produces (causes) discourse with cohesive devices.

Cohesive devices are not necessary for coherence. If the presence or absence of semantic units such as topics cannot guarantee coherence, there is little reason to think that lexicogrammatic units will be guarantors either. Cohesive devices have been identified as lexicogrammatic units whose presence guarantees coherence (Halliday & Hasan, 1976). Despite such claims, coherent discourse can exist without the use of cohesive devices.

Little disagreement exists in the literature on what cohesive devices are. Halliday and Hasan (1976) identify five forms these devices can take: reference, substitution, conjunction, ellipsis, and lexical cohesion. Most authors (Brown & Yule, 1983; Gutwinksi, 1976; Jackson, Jacobs & Rossi, 1986; Moe & Irwin, 1986) seem to concur, although others argue for more abstract principles such as the "prominence" created by verb tense (Longacre, 1983) or the "elaboration" of inferences created by a text (Hobbs, 1979).

Debate does exist over what these textual devices do in discourse. Cohesive devices are claimed to create "cohesion"—textual linkages between words, phrases, and/or sentences (Halliday & Hasan, 1976); to provide pragmatic linkages between propositions (van Dijk, 1977a); and to aid in information processing, inference making, and conversational management (Badzinski, 1985). The common denominator here is that such devices serve as *cues* for the subsequent interpretation of discourse. In other words, cohesive devices signal the need to engage in a cognitive search for connections between the elements of the discourse. This *interpretation* claim is at odds with the typical analysis of cohesive devices. Typically, proponents of the "cohesive devices cause coherence" perspective argue that such devices "work" because words "refer" to earlier words or concepts in the discourse. However, the ability of such cohesive devices to guide us to interpretation of meaning requires that we, as processors of the discourse, *assume* that the discourse is coherent so we know to *search for* a proper reference in *memory* (Jackson, Jacobs, & Rossi, 1986; Morgan, 1978; Morgan & Sellner, 1980). In themselves, these devices do not create semantic linkages. At most, cohesive devices signal connectivity, relatedness, and pertinence—not, as we have already argued, coherence.

In the absence of cohesive devices, discourse can still be considered meaningful (Gutwinksi, 1976; Jackson, Jacobs, & Rossi, 1986; Keenan et al., 1984; van Dijk, 1977b) because discourse processors are willing to make inferences in order to produce judgments of coherence (Brown & Yule, 1983).

For example, the following exchange reported in Brown and Yule (1983, p. 196) is devoid of cohesive devices, yet most would judge it coherent:

A: There's the doorbell.
B: I'm in the bath.

We *infer* a relationship between A's and B's utterances even though no explicit cohesive device ties the two utterances. Descriptive passages in text are frequently devoid of such markers and yet are deemed coherent (Garnham et al., 1982). If cohesive devices were important semantic units, their absence should affect comprehension by increasing processing time, which does not always occur (Garrod & Sanford, 1981). Furthermore, if such devices were a necessary condition for coherence, then one might expect their frequency of use in discourse to be quite high. Warner (1985) reports, however, that in one sample text of 325,000 words only about 1,890 (.6%) of them were cohesive devices other than temporal connectives. Therefore, a judgment about the meaningfulness of discourse is available without the overt employment of cues to guide that judgment.

Cohesive devices are not sufficient for coherence. Even if every possible cohesive device were employed in a given discourse, unless the perceiver of that discourse comprehends the meaning of those devices, the discourse will not be judged coherent. Cohesive devices must have meaning for the processor of the discourse prior to their being effective in guiding discourse interpretation. Further, if the entire discourse were nothing more than a series of cohesive devices (e.g. "Well, anyway, and then . . ."), one would be hard pressed to judge that discourse as being meaningful (i.e., coherent).

Not only are cohesive devices limited in their effectiveness by the world knowledge of the discourse processor, but the presence of cohesive devices makes no guarantee of the meaningfulness of a conversation. We have argued that these devices are simply cues that initiate a search for connections. However, what is connected must be able to be found sensible by the processor (Petofji, 1985; van Dijk, 1977a). Cohesive devices aid in this sense-making process, but do not guarantee it (Badzinski, 1985). Bower and Cirilo (1985) note that *working memory* is integral to the process of establishment of meanings of coreferents in the process of comprehension. Such interpretation is facilitated by appropriate serial order, common goals, and common world knowledge in much the same way topic interpretation is facilitated (see, e.g., Keenan et al., 1984). In fact, cohesive devices may even detract from a coherent interpretation because appropriate world knowledge cannot be brought to bear (Bransford, 1979; Brown & Yule, 1983). For example, the use of conjunctions at inappropriate points in a conversation could "miscue" persons to search for interpretations in inappropriate places (Jackson, Jacobs & Rossi, 1986).

Therefore, the presence of cohesive devices alone will not guarantee a judgment that discourse is coherent. Furthermore, the absence of such devices does not prohibit discourse from being coherent. Cohesive devices are neither necessary nor sufficient for coherence (Jackson & Jacobs, 1986; Langleben, 1983; van Dijk, 1977a, 1977b, 1985).

Structurally Correct Discourse Is Not Coherence

Some of the literature on the nature of coherence argues that structurally correct discourse (syntactic appropriateness, and so on) yields coherent discourse.

Structurally correct discourse is not necessary for coherence. If judgments of coherence, however, depend on structural correctness, then most everyday conversations, which exist in a world of interruption, distraction, contradiction, and inference, would be found incoherent. Discourse is often *not* syntactically correct, yet this condition does not prevent a judgment of coherence (Clancy, 1972; Ochs, 1977). Coherence does not reside in syntax, which is solely a rule-governed structural component of discourse that yields recognizable patterns (Carroll, 1986). Syntax makes an implicit semantic link explicit. However, if people can mean more than they say (Grice, 1975), explicit links are not necessary for coherence. If correct syntax were necessary for coherence, then alterations in syntax should yield alterations in perceptions of coherence. However, we often do not detect variations in syntax when the functional relations between components of sentences are maintained (Sachs, 1967). Syntactic information is primarily employed *only* until a semantic interpretation of a clause is derived (Jarvella, 1971). The meaning of sentences is remembered even when the syntactic structure of those sentences is not, indicating that comprehension is a semantically driven process rather than a syntactically driven one (Fillenbaum, 1966). Phillips (1985) notes that "traditional grammar . . . cannot account for intersentential cohesion. Still less can it be expected to explain large scale structures extending over long texts" (p. 31).

An insistence that correct structure is required for coherence limits the number of relations possible between speech acts (Ferrara, 1985; van Dijk, 1977a); that is, questions could be followed only by answers, when it is evident that they often (and coherently) are not (Nofsinger, 1976). For example, Merritt (1976) notes the extensive use of *questions* following *questions* in service encounters. The well-formedness of utterances that allows for coherence to be found does not rest on syntax alone. Context can determine well-formedness (Brockway, 1981). Nonsyntactic macrostructures that identify a discourse as a particular kind of communication—a narrative versus a business letter—can determine well-formedness. Therefore, if well-formedness can obtain in the absence of correct structure, then its absence will not preclude judgments of coherence.

Structurally correct discourse is not sufficient for coherence. The implicit assumption behind the claim that correct structure guarantees coherence is that meaning resides in the words themselves. Therefore, all one must do is organize words according to syntactic rules and the resulting sentences will be meaningful. Lewis Carroll (1982/1897) knew better when he wrote: "'Twas brillig in the slithey toves/Did gyre and gimble in the wabe. . . "(p.134). Here is structure without coherence. Carroll took advantage of the fact that meaningless words could be "correctly" connected to yield the appearance of meaningfulness. Even when words are employed to which persons can attach meaning, syntactically correct utterances do not guarantee coherent discourse. Individual words might have meaning and they may seem to be ordered according to syntactic rules, but the discourse itself may lack meaningfulness.

Factors other than structure are needed for judgments of coherence. Discourse is situated in contexts of various kinds: neighboring discourses in which the current one may be embedded; perceived task requirements; the situation itself; and the interests, attitudes, and preexisting knowledge of the comprehender (Spiro, 1980). Any or all of these contexts may supplant or determine the need for correct structure (Kieras, 1978; Schegloff & Sacks, 1973). Communicative outcomes are not solely dependent on correct structure. Politeness codes certainly dictate structure that may be syntactically odd (Brown & Levinson, 1978). Furthermore, people must be able to recover syntactic structure in printed discourse or be properly temporally cued (prosodically) when listening in order to find coherence (Adams, 1980). Correct syntax therefore is insufficient for judgments of coherence.

Summary

Coherence, then, is not solely dependent on the presence or absence of relevance, topics, cohesive devices, or structure. Incoherent discourse may or may not be found to be relevant. On-topic comments may be a sign of relatedness and not coherence. Cohesive devices may serve as cues for coherence, but that judgment may well depend on the presence of other factors. Correct structure may be made to appear coherent without coherence being found. Coherence can exist despite the arbitrary presence or absence of any of these factors.

WHAT COHERENCE IS

By arguing that coherence is not relevance, topics, cohesive devices, or structure, we have eliminated most prior approaches to understanding conversational coherence. Though this outcome was intentional, we worked in the hope that coherence, *as a distinct construct*, could be differentiated from similar, though not isomorphic, terms. In this section, we explore the nature of coherence. The thesis of our argument is that coherence is an *evaluative judgment of meaningfulness* of discourse. This judgment is a product of cognitive processing of the discourse and should not be equated with comprehension of the discourse. In essence, we will argue that coherence does not reside in the discourse but resides in the output of mental operations conducted on the discourse. To do so, we need to distinguish between the process of those mental operations and the judgments that result.

Coherence Is an Evaluative Judgment

We have rejected definitions of coherence as a feature of the text because *none* of these features is possible without cognitive processing. Relevance and cohesive devices require cognitive searches under a *presumption* the discourse is coherent. Syntax is not retained in mental representations of discourse after semantic meaning is extracted. Thus the process of interpreting discourse is a cognitive one. However, the determination of coherence of the discourse occurs *after* processing has been initiated. Specifically, we will argue that coherence is an output of this comprehension process and that output is in the form of an evaluative judgment.

Coherence Is a Judgment, Not a Process

Those scholars arguing for a cognitive perspective on coherence tend to confuse *comprehension* with *coherence*. Comprehension is a *process* that involves parsing discourse, assigning it meaning, drawing inferences, and storing whatever aspects of it one wishes into memory. Bransford, McCarrell, Franks, and Nitsch (1977) write that "understanding involves *relationships;* it is an activity rather than a *thing*" (p. 438). Ortony (1978) defines comprehension as a process that relates input information to contextual information. Comprehension is an *act* not an *object*. By contrast, coherence is not defined as a *process* in any literature we are familiar with. Generally, discourse is viewed as coherent or incoherent; that is coherence is a "state" of being (often viewed in dichotomous terms). Thus discourse is *characterized* as coherent or incoherent, often by the very same persons who are explicitly or implicitly arguing that the process of comprehension is isomorphic with the state of coherence. For example, van Dijk (1977a, 1977b, 1985) defines coherence in terms of the creation of propositions that link semantic content of text together for purposes of comprehension. This view of coherence does not differentiate comprehension from coherence and ignores the process versus state distinction. In this view, coherent discourse is discourse that is comprehended, and comprehended discourse is discourse that is coherent.

We admit that discourse cannot have meaning in the absence of cognition; the meaning of discourse does not reside in the symbols but instead in what a perceiver believes those symbols to represent. Just because symbols have been assigned meaning, however, does *not* imply that the discourse is judged to be coherent. Coherence is an *evaluation* of the state of some piece of discourse; it is a judgment that is related to processes of comprehension though it is an *output* of such processes rather than being isomorphic with them.

Some researchers argue that the process of comprehension results in a judgment of coherence. For example, Widdowson (1978) argues that only through *recognition* (e.g., comprehension) of the actions underlying utterances do we judge discourse to be coherent. Widdowson's view is similar to that of Jackson et al's (1986), in which identification of the purposes, plans, activities, and relations between and of communicators is a precondition for coherence. Hobbs (1982) outlines much the same position for a line of coherence research that revolves around use of planning mechanisms; that is, in the planning framework, an "utterance is coherent insofar as it can be seen as an action in the implementation of some plan" (p. 226). Garnham et al. (1982) argue that the creation of a unitary representation that integrates all information in a given discourse is a necessary condition for a judgment of coherence. Consequently, these researchers tend to focus on how persons build mental representations of discourse (comprehend it), rather than on how comprehension *relates* to coherence. In this same manner, other researchers argue that the *purpose* of comprehension is to form a coherent representation of a text (Keenan et al., 1984).

While we agree with the judgmental nature of coherence, we disagree that comprehension must occur *prior* to determining that discourse *is* coherent. For example, individuals are capable of assessing discourse as coherent even when they are unable to assign specific meaning to it. When we hear a foreign language we do not speak, we do not judge the speaker as incoherent when we are unable to comprehend utterances. Similarly, a communication professor attending a conference on nuclear physics is unlikely to judge paper presentations as incoherent when his or her attempts to process the presentations and achieve meaning fail. If anything, in these instances it is likely that we judge the speaker coherent and ourselves as incapable of comprehension. In other words, comprehension is not necessary for a judgment of coherence.

What is the relationship between comprehension and coherence? Comprehension will, in all likelihood, facilitate judgments of coherence. We are willing to hypothesize that all other things being equal, the more difficulty a person has in comprehending a conversation, the less coherent that conversation will be judged. However, this hypothesis hinges on a number of critical factors, all placed in that innocuous phrase "all other things being equal." For example, if we attribute responsibility to ourselves (rather than the speaker or speakers) for the failure to comprehend the discourse, it is likely we will judge the discourse coherent even though we are unable to comprehend it. If, on the other hand, we blame the speaker for our inability to comprehend, we are likely to judge the discourse incoherent. Noticeably, in the examples of the foreign language speaker and the nuclear physics speaker, we are likely to assign responsibility to ourselves and hence judge the discourse coherent. Thus the assigned locus of responsibility influences judgments of coherence such that comprehension is not a *necessary* cause of coherence.

Is comprehension, then, a sufficient condition for coherence? Is it the case that *if* you comprehend, you *will* judge the discourse as minimally coherent? Again, we are willing to admit the positive correlation between comprehension and coherence, but we would like to temper the *causal* interpretation of this relationship. In fact, we would argue that difficulty in comprehension will stimulate the perceiver of discourse to attempt to develop a "coherent" interpretation of it (Charolles, 1983). The degree of success in these endeavors will affect the coherence perceived in the discourse as will the degree of effort needed for such endeavors. Therefore, if one views the comprehension process as *including* attempts to reformulate the text such that it *can* be perceived as coherent, then comprehension is a sufficient condition for coherence. However, such a procedure confounds cause and effect. The actual cognitive processing is this: (1) Difficulty in comprehension leads to (2) judgment (temporary) of incoherence, which leads to (3) perception that self has failed in comprehending text, leading to (4) desire to comprehend text, which leads to (5) reformulation of meaning of text, and so on and so on until a judgment of coherence results. In such a case, the *initial* judgment of coherence is the "cause" of further comprehension attempts, just as these comprehension attempts then lead to further assessment of the degree of coherence of the text.

Perhaps a more critical issue to address in the potential sufficient role of comprehension in the production of judgments of coherence concerns the presumption that when comprehension is mentioned, it is somehow the same for all perceivers. If one admits different interpretations are possible in the comprehension process, then it is likely that a given discourse can be judged as having varying degrees of coherence by different individuals. In such a case, the process of comprehension is occurring and indeed may be occurring at "equal levels." However, the nature of the exact mental representations may differ in structure, form, or consonance with the discourse or may require more or less effort in their derivation such that no expectations of similarity in coherence judgments should or would be expected. Thus comprehension is not a sufficient condition for coherence, though it is positively correlated with it.

Coherence evaluates meaningfulness of discourse. The related nature of comprehension and coherence comes about because comprehension is a process that involves the assignment of meaning, whereas coherence is a judgment of the meaningfulness of discourse. Meaningfulness, as a judgment, is an assessment of whether utterances are conveying information *regardless* of whether one is capable of deciphering that information. Typically, persons are reluctant to judge discourse as completely incoherent, often engaging in considerable cognitive work to produce even a somewhat coherent interpretation of the discourse (Charolles, 1983).

Coherence Is Discourse and Knowledge Structure Consonance

As coherence is the evaluation of the *state* of a given discourse reflecting its judged meaningfulness, the process by which this judgment arises and is affected is important. We will argue that meaningfulness is determined through the application of knowledge structures in the comprehension process; their *consonance* with the discourse will generate the judgment of coherence. That is, knowledge structures consonant with the discourse (to *some* degree) are necessary if discourse is to be perceived to be coherent (to *any* degree). We will build our defense for the need for knowledge structures in the making of judgments of coherence by first arguing that inferences are required in discourse comprehension and that such inferential processes must make use of knowledge structures.

Discourse comprehension requires the making of inferences. It is relatively well accepted that differences exist between a speaker's meaning for an utterance and the "actual" meaning of that utterance. Grice (1969) notes that what a speaker means by an utterance may not be closely related to the literal meaning of that utterance at all. Searle's (1975) discussion of indirect speech acts explicitly relies on the idea that "the speaker communicates to the hearer more than he actually says" (p. 60). For example, left largely implicit in utterances are the interpersonal aspects of meaning (Hildyard & Olson, 1978). Furthermore, people abstract meanings from utterances that are not directly available in the symbols used in those utterances. People often know more than an utterance specifies directly (Kintsch, 1972) and often report information and ideas not directly stated in discourse (Bransford & Franks, 1971; Bransford, Barclay, & Franks, 1972; Brewer, 1977; Harris, 1974; Johnson, Bransford, & Solomon, 1973). Thus more is meant and more is comprehended than is usually uttered.

The physical provision of a set of symbols, *of and by themselves*, is *insufficient* for assigning meaning to an utterance. Information beyond the symbols themselves is required for assignment of meaning when, for example, we refer to a specific person as "the curly top" or to a specific location as "the bar" (Anderson & Shifrin, 1980). Inferences explain "how it is possible to mean (in some general sense) more than what is actually said" (Levinson, 1983, p. 97). Inferences "bridge the gap" between otherwise seemingly unrelated utterances. Bridging is seen by many to be the necessary condition for comprehension (Clark, 1977). For example:

(1) John was drunk.
(2) Mary was angry.

These two utterances are unrelated *except* through inferential processes that lead us to believe that Mary was angry *because* John was drunk. Causal inferences needed to link story statements are made by readers of text (Black, Turner, & Bower, 1979; Haberlandt & Bingham, 1978; Thorndyke, 1976). Such bridging improves recall of discourse and retelling usually evidences the gap filling through the use of explicit connectives (Black & Bern, 1981). Given that we *expect* others to produce coherent discourse, we bridge gaps in discourse through inferential processes aimed at achieving an interpretation we can judge coherent, if possible.

One such inferential process involves the establishment of meaning relations *between* symbols employed in the discourse. The literature on coherence and discourse comprehension tends to focus exclusively on these types of inferential relations (see, e.g., Bellert, 1970; Clark, 1977). For example, Levinson (1983) writes that "above all, understanding an utterance involves the making of *inferences* that will connect what is said to what is mutually assumed or what has been said before" (p. 21). As noted by Levinson, the typical sources for the formation of meaning relations develop through use of background knowledge or through the utterance history of the discourse as it unfolds. Most of the inferences individuals make when comprehending discourse stem from background knowledge of the world (Graesser & Clark, 1985). However, the utterance history of the discourse permits individuals to distinguish between *given* and *new* information in an unfolding discourse (Clark & Haviland, 1977; Halliday, 1967; Vande-Kopple, 1982). Clark (1977) argues that new information is bridged to given information such that the shortest possible bridge (inference) is developed that is consistent with the given/new contract. Cohesive devices are understood through inferential processes that search a memory representation of the discourse for meaning (i.e., bridging). For example, referents for definite noun phrases are identified through inferential activities explained by the bridging assumption (Haviland & Clark, 1974). When two utterances need to be linked for their semantic meaning, certain inferences will be made relatively automatically; others will lead to additional processing time (Brown & Yule, 1983; Sanford & Garrod, 1981). Automatic inferences are those supplied through preexisting knowledge structures, that is, background knowledge. Those inferences requiring additional processing time need to be *deduced* (Bellert, 1970) from the semantic meaning of the utterance. Thus meaning relations are inferred from background knowledge and the history of utterances in the discourse.

Second, contextual inferences are made. Any discourse occurs within a context. This context permits inferences to be made about that discourse. For example, the formality of a situation may evoke different inferences. It is our contention that more than just inferences based on *meaning* relations of the discourse are made. Certainly, these contextual inferences might inform inferences related to meaning of any part of the discourse, constraining or expanding meaning in response to contextual expectations. However, the *inability* to generate inferences of *meaning* relations does not inhibit one's ability to generate inferences about the discourse from contextual sources.

Third, speaker inferences are made. Such inferences are not widely discussed in the coherence or discourse comprehension literature (for a notable exception, see Clark, 1975); however, producers of discourse are often the object of inferential processing of their role, speaking style, appearance, and so on. In other words, knowing that a speaker is making a presentation at a nuclear physics convention might lead to the expectation that the speaker is a nuclear physicist. This role category, then, permits individuals to make inferences that relate to the discourse. For example, many technical words might be anticipated; perhaps "large" words would be expected as well. These inferences stemming from a speaker's role might also inform inferences of meaning relations between elements of the discourse, though the inability to generate meaning relations does not inhibit one's ability to generate discourse inferences stemming from a speaker's role.

Fourth, attributional inferences are made. Clark (1977) notes that attributional processes guide many of the inferences people make when comprehending discourse. In other words, inferences are being made about the reasons and causes of a person's behavior.

In essence, comprehension of discourse is an inferential process. Inferences can involve meaning relations, context, speakers, and attributions. Each inferential source may interact with the others, though inability to generate inferences from one source does not inhibit the ability to generate inferences from another source. Regardless of the source of inferences about the discourse, the act of comprehending the discourse necessarily entails the generation of inferences.

Inference making requires the use of knowledge structures. Different types of inferences employ different background knowledge for their generation. Although many different types of knowledge structures could be employed, most fall under the heading of a schema. "A schema is a cognitive structure that consists in part of the representation of some defined stimulus domain. The schema contains general knowledge about that domain, including a specification of the relationships among its attributes, as well as specific examples or instances of the stimulus domain" (Taylor & Crocker, 1981, p. 91). In other words, schemata organize knowledge, providing expectations about incoming information, means of interpreting information, suggestions for gathering information, and bases for activating actual behavior sequences.

Schemata aid in the inference-making process by suggesting the relative importance of concepts in the discourse and guiding the short-term memory and working memory systems in the selection, chunking, and discarding of information. For example, words that are *expected* are identified more readily (Bower & Cirilo, 1985), and when words are missing, an appropriate schema from the knowledge store is activated to suggest an interpretation (Waern, 1982). Furthermore, schematic discourse processing will provide information to connect meanings in texts (Bransford & McCarrell, 1974; Dooling & Lachman, 1971; Johnson, 1970; Sanford & Garrod, 1981; Spiro, 1977).

A mind that is a blank slate is unable to comprehend unless the structure for comprehension is being provided simultaneously with the discourse. Persons lacking the requisite knowledge structures who are placed in situations in which such structures are not provided typically feel "lost" because the discourse is not comprehensible to them; they are unable to abstract meaning because they have no foundation on which to assign meaning and bridge gaps.

For example, a student attending class for the first time during the sixth week of a term is generally faced with this problem. When discourse employs words and concepts unfamiliar to the perceiver, *significantly* fewer inferences are generated during comprehension (Graesser, 1981). Text-based, (i.e., bottom-up) inferences are insufficient by themselves to guarantee the generation of inferences that permit understanding of the discourse (Bower & Cirilo, 1985; Krulee, Fairweather, & Bergquist, 1979).

Without the *automatic* inferences *provided* by the use of knowledge structures, the text alone may be inadequate for generating the required inferences. Unique to a top-down processing point of view is the dual nature of inferences inherent to discourse comprehension. One set of inferences is employed to "fill out" the schema. A second set of inferences is *provided* by the schema as default values to help bridge gaps between semantic meanings of utterances. Without the automatic inferences provided to bridge gaps, comprehension suffers. For example, inference generation is difficult and error-prone when reasoning with formal syllogisms (Johnson-Laird, 1983) or when reading texts on topics that are unfamiliar to an individual who "does not have an adequate background knowledge for interpreting and integrating the words, topics, and concepts in the text" (Graesser & Clark, 1985, p.54). Most discourse permits a very large number of inferences to be generated (Charniak, 1975; Clark, 1975), though the limitations on our processing capabilities reduce the number actually generated (Singer, 1980). The literature suggests that only "important" inferences are drawn in text comprehension where relevance is the criterion for importance (Crothers, 1978). These inferences are relevant because they often are required for conceptual connectivity between utterances (Graesser & Clark, 1985).

Graesser and Clark (1985) identify a number of principles that guide whether inferences will be generated during comprehension, including principles of connectivity, cohesion, preservation, functionality, and automaticity. These principles may reflect the desire to decrease cognitive energy when possible, employ top-down processing when possible, and generate a comprehensible model of the discourse. The organization of the discourse also influences inference generation, with thematically organized texts providing quantitatively more inferences during comprehension and altering the *nature* of those inferences (Schnotz, 1985). In general, inferences necessary for comprehension such that the discourse will be judged more coherent tend to be generated (Hildyard & Olson, 1978; Singer, 1980; Stein & Nezworski, 1978).

Schematic processing influences comprehension of the text. The schema instantiated during comprehension of the discourse will affect what inferences are made, what information is retained, and the meaning one assigns to the discourse. Many studies have indicated that altering one's perspective, approach, or viewpoint on some event or text leads to an alteration in comprehension and memory of that text or event (Anderson, Spiro, &

Anderson, 1978; Anderson, Reynolds, Schallert, & Goetz, 1977; Bower, 1978; Pichert & Anderson, 1977; Schallert, 1976). Such alterations can lead to distortions that interfere with accurate recall of the discourse (Owens, Bower, & Black, 1979). Schematic-based processing also permits one to develop inferences about the ordering of events. Though stories with their paragraphs randomly ordered take people longer to read, *summaries* of these stories are no different than when the paragraphs follow the schematic order (Kintsch & van Dijk, 1975). Such reorganization of the discourse to "match" the schema is common (Kintsch, Mandel, & Kozminsky, 1977; Stein & Nezworski, 1978).

The meaning one extracts from discourse will depend, however, on the schema employed to comprehend it. Zadny and Gerard (1974) provided a vivid demonstration of how meaning is dependent on schematic processing. These researchers made a videotape of two persons searching through an apartment. Subjects in the study were variously told that they would see a videotape of persons (1) preparing for a drug bust by removing their illicit drugs, (2) engaging in burglary, or (3) waiting for friends. Events and features relevant to the schema employed for processing were better remembered, indicating that the schema that is *activated* affects the comprehension that occurs.

Discourse can be consistent, neutral, or inconsistent with the schema instantiated for comprehension. Consistent and neutral discourse matches the schema or is irrelevant to it and hence is easily integrated. Furthermore, neutral events permit precisely the distortions in interpretations that interfere with accuracy in representation of the discourse (Owens et al., 1979). Inconsistent information does not necessarily lead to *rejection* of the schema. Mildly inconsistent information may not be noticed because of perceptual distortions. Relatively infrequent inconsistencies will tend to be "tagged" for further processing (Graesser, Gordon, & Sawyer, 1979; Graesser, Woll, Kowalski, & Smith, 1980) or elaborated and "explained away" (Hastie, 1981). In other words, people tend to make the discourse fit the schema they are employing to comprehend it. The impact of such a "distortion" procedure is great. For example, Langer and Abelson (1974) prepared an audiotape of an interaction, instructing one group of listeners that it was a tape of a job interview and another group that it was a psychiatric intake interview. Therapists served as subjects in the study. Particularly disheartening in Langer and Abelson's results is that the therapists distorted the background information on the "to-be-committed" person in the psychiatric interview to be consistent with their schema, leading to findings of more "pathology" in the behavior of this person. Thus two different schemata were employed to process this discourse with significantly different outcomes in terms of assessment of the mental health of the interviewee.

Multiple schemata potentially could be employed (either simultaneously or by different persons) to facilitate comprehension of discourse. However, what does a person do when faced with discourse to which he or she cannot attach a schema permitting inferences of its meaning relations? Reconsider the case of the communication professor at the physicists' convention listening to a paper presentation, trying to attach various schemata in the hope that one might permit some set of inferences about the meaning of the discourse. A situation schema (convention paper presentations) and a person prototype (nuclear physicist) might be instantiated so that various expectations about the discourse might be generated. Not only might such schemata lead to predictions that technical jargon and big words will be used by the presenter, but expectations will also be generated about the ability of the communication professor to understand the deeper meaning of the discourse. If the communication professor does not comprehend the presentation, he or she assumes responsibility and does not assess the speaker as incoherent. In other words, the schemata we activate for interpretation of discourse generate expectations that lay the foundation for attributions of responsibility for lack of comprehensibility.

Consonance between knowledge structures and discourse produces coherence. We have been arguing that discourse comprehension *requires* the making of inferences, that such inferences cannot be made solely on the basis of the text, that knowledge structures are required in the inferential process, and that these knowledge structures affect one's comprehension of the discourse. As a result, we would argue that the perceived degree to which the instantiated knowledge structures (and their resultant expectations) match the perceived nature of the discourse is the degree to which we will judge the discourse coherent. In specific, the judgment of coherence is made on the degree to which the discourse (as perceived) is organized consonant with the knowledge structure(s) employed in comprehension.

Research on shifting points of view in storytelling is supportive of our argument. Narratives in which the relation between the narrator and the action in the story is shifting are seen as less coherent than narratives that maintain a consistent relation between the narrator and the action (Black, Turner, & Bower, 1979). The reason for such a decrease in coherence stems from the disruption of schematic processing of the discourse. Schemata tend to assume a consistent point of view for the circumstance in which they are instantiated; shifting the point of view necessitates revising the schema or instantiating new schemata. Such a process disrupts the ability to obtain high consonance between the perceived structure of the discourse and schematic expectations and knowledge.

This production of a coherence judgment does not hinge on whether *meaning* is assigned to the discourse *unless* schematic processing generates an expectation that the meaning *should be* extractable. If the schema(ta) employed for processing the discourse are such that meaning relations are not attempted and the lack of that attempt is due to the *schema,* suggesting one should not *expect* to be able to extract meaning, then consonance does exist between the knowledge structures and the "incomprehensible" or noncomprehended discourse (presuming other features of the discourse match expectations). For example, we judge the presentation by the nuclear physicist as coherent because the situational, person, and role schema we employ suggest to us that we should *not* be able to comprehend the physicist because of use of technical jargon. As long as we perceive that such attributes characterize the discourse, then our schematic expectations match our perceptions of the discourse or, in other words, we have consonance between our schema and the discourse (as perceived).

Does such an approach to the process by which a judgment of coherence is produced explain why it is so difficult to obtain judgments of discourse as absolutely incoherent? We believe this schematic consonance approach can explain such an outcome. First, individuals have many schemata that can be instantiated in any given instance for purposes of processing discourse. Though some schemata may be more appropriate than others, "distortion" (or "construction") processes seem to provide a fairly strong assurance of at least minimal coherence. The tendency to correct distortions, however, decreases as the number and importance of violations increase (Bower & Cirilo, 1985). Second, individuals are capable of flexibly adapting schemata to given circumstances, combining them in unique ways to handle seemingly novel situations (Schank, 1982). Thus a judgment of incoherence would only result, in this perspective, if *no* activated schemata were consonant to any degree with the perceived nature of the discourse.

So why did my colleague in the communication department refer to a paper presenter at a convention as incoherent? We would argue that this judgment was a result of the following conditions: (1) the convention was a communication convention; (2) the colleague is a knowledgeable, respected professor of communication; (3) the colleague instantiated schemata requiring meaning relations be established; (4) the instantiated schemata led to the expectation that the colleague *should have* been able to comprehend the discourse to a significant degree; (5) the discourse could not be minimally comprehended as to its meaning relations; (6) the locus of responsibility for the failure was placed on the shoulders of the presenter; consequently, (7) the presenter was judged incoherent in his or her presentation. In other words, it was the lack of consonance between schematic knowledge (including expectations) and the perceived nature of the discourse that led to the judgment of incoherence.

It is possible that discourse judged incoherent at one time may be judged as coherent at another. The first author recalls a numerical analysis course, one part of which never made a great deal of sense despite expectations that it should. At the time of presentation, the discourse about a given approximation procedure seemed incoherent. Two years later in another mathematics class, the meaning of that "incoherent" discourse became clear upon the receipt of new information. Thus a judgment of incoherence is not necessarily permanent.

It is also possible that when discourse is judged fairly coherent that the meaning the speaker intended to convey was not the meaning the receiver of the discourse assigned. Persons uttering a remark, and those interpreting it, need not employ the same schemata for generation of meaning relations. That is why, for example, two students can attend the same lecture and arrive at very different interpretations of what was said without necessarily varying in their judgments of coherence.

Certainly, however, a perceiver of discourse who lacks the requisite knowledge structures will tend to judge discourse (or parts thereof) as incoherent even while others, who have the requisite knowledge structures, judge the discourse as coherent (Bellert, 1970). Judgments of incoherence are based on beliefs that the discourse should have been coherent: The perceiver is not cognizant that he or she lacks the requisite knowledge structures. The key to all judgments of coherence is simply the degree of consonance between activated schemata (along with their resultant expectations) and the perceived nature of the discourse.

Coherence Does Not Reside in the Text

Our definition of coherence as a judgment and the process by which we argue that the judgment will be made has a necessary and immediate implication: Coherence does not reside in the text, but instead resides in the mind of the perceiver of the text. Consequently, some apparently coherent (from the sender's perspective) discourse may be found to be incoherent by receivers who are incapable of doing the requisite processing or are missing some part of the context (background information, goal orientation, situational constraints). On the other hand, some apparently incoherent discourse may be found coherent because the receiver can fill in "missing" information. The determination of coherence, however, does not require extraction of similar meanings by different perceivers of the discourse. Finding discourse coherent does not guarantee mutual understanding, but it certainly facilitates it; judgments that discourse is relatively incoherent are likely to inhibit mutual understanding.

Searching in the discourse for coherence, though, is likely to reveal more about the searcher's own knowledge structures than about the discourse structure itself. Coherence is the output of a cognitive process; it is a judgment of meaningfulness, not meaning. Coherence *evaluates* the *state* of a text and does not describe the actual concrete reality of the text. Simply stated, coherence does not reside in the text, it resides in the mind.

WHEN COHERENCE WILL BE

Much of our criticism of past literature on coherence concerns the confusion between coherence and elements of the text as cause and effect. Other scholars have viewed cohesive devices, relevance, topical relevance, and structure as causes of coherence. By contrast, we see such textual features as outcomes of persons' attempts to have their discourse judged as coherent. We believe that these features can serve as cues that can be manipulated to aid perceivers in accessing appropriate knowledge structures for comprehending the discourse. The success of such cueing attempts will depend not only on the cues employed, but also on the existence of the knowledge structures in the perceivers, the ability of the cues to access those structures, and the actual correspondence of the content of those structures to the perceived nature of the discourse. This section will explore the interrelationship of textual features and judgments of coherence, focusing on how individuals might produce discourse such that perceivers would be more likely to judge it coherent.

Interlocutors Can Try to Cue Others to Perceive the Discourse as Coherent

It is likely that individuals will actively assist those they interact with to perceive discourse as coherent. Attempting to make relevant remarks, employing cohesive devices, using topical references, and employing correct structure are four general cueing approaches available to persons, but the choice of a specific cue within any of these categories is based on an assessment of its probable effectiveness. The purpose of a cue is to help a perceiver instantiate appropriate knowledge structures for a generation of inferences in the hope that consonance will be achieved between those structures and the perceived nature of the discourse. For cues to be effective, they must be associable with an appropriate knowledge structure such that consonance occurs between that structure and the discourse (as perceived).

Many potential cues exist. For example, cohesive devices have been argued to serve an information-processing function by cueing appropriate knowledge structures for processing of discourse (Badzinski, 1985; Planalp & Tracy, 1980). Cohesive devices provide repetition of references to the same concepts in different utterances. Such referential cohesion helps cue appropriate knowledge structures (Jackson, Jacobs, & Rossi, 1986), resulting in improved recall of the text (de Villiers, 1974; Kintsch, Kozminsky, Streby, McKoon, & Keenan, 1975; Manelis & Yekovich, 1976). In essence, cohesive devices aid in the generation of inferences by reducing the cognitive energy needed to process the discourse (Black & Bern, 1981; Haviland & Clark, 1974; Hildyard & Olson, 1978; Singer, 1976, 1980). The use of cohesive devices permits a more highly integrated representation of the discourse in memory that makes the discourse simultaneously easier to process and easier to recall (Goetz & Armbruster, 1980).

Topical relevance can serve as a cue to knowledge structure instantiation and use (Krulee et al., 1979). As the thematic structure of the discourse increases, comprehension and recall tend to increase (Garnham et al., 1982; Kintsch & Greene, 1978; Mandler & Johnson, 1977; Masson & Alexander, 1981; Stein & Nezworski, 1978; Vande-Kopple, 1982). Brown and Yule (1983) note that "one function of thematisation at the text level may be to activate a particular scenario representation for the reader" (p. 246). Topics that occur in discourse are associated with a variety of grammatical tactics (Bates & MacWhinney, 1982), including word order, sentence subject, and the use of definite articles. Fletcher (1984), for example, has demonstrated that as topic continuity increases, use of full noun phrases decreases, whereas the more linguistically marked a referent, the higher the chance of a topic change. Such linguistic cues to topical relevance can signal processors of discourse to instantiate new schemata.

Syntax can serve as a cue for instantiation of appropriate knowledge structures and inferences. "Syntax is the primary means by which we can specify the intended relation among words" (Adams, 1980, p. 18). Obscured or distorted sentence structure creates difficulties in discourse processing in terms of comprehension and recall (Anglin & Miller, 1968; Oaken, Wiener, & Cromer, 1971). Such difficulties are likely a result of miscueing of knowledge structures and/or are significant enough distortions that instantiated structures significantly disconfirm expectations. Syntactic cues in discourse can signal what is given information and what is new information through the use of definite versus indefinite articles (Bower & Cirilo, 1985). Consequently, appropriate syntax is a cue persons can employ to aid perceivers in accessing knowledge structures that can stand in consonance to the discourse—a circumstance, we argue, that will be more likely to produce a judgment of coherence.

Other linguistic features can also serve as cues for instantiation and maintenance of knowledge structures. Preindexing (Beach & Dunning, 1982) is employed to "set up" and "preorganize" sequences of talk, thus providing a *cue* to instantiate certain schemata for processing upcoming discourse. Maintaining a consistent point of view in a narrative aids discourse processing because shifts between schemata or between roles in schemata or between instantiations of schemata are not required (Black et al., 1979). Causally relating events also improves memory for discourse (Mandler & Johnson, 1977). Thus numerous potential cues exist that discourse producers can employ to assist perceivers in processing discourse by helping guide the selection and instantiation of knowledge structures. The cues are simply aids for comprehension in the hope that a cued schema will be consonant with the discourse. Nevertheless, the cue may or may not work; the schema that is cued may or may not be consonant with the discourse; schemata may be activated in the absence of such cues; these schemata may or may not be consonant with the discourse. Cueing, therefore, is a tactic for which no guarantee of success is made.

Cues are not equally shared. Any given cue can be placed along a continuum of frequency of cooccurrence across discourse users. An individual could have a cue that was highly associated with a particular knowledge structure for him or her that is not shared by many others, or, at the opposite extreme, this cue could be nearly universally shared by others in a culture. For example, individuals in an intimate relationship may share a set of cues not available to persons outside the relationship as well as maintain a set of cues that persons outside the relationship would also find highly associated to given knowledge structures.

Certain cues frequently occur simultaneously in the discourse of a culture such that these cues are likely to be culturally shared. For example, high consistency exists among discourse processors in their grammatical segmentation of utterances (Scholes, 1971). As a consequence, culturally shared cues are likely to be more effective for accessing appropriate knowledge structures, thus more likely to generate a judgment of coherence. In fact, Gumperz (1982) argues that a set of culturally shared cues is necessary for effective conversational interaction. While we would not go to such an extreme, we do note that *if* cueing is necessary in a given instance, then cues that are not entirely idiosyncratic will be the only effective ones.

Cues can vary in their degree of association to knowledge structures. For one individual to cue another successfully, the cues must have associative value with the other's knowledge structures. The associative value of cues can vary. First, a cue can be strongly or weakly associated with a given knowledge structure. A weakly associated cue may fail to lead to the instantiation of the desired knowledge structure or of *any* structure, for that matter (de Beaugrande, 1980). Typically, persons watch for intersections (Charniak, 1975) or coincidences (Woods, 1978) of cues so that an appropriate knowledge structure can be selected prior to the discourse being lost for lack of an interpretive device. When the cue is strongly associated with a structure, memory for discourse increases dramatically (Anderson et al., 1978; Bransford & Johnson, 1972; Dooling & Lachman, 1971).

Second, a given knowledge structure can have few or many cues that might be associated with it. Many different cues might encourage a discourse processor to access one knowledge structure, while only a limited number of cues might be available for other knowledge structures. Locating appropriate cues would be more difficult the smaller the constellation available.

Third, a given cue can be attached to multiple knowledge structures. In such instances, the processing of discourse can lead to ambiguities in its interpretation because the cues tap more than one schema (Graesser & Nakamura, 1982), permitting different schemata or multiple (and not necessarily consistent) schemata to be simultaneously activated. The more a cue is attached to multiple knowledge structures, the less it discriminates between those structures. A discourse processor perceiving such a cue may be *unsure* of which knowledge structure of the many possible to activate.

Cues can vary in effectiveness. The presence of cues does not guarantee either comprehensibility or a judgment of coherence; the cued schema must still be consonant with the discourse (Jackson, Jacobs, & Rossi, 1986). The lack of effective cues can lead to problems in communication. Studies of intercultural communication (Gumperz, 1979; Gumperz & Kaltman, 1980) discuss the problems when interactants "read cues" differently. Gumperz (1982) writes that

> when all participants understand and notice the relevant cues, interpretive processes are then taken for granted and tend to go unnoticed. However, when a listener does not react to a cue or is unaware of its function, interpretations may differ and misunderstandings may occur. (p. 132)

de Beaugrande (1980) argues that determinate cues are superior to typical cues, which in turn are superior to accidental cues for helping perceivers access appropriate knowledge structures. In this section, we will attempt to outline possible routes to identifying determinate cues.

The most effective cue across many perceivers would be one that is culturally shared and highly associated with only one knowledge structure that is also culturally based. Typically, explicit identification of a culturally shared topic is such a cue. The effectiveness of explicit identification of a culturally shared topic can be seen in Bransford and Johnson's (1972) research. The following paragraph was employed in one of the studies these researchers report:

> The procedure is actually quite simple. First you arrange things into different groups. Of course, one pile may be sufficient depending on how much there is to do. If you have to go somewhere else due to lack of facilities, that is the next step, otherwise you are pretty well set. It is important not to overdo things. That is, it is better to do too few things at once than too many. In the short run this may not seem important but complications can easily arise. A mistake can be expensive as well. At first the whole procedure will seem complicated. Soon, however, it will become just another facet of life. It is difficult to foresee any end to the necessity for this task in the immediate future, but then one can never tell. After the procedure is completed, one arranges the materials into different groups again. Then they can be put into their appropriate places. Eventually they will be used once more and the whole cycle will then have to be repeated. However, that is part of life. (p.400)

When subjects in Bransford and Johnson's experiment were provided with an explicit topic identifier (e.g., "washing clothes"), the differences in recall and comprehension were stark. The issue with such a text is not that individuals lack the appropriate schema; rather, the "bottom-up" textual cues are sufficiently equivocal so as not to "suggest" activation of that schema. Thus a culturally shared cue that is strongly associated to the desired knowledge structure will probably be the most effective cue a discourse producer could employ.

The least effective cues are those that are not shared with the perceiver, those that are weakly associated with knowledge structures in the perceiver, or those that are associated with multiple knowledge structures, some of which the discourse producer wishes *not* to instantiate. If cues are associated to "improper" (from the discourse producer's point of view) knowledge structures, then the fit of the accessed knowledge structure to the discourse is likely to be poor, leading to a judgment of incoherence on the part of the discourse perceiver. Similarly, if the cues are only weakly associated to the proper knowledge structures, these structures are less likely to be accessed by the discourse perceiver. Consequently, knowledge structures more strongly associated with that cue are likely to be employed, again leading to possible judgments of incoherence on the part of the discourse perceiver.

Basically, cues cannot be effective unless the perceiver of the discourse has a strong association between the cues and the knowledge structure the discourse producer wishes the perceiver to access *and* the accessed knowledge structure is consonant with the discourse. Even in the face of *very effective* cues, no guarantee exists of (1) the perceiver *having* the cued knowledge structure, (2) the cues *accessing* the desired knowledge structure, or (3) the cued knowledge structure being consonant with the discourse.

Ineffective cueing can be self-correcting. When perceivers in interactive contexts become aware that they have been miscued, have failed to be cued, or that their own knowledge structures are incomplete, they can indicate these problems to their cointeractants. The use of clarification requests is one example that problems in discourse processing are occurring. On the other hand, discourse perceivers need not overtly indicate miscueing, but can move to repair on their own. "It is certainly possible for subjects to 'change their minds' as a story proceeds, to decide that they have gotten off on the wrong track, and to revise their notions of what the story is about" (Mandler, 1978, p.15). In other words, both bottom-up and top-down approaches are available to handle miscueing. It is likely that top-down repairs are preferred to bottom-up approaches as they are more efficient (Ringle & Bruce, 1982) and permit the perceiver and producer to "save face."

Not only the perceiver of discourse is capable of recognizing miscued or incomplete knowledge structures for comprehending discourse. The discourse producer is also capable of making these judgments. When miscueing is unintentional and recognized by the discourse producer, he or she can then provide additional cues or information to aid the perceiver in processing the discourse. Self-initiated textual repairs are examples of such producer-generated attempts to cue the perceiver better (Schegloff, Jefferson, & Sacks, 1977). Inappropriate discourse behaviors (e.g., unusual topic shifts or topic extensions, "incoherent" follow-up questions) are typical indices to the producer of the discourse that the perceiver has been miscued and does not recognize this fact.

Even with perceivers and producers monitoring the discourse to determine the effectiveness of the cues in accessing knowledge structures, not all ineffective cues will be detected or corrected. Such lack of notice and disregard occurs because of the "trivial" nature of many miscues or ineffective cues (Ringle & Bruce, 1982). Thus ineffective cueing can be, though is not necessarily, self-correcting.

IMPLICATIONS

We have argued that coherence is an evaluative judgment of the meaningfulness of discourse that comes about when activated knowledge structures are consonant with the perceived nature of the discourse. Interlocutors can attempt to cue knowledge structures in the perceiver, though such cueing does not guarantee a judgment of coherence. At this point, we are ready to examine two implications of our perspective. The first implication examines the nature of a coherent conversation, the second examines the potential impermanence of any such judgment.

A Coherent Conversation Occurs When Participants Access Knowledge Structures that Are Consonant with the Discourse

When interlocutors access knowledge structures (whether cued or not) that are consonant with the perceived nature of the conversation, they will arrive at a judgment of coherence. However, these judgments do not imply that the same meanings have been extracted from the conversation by the participants. Interlocutors can access different knowledge structures, each of which might be consonant with the discourse. Misunderstandings are a common result of accessing such differential, though more or less equally consonant, knowledge structures. Consequently, misunderstandings between persons can stem from coherent discourse.

We believe an incoherent conversation occurs when any participant or perceiver is unable to access a knowledge structure that is consonant with the discourse. Thus if one participant in a dyadic interaction judges that conversation incoherent, we would argue it is incoherent—to that perceiver. In other words, coherence does not reside in the conversation but in the mind of the perceiver. A coherent conversation is no more and no less than a person's judgment of the consonance between expectations and perceived actuality.

Discourse Perceived as Incoherent Today May Be Perceived as Coherent Tomorrow

People are able to remember their conversational interactions to a greater or lesser degree. Conversations judged coherent tend to be integrated into the preexisting knowledge store, whereas ones judged relatively less coherent are often "tagged" for further processing. If sufficient information from such a conversation is stored in memory, then it is possible that this interaction can be reflected on at some future point. Such reflections might lead to reinterpretation if the reflection accesses different or newly acquired knowledge structures. The implication is that the coherence of a given piece of discourse or a given conversation is not permanent; it potentially can be in a continous state of change. However, we do note that once a judgment of coherence is made (upon an initial assessment or a reassessment) that further processing is unlikely. Integration of that specific instance into the schema(ta) used to comprehend it is likely to prevent that specific information being available for further processing. The opportunity for reprocessing to even occur, however, stems from the fact that coherence does not reside intact in discourse or in any memory structure.

A Final Remark

As we have argued, coherence is an evaluative judgment of meaningfulness that stands in relation to, but is not an overt piece of, a given conversation or text. Given that we operate under a *presumption* that persons are trying to produce discourse that will be judged to be coherent, any judgment of incoherence is likely to propel us to attempt to realign knowledge structures (if possible) so that the assumed cooperative nature of conversational interaction is maintained. In other words, our judgments of coherence are colored by our *expectation* that discourse is meaningful. It is this *presumption* of meaningfulness that provides the "glue" that adheres thoughts to each other, suggesting that connections should be possible. The judgment of coherence indicates that we believe that what is said is meaningful, that utterances adhere to one another in some meaningful manner. In essence, the judgment of coherence is the adhesive of discourse.

REFERENCES

Adams, M. J. (1980). Failures to comprehend and level of processing in reading. In R. J. Spiro, B. C. Bruce, & W. F. Brewer (Eds.), *Theoretical issues in reading comprehension: Perspectives from cognitive psychology, linguistics, artificial intelligence, and education* (pp. 9-32). Hillsdale, NJ: Lawrence Erlbaum.

Anderson, R. C., Reynolds, R. E., Schallert, D. L., & Goetz, E. T. (1977). Frameworks for comprehending discourse. *American Educational Research Journal, 14*, 367-381.

Anderson, R. C., & Shifrin, Z. (1980). Discourse and linguistic theory. In R. J. Spiro, B. C. Bruce, & W. F. Brewer (Eds.), *Theoretical issues in reading comprehension: Perspectives from cognitive psychology, linguistics, artificial intelligence, and education* (pp. 331-348). Hillsdale, NJ: Lawrence Erlbaum.

Anderson, R. C., Spiro, R., & Anderson, M. C. (1978). Schemata as scaffolding for the representation of information in connected discourse. *American Educational Research Journal, 15*, 433-440.

Anglin, J. M., & Miller, G. A. (1968). The role of phrase structure in the recall of meaningful verbal material. *Psychonomic Science*, 10, 343-344.

Badzinski, D. (1985, November). *The functions that cohesive devices serve in conversation.* Paper presented at the annual meeting of the Speech Communication Association, Denver.

Bates, E., & MacWhinney, B. (1982). Functionalist approaches to grammar. In L. Gleitman & E. Wanner (Eds.), *Language acquisition: The state of the art.* (pp. 173-218). New York: Cambridge University Press.

Beach, W. A., & Dunning, D. G. (1982). Preindexing and conversational organization. *Quarterly Journal of Speech, 68,* 170-185.

Bellert, I. (1970). On a condition for the coherence of texts. *Semiotica, 2,* 335-363.

Black, J. B., & Bern, H. (1981). Causal coherence and memory for events in narratives. *Journal of Verbal Learning and Behavior, 20,* 267-275.

Black, J. B., Turner, T. J., & Bower, G. H. (1979). Point of view in narrative comprehension. *Journal of Verbal Learning and Verbal Behavior, 18,* 187-198.

Bower, G. H. (1978). Experiments on story comprehension and recall. *Discourse Processes, 1,* 211-231.

Bower, G. H., & Cirilo, R. K. (1985). Cognitive psychology and text processing. In T. A. van Dijk (Ed.), *Handbook of discourse analysis: Vol. 1. Disciplines of discourse* (pp. 71-105). London: Academic Press.

Bransford, J. D. (1979). *Human cognition: Learning, understanding.* Belmont, CA: Wadsworth.

Bransford, J. D., Barclay, J. R., & Frank, J. J. (1972). Sentence memory: A constructive versus interpretive approach. *Cognitive Psychology, 3,* 193-209.

Bransford, J. D., & Franks, J. J. (1971). The abstraction of linguistic ideas. *Cognitive Psychology, 2,* 331-350.

Bransford, J. D., & Johnson, M. K. (1972). Contextual prerequisites for understanding: Some investigations of comprehension and recall. *Journal of Verbal Learning and Verbal Behavior, 11,* 717-726.

Bransford, J. D., & McCarrell, N. S. (1974). A sketch of a cognitive approach to comprehension. In W. B. Weimer & D. S. Palermo (Eds.), *Cognition and the symbolic processes.* Hillsdale, NJ: Lawrence Erlbaum.

Bransford, J. D., McCarrell, N. S., Franks, J. J., & Nitsch, K. E. (1977). Toward unexplaining memory. In R. Shaw & J. Bransford (Eds.), *Perceiving, acting, and knowing* (pp. 431-466). Hillsdale, NJ: Lawrence Erlbaum.

Brewer, W. F. (1977). *Memory for the pragmatic implications of sentences* (Report No. 65). Urbana: University of Illinois at Urbana-Champaign, Center for the Study of Reading.

Brockway, D. (1981). Semantic constraints on relevance. In H. Parret, M. Sbisa, & J. Bershueren (Eds.), *Possibilities and limitations of pragmatics: Proceedings of the Conference on Pragmatics, Urbino, July 8-14, 1979* (pp. 57-78). Amsterdam: Benjamins.

Brown, P., & Levinson, S. C. (1978). Universals in language usage: Politeness phenomena. In E. M. Goody (Ed.), *Questions and politeness: Strategies in social interaction* pp. (56-289). New York: Cambridge University Press.

Brown, P., & Yule, G. (1983). *Discourse analysis.* Cambridge: Cambridge University Press.

Carroll, D. W. (1986). *Psychology of language.* Monterey, CA: Brooks/Cole.

Carroll, L. (1982/1897). *Alice's adventures in wonderland* and *Through the looking glass.* Oxford: Oxford University Press.

Chafe, W. L. (1976). Giveness, contrastiveness, definiteness, subjects, topics, and point-of-view. In C. Li (Ed.), *Subject and topic* (pp. 25-55). New York: Academic Press.

Charniak, E. (1975, June). Organization and inference in a framelike system of common knowledge. In R. Schank & B. Nash-Webber (Eds.), *Theoretical issues in natural language processing: An interdisciplinary workshop in computational linguistics, psychology, and artificial intelligence.* Massachusetts Institute of Technology.

Charolles, M. (1983). Towards a heuristic approach to text-coherence problems. In F. Neubauer (Ed.), *Coherence in natural language texts* (pp. 1-16). Hamburg: Buske.

Clancy, P. (1972). Analysis of a conversation. *Anthropological Linguistics, 14,* 78-86.

Clark, H. H. (1975, June). Bridging. In R. Schank & B. Nash-Webber (Eds.), *Theoretical issues in natural language processing: An interdisciplinary workshop in computational linguistics, psychology, linguistics, and artificial intelligence* (pp. 188-193). Massachusetts Institute of Technology.

Clark, H. H. (1977). Bridging. In P. N. Johnson-Laird & P. C. Wason (Eds.), *Thinking: Readings in cognitive science* (pp. 411-419). Cambridge: Cambridge University Press.

Clark, H. H., & Haviland, S. E. (1977). Comprehension and the given-new contract. In R. O. Freedle (Ed.), *Discourse production and comprehension* (pp. 1-40). Norwood, NJ: Ablex.
Coulthard, M. (1977). *An introduction to discourse analysis.* London: Longman.
Crothers, E. J. (1978). Inference and coherence. *Discourse Processes, 1,* 51-71.
Crow, B. K. (1983). Topic shift in couple's conversations. In R. Craig & K. Tracy (Eds.), *Conversational coherence: Form, structure, and strategy* (pp. 136-156). Newbury Park, CA: Sage.
Dascal, M., & Katriel, T. (1979). Digressions: A study in conversation coherence. *PTL: A Journal for Descriptive Poetics and Theory of Literature, 4,* 203-232.
de Beaugrande, R. (1980). *Text, discourse, and process: Toward a multidisciplinary science of texts.* Norwood, NJ: Ablex.
de Villiers, P. A. (1974). Imagery and recall of connected discourse. *Journal of Experimental Psychology, 103,* 63-168.
Dooling, D. J., & Lachman, R. (1971). Effects of comprehension on retention of prose. *Journal of Experimental Psychology, 88,* 216-222.
Ferrara, A. (1985). Pragmatics. In T. A. van Dijk (Ed.), *Handbook of discourse analysis: Vol. 2. Dimensions of discourse* (pp. 137-157). London: Academic Press.
Fillenbaum, S. (1966). Memory for gist: Some relevant variables. *Language and Speech, 9,* 217-277.
Fiske, S. T., & Taylor, S. E. (1984). *Social cognition.* Reading, MA: Addison-Wesley.
Fletcher, C. R. (1984). Markedness and topic continuity in discourse processing. *Journal of Verbal Learning and Verbal Behavior, 23,* 487-493.
Frederiksen, C. H. (1977). Structure and process in discourse production and comprehension. In M. A. Just & P. A. Carpenter (Eds.), *Cognitive processes in comprehension* (pp. 313-322). Hillsdale, NJ: Lawrence Erlbaum.
Garnham, A., Oakhill, J. V., & Johnson-Laird, P. N. (1982). Referential continuity and the coherence of discourse. *Cognition, 11,* 29-46.
Garrod, S. C., & Sanford, A. J. (1981). Bridging inferences and the extended domain of reference. In J. Long & A. Baddeley (Eds.), *Attention and performance IX* (pp. 331-346). Hillsdale, NJ: Lawrence Erlbaum.
Goetz, E. T., & Armbruster, B. B. (1980). Psychological correlates of text structure. In R. J. Spiro, B. C. Bruce, & W. F. Brewer (Eds.), *Theoretical issues in reading comprehension: Perspectives from cognitive psychology, linguistics, artificial intelligence, and education* (pp. 201-220). Hillsdale, NJ: Lawrence Erlbaum.
Graesser, A. C. (1981). *Prose comprehension beyond the word.* New York: Springer.
Graesser, A. C., & Clark, L. F. (1985). *Structures and procedures of implicit knowledge.* Norwood, NJ: Ablex.
Graesser, A. C., Gordon, S. E., & Sawyer, J. D. (1979). Memory for typical and atypical actions in scripted activities: Test of a script pointer + tag hypothesis. *Journal of Verbal Learning and Verbal Behavior, 18,* 319-332.
Graesser, A. C., & Nakamura, G. V. (1982). The impact of a schema on comprehension and memory. In G. H. Bower (Ed.), *The psychology of learning and motivation* (Vol. 16, pp. 59-109). New York: Academic Press.
Graesser, A. C., Woll, S. B., Kowlaski, D. J., & Smith, D. A. (1980). Memory for typical and atypical actions in scripted activities. *Journal of Experimental Psychology: Human Learning and Memory, 6,* 503-513.
Grice, H. P. (1969). Utterer's meaning and intentions. *Philosophical Review, 78,* 147-177.
Grice, H. P. (1975). Logic and conversation. In P. Cole & J. L. Morgan (Eds.), *Syntax and semantics: Vol. 3. Speech acts* (pp. 41-58). New York: Academic Press.
Grice, H. P. (1978). Further notes on logic and conversations. In P. Cole (Ed.), *Syntax and semantics: Vol. 9. Pragmatics* (pp. 113-127). New York: Academic Press.
Gumperz, J. J. (1979). The sociolinguistic basis of speech act theory. In J. Boyd & S. Ferrara (Eds.), *Speech act ten years after.* Milan: Versus.

Gumperz, J. J. (1982). *Discourse strategies.* Cambridge: Cambridge University Press.
Gumperz, J. J., & Kaltman, H. (1980). In B. R. Caron, M.A.B. Hoffman, N. Silva, J. Van Oosten, D. K. Alford, K. A. Hunold, M. Macauley, & J. Manley-Buser (Eds.), *Proceedings of the Sixth Annual Meeting of the Berkeley Linguistic Society* (pp. 44-65). Berkeley, CA: Berkeley Linguistics Society.
Gutwinksi, W. (1976). *Cohesion in literary texts.* The Hague: Mouton.
Haberlandt, K., & Bingham, G. (1978). Verbs contribute to the coherence of brief narratives: Reading-related and unrelated sentence triples. *Journal of Verbal Learning and Verbal Behavior, 17,* 419-429.
Halliday, M. (1967). Notes on transitivity and theme in English: II. *Journal of Linguistics, 3,* 199-244.
Halliday, M., & Hasan, R. (1976). *Cohesion in English.* London: Longman.
Harris, R. J. (1974). Memory and comprehension of implications and inferences of complex sentences. *Journal of Verbal Learning and Verbal Behavior, 13,* 626-637.
Hastie, R. (1981). Schematic principles in human memory. In E. T. Higgins, C. P. Herman, & M. P. Zanna (Eds.), *Social cognition: The Ontario Symposium* (Vol. 1, pp. 39-88). Hillsdale, NJ: Lawrence Erlbaum.
Haviland, S. E., & Clark, H. H. (1974). What's new: Acquiring new information as a process in comprehension. *Journal of Verbal Learning and Verbal Behavior, 13,* 512-521.
Hildyard, A., & Olson, D. R. (1978). Memory and inference in the comprehension of oral and written discourse. *Discourse Processes, 1,* 91-117.
Hobbs, J. R. (1979). Coherence and co-reference. *Cognitive Science, 3,* 67-90.
Hobbs, J. R. (1982). Towards an understanding of coherence in discourse. In W. G. Lehnert & M. H. Ringle (Eds.), *Strategies for natural language processing.* Hillsdale, NJ: Lawrence Erlbaum.
Hobbs, J. R. (1983). Why is discourse coherent? In F. Neubauer (Ed.), *Coherence in natural language texts* (pp. 29-70). Hamburg: Buske.
Hopper, R. (1981). The taken-for-granted. *Human Communication Research, 7,* 195-211.
Irwin, J. W. (1986b). Cohesion and comprehension: A research review. In J. W. Irwin (Ed.), *Teaching cohesion comprehension* (pp. 31-43). Newark, DE: International Reading Association.
Jackson, S., Jacobs, S., & Rossi, A. M. (1986, June). *Conversational relevance: Three experiments on pragmatic connectedness in conversation.* Paper presented at the annual meeting of the International Communication Association, Chicago.
Jacobs, S., & Jackson, S. (1983). Speech act structure and conversation: Rational aspects of pragmatic coherence. In R. T. Craig & K. Tracy (Eds.), *Conversational coherence: Form, structure, and strategy* (pp. 47-66). Newbury Park, CA: Sage.
Jarvella, R. J. (1971). Syntactic processing of connected speech. *Journal of Verbal Learning and Verbal Behavior*, 10, 409-416.
Johnson, M. K., Bransford, J. D., & Solomon, S. K. (1973). Memory for tacit implications of sentences. *Journal of Experimental Social Psychology, 98,* 203-205.
Johnson, R. E. (1970). Recall of prose as a function of the structural importance of the linguistic units. *Journal of Verbal Learning and Verbal Behavior, 9,* 12-20.
Johnson-Laird, P.N. (1983). *Mental models.* Cambridge, MA: Harvard University Press.
Keenan, J. M., Baillet, S. D., & Brown, P. (1984). The effects of causal cohesion on comprehension and memory. *Journal of Verbal Learning and Verbal Behavior, 23,* 115-126.
Kieras, D. E. (1978). Good and bad structure in simple paragraphs: Effects of apparent theme, reading time, and recall. *Journal of Verbal Learning and Verbal Behavior, 17,* 13-28.
Kintsch, W. (1972). Notes on the structure of semantic memory. In E. Tulving & W. Donaldson (Eds.), *Organization of memory* (pp.247-308). New York: Academic Press.
Kintsch, W., & Greene, E. (1978). The role of culture specific schemata in the comprehension and recall of stories. *Discourse Processes, 1,* 1-13.

Kintsch, W., Kozminsky, E., Streby, W. J. McKoon, G., & Keenan, J. M. (1975). Comprehension and recall of texts as a function of content variables. *Journal of Verbal Learning and Verbal Behavior, 14,* 196-214.
Kintsch, W., Mandel, T., & Kozminsky, E. (1977). Summarizing scrambled stories. *Memory and Cognition, 5,* 647-552.
Kintsch, W., & van Dijk, T. A. (1975). Recalling and summarizing stories [Comment on Se rappelle et on resumes des histoires]. *Languages, 40,* 98-116.
Krulee, G. K., Fairweather, P. G., & Berquist, S. R. (1979). Organizing factors in the comprehension and recall of connected discourse. *Journal of Psycholinguistic Research, 8,* 141-163.
Labov, W. (1972). *Sociolinguistic patterns.* Philadelphia: University of Pennsylvania Press.
Langer, E. J. (1978). Rethinking the role of thought in social interaction. In J. H. Harvey, W. Ickes, & R. F. Kidd (Eds.), *New directions in attribution research* (Vol. 2, pp. 36-58). Hillsdale, NJ: Lawrence Erlbaum.
Langer, E. J., & Abelson, R. P. (1974). A patient by any other name . . . clinician group differences in labeling bias. *Journal of Consulting and Clinical Psychology, 42,* 4-9.
Langleben, M. (1983). An approach to the microcoherence of a text. In F. Neubauer (Ed.), *Coherence in natural language texts* (pp.71-98). Hamburg: Buske.
Lesgold, A. M. (1972). Pronominalization: A device for unifying sentences in memory. *Journal of Verbal Learning and Verbal Behavior, 11,* 316-323.
Levinson, S. C. (1983). *Pragmatics.* Cambridge: Cambridge University Press.
Levy, D. M. (1979). Communicative goals and strategies. Between discourse and syntax. In T. Givon (Ed.), *Syntax and semantics: Vol. 12. Discourse and syntax* (pp. 183-210). New York: Academic Press.
Longacre, R. E. (1983). Vertical threads of cohesion in discourse. In F. Neubauer (Ed.), *Coherence in natural language texts* (pp. 99-114). Hamburg: Buske.
Mandler, J. M. (1978). A code in the node: The use of a story schema in retrieval. *Discourse Processes, 1,* 14-35.
Mandler, J. M., & Johnson, N. S. (1977). Remembrance of things parsed: Story structure and recall. *Cognitive Psychology, 9,* 111-151.
Manelis, L., & Yekovich, F. R. (1976). Repetitions of propositional arguments in sentences. *Journal of Verbal Learning and Verbal Behavior, 15,* 301-312.
Masson, M. E., & Alexander, J. H. (1981). Inferential processes in sentence encoding and recall. *American Journal of Psychology, 94,* 399-416.
Maynard, D. W. (1980). Placement of topic changes in conversation. *Semiotica, 30,* 263-290.
McLaughlin, M. L. (1984). *Conversation: How talk is organized.* Newbury Park, CA: Sage.
Merritt, M. (1976). On questions following questions in service encounters. *Language in Society, 5,* 315-357.
Moe, A. J., & Irwin, J. W. (1986). Cohesion, coherence and comprehension. In J. W. Irwin (Ed.), *Teaching cohesion comprehension* (pp.3-8). Newark DE: International Reading Association.
Morgan, J. L. (1978). Toward a national model of discourse comprehension. In D. L. Waltz (Ed.), *Theoretical issues in natural language processing—2* (pp. 109-114). New York: Association for Computing Machinery.
Morgan, J. L., & Sellner, M. B. (1980). Discourse and linguistic theory. In R. J. Spiro, B. C. Bruce, & W. F. Brewer (Eds.), *Theoretical issues in reading comprehension: Perspectives from cognitive psychology, linguistics, artificial intelligence, and education* (pp. 165-200). Hillsdale, NJ: Lawrence Erlbaum.
Nofsinger, R. E. (1975). The demand ticket: A conversational device for getting the floor. *Speech Monographs, 42,* 1-9.
Nofsinger, R. E. (1976). On answering questions indirectly: Some rules in the grammar of doing conversation. *Human Communication Research, 2,* 172-181.
Norman, D. A. (1981). Categorization of action slips. *Psychological Review,* 88, 1-15.

Oaken, R., Weiner, M., & Cromer, W. (1971). Identification, organization and reading comprehension for good and poor readers. *Journal of Educational Psychology, 62,* 71-78.

Ochs, E. (1977). Planned and unplanned discourse. In T. Givon (Ed.), *Syntax and semantics: Vol. 12. Discourse and syntax* (pp.51-80). New York: Academic Press.

Ortony, A. (1978). Remembering, understanding and representation. *Cognitive Science, 2,* 53-69.

Owens, J., Bower, G. H., & Black, J. B. (1979). The "soap opera" effect in story recall. *Memory and Cognition, 7,* 185-191.

Palmer, M. T., & Badzinski, D. (1985, November). *Natural processing units in discourse: Topics or not topics, that is the question.* Paper presented at the annual meeting of the Speech Communication Association, Denver.

Petofji, J. (1985). Lexicon. In T. A. van Dijk (Ed.), *Handbook of discourse analysis: Vol. 2. Dimensions of discourse* (pp. 87-101). Orlando, FL: Academic Press.

Phillips, M. (1985). *Aspects of text structure.* New York: Elsevier.

Pichert, J. W., & Anderson, R. C. (1977). Taking different perspective on a story. *Journal of Educational Psychology, 69,* 309-315.

Planalp, S., & Tracy, K. (1980). Not to change the topic but . . .: A cognitive approach to the management of conversation. In D. Nimmo (Ed.), *Communication yearbook* (Vol. 4, pp. 237-258). New Brunswick, NJ: Transaction.

Reichman, R. (1978). Conversational coherency. *Cognitive Science, 2,* 283-327.

Ringle, M. H., & Bruce, B. C. (1982). Conversational failure. In W. G. Lehnert & M. H. Ringle (Eds.), *Strategies for natural language processing* (pp. 203-221). Hillsdale, NJ: Lawrence Erlbaum.

Sachs, J. (1967). Recognition memory for syntactic and semantic aspects of connected discourse. *Perception and Psychophysics, 2,* 437-442.

Sanders, R. E. (1983). Tools for cohering discourse and their strategic utilization: Markers of structural connections and their meaning relations. In R. T. Craig & K. Tracy (Eds.), *Conversational coherence: Form, structure, and strategy* (pp. 67-80). Newbury Park, CA: Sage.

Sanford, A. J., & Garrod, S. C. (1981). *Understanding written language: Explorations of comprehension beyond the sentence.* Chichester: John Wiley.

Schallert, D. C. (1976). Improving memory for prose: The relationship between depth of processing and context. *Journal of Verbal Learning and Verbal Behavior, 15,* 621-632.

Schank, R. C. (1977). Rules and topics in conversation. *Cognitive Science, I,* 421-441.

Schank, R. C. (1982). *Dynamic memory: A theory of reminding and learning in computers and people.* Cambridge: Cambridge University Press.

Schegloff, E. A., Jefferson, G., & Sacks, H. (1977). The preference for self-correction in the organization of repair in conversation. *Language, 53,* 361-382.

Schegloff, E. A., & Sacks, H. (1973). Opening up closings. *Semiotica, 8,* 389-327.

Scholes, R. J. (1971). *Acoustic cues for constituent structure.* The Hague: Mouton.

Schnotz, W. (1985). Selectivity in drawing inferences. In G. Rickheit & H. Strohner (Eds.), *Inferences in text processing.* (pp.287-326). Amsterdam: North-Holland.

Schwarz, M.N.K., & Flammer, A. (1981). Text structure and title-effects on comprehension and recall. *Journal of Verbal Learning and Verbal Behavior, 20,* 61-66.

Searle, J. R. (1975). Indirect speech acts. In P. Cole & J. L. Morgan (Eds.), *Syntax and Semantics: Vol. 3. Speech acts* (pp. 59-82). New York: Academic Press.

Singer, M. (1976). Context inferences in comprehension of sentences. *Canadian Journal of Psychology, 30,* 39-46.

Singer, M. (1980). The role of case-filling inferences in coherence of brief passages. *Discourse Processes, 3,* 185-201.

Sorensen, V. (1981). Coherence as a pragmatic concept. In H. Parrett, M. Sbisa, & J. Bershveren (Eds.), *Possibilities and limitations of pragmatics: Proceedings of the conference on pragmatics, Urbino, July 8-14, 1979* (pp. 657-682). Amsterdam: Benjamins.

Spiro, R. J. (1977). Remembering information from text: Theoretical and empirical issues concerning "state of schema" reconstruction hypothesis. In R. C. Anderson, R. J. Spiro, & W.

E. Montague (Eds.), *Schooling and the acquisition of knowledge* (pp.137-165). Hillsdale, NJ: Lawrence Erlbaum.

Spiro, R. J. (1980). Constructive processes in prose comprehension and recall. In R. J. Spiro, B. C. Bruce, & W. F. Brewer (Eds.), *Theoretical issues in reading comprehension: Perspectives from cognitive psychology, linguistics, artificial intelligence, and education* (pp. 245-278). Hillsdale, NJ: Lawrence Erlbaum.

Stein, N. L., & Nezworski, T. (1978). The effects of organization and instructional set on story memory. *Discourse Processes, I,* 177-194.

Taylor, S. E. (1980). The interface of cognitive and social psychology. In J. Harvey (Ed.), *Cognition, social behavior, and the environment* (pp. 189-211). Hillsdale, NJ: Lawrence Erlbaum.

Taylor, S. E., & Crocker, J. (1981). Schematic bases of social information processing. In E. T. Higgins, C. P. Herman, & M. P. Zanna (Eds.), *Social Cognition: The Ontario Symposium* (Vol. 1, pp. 89-134). Hillsdale, NJ: Lawrence Erlbaum.

Thorndyke, P. W. (1976). The role of inferences in discourse comprehension. *Journal of Verbal Learning and Verbal Behavior, 15,* 436-446.

Tracy, K. (1982). On getting the point: Distinguishing "issues" from "events," an aspect of conversational coherence. In M. Burgoon (Ed.), *Communication yearbook* (Vol. 5, pp. 279-301). New Brunswick, NJ: Transaction.

Tracy, K. (1984a, May). *The obligation to be irrelevant.* Paper presented at the annual meeting of the International Communication Association, San Francisco.

Tracy, K. (1984b). Staying on topic: An explication of conversational relevance. *Discourse Processes, 7,* 447-464.

Tracy, K. (1985). Conversational coherence: A cognitively grounded rules approach. In R. L. Street, Jr., & J. N. Cappella (Eds.), *Sequence and pattern in communication behavior* (pp. 30-49). London: Edward Arnold.

Tracy, K., & Moran, J. (1982, November). *Competing goals and conversational extensions.* Paper presented at the annual meeting of the Speech Communication Association, Louisville, KY.

Tracy, K., & Moran, J. (1983). Conversational relevance in multiple-goal settings. In R. T. Craig & K. Tracy (Eds.), *Conversational coherence: Form, structure, and strategy* (pp. 116-135). Newbury Park, CA: Sage.

Vande-Kopple, W. J. (1982). The given-new strategy of comprehension and some natural expository paragraphs. *Journal of Psycholinguistic Research, II,* 501-520.

van Dijk, T. A. (1977a). *Text and context: Explorations in the semantics and pragmatics of discourse.* London: Longman.

van Dijk, T. A. (1977b). Semantic macro-structures and knowledge frames in discourse comprehension. In M. A. Just & P. A. Carpenter (Eds.), *Cognitive processes in comprehension* (pp. 3-32). Hillsdale, NJ: Lawrence Erlbaum.

van Dijk, T. A. (1979). Relevance assignment in discourse comprehension. *Discourse Processes, you fill this xxx? On some interpretation processes. In A. Flammer &*
A. Kintsch (Eds.), Discourse processes (pp.152-162). New York: Elsevier Science Publishers.

Warner, R. G. (1985). *Discourse connectives in English.* New York: Garland.

Widdowson, H. G. (1978). *Teaching language as communication.* Oxford: Oxford University Press.

Wilson, D., & Sperber, D. (1981). On Grice's theory of conversation. In P. Werth (Ed.), *Conversation and discourse: Structure and interpretation* (pp. 154-178). New York: St. Martin's.

Woods, W. (1978). Knowledge-based natural language understanding. In W. Woods, & R. Bachman (Eds.), *Research in natural language understanding* (pp. 4-35). Cambridge: Bolt Beranek, & Newan (Quarterly Progress TR1, 3742).

Zadny, J., & Gerard, H. B. (1974). Attributed intentions and informational selectivity. *Journal of Experimental Social Psychology, 10,* 34-52.

On Coherence Judgments and Their Multiple Causes: A View from the Message-Variable Paradigm

JAMES J. BRADAC
University of California, Santa Barbara

BEING something of a social cognitivist (e.g., Bradac, 1983; Berger & Bradac, 1982), I am attracted to the metatheoretical underpinnings of the Kellermann and Sleight essay on coherence: There are knowledge structures and information in the universe, and meaningfulness arises when the former interacts with the latter. And I am attracted to the strong stand that the authors take, for it is clear and forthright; it gives us something definite to react to: "Coherence does not reside in the text, but instead resides in the mind of the perceiver of the text" (p. 116). It seems to me that this view represents a bold alternative to the position that meanings are in "texts"(symbolic artifacts of whatever type), a position taken by "New" literary critics on the one hand (e.g., Empson, 1947) and conversational analysts on the other (e.g., Schenkein, 1977). But I am a chronic skeptic (and a contextualist, e.g., McGuire, 1983), so I choose to ask this question: Under what circumstances are the "meanings-are-in-texts" position and the "meanings-are-in-minds" position alternately plausible in fact? Additionally, it may be useful to distinguish what is essential and novel in Kellermann and Sleight's chapter from what is inessential, derivative, familiar, and so on. It should be noted at the outset that I regard the Kellermann and Sleight work as substantially more than merely an example of nominalistic gaming, an instance of definitional parrying, or an exercise in verbal purification. Their ruminations over the meaning of "coherence" are theoretically motivated. They attempt to explicate this concept with the purpose of arguing for a

Correspondence and requests for reprints: James J. Bradac, Communication Studies, University of California, Santa Barbara, Santa Barbara, CA 93106.

Communication Yearbook 12, pp. 130-145

particular mechanism that underlies judgments of conversational coherence or incoherence, namely, knowledge structures yielding expectations that can be violated or fulfilled.

ABOUT: WHAT COHERENCE IS NOT

Kellermann and Sleight suggest that the literature on coherence is confusing mainly because different people use the term *coherence* in different ways. This terminological diversity is not surprising, because a very diverse set of scholars representing a very diverse set of theories, models, and paradigms have become interested in problems of "coherence": teachers of composition (Bamberg, 1983), linguists (Halliday & Hasan, 1976), interpersonal communication researchers (Sanders, 1986), and cognitive scientists (Schank et al., 1982), to name some. Disciplinary diversity and definitional diversity go hand in hand. Many other interesting concepts are defined variously; the situation is not unique to "coherence": linguistic complexity (Burling, 1986; Fodor, Bever, & Garret, 1974), compliance gaining (Baxter, 1984; Miller, Boster, Roloff, & Seibold, 1977), and intelligence (Eysenck, 1979; Sternberg, 1977), for example. Definitional or conceptual diversity can be annoying, but it can also be a virtue because via cross-disciplinary triangulation (Webb, Campbell, Schwarz, & Sechrest, 1966) researchers can gradually embrace richer and deeper conceptualizations. The guiding assumption of previous research in discourse connectedness has been that analysts can more or less objectively determine a given text's level of coherence by examining textual attributes, for example, use of (versus nonuse of) cohesive devices (Halliday & Hasan, 1976), and Kellermann and Sleight suggest that this assumption is incorrect. They suggest alternatively that coherence determination is a thoroughly subjective matter, that it is a judgment.

More particularly, Kellermann and Sleight, following Grice (1975), argue that "relevance, topical relevance, cohesive devices, and syntactic structure are neither necessary nor sufficient conditions for coherence" because they "do not provide adequate grounds for understanding how *judgments* of coherence are determined" (p. 98). They suggest further that it is a mistake to *equate* relevance, syntactic structure and so on with coherence, as some persons have done.

Implicit in Kellermann and Sleight's objection to the attribute-coherence equation is the notion that this sort of micro-level coherence should not be *confused with* macro-level coherence (a global judgment of meaningfulness), that the two are conceptually distinct. Kellermann and Sleight are not particularly *interested* in coherence of the microscopic sort. But it is the case that others are and will continue to be. There is certainly nothing wrong with or even confusing about postulating syntactic coherence or coherence at the level of relevance. That is, researchers can ask meaningful questions about how particular kinds of microstructures cohere, and they can offer rules (or, on a larger scale, theories) that ostensibly generate coherent microstructures.

Kellermann and Sleight further suggest that micro-level coherence is neither a necessary nor a sufficient *cause* of macro-level coherence—that a well-formed sentence, for example, will not necessarily yield a global judgment of high meaningfulness, nor is it sufficient to cause such a judgment. It is difficult to object to this claim. But why should the connection between judgments of coherence or meaningfulness and textual features be subjected to the unusually stringent criteria of necessity and sufficiency? We do not use this sort of language when talking about other message-variable judgment connections. Rather, we use the language of *likelihood* or *probability*: Lexical diversity *tends* to be associated positively with judgments of communicator status (Bradac, Bowers, & Courtright, 1979; Bradac & Wisegarver, 1984). Similarly, it would be useful to conceptualize the relationship between perceived coherence and textual features (well or poorly formed sentences, relevant or irrelevant remarks, and so on) as a probabilistic one.

From a probabilistic perspective, one could ask this: Does a high level of syntactic incoherence throughout a message tend to produce judgments of low overall meaningfulness? Under what conditions might this relationship hold? Or do utterances that message recipients perceive to be irrelevant to message senders' beliefs regarding what the topic is tend to produce in recipients judgments of low coherence (Bowers, Elliott, & Desmond, 1977; Bradac, Friedman, & Giles, 1986)?

A probabilistic model would legitimize researchers' examination of connections between micro-level coherence and coherence at the macro level. Of course, Kellermann and Sleight could (and might) claim that increases in topical coherence, cohesive devices, syntactic coherence, and so forth will *not* tend to produce increases in judgments of overall coherence. They might reassert the interesting claim that a connection between micro coherence and macro coherence exists strictly at the level of *en*coding, that instances of micro coherence reflect a communicator's desire to be coherent at the macro level. But the issue becomes an empirical one motivating a reasonable search for the possibility of association under some conditions, instead of a demand for guarantees. The implicit rejection of probabilism that undergirds Kellermann and Sleight's arguments regarding what coherence is not leads to a rejection of potentially interesting research on micro coherence and judgments of global meaningfulness (e.g., research similar to Ball, Giles, & Hewstone, 1986; Peterson, 1986; Tracy, 1983).

Thus it may not be maximally useful to claim, for example, that "structurally correct discourse is not coherence" (p. 104). It may be more useful to claim that a syntactically "correct" sentence may cohere in ways indicated by syntactic rules, that this coherence may (or may not) be perceived by specialists (linguists) and nonspecialists alike, that this coherence may (or may not) be related to the perceived coherence of larger units, and that this coherence may (or may not) be related to global judgments of meaningfulness. Undoubtedly, it will be important for future theorists and researchers to be clear about the level and type of coherence they are examining. Similarly, it may not be maximally useful for Kellermann and Sleight to assert that since "coherence is not relevance, topics, cohesive devices, or structure, we have effectively eliminated most prior approaches to understanding conversational coherence" (p. 105). Such "elimination" would indeed be a case of throwing out the baby with the bath water! The study of relevance, syntactic structure, and so on may shed additional light (as it has shed important light) on the phenomenon of coherence if researchers and theorists keep their levels and types straight.

ABOUT: WHAT COHERENCE IS

After arguing against various views of coherence, Kellermann and Sleight offer their conceptualization: "coherence is an evaluative judgment of meaningfulness of discourse" (p. 105) resulting from "consonance between expectations about the discourse and the actual [text]" (p. 116, emphasis deleted). A coherence judgment is correlated with comprehension of a text, but it is not caused by such comprehension; assignment of meaning to a text and a judgment of meaningfulness are correlated but independent activities. Meaningfulness "is determined through the application of knowledge structures in the comprehension process; their *consonance* with the discourse will generate the judgment of coherence" (pp. 108-109).

There are many things to say about this view of coherence. First, I will discuss at some length the coherence = evaluative judgment equation. Then I will examine the claim that comprehension is not causally linked to judgments of coherence; this will entail a broader discussion of causal factors in the production of coherence judgments. Finally, I will focus upon the proximate cause of coherence judgments invoked by Kellermann and Sleight: their notion of expectations.

Coherence as an Evaluative Judgment

Of the several interesting moves made in the Kellermann and Sleight work, the claim that coherence is a judgment seems to me to be the *most* interesting one: Coherence shifts from a textual attribute to a state of mind (see also Bradac, Martin, Elliott, & Tardy, 1980; Williams, 1985). This shift has many implications. At the outset, it is worth unpacking the meaning of *evaluative judgment*. This particular theoretical entity has special properties that may differ from the specific entity that interests Kellermann and Sleight. At various places in their statement regarding what coherence is, the authors write as though they *are* centrally interested in evaluations made by message recipients; for example, in their all too brief discussion of responsibility for meaningfulness—if a message producer is seen as being responsible for a meaningless message, he or she is blamed. At various other places, however, Kellermann and Sleight seem to be interested primarily in descriptive attributions reflecting message recipients' perceptions of communication events: for example, when the message recipient attributes high coherence to the event because there is a fit between the produced message and the perceived psychological state of the communicator. Although perception and judgment influence each other constantly in everyday life, they are potentially theoretically distinct (Brunswick, 1956; Street & Hopper, 1982) and ought not to be conflated. Messages (texts) are both perceived and evaluated: I perceive a speaker switching from French to English and I evaluate this positively (as a polite act of accommodation; Genessee & Bourhis, 1982).

Perceived meaninglessness seems likely to have negative evaluative consequences in many communication contexts; on the other hand, perceived meaningfulness seems likely to have positive consequences. But note that the conscious perception of meaningfulness is probably exceedingly rare; acts that are coherent are processed "mindlessly" (Langer, 1978) because, as Kellermann and Sleight suggest, we typically *expect* acts to make sense in context. So, most instances of coherent behavior seem unlikely to produce any sort of evaluative reaction. Additionally, because of these same expectations (and because of the resourcefulness and creativity of message recipients), perceived meaninglessness is probably also a rare state, although less rare than perceived meaningfulness. So, if these are rare perceptual events, evaluative reactions based upon coherence perceptions probably represent a small piece of the message-evaluative judgment pie—compared to, say, evaluations reflecting speech rate variation (Brown, Giles, & Thackerar, 1985), accent differences (Ryan & Bulik, 1982), or levels of vocabulary diversity (Bradac, Konsky, & Davies, 1976).

Related to the issue of rareness, it may be instructive to note that studies of message evaluation designed to explore the underlying dimensions of judgment have not yielded factors reflecting a judgment of meaningfulness.

Zahn and Hopper's (1985) survey of message evaluation studies did uncover evaluative dimensions relevant to this discussion that reflected message *source* characteristics almost exclusively. Perhaps message recipients tend very strongly to think of message sources when evaluating communication events; perhaps it is less usual to focus on the message as an object detached from the source or to focus on the situation in which the message was produced. Something like the "fundamental attribution error" may exist in the realm of message evaluation (Nisbett & Ross, 1980). Perhaps persons will not usually think in terms of incoherent messages, but in terms of incoherent sources because a separate meaningfulness factor is not apparent (although, as suggested above, perceived meaninglessness may be rare).

Although the distinct entities of perceived coherence/incoherence and of judged meaningfulness/meaninglessness may be rare, for some purposes they are important. In scholarly realms, theories and methodologies that have been learned by the scrutinizers of texts will affect their perceptions of coherence and their judgments of well-formedness or meaningfulness. Their perceptions and evaluations are not "naive" and they may differ from the perceptions and evaluations of untutored message recipients in everyday life. For example, linguists may judge certain putative sentences as grammatical as a result of their theoretical preconceptions, whereas nonlinguists who do not share these preconceptions may judge the same language structures as ungrammatical (Bradac et al., 1980). In this case, one could regard the theory as a knowledge structure that produces judgments of coherence, a view that is consistent with Kellermann and Sleight. This analysis calls attention to the fact that linguists, conversational analysts, literary critics, and the like do not *neutrally* uncover instances of coherence or incoherence that are *in* the text. Rather, their claims regarding coherence reflect perceptions and judgments of texts that are subject to a variety of potentially relevant and *ir*relevant influences (see Bradac et al., 1980). Judgments of textual coherence are influenced by a variety of textual and nontextual features, an observation that leads to the next issue.

Causal Factors in Judgments of Coherence

Kellermann and Sleight distinguish between *comprehension* and *coherence,* suggesting that the former term represents a process, whereas the latter represents a state—a judgment of meaningfulness. Comprehension is not isomorphic with coherence. Comprehension entails grasping the point of a message (Schank et al., 1982) or extracting from it propositions. Essentially, it is a self-perception of the extent to which an understanding has been achieved regarding important, salient, or relevant textual features. So the question becomes: What is the connection between this self-perception regarding understanding and an evaluation of meaningfulness? Kellermann and Sleight state (not surprisingly) that comprehension is neither a necessary nor a sufficient cause of coherence judgments, but that "comprehension will, in all likelihood, facilitate judgments of coherence" (p. 107). Here, they shift to the kind of probabilistic logic that they avoided in their discussion of what coherence is not. One can ask: What factors facilitate comprehension? And, in the spirit of what I just said, one can suggest such things as conformity to syntactic rules, globally relevant remarks, and so on. This suggests a causal model in which structure, relevance, cohesive devices, and so on, lead to comprehension, which leads to judgments of coherence. Thus if I perceive a speaker to be using strange syntax (e.g., "Sent the man a books gardens about his wife to a small city from Chicago near." Bradac et al., 1980), I may perceive that I do not fully comprehend his point or proposition, and, accordingly, I may evaluate his discourse as relatively low in coherence. The question becomes, What are the relative strengths of the various causal links? What factors can intensify or attenuate the magnitudes of association? What other causal associations exist?

The question regarding intensification or attenuation of magnitudes suggests that, in some cases, the connection between comprehension and coherence judgments will be low; other factors may more strongly influence such judgments. One such factor suggested by Kellermann and Sleight (although they do not use this term) is *recognition:* I may recognize that a speaker is speaking French, but because I do not speak this language I will not comprehend this individual's discourse.

Thus the link between recognition and coherence is strong, whereas the link between comprehension and coherence is weak. It seems likely that the mediating variables of recognition and comprehension are related in the following way: When comprehension is high, recognition will tend strongly to be high also (if I comprehend something I will recognize it); when recognition is low, comprehension will tend strongly to be low also (I cannot comprehend something without recognizing it); when comprehension is low, recognition is free to vary (even if I do not comprehend something I may recognize it); when recognition is high, comprehension is free to vary (even if I recognize something, I may not comprehend it).

A third mediating variable is suggested by Kellermann and Sleight—namely, responsibility for comprehension. The logic can be extended to include responsibility for recognition—a belief regarding recognition's cause. The interesting idea that Kellermann and Sleight offer is that if comprehension is low, the noncomprehender can assign responsibility (blame) to self or to the communicator. Self-blame may result in the judgment that the message is coherent despite low comprehension, whereas blame of the other may force attribution of low comprehension to an incoherent performance or deliberate effort (speaking French or high physics) by the communicator.

This idea can be usefully extended. For one thing, it may be the case that in some circumstances the noncomprehending message recipient may view the *situation* as being responsible for noncomprehension; that is an external attribution may be made regarding environmental factors. For example, "The crowd was really noisy, so the speech was difficult to follow." It is not clear (to me at least) just how this situational attribution would affect coherence judgments. Perhaps such judgments would be suspended or would be contingent upon other factors, such as the premessage credibility of the source.

The relationship between assignment of recognition or comprehension responsibility and coherence judgments is a complex one. Some reflections include the following: High attributed responsibility, low comprehension, and low estimates of coherence may not be strongly linked. *Recognition* of the message as an instance of a type may compel a coherence judgment quite apart from the assignment of responsibility. Low comprehension, which is attributed to the communicator, may produce a judgment of low coherence primarily in circumstances in which the message recipient believes that the state of low comprehension is inconsistent with the communicator's plan to create comprehension in the message recipient and where a situational attribution cannot be made with ease. Some instances of low comprehension may be attributed to a communicator state ("he was nervous") whereas others may be attributed to a trait or disposition ("he is insane"). The message recipient's prediction regarding future levels of coherence may hinge on whether a situational or dispositional inference is made, and within a communication event, initial situational or dispositional inferences regarding comprehensibility may affect later estimates of coherence. Our modeling of the relationship between responsibility and coherence must also include a group of variables that mediate comprehension, recognition, attributed responsibility, and coherence judgments, for example, perceived communicator plan or intention. It is further possible that recognition and comprehension in some cases may be linked to coherence judgments without the mediation of attributed responsibility, as when a person simply passively observes two persons interacting in a foreign language apparently comprehending each other.

Thinking about judgments of coherence in light of the preceding discussion of comprehension, recognition, and responsibility and in light of the earlier discussion of probabalistic connections between the likes of syntactic coherence and judgments of meaningfulness suggests to me that the problem of coherence can be placed squarely in the domain of message variable research. Work in this area is centrally concerned with the antecedents for and consequences of message variation (Bradac & Wiemann, 1986). The guiding assumption is that social psychological states and traits affect the encoding of messages and that once encoded, messages have social psychological consequences. Another assumption is that objectively identifiable message features, for example, level of lexical diversity, have subjective consequences and determinants (in tacit accordance with the Brunswick lens model, 1956). On the face of it, the latter assumption is at odds with the guiding assumption of the Kellermann and Sleight chapter, namely, that subjectivity is the name of the coherence game. But a closer analysis suggests that "objective" message features are intersubjectively verifiable constructions that reflect the researcher's special theory or method; the researcher's "objective" claims about a text or message are mediated by his or her technical knowledge (and by other social-psychological variables). Yet persons sharing this knowledge can create or discover messages that represent features of interest, and the antecedents for and consequences of these features can be investigated publicly and empirically. So, if two researchers share a conception of syntactic well-formedness, they can use this conception independently to generate messages that are high and low in terms of this feature, and they can independently compare the effects of messages exhibiting high and low-syntactic well-formedness upon judgments of global coherence or meaningfulness.

Placing the coherence problem in the message-variable domain also calls attention to the potential value of examining factors that are antecedent to the creation of messages that produce judgments of high or low coherence. Kellermann and Sleight make the intriguing suggestion that the use of cohesive devices reflects a communicator's desire to appear coherent; cohesive devices may reflect a particular encoding strategy in short. But, of course, there are many encoding strategies that could be examined.

A causal model that summarizes the various strands of the preceding discussion shows social psychological variables leading to encoded message features, which lead to comprehension and recognition, which implicate responsibility and other social psychological variables to result in judgments of coherence.

This model (which does not specify all possible paths) is similar in form to other models inhabiting the message-variable domain (e.g., Bradac et al., 1980; Street & Hopper, 1982).

Violating and Fulfilling Expectations

One of the important social-psychological variables mediating message variables on the one hand and coherence judgments on the other is undoubtedly "expectancies," as Kellermann and Sleight suggest. In terms of the previous model "expectancies" is probably most reasonably inserted prior to recognition and comprehension as in "encoding strategies give rise to expectancies, which lead to recognition and comprehension." Of course, in some circumstances, expectancies will exist prior to exposure to the text, giving rise to particular encoding strategies.

"Expectancies" reflect person-message-situation schemata that have been learned by message recipients—knowledge structures pertaining to communication events. Knowledge structures exist at a micro level, as when one anticipates a recurrent phrase, and at a macro level, as when one anticipates a political speech. According to Kellermann and Sleight, "knowledge structures in consonance with the discourse (to *some* degree) are necessary if discourse is to be perceived as coherent" (p. 109). Discourse will tend to be perceived as coherent because "people tend to make the discourse fit the [knowledge structure] they are employing to comprehend" the discourse (p. 109). Discourse that is not adjustable in this way and that is dissonant with expectations will tend to be perceived as incoherent. Communicators use cohesive devices, well-formed sentences, and so forth as cues that assist message recipients in accessing appropriate knowledge structures: "For cues to be effective, they must be associable with an appropriate knowledge structure such that consonance occurs between that structure and the discourse" (p. 117). Such cues "permit access to schematic knowledge that increases the opportunity for consonance to occur between the knowledge structures and the perceived discourse" (p. 118). So, using textual attributes as an example, the authors are suggesting that knowledge structures mediate the relationship between textual attributes (cues) and judgments of coherence. But other kinds of knowledge structures must also be invoked in order to explain the coherence judgment, for example, knowledge of syntactic structures of the language in question. Such knowledge of syntactic structures might be described as rules reflecting the linguistic knowledge of "naive grammarians," that is untutored speakers of the language (Bradac et al., 1980). In a much more unusual case, these structures might reflect the special syntactic theories of linguists (see Moscovici & Hewstone, 1983). Thus an expectation of a particular kind of discourse (which could be subsequently violated or confirmed) might be rooted in knowledge that allows judgments of syntactic well-formedness.

This claim suggests that it would be premature to disregard or to minimize the role of message variables such as syntactic form in the production of coherence judgments; such variables have effects by virtue of their interaction with special forms of knowledge, for example, syntactic rules; they do more than cue the kinds of knowledge structures that Kellermann and Sleight have described. On the other hand, the kind of communication event schema that these scholars call attention to is interesting and seems likely to be important as a theoretical construct in the area of coherence. This sort of knowledge structure may indeed be crucially related to the kinds of expectancy confirmations or disconfirmations that the authors believe to be related to coherence judgments.

In future efforts it will be useful to specify the essential components of communication event schemata; as Kellermann and Sleight imply, perhaps perceived intentions, knowledge of message genres, and knowledge of communication context types may be important. There may exist, in any given culture or subgroup, intention-genre-context clusters that constitute discrete schemata, which are used by message recipients to interpret messages and to render coherence judgments. The expectancy violations that cause judgments of message incoherence may reflect a discrepancy between a particular cluster initially invoked cognitively by the message recipient and message features subsequently processed by him or her.

EXTENDING THE ARGUMENT

The concept of "coherence judgment," which is central to the Kellermann and Sleight work, suggests two extensions that may be useful to researchers and theorists in this area.

The Ubiquity of Coherence

As Kellermann and Sleight observe, a judgment of incoherence is a comparatively rare event; a recent study by Peterson (1986) supports this claim. This expectation may be related to the more general tendency for humans to see pattern everywhere, even when events or outcomes are certifiably random (Wright, 1962). But if communicative acts are rarely viewed as incoherent, they are probably fairly frequently seen as puzzling, weird, inappropriate, and surprising. Saying this may or may not be equivalent to saying that some messages are perceived as being slightly coherent or somewhat incoherent, viewing coherence as a continuous variable. Perhaps judgments of "slight coherence" are rarely made; perhaps more often a message is perceived as being coherent but its creator is judged to be an odd person or in an unusual frame of mind. In fact, to reiterate what I said earlier, a judgment of message coherence may be extremely rare in everyday life. It may be that only experts with special theories scrutinize messages for the purpose of rendering coherence judgments.

How is it so many roads lead to Rome in the case of coherence? To find an answer following Kellermann and Sleight's logic, we should be asking questions like these: Do message recipients in everyday life think about message coherence? What are the dimensions of coherence that exist for them? What factors stimulate naive thinking about coherence? What message variables affect such thinking? How do comprehension and recognition relate to coherence judgments? How do textual attributes, for example, syntactic well-formedness, affect comprehension and recognition in various contexts? And how do these attributes affect coherence judgments?

Also, assuming that the search for coherence judgments in everyday life proves fruitful—that it is determined that naive, untutored persons *do* make global judgments of communication coherence in significant contexts despite the likely infrequency of such judgments—it will be useful at some point to view "coherence judgment" as an *independent* variable to investigate what sorts of attributions or behaviors follow when a judgment of low (or high) coherence is made. What are the communicative consequences of viewing someone's message as high or low in coherence? What are the consequences of making a dispositional inference? That is, this person tends to produce relatively coherent or incoherent messages, so what sort of person is he? One consequence of coherence judgments that might be worth pursuing is "attributional confidence" (Clatterbuck, 1979; Gudykunst, 1985) or degree of subjective certainty or uncertainty regarding communicators (Berger & Bradac, 1982; Berger & Calabrese, 1975). For example, it seems likely that in initial-impression contexts a judgment of high message incoherence will be associated with a sense of high subjective uncertainty regarding the message sender's cognitions and behaviors. And high uncertainty on the part of the message recipient may result in his or her engaging in high levels of information seeking vis-à-vis the message sender, in low levels of intimacy toward the message sender, and in lower levels of liking for this person (Berger & Calabrese, 1975). Thus, axiomatically, it may be the case that low message coherence results in low liking, low intimacy, and high information seeking.

Text Versus Mind in Coherence Judgments

Kellermann and Sleight's move to locate coherence in the mind of the message recipient suggests interesting possibilities. For one thing it calls our attention to extreme and unusual cases—at least, I hope they are unusual—in which message recipients form judgments of high or low coherence based upon the barest fact that a message is being provided by a person in a situation, but regardless of substantive or stylistic attributes of the text. The text is the merest of triggers. Perhaps deviant composition teachers do this when reading essays from very bad (or very good) pupils. Even more extremely, perhaps psychotic individuals form coherence judgments on the basis of no text at all, at least no text perceivable by others. These would be delusions of coherence. Dialectically one can imagine the other extreme, in which coherence judgments are 99.9% text driven. Perhaps a case in point would be a message analyst who has the simplest imaginable theoretically motivated scheme for coherence, which consists of two categories; text units are then mechanically assigned to one or the other category and a frequency count emerges. This count is compared to other frequency counts emerging from other texts, which yields a picture of relative textual coherence.

Probably in everyday life, when judgments of coherence occur, they reflect situations less extreme than those just depicted; they are "caused" by both textual attributes and components of mind. An interesting general question from a contextualist view is: Under what circumstances will coherence judgments be text driven and under what circumstances will such judgments be driven by mind? In other words, when will textual attributes or message variables be strong influences upon coherence judgments and when will communication event schemata carry most of the judgmental weight? A theory of coherence judgments is needed to call our attention to the relevant factors, but previous research and theory in other areas of endeavor suggest some possibilities. For example, work by Kruglanski and others suggests that communication event schemata may be especially influential when the message recipient has a high need for cognitive structure and a low fear of judgmental invalidity; conversely, textual attributes are likely to be relatively influential when there is a low need for cognitive structure and fear of invalidity is high (Kruglanski, 1980; Kruglanski & Freund, 1983). Or, from a different perspective, persons experiencing high subjective self-awareness may be strongly affected by textual features in forming coherence judgments, whereas persons experiencing high objective self-awareness may be strongly affected by communication event schemata (Carroll, Bever, & Pollack, 1981; Duval & Wicklund, 1972). Or from still a different perspective, message features other than those that are directly related to coherence judgments may affect the relative impact of text versus mind. For example, some forms of language may lead message recipients to be highly attentive to the details of message substance and form, such as high-intensity language (Bowers, 1963), "powerful" lexical items (O'Barr, 1982), and linguistic features indicating the speaker's membership in negatively evaluated "out groups" (Turner & Giles, 1981). And, finally, aspects of the communication situation may force the message recipient to be highly attentive to textual details, as when the message sender says, "Listen carefully to what I am about to say." ("I listened carefully and it made no sense!")

It will probably be useful in future work on coherence to avoid taking either the "in-the-text" or the "in-the-mind" positions, taking instead the position that we can uncover a range of interesting social psychological communication factors that variously affect the strength of association between both text and mind and judgments of coherence.

CONCLUSION

I have suggested that the pivotal concept in Kellermann and Sleight's chapter is "coherence judgment," and that by invoking this concept, and despite their claim to the contrary, these scholars place coherence theory and research squarely in the message-variable paradigm. The question becomes: Which textual attributes or message variables affect judgments of coherence under what schematic conditions? This question is analogous to other questions pertaining to message effects: Which features of language produce judgments of high and low communicator power (Bradac & Mullac, 1984) or high and low communicator dynamism (Mulac, Lundell, & Bradac, 1986)? Another important question is: What sorts of situational/cognitive variables constitute important antecedents of message factors associated with coherence judgments? This question parallels questions such as these: What aspects of perceived situations affect message style? (Giles & Hewstone, 1982). Under what conditions will communicators converge to the dialect of their conversational partner, and under what conditions will they diverge instead? (Giles & Smith, 1979). It is important to note, as Kellermann and Sleight suggest, that the search for antecedents and consequences of coherence-related message variables will entail examining cognitive variables such as expectancy violations and fulfillments.

I have suggested also that it is probably premature to discount the role of textual attributes in the production of coherence judgments, including the particular features that "are not" or do not "guarantee" coherence according to Kellermann and Sleight: syntactic well-formedness, cohesive devices, and so on. Instead, it may be desirable to probe the circumstances under which these and other message variables may influence coherence judgments and the circumstances under which such judgments may be influenced otherwise, by communication event schemata. But perhaps the most basic question pertains to the reality of coherence judgments: Do persons in everyday life indeed make judgments of coherence in the way that they make judgments of communicator power, status, solidarity, and attractiveness, for example (Giles & Ryan, 1982)? Or is judged coherence instead a variable operating primarily in the domain of experts examining special theories in the way that judgments of sentence well-formedness are typically made by linguists, not naive message recipients? Also, how do coherence judgments relate dimensionally to other sorts of judgments that persons make of communicators? Probably before the idea of coherence judgment is taken much further conceptually, it will be useful to explore empirically the nature of this judgmental act. Such an exploration would constitute a study of ecological validity, which would cohere nicely with the conceptual approach of Kellermann and Sleight.

REFERENCES

Ball, P., Giles, H., & Hewstone, M. (1986). Interpersonal accommodation and situational construals. In H. Giles & R. N. St. Clair (Eds.), *Recent advances in language, communication, and social psychology*. Hillsdale, NJ: Lawrence Erlbaum.

Bamberg, B. (1983). What makes a text coherent? *College Composition and Communication, 34*, 417-429.

Baxter, L. A. (1984). An investigation of compliance-gaining as politeness. *Human Communication Research, 10*, 427-456.

Berger, C. R., & Bradac, J. J. (1982). *Language and social knowledge: Uncertainty in interpersonal relations*. London: Edward Arnold.

Berger, C. R., & Calabrese, R. J. (1975). Some explorations in initial interaction and beyond: Toward a development theory in interpersonal communication. *Human Communication Research, 1*, 99-112.

Bowers, J. W. (1963). Language intensity, social introversion, and attitude change. *Speech Monographs, 30*, 345-352.

Bowers, J. W., Elliott, N. D., Desmond, R. J. (1977). Exploring pragmatic rules: Devious messages. *Human Communication Research, 5*, 235-242.

Bradac, J. J. (1983). The language of lovers, flovers, and friends: Communication in personal social relations. *Journal of Language and Social Psychology, 2*, 141-162.

Bradac, J. J., Bowers, J. W., & Courtright, J. A. (1979). Three language variables in communication research: Intensity, immediacy, and diversity. *Human Communication Research, 5*, 257-269.

Bradac, J. J., Bowers, J. W., & Courtright, J. A. (1980). Lexical variations in intensity, immediacy, and diversity: An axiomatic theory and causal model. In R. N. St. Clair & H. Giles (Eds.), *The social and psychological contexts of language* (pp. 193-223). Hillsdale, NJ: Lawrence Erlbaum.

Bradac, J. J., Friedman, E., & Giles, H. (1986). A social approach to propositional communication: Speakers lie to hearers. In G. McGregor (Ed.), *Language for hearers* (pp. 127-151). Oxford: Pergamon.

Bradac, J. J., Konsky, C. W., & Davies, R. A. (1976). Two studies of the effect of lexical diversity upon judgments of communicator attributes and message effectiveness. *Communication Monographs, 43*, 70-79.

Bradac, J. J., Martin, L. W., Elliott, N. D., & Tardy, C. H. (1980). On the neglected side of linguistic science: Multivariate studies of sentence judgment. *Linguistics, 18*, 967-995.

Bradac, J. J., & Mulac, A. (1984). A molecular view of powerful and powerless speech styles: Attributional consequences of specific language features and communicator intentions. *Communication Monographs, 51*, 307-319.

Bradac, J. J., & Wiemann, J. W. (1986). *The scope of message variables in communication research*. Paper presented at the annual meeting of the Speech Communication Association, Chicago.

Bradac, J. J., & Wisegarver, R. (1984). Ascribed status, lexical diversity, and accent: Determinants of perceived status, solidarity, and control of speech style. *Journal of Language and Social Psychology, 3*, 239-255.

Brown, B. L., Giles H., & Thackerar, J. N. (1985). Speaker evaluations as a function of speech rate, accent, and context. *Language and Communication, 5*, 207-220.

Brunswick, E. (1956). *Perception and the representative design of psychological experiments* (2nd ed.). Berkeley: University of California Press.

Burling, R. (1986). The selective advantage of complex language. *Ethology and Sociobiology, 7*, 1-16.

Carroll, J. M., Bever, T. G., & Pollack, C. R. (1981). The non-uniqueness of linguistic intuitions. *Language, 57*, 368-383.

Clatterbuck, G. W. (1979). Attributional confidence and uncertainty in initial interaction. *Human Communication Research, 5*, 147-157.

Duval, S., & Wicklund, R. A. (1972). *A theory of objective self-awareness*. New York: Academic Press.

Empson, W. (1947). *Seven types of ambiguity* (2nd ed.). New York: New Directions.

Eysenck, H. J. (with D. W. Fulker) (1979). *The structure and measurement of intelligence*. New York: Springer-Verlag.

Fodor, J. A., Bever, T. G., & Garrett, M. F. (1974). *The psychology of language: An introduction to psycholinguistics and generative grammar*. New York: McGraw-Hill.

Genessee, F., & Bourhis, R. Y. (1982). The social psychological significance of code switching in cross-cultural communication. *Journal of Language and Social Psychology, 1*, 1-27.

Giles, H., & Hewstone, M. (1982). Cognitive structures, speech, and social situations. Two integrative models. *Language Sciences, 4*, 187-219.

Giles, H., & Ryan, E. B. (1982). Prolegomena for developing a social psychological theory of language attitudes. In E. B. Ryan & H. Giles (Eds.), *Attitudes toward language variation: Social and applied contexts* (pp. 208-223). London: Edward Arnold.

Giles, H., & Smith, P. M. (1979). Accommodation theory: Optimal levels of convergence. In H. Giles & R. N. St. Clair (Eds.), *Language and social psychology* (pp. 45-65). Oxford: Basil Blackwell.

Grice, H. P. (1975). Logic and conversation. In P. Cole & J. L. Morgan (Eds.), *Syntax and semantics: Vol. 3. Speech acts* (pp. 41-58). New York: Academic Press.

Gudykunst, W. B. (1985). A model of uncertainty reduction in intercultural encounters. *Journal of Language and Social Psychology, 4*, 79-98.

Halliday, M., & Hasan, R. (1976). *Cohesion in English*, London: Longman.

Kruglanski, A. W. (1980). Lay epistemo-logic-process and contents: Another look at attribution theory. *Psychological Review, 87*, 70-87.

Kruglanski, A. W., & Freund, T. (1983). The freezing and unfreezing of lay inference: Effects on impressional primacy, ethnic stereotyping, and numerical anchoring. *Journal of Experimental Social Psychology, 19*, 448-468.

Langer, E. J. (1978). Rethinking the role of thought in social interaction. In J. H. Harvey, W. J. Ickes, & R. F. Kidd (Eds.), *New directions in attribution research* (Vol. 2, pp. 35-58). Hillsdale, NJ: Lawrence Erlbaum.

McGuire, W. J. (1983). A contextualist theory of knowledge: Its implications for innovation and reform in psychological research. In L. Berkowitz (Ed.), *Advances in experimental social psychology* (Vol. 16, pp. 1-47). Orlando, FL: Academic Press.

Miller, G. R., Boster, F., Roloff, M., & Seibold, D. (1977). Compliance-gaining message strategies: A typology and some findings concerning effects of situational differences. *Communication Monographs, 44*, 37-51.

Moscovici, S., & Hewstone, M. (1983). Social representations and social explanation: From the "naive" to the "amateur" scientist. In M. Hewstone (Ed.), *Attribution theory: Social and functional extensions* (pp. 98-125). Oxford: Basil Blackwell.

Mulac, A., Lundell, T. L., & Bradac, J. J. (1986). Male/female language differences and attributional consequences in a public speaking situation: Toward an explanation of the gender-linked language effect. *Communication Monographs, 53*, 115-129.

Nisbett, R. E., & Ross, L. (1980). *Human inference: Strategies and shortcomings of social judgment*. Englewood Cliffs, NJ: Prentice-Hall.

O'Barr, W. M. (1982). *Linguistic evidence: Language, power, and strategy in the courtroom*. New York: Academic Press.

Peterson, J. (1986). *Conversational coherence: An examination of topical relevance, cohesion, and communicative competence*. Unpublished master's thesis, University of California, Santa Barbara.

Ryan, E. B., & Bulik, C. M. (1982). Evaluations of middle-class speakers of standard American and German-accented English. *Journal of Language and Social Psychology, 1*, 51-62.

Sanders, R. E. (1986). *Cognitive foundations of calculated speech*. Albany: State University of New York Press.

Schank, R. C., Collins, G. C., Davis, E., Johnson, P. N., Lytmen, S., & Reiser, B. J. (1982). What's the point? *Cognitive Science, 6*, 255-275.

Schenkein, J. (Ed.). (1977). *Studies in the organization of conversational interaction*. New York: Academic Press.

Sternberg, R. J. (1977). *Intelligence, information processing, and analogical reasoning: The componential analysis of human abilities*. Hillsdale, NJ: Lawrence Erlbaum.

Street, R. L., Jr., & Hopper, R. (1982). A model of speech style evaluation. In E. B. Ryan & H. Giles (Eds.), *Attitudes towards language variation: Social and applied contexts* (pp. 175-188). London: Edward Arnold.

Tracy, K. (1983). The issue-event distinction: A rule of conversation and its scope condition. *Human Communication Research, 9*, 320-334.

Turner, J. C., & Giles, H. (1981). *Intergroup behavior*. Oxford: Basil Blackwell.

Webb, E. J., Campbell, D. T., Schwarz, R. D., & Sechrest, L. (1966). *Unobtrusive measures*. Chicago: Rand McNally.

Williams, J. D. (1985). Coherence and cognitive style. *Written Communication, 2*, 473-491.

Wright, J. C. (1962). Consistency and complexity of response sequences as a function of schedules of noncontingent reward. *Journal of Experimental Psychology, 63*, 601-609.

Zahn, C. J., & Hopper. R. (1985). Measuring language attitudes: The Speech Evaluation Instrument. *Journal of Language and Social Psychology, 4*, 113-123.

About Coherence

SALLY JACKSON
SCOTT JACOBS
University of Oklahoma, Norman

KELLERMANN and Sleight's essay on coherence addresses *the* central issue for theories of the organization of discourse. A real strength of the essay is the authors' appreciation of the fact that progress in this area depends on a clear conceptualization of just what coherence is and is not and on outlining a theoretically motivated program of research. Given the state of the research on coherence, they clearly point out that what is needed at this time is not necessarily more research, but certainly more careful thinking about the nature of the phenomenon and the puzzles it presents.

Kellermann and Sleight's theoretical position is that judgments of coherence are judgments of the meaningfulness of discourse. But the point of this claim is not just to *define* coherence in more primitive terms. Since we have no clear conception of what meaningfulness is, such a definition would add little clarity. Rather, the point is to introduce a cognitive approach to coherence in which the properties of coherence will be explained by the principles of cognitive processing.

Kellermann and Sleight repeatedly emphasize that "coherence does not reside in the text, but instead resides in the mind of the perceiver of the text" (p. 116). If all they were saying was that constructs like coherence and meaningfulness presuppose mental processes on the part of human beings, we might fairly dismiss them. No discourse analyst in the 1980s would seriously suggest that discourse comprehension or any related process can operate independently of contextual assumptions, background knowledge, and inferential work by perceivers (Jacobs, 1985). But Kellermann and Sleight's position does more than this light work.

Their position departs from other approaches by shifting the explanation of coherence from features of text presumed to be "objective" (and available

Correspondence and requests for reprints: Sally Jackson, Department of Communication, 780 Van Vleet Oval, University of Oklahoma, Norman, OK 73019.

Communication Yearbook 12, pp. 146-156

uniformly to perceivers), to characteristics of individuals' subjective experience. This shift offers the possibility of accounting for individual variability in judgments of the same text—people with different background knowledge may arrive at quite different meanings, assuming that they find the text meaningful at all. Likewise, their position emphasizes the fallibility of judgments of coherence: There is no "correct" underlying meaning of a text, nor is there anything in the "material symbols" of a text that guarantees or rules out any particular meaning apart from the ways in which a perceiver processes those symbols.

Of course, the risk inherent in such a position is that it may *over*emphasize individuality in discourse production and comprehension. Theories of discourse processing must explain *both* the phenomenon of individuality and the phenomenon of sociality. The massive fact that we *do* arrive at common interpretations of discourse is a problem for approaches that begin with the assumption that communication is fundamentally an individual-level process. It seems likely to us that the Kellermann and Sleight position, if extended into detailed substantive analysis, would wind up postulating special "knowledge structures" having to do with conventions and rules of language use that currently lead to discussions of "social structures" and so-called objective features of texts.

The metatheoretical advantages of individualism and sociality in the explanation of communication phenomena could be debated endlessly. That is not our purpose in this essay. We accept the general legitimacy of a cognitive approach and, like Kellermann and Sleight, think such an approach has a great deal of promise. We wish to focus on the specific claims about cognition and discourse made by Kellermann and Sleight. Following Kellermann and Sleight, we will target conceptual issues, considering in turn the relationship between coherence and comprehension, the relationship between coherence and relevance, and the relationship between coherence and knowledge structures.

COHERENCE AND COMPREHENSION

Most of the appeal of the claim that coherence is a judgment of the meaningfulness of discourse comes from the suggestion that principles of coherence are going to depend on principles of comprehension. We think that Kellermann and Sleight are right to draw this connection.

It seems to us, however, quite paradoxical to say, on the one hand, that judgments of coherence are judgments of meaningfulness but then to say, on the other hand, that one can judge as coherent a stretch of discourse that is incomprehensible. Kellermann and Sleight develop this paradox when they say that "coherence is an output of this comprehension process" (p. 106), but then insist that "comprehension is not necessary for a judgment of coherence"

(p. 107) and deny that "comprehension must occur *prior* to determining that discourse *is* coherent" (p. 107). Granted that comprehension is a process and coherence is a product (so the two are not the same), one would still like to argue that coherence is a product of the comprehension process.

Kellermann and Sleight justify their seemingly paradoxical position with detailed argument based on examples. They argue for the clear separation of coherence and comprehension on the grounds that discourse may be judged coherent even though not comprehended:

> Individuals are capable of assessing discourse as coherent even when they are unable to assign specific meaning to it. When we hear a foreign language we do not speak, we do not judge the speaker as incoherent when we are unable to comprehend utterances. Similarly, a communication professor attending a conference on nuclear physics is unlikely to judge paper presentations as incoherent when his or her attempts to process the presentations and achieve meaning fail. (p. 107)

But the argument they build from these examples appears to rest on a subtle version of a familiar fallacy: Just because we fail to prove *not-X* does not mean that we can conclude *X*. All we can conclude is that we do not know whether *X* or *not-X*. Kellermann and Sleight seem to conclude *X* from a failure to prove *not-X,* since their examples show only that listeners fail to judge these cases to be *in*coherent. That result does not mean we can conclude that listeners judge such cases to be *coherent*. Most people would simply say that a listener *could not determine* whether the conversation between the foreign language speakers or the presentation by the nuclear physicist was coherent or incoherent.

People may *presume* that the discourse is coherent. Kellermann and Sleight appear correct in adopting the position that people communicate with a "coherence expectation" (p. 107). But to *presume* that discourse is coherent is not the same thing as to *determine* that the discourse is coherent. All too often Kellermann and Sleight equivocate in the way that they use terms like *judgment*. For example, they state that "comprehension will, in all likelihood, facilitate judgments of coherence" (p. 107), but then they state elsewhere that an "initial judgment of coherence is the 'cause' of further comprehension attempts" (p. 108). In the former statement, they use judgment to mean decision or assessment; in the latter statement, they use judgment to mean presumption or expectation. And they often use "assess" in place of "judge" where they should use "presume" (as in the passage just quoted).

All this paradoxical talk about the relationships among coherence, meaningfulness, and comprehension can be avoided if we keep straight the distinction between a presumption and an actual assessment. Hopper's (1981) discussion of the taken-for-granted makes a strong case for this sort of distinction. In doing so, one can say that yes, people do process discourse on the presumption of its coherence and this presumption does operate prior to the comprehension of the discourse. In fact, as Sanders (1983) points out, the presumption of coherence is necessary to drive the search for meaningfulness. But one can also say that no, people will not decide that discourse is coherent if they decide that it is incomprehensible. This preserves the intuitively obvious point that discourse that does not make sense cannot be coherent and that discourse that does make sense must also be coherent.

Kellermann and Sleight's examples do establish an important point: Failure to comprehend a text gives rise to a judgment of incoherence only when the text—and not the perceiver—is assigned responsibility for that failure. But here we would say that the texts are *presumed* coherent, not *judged* coherent. Furthermore, it should be seen that even the presumption of coherence depends upon a presumption of comprehensibility. With the foreign language speakers or the nuclear physicist, a listener presumes that the conversation is comprehensible to persons possessing the requisite background knowledge. Without the presumption of comprehensibility, the presumption of coherence would also collapse.

One might, in defense of Kellermann and Sleight's position, point to examples such as the Bransford and Johnson (1972) passage about doing laundry (see p. 120). One might read such a passage without really understanding it, but still assess it to be coherent enough.

At first glance, this example does seem to support the Kellermann and Sleight position. But we should keep in mind that comprehension can occur at many different levels. When we say that discourse is coherent, it is coherent with respect to some level of representation of the text. Bransford and Johnson's (1972) description is recognizably a description of an orderly procedure of some sort, though what kind of procedure is not apparent without a title or other topic cue. And the description sounds coherent at that depth of comprehension.

Or consider a similar case. Kellermann and Sleight suggest that structure alone does not lead to coherence, but their argument rests on the assumption that there is only one level at which texts can be comprehended and judged coherent. They suggest that Lewis Carroll's (1960) poem, *Jabberwocky*, contains "structure without coherence" so that meaningless words are "connected to yield the appearance of meaningfulness" (Kellermann & Sleight, p. 105):

> 'Twas brillig, and the slithey toves
> Did gyre and gimble in the wabe:
> All mimsy were the borogoves,
> And the mome raths outgrabe.

Certainly we can agree with Alice's assessment: "It seems very pretty, but it's *rather* hard to understand! Somehow it seems to fill my head with ideas—only I don't exactly know what they are!" (Carroll, 1960, p. 196). But compare the poem to an *un*structured version:

Brillig, and 'twas toves slithey the
Did in gyre gimble the and wabe:
Mimsy the all, were borogoves
Raths and mome the outgrabe.

Carroll's poem may not be as meaningful as, say, Eliot's *The Wasteland*, but it *is* meaningful at *some* level. And that's just as it should be, if Kellermann and Sleight are correct about the really central issues, because it also happens that *Jabberwocky* is pretty clearly consonant with some basic knowledge structures about poems and grammatical relations—and such consonance, according to Kellermann and Sleight, is what produces coherence.

The point of all this is not to challenge the basic claim that a judgment of coherence is a judgment of the meaningfulness of discourse. In fact, we believe that the position on coherence and comprehension that we have outlined is quite consistent with the general thrust of Kellermann and Sleight's position. What we have tried to argue is that neither the theoretical perspective behind their position nor the examples presented in their essay force the paradoxical position they take about coherence and comprehension. If we distinguish presumption from judgment and remember that there are multiple levels for representing discourse, the examples support a much more straightforward position on the relation between coherence and comprehension.

COHERENCE AND RELEVANCE

Contrary to most theories of discourse coherence, which assume some kind of close conceptual connection between coherence and relevance, Kellermann and Sleight argue: "Coherence is different from relevance; the presence or absence of one does not signal the presence or absence of the other" (p. 99). To support this position, they claim that relevance and coherence are not "isomorphic in meaning" and cite examples in which units of discourse are incoherent but relevant or elements of discourse are coherent but irrelevant (pp. 99-100).

But their position has force only by virtue of their arguing from a false dichotomy: There are many alternatives to coherence and relevance either being conceptually connected by virtue of the two concepts meaning the same thing or not being connected at all. Moreover, when we ask how the concepts might be connected, we have to be clear about just how we are using these terms: the coherence of what and the relevance of what to what.

Contrast the Kellermann and Sleight alternative with the traditional position on this issue (see McLaughlin, 1984, pp. 36-38; Jackson, Jacobs, & Rossi, 1987, p. 323): Coherence is the way in which the elements of a unit of discourse are organized into a whole; relevance is the way in which an element in the whole contributes to that unified patterning. So, coherence is a global property at the level of the whole unit; relevance is a property at the level of the elements of that whole. The two concepts do not mean the same thing, but they are connected. The coherence of a whole unit grows out of the way in which the elements are organized into relevant component parts; and the relevance of any element is always anchored to a unified representation.

Many of Kellermann and Sleight's counterexamples simply have no bearing on this position. In one example, they are talking about the coherence and relevance of a whole unit (the incoherence of a convention presentation and the relevance of that presentation to the paper on which it is based). In another example, they are talking about the coherence and relevance of one element of a broader unit (a comment that is coherent, but irrelevant to the conversation as a whole). The examples are irrelevant to the issue of whether it is possible for a whole unit to be coherent but the elements of that unit to be irrelevant, or for a whole unit to be incoherent but the elements of that unit to be relevant.

To establish that a text can be irrelevant, but coherent, Kellermann and Sleight also offer the example of "a 'boring' storyteller" who "'clutters' up the story with unnecessary, trivial details." They argue: "These details do not affect the *coherence* of the discourse, rather they affect perceptions of the relevance of parts of the discourse" (p. 99).

Actually, the assertion that unnecessary details do not affect the coherence of the discourse requires considerable qualification. Surely, if enough boring details were added, they would eventually overwhelm the "pertinent" information, making it difficult to find the "sense" of the story. Notice also that Kellermann and Sleight still call these so-called irrelevant elements "details." You couldn't call these elements "details" unless they had some relevance to something they were details *of*. The relevance may not be as strong as other possible contributions, or, perhaps, the relevance exists only with respect to a level of comprehension that is not as deep as a reader would prefer. But we should be careful not to slip into absolutist, either/or kinds of judgments here.

Coherence should be conceptualized as a global property that does not necessarily appear or disappear with the (ir)relevance of any single element or group of elements in a text. And just as we need to keep in mind that there are different levels of comprehension of discourse, we should also keep in mind that there are degrees of relevance (Jackson et al., 1987; Tracy, 1984), and there will be degrees of coherence.

Kellermann and Sleight claim (correctly, we think) that utterance-to-utterance linkage cannot be the basis for coherence. But, as we have tried to suggest, that does not imply that the coherence of a text has nothing to do with the relevance of the elements within the text. The idea that local relevance can create coherence is in error in that this conception misses what an utterance or sentence *must be related to* in order for coherence to appear. The relevance of an utterance or sentence is *not* to prior utterances or sentences, but to a conceptual model built from the prior discourse. That is why conversations like the one Jacobs (1985, p. 315) cites from *The Music Man* can be hard to follow even though each utterance is sequentially related to the topic addressed in the previous utterance. There is no anchoring in a unified overall representation.

On our view, coherence and relevance are closely interconnected. The coherence of discourse is conditioned on enough of the elements being strongly relevant to a unified, meaningful representation of the discourse in order for a global perception of coherence to appear at some level. And, unless there is some level of meaningfulness to represent the discourse as a whole, no element (utterance or sentence) can be said to be relevant to the discourse. This way of thinking about relevance and coherence can also clear up some of the residual vagueness in defining coherence in terms of "meaningfulness." It is not enough for the elements of the discourse to be individually meaningful in just any way; their meaning must be pertinent to the overall meaning of the discourse, and this overall meaning must amount to some unified, consistent representation or model.

COHERENCE AND CONSONANCE WITH KNOWLEDGE STRUCTURES

According to Kellermann and Sleight, judging a text coherent requires that there be "consonance" between text and "knowledge structures." Here Kellermann and Sleight are vulnerable, to some extent, to the same criticism they level at other researchers in the area by leaving implicit their definition of "knowledge structure" and by giving only a vague and suggestive explanation of "consonance."

Kellermann and Sleight offer partial clarification of the notion of consonance: "A coherent conversation is no more and no less than a person's judgment of consonance between expectations and perceived actuality" (p. 122). So consonance has something to do with meeting expectations. But that is not nearly clear enough for our purposes, especially since it is obvious that consonance is not *simply* consistency with expectations. Discourse that violates our expectations is not incoherent—or at least, not incoherent by virtue of violating our expectations. Imagine that Ronald Reagan were to give a speech calling for large tax increases to finance national health insurance. That would certainly violate expectations, but the speech might also be judged perfectly coherent.

Nor does a conversation that fulfills expectations always appear coherent. Consider the case of schizophrenic talk. If one can have a "knowledge structure" relevant to convention papers presented by nuclear physicists, then presumably one can also have a "knowledge structure" for schizophrenic talk. This knowledge structure should generate certain expectations about how schizophrenic talk will sound, one of the expectations being that it will sound incoherent. If we take Kellermann and Sleight literally, they wind up claiming that schizophrenic talk will sound coherent if it fits our expectations that it will be incoherent. Consonance, then, must mean something other than "fit with expectations." But what?

In much the same way, the notion of knowledge structure is also left open ended and indefinite. Unless we can specify the content of knowledge structures, there is little virtue in pointing out that knowledge structures are important to comprehension and coherence. We find ourselves echoing two cognitive scientists (Schank & Abelson, 1977), who made the same complaint fully 10 years ago:

> There is a very long theoretical stride . . . from the idea that highly structured knowledge dominates the understanding process, to the specification of the details of the most appropriate structures. It does not take one very far to say that schemas are important: one must know the content of the schemas. To be eclectic here is to say nothing. If one falls back on the abstract position that only form is important, that the human mind is capable of developing knowledge structures of infinitely varied content, then one sacrifices the essence of the structure concept, namely the strong expectations which make reality understandable. In other words, a knowledge structure theory must make a commitment to particular content schemas. (p.10)

To some extent, the vagueness of the central theoretical terms may reflect only the fact that Kellermann and Sleight are *arguing for the development of a certain kind of position* rather than actually *developing a position.* We can anticipate, however, a theoretical pothole toward which Kellermann and Sleight seem to be headed. Behind the vague talk of consonance with knowledge structures is a picture of discourse processing as a kind of template-matching triggered by objective cues in the text.

Kellermann and Sleight seem to picture a person trying to comprehend texts by identifying some cues in the text that activate knowledge structures strongly associated with those cues ("bottom-up processing") and then fitting the knowledge structure over the rest of the text ("top-down processing"). The problem we see in this position is that this picture bypasses a step that has to be there: the process by which perceivers construct models or particular representations of the discourse. The main thrust of our discussion so far has been that positing a model or representation of the text is essential to understanding issues of meaningfulness, relevance, and coherence. Textual cues and preorganized knowledge structures triggered by these cues are not adequate to account for these features of text processing; a cognitive approach must offer some account of how cues and knowledge structure are used to construct models of discourse.

It might be thought that a model is just what you get when you activate or instantiate a schema. But this is exactly the error that Kellermann and

Sleight's approach invites. Constructing a model is a different sort of process than is template matching. For one thing, a model need not be composed of the sort of categorical knowledge we expect as the content of a schema, but may represent a novel construction based on some sort of integration of any number of schemata. For another thing, a model would not be seen as being *selected* on the basis of objective cues, but would be seen instead as *constructing* some of the very things Kellermann and Sleight refer to as cues—things like topic and point of view. At some level, we would want to say that schemata constrain the models people can build, but which schemata get "activated" also depends on what model can finally be constructed to make sense of the discourse. So, the problem is not just one of "activating" schemata with "cues," but one of constructing unified models that are simultaneously consistent with schematic structures of knowledge and with the particulars of text and context.

Attempting to explain the details of discourse comprehension in terms of a matching of discourse and knowledge structure will almost certainly be futile. For knowledge structures alone to explain the brute facts of discourse comprehension, we would have to accept the idea of an infinite number of knowledge structures, and eventually to deal with the fact that the knowledge structure required in order to comprehend is not necessarily available prior to the act of comprehension. People are able to comprehend an infinite number of passages that refer to particularized, idiosyncratic, and otherwise novel situations. To suggest that schemata are directly imposed on discourse is to suggest that these novel situations are prerepresented in knowledge structures stored in memory. This is impossible—just as it is impossible for people to have stored in memory all of the possible sentences of a language—not only because the human mind cannot store an infinite number of structures, but also because it is not possible for such structures to be learned (and so prerepresented) prior to the situations in which they will be required for comprehension. Instead, there must be some way of generating novel representations from a finite number of schemata, as the need arises.

It might be thought that this problem could be handled simply as a process of general categories generating an infinite number of particular cases. For some cases, that solution seems plausible—for example, seeing Bransford and Johnson's (1972) passage on doing laundry as a particular instantiation of a "laundry script." But this line of reasoning soon exhausts itself. Consider another experimental text from Bransford and Johnson (1972):

> If the balloons popped, the sound would not be able to carry since everything would be too far away from the correct floor. A closed window would also prevent the sound from carrying since most buildings tend to be well insulated. Since the whole operation depends on a steady flow of electricity, a break in the middle of the wire would also cause problems. Of course the fellow could shout, but the human voice is not loud enough to carry that far. An additional problem is that a string could break on the instrument. Then there could be no

> accompaniment to the message. It is clear that the best situation would involve less distance. Then there would be fewer potential problems. With face to face contact, the least number of things could go wrong.

People do not understand this passage without some additional help in activating the proper knowledge structures, which seems to support the Kellermann and Sleight position. The passage becomes much clearer if accompanied by a picture showing a man with a guitar standing on a city sidewalk, singing into a microphone connected by wires to loudspeakers that are supported by helium balloons floating near the top window of a high-rise apartment building. In this way, the man can serenade a woman leaning out of the window of the building. But what kind of knowledge structure is instantiated by a picture of a man serenading a woman in a high-rise building, using loudspeakers lofted by helium balloons?

Certainly, it is not helpful to posit a "man serenading a woman in a high-rise building using loudspeakers lofted by helium balloons" script. No such script could be said to exist prior to encountering this very novel situation. Nor is it helpful to try to assimilate the text to a more general "man serenading a woman" script. Such a script would not fit over the text in any reasonable sense of the word *fit*. The problem is that understanding this passage is outside the range of the sort of categorical knowledge one might have prior to reading the passage. If we wish to think of readers as having a knowledge structure dealing with high-rise serenading using balloons, we must be prepared to grant that it is something built from the story, and that something is what we call the model.

If we are willing to assume that people come up with scripts and schemas and whatnot on an ad hoc basis to comprehend any particular text, we have not really explained comprehension in terms of knowledge structures. On the other hand, if we commit to specific content for the knowledge structures we think people have, it becomes apparent that these structures are not simply fitted over discourse, but must be used to build representations of text that are more than just concrete versions of a script or schema.

Of course, that leaves us with the engaging yet unanswered question of *how* people use text and knowledge structure to build these models. That is a question a cognitive approach might try to answer.

REFERENCES

Bransford, J. D., & Johnson, M. K. (1972). Contextual prerequisites for understanding: Some investigations of comprehension and recall. *Journal of Verbal Learning and Verbal Behavior, 11*, 717-726.

Carroll, L. (1960). *The annotated Alice* (M. Gardner, intro. and notes). New York: Bramhall House.

Hopper, R. (1981). The taken-for-granted. *Human Communication Research, 7*, 195-211.

Jackson, S., Jacobs, S., & Rossi, A. M. (1987). Conversational relevance: Three experiments on pragmatic connectedness in conversation. In M. L. McLaughlin (Ed.), *Communication yearbook* (Vol. 10, pp. 323-347). Newbury Park, CA: Sage.

Jacobs, S. (1985). Language. In M. L. Knapp & G. R. Miller (Eds.), *Handbook of interpersonal communication* (pp. 313-343). Newbury Park, CA: Sage.

McLaughlin, M. L. (1984). *Conversation: How talk is organized.* Newbury Park, CA: Sage.

Sanders, R. (1983). Tools for cohering discourse and their strategic utilization: Markers of structural connections and meaning relations. In R. T. Craig & K. Tracy (Eds.), *Conversational coherence: Form, structure, and strategy* (pp. 67-80). Newbury Park, CA: Sage.

Schank, R., & Abelson, R. (1977). *Scripts, plans, goals and understanding: An inquiry into human knowledge structures.* Hillsdale, NJ: Lawrence Erlbaum.

Tracy, K. (1984, May). *The obligation to be irrelevant.* Paper presented at the annual meeting of the International Communication Association, San Francisco.

3 A Dialectical Analysis of the Tensions, Functions, and Strategic Challenges of Communication in Young Adult Friendships

WILLIAM K. RAWLINS
Purdue University

This monograph synthesizes selected findings from an ongoing program of empirical and theoretical research regarding the nature and functions of communication in young adult friendships. It argues that friendship involves inherent dialectical tensions as a specific category of interpersonal relationship within American culture, in the actual communicative practices of friends, and within and across developmental periods of the life cycle. First are delineated four basic elements of the dialectical perspective employed to analyze the communication of friends: totality, contradiction, motion, and praxis. Next, an extensive examination of dialectical principles inherent in the communicative management of friendship occurs. The principles are then used to develop an intelligible frame for the practices and predicaments of managing young adult friendships communicatively with particular attention to gender, marriage, and work exigencies. Implications for the study of interpersonal communication in general and friendship in particular are discussed.

I begin by delineating four basic elements of the dialectical perspective employed to analyze the communication of friends—totality, contradiction, motion, and praxis. Next, I move to an extensive examination of dialectical principles inherent in the communicative management of friendship. Contextual dialectics involve the dialectic of the private and the public, and the dialectic of the ideal and the real. Interactional dialectics include the dialectics of the freedom to be independent and the freedom to be dependent, affection and instrumentality, judgment and

Correspondence and requests for reprints: William K. Rawlins, Communication Department, Purdue University, Room 301A, West Lafayette, IN 47907.

Communication Yearbook 12, pp. 157-189

acceptance, and expressiveness and protectiveness. I then use these principles to develop an intelligible frame for the practices and predicaments of managing young adult friendships communicatively with particular attention to gender, marriage, and work exigencies. The essay concludes with implications of this research for the study of interpersonal communication in general and friendship in particular.

A DIALECTICAL PERSPECTIVE

The term *dialectic* implies several meanings. Originally, for ancient Greek philosophers, it was a logical, conversational procedure for the invention and evaluation of ideas (Benjamin, 1983). Over subsequent centuries, however, the word has indexed a variety of ontological, epistemological, and methodological conceptions including the objective idealism of Hegel, Engels's "dialectics of nature," and the Frankfurt School's critical analyses of mass culture. Accordingly, one must specify how the term is being used. The present dialectical perspective regards social processes and incorporates four basic elements common to numerous dialectical formulations. These core aspects are totality, contradiction, motion, and praxis. The order for examining these features is arbitrary since linear exposition unavoidably violates dialectical circularity and interrelatedness.

Totality

Dialectical totality hinges on relatedness and contextuality. Discrete "things" are inconceivable from a dialectical perspective; what comprises reality are relations and relations among relations. Ball (1979) observes, "Dialectics does not begin with abstract theoretical entities which it then tries to relate, but with a processual conception of reality as consisting of relationships" (p. 788). What appear as distinct phenomena achieve their unity only in reference to other phenomena, which exist only in relation to others. Structural interconnection underlies surface distinctions (Kieve, 1983).

Dialectical analyses originate from the vantage point of a dynamic totality and not elements (Israel, 1979). Still, the reciprocal interrelationship between wholes and parts in the composition of a given social domain is a primary concern for dialectical thinkers (Mirkovic, 1980; Bopp & Weeks, 1984). Wholes have no concrete existence without the relationships among parts, and the constitutive nature of parts derives from their relationship to a whole. Separating them constitutes a temporary analytical or abstract move.

Dialectical totalities are not static or fixed but are in constant movement and alternation between contextualizing and being contextualized. Since dialectical inquiries and the social formations they attempt to investigate change in different contexts, it is essential to situate the phenomena of interest in their spatio-temporal cultural setting. Moreover, their organizing principles do not imply harmony (Israel, 1979). As such, a dialectical totality is a "negative totality" composed of inherent contradictions and consequently undergoing continuous development (Marcuse, 1964). This contradictory essence of totalities is integral to the discussion of dialectics.

Thus I conceive any component or aspect of friendship as existing in connection with all of the others. For example, the nature and extent of two friends' displays of affection interact with their personal circumstances, shared patterns of instrumentality, independence and dependence, judgment and acceptance, and candor and restraint. Each of these activities both contextualizes and is contextualized by the other practices. As a result, in a given public situation one friend's affectionate behaviors may contradict the other's need for independence or restraint. This friend's response may offend prior expectations, which then could reverberate throughout virtually every area of the relationship. Accordingly, the partners might negotiate new practices that limit public displays of caring but simultaneously generate a new mode of private argument within the friendship. Ironically, both developments may prove inadequate in another life situation the friends might face together.

Contradiction

Contradiction, the coexistence and conflict of interpenetrated opposites, pervades dialectical thinking. Marquit (1981) stipulates that any concrete unity is composed of the active interconnection of dialectical opposites which are simultaneously "mutually conditioning" and "mutually excluding" (p. 308). "Mutually conditioning" means the occurrence or essence of a given feature of reality is premised upon its opposite. Privacy presupposes publicity and vice versa. Similarity between entities is conceivable only because different objects are being compared. "Mutually excluding" describes the relation of negation that constitutes any feature of reality as the opposite extreme of a given continuum from another. Justice is recognized as the negation of injustice (mutually excluding) simultaneously with its identification with injustice as two opposite poles constituting possible forms of moral praxis (mutually conditioning).

Dialectical contradictions are viewed as intrinsic features of social life, not to be confused with logical contradictions that are merely formal expressions of contradictory essences failing to embody their objective content (Marquit, 1981; Mirkovic, 1980). Even so, gradations of dialectical opposites have been identified (Israel, 1979), such as contradictory opposites that are mutually exclusive and exhaustive (e.g., life and death), contradictory opposites that are mutually exclusive but not exhaustive (e.g., independence and dependence), and opposites that are complementary (e.g., giving and receiving help). Therefore, the mutually conditioning and excluding qualities of social life's contradictory features assume various forms and gradations in the actual accomplishment of social interaction.

In short, contradictory tendencies are not to be explained away or dissolved by formal logic but recognized as bases for constructing explanations. The concrete composition and accomplishment of social formations in space and time suggest certain possibilities. First, one can examine a given social entity for the contradictions evident within the entity and those occurring between the particular formation and external units contextualizing it. Such contradictions have been termed "inner" or "internal," and "outer" or "external," contradictions, respectively (Riegel, 1976; Bopp & Weeks, 1984). Two friends experience the former type when attempting to manage the contradictory requirements of expressive versus protective communication within their relationship. By comparison, external contradictions develop when the constraints of one person's marriage or job undermine freedoms negotiated with his or her friend.

Next, contradictions in time can be identified. Riegel (1976) has stressed the importance of synchrony and asynchrony and tensions between these temporal relations as a critical factor in human development. For example, certain friendships thrive when the partners occupy similar or complementary stages in the life cycle. Yet if the friends develop personally at excessively uneven rates, the resulting behavioral and/or attitudinal oppositions may reconstitute the bond.

Third, dialectical thinkers have distinguished between principal and secondary contradictions as well as primary and secondary aspects of contradictions (Mao Tse-Tung, 1966; Israel, 1979). In ongoing dyads, managing specific contradictions such as independence versus dependence may greatly outstrip the effort or attention accorded others, which consequently are less significant in defining the friends' communication. Moreover, a particular aspect of a contradiction, like dependence, may so thoroughly characterize two friends' interaction patterns that either friend's independence is a secondary concern. Finally, emergent contradictions are generated throughout the development of social formations (Benson, 1973). Conflicting tensions not readily apparent in a given guise of a friendship may surface as vital constitutive features when personal factors or the circumstances of the friendship change.

Motion

Movement, activity and change are fundamental properties of social life in a dialectical perspective; stability requires accounting for and explanation. Accordingly, an entity or system that appears unchanging or stable is conceived of as a "temporarily equilibrated form in transition" (Bopp & Weeks, 1984, p. 52). While everything varies, what seems constant is simply changing at a slower rate; or as Israel (1979) states, "Structure is a property of process" (p. 117).

This being so, contradictions comprise the basis for perceived stability as well as change. The relative intensities of opposites constituting a given totality are responsible for the comparative stability of the system (Marquit, 1981). One must examine various levels of the interconnection and mutual antagonism of opposites to understand how a social formation is simultaneously composing and changing itself and which aspect of this ongoing process is ascendant at a specific juncture. However, stability does not necessarily connote "a static balance or equilibrium of forces or tendencies" (Marquit, 1981, p. 312). Should new contradictions emerge or the relative intensities of contradictory poles significantly alter, the system may behave differently or transform itself (Marquit, 1981).

Analysis of the interrelated processes of change and stability have yielded two generic accounts, termed here *dialectics of transcendence and transformation,* and *dialectics of encapsulation.*

Dialectics of Transcendence and Transformation

Frequently associated with dialectical theorizing is the triad of terms thesis-antithesis-synthesis. This conception of historical development and change derives from the dialectical law of the negation of the negation. In this view change involves "the replacement of the old by the new (negation), and the re-replacement of the new by the newer still (negation of the negation)" (Wozniak, 1975, p. 34). The product of this process exists at a higher level of development. This emergent stage of a social form is premised upon prior manifestations, preserving some of their aspects while eliminating others (Israel, 1979). But it cannot be reduced to previous stages or lower levels because it "operates in accordance with its own principles of organization, its own modes of expression" (Ball, 1979, p. 791).

The process of the negation of the negation results in dialectical transcendence (Israel, 1979). The new social formation resolves its generative contradictions by elevating them to a fresh form, itself constituted by an ongoing process of embracing and resolving subsequent contradictions (Kieve, 1983). Contradictions are therefore preserved and development continues incessantly (Wozniak, 1975; Sayers, 1982).

In friendship, for example, dialectical relationships persist between affection and instrumentality. A friendship might begin because two people like each other's personal qualities and simply enjoy spending time together (thesis). As time passes, each friend may begin to use the other as a convenient source of labor and/or materials, which negates the conception of friendship as an end-in-itself (antithesis). Even so, these new practices may activate more comprehensive changes throughout the friendship, which in turn negate the utilitarian ethic as primarily constituting the friendship. Thus the organizing principles of the friendship are expanded and reconstituted to include both affection and instrumentality as practices that complement each other (synthesis). But this new level of organization involves inherent contradictions that will incite further changes in the friendship.

Authors have remarked upon the tendency for such dialectical formulations to suggest constant growth and upward development (Altman, Vinsel, & Brown, 1981). The idealistic cast of such conceptions is probably traceable to Hegel's (1966) teleological, dialectical idealism. Even so, such principles do not help explain apparently stagnant or hyperstable social formations. For these purposes other conceptions are useful.

Dialectics of Encapsulation

Handelman (1984) has described dialectical processes that, contrasting to those considered here, are "closed and regenerative." Handelman argues:

> The encapsulated dialectic is predicted on a major thesis and its relationship to a minor antithesis, such that the latter is subsumed by or encapsulated within, the former. Then the emergence of antithesis revalidates the thesis instead of generating a new synthesis. (p. 268)

While process and motion are ongoing in such a situation, the transformations are minimal.

Handelman's formulation registers the potential for uneven or truncated development inhering in contradictions with clearly superordinate and subordinate aspects. Such balanced inequality may rigidify or overdetermine the behavior of a social system. Mao Tse-Tung (1966) observes, "The principal aspect is the one playing the leading role in the contradiction. The nature of a thing is determined mainly by the principal aspect of a contradiction, the aspect that has gained the dominant position" (p. 54). Clearly, the analysis of principal and secondary contradictions as well as aspects or poles of specific contradictions is vital for understanding dialectical motion.

In contrast to the previous example, a friendship might commence because two individuals like each other as an end-in-itself (thesis). Events occur that reveal the friends to be mutually useful. However, the friends insist on minimal use of each other or experience their favors as insignificant in comparison with their greater involvement with each other's being (minor antithesis). As a result, the relationship continues to reconstitute itself as primarily based on affection with instrumental actions merely functioning to reinforce that conception (minimally modified thesis).

Motion also involves the "Law of Transformation of Quantitative Changes into Qualitative Changes and Vice Versa "(Marquit, 1981, p.311). Quantitative changes in the comparative intensity of poles of particular contradictions, like affection versus instrumentality, may result in qualitative change in the nature of these contradictions. There must be sufficient antagonism and opposition between contradictory aspects of a social sphere to fuel change, as in the example in which affection and instrumentality were strongly countervailing poles. If the opposites are too lopsided in intensity, however, the process may be encapsulating, as in the example in which affection clearly dominated. But should a certain number of principal contradictions comprising a given relationship change, they can alter the qualitative arrangement or configuration of contradictions constituting a friendship, thereby changing its essential nature (Marquit, 1981).

Praxis

The final feature of the present dialectical perspective—praxis—regards the reflexive constitution of human beings and their social worlds. People are conceived as producers and products of their own actions. The active, conscious, human subject acts to produce contexts, which in turn function to produce the subject as an object. The subject molds and is molded by his or her social context.

Accordingly, social formations presented as given at any moment are the products of prior human activity. Though the objective constraints of the status quo can transform individuals, individuals can act to transform the status quo (Berger & Luckman, 1966). As Rossi (1983) maintains, neither the human subject nor social structure "are constituted or even conceivably independent of each other" (p. 320). Rather, individualized persons compose themselves through praxis in concrete social situations over time. They are constituted through interaction in their active management of, and communication within, relationships as their actual, lived histories affect and inform their present actions. Consequently, Israel (1979) argues that persons should not be analyzed "in terms of properties, traits, and substances, but in terms of interactions and situations" (p. 59).

The notion of praxis focuses attention on the active choices friends make in the face of objective constraints existing in their temporally and spatially specific social circumstances. For example, an individual may have to decide whether to acknowledge publicly a privately valued friend who may not fit the expectations of his or her spouse, other friends, or colleagues. However, a praxic view also emphasizes that one's spouse, friends or work associates also derive from choices the individual has made and now manifest themselves as objective and concrete limitations upon choice. Further, how one elects to treat one's friend will result in changes in the composition of the friendship, which will change or limit one's options for communicating with the friend at another social juncture.

The praxic accomplishment of individualized human existence involves a dialectical enactment of the tension between "the subject structuring aspect of the social structure" objectifying persons and their knowledge-based "conscious activity" revealing them to be subjects (Rossi, 1983, p. 320). Accordingly, we engage ourselves and other people as partly objective and partly subjective.

A Dialectical Perspective on Friendship: Summary

A dialectical perspective, with totality, contradiction, motion, and praxis as its critical components, has implications for the analysis of communication in friendship. According to this view, configurations of contradictions compose and organize friendships through an ongoing process of change. However, questions arise: What appear to be the principal or secondary contradictions or aspects of contradictions constituting certain friendships? What contradictions are created by the friends' attempts to manage strategically the incompatible requirements of their relationship? What contradictions are activated by or contribute to a friendship's nesting within or vis-à-vis other social spheres, ranging from local relationships and subcultures to larger cultural orders? An investigator may glimpse the contours of such arrangements by examining how the communicative management of friendship is situated hierarchically in social space and over time. Studying the synchrony or asynchrony of temporal sequences also provides perspective on the contradictions constituting friendships. Riegel (1976) argues that synchronization is "the most critical issue in dialectical theory" (p. 693). He views asynchronies as responsible for most crises in human development and resultant change. Accordingly, short- and long-term changes in both individuals and their relationships must be examined in relation to both rapid and drawn-out cultural developments.

The time grain of these various processes and the extent of their coordination or disorder are key factors in a dialectical analysis. Thus dialectical inquiries are intrinsically historical investigations concerned with the developmental and historical specificity of the process in question (Rossi, 1983). How are human beings consciously acting in this concrete situation and what implications do their actions have for the ongoing constitution of their social worlds in which friendships function as a particular part?

DIALECTICAL PRINCIPLES INHERENT IN THE COMMUNICATIVE MANAGEMENT OF FRIENDSHIP

Communicating within friendships involves inherent dialectical features. Two broad analytical classes, contextual and interactional dialectics, are examined next, though in actuality these principles extensively interconnect in the communication of friends.

Contextual Dialectics

Contextual dialectics derive from the place of friendship in the prevailing social order of American culture. They describe cultural conceptions that frame and permeate interaction within specific friendships yet are conceivably subject to revision as a result of significant changes in everyday practices. We will consider the dialect of the private and the public and the dialectic of the ideal and real, while suggesting their theoretical and practical interdependence.

The Dialectic of the Private and the Public

This principle articulates the tensions produced by friendship occupying experiential and behavioral continua encompassing private and public realms. The interweaving of these generic, discursive contexts presents significant challenges and opportunities requiring various strategies of communicators.

Within the observable public matrix of American interpersonal relationships, friendship occupies a marginal position. Unlike kin, it is not a certifiable blood relationship. It lacks the religious and legal warrants and the culturally sanctioned procreative function of marriage. It is generally regarded differently from the possessive and sexual nature of romantic love (Brain, 1976). Neither is friendship objectively defined by economic contracts as are work or professional relationships. Basically, friendship has no clear normative status within publicly constituted hierarchies of role relationships; yet it may compete with, complement, substitute for, or fuse with these other types of social bonds (Hess, 1972). In short, the degree of public recognition of friendship as a category of interpersonal relationship renders it an "institutionalized non-institution" (Paine, 1969, p. 514).

Contrasting with friendship's vagrant position in the public realm is its peculiar moral character as a private bond. Friendship cannot be imposed on people; it is an ongoing human association voluntarily developed and privately negotiated. Consequently, the rights and obligations of friendships can transcend formal, objective, or material institutional requirements and statuses (Paine, 1969). This autonomous quality makes friendship potentially more "pure" than are relationships governed by wider social structures like labor and power, especially if the friends experience those structures as threatening essential human values (Eisenstadt, 1974). Disturbingly, however, sinister, nihilistic, or violent values may also characterize a given friendship's private morality. Appropriate behavior is determined within the friendship and is upheld principally by each individual's affection for and/or loyalty and commitment to the other. Personal responsibility and trust are the lynchpins of this private order, which may be as evanescent as human caprice or as enduring as human dedication allows.

In its dialectical character, combining public marginality and private morality, friendship weaves in and out of the larger social order like a "double agent," fulfilling both individual and social functions. Sometimes friends wear "feathers" borrowed from other culturally sanctioned roles so that their relationship is viewed publicly as acceptable (Parsons, 1915). For example, this costuming occurs frequently in adult cross-sex friendships in which one or both parties are married to others (Rawlins, 1982). Such a publicly acknowledged cross-sex friendship may threaten the culturally endorsed marriage relationship in others' eyes, whereas defining the bond as a professional one would not. Ironically, although this "disguised" cross-sex friendship might be pursued primarily as a self-serving release from the pressures of an overweening marriage, it may, at the same time, function to strengthen that socially favored bond.

In contrast, cultivating the private morality and manners of a friendship within, for example, ostensibly political or professional relationships, often allows for the special treatment of one's friend or standards of evaluation that differ from public statements. Such arrangements may result in friends as happier clients or constituents, or even more valid appraisals of an individual's performance because of the added concern and insight of one's friend. However, "greasing the wheels" in this fashion can also undermine fair practice and publicly accountable procedures.

Thus the liberating potential of friendship for two individuals might be regarded as its subversive potential from a broader social perspective. Conversely, behaviors that civic-minded people could view as preserving public decorum, friends might perceive as stultifying their freedom of action and expression. Because friendships are constrained but not determined by public roles or institutions, tensions between public and private comportment persist. A given friendship may duplicate culturally encouraged actions but for idiosyncratic reasons. And some partners may conduct themselves in the personalized manner of friends, but clearly for publicly redeemable purposes. The ongoing rhetorical challenge to friends, therefore, is to develop and share private definitions and practices while orchestrating social perceptions of their relationship (Paine, 1969).

The dialectic of the private and the public delineates a critical facet of managing friendship. These terms not only reference realms of actual behavior and experience but also comprise interpretive categories used rhetorically by commentators in the service of moral visions (Wells, 1985). Different cultural moments privilege one sphere over the other. During the reign of an "ideology of intimacy," for example, private and personal relationships like friendship are celebrated for their potential to confirm individuals' self-conceptions (Sennett, 1978). From this ideology, Suttles (1970) argued that a primary basis for friendship was negotiated remissions from public expectations. He observed, "Friendship demands a verifiable self and it cannot be one that complacently complies with public propriety" (p. 107). Still, as Naegele (1958) commented, such an exclusive conception of friendship negates certain readings of the meanings of democracy. Accordingly, in more public-spirited times, Bellah, Madsen, Sullivan, Swidler, and Tipton (1985) have praised civic friendships for facilitating the larger community by serving the social order and derided private relationships for their "therapeutic" cast.

Thus friendship's role as a double agent is categorically vulnerable in American culture. Within a particular dyad, a friend can be criticized or congratulated for asserting a public or private aspect of the relationship in a given situation. Simultaneously, depending on the cultural mood of the day, that same person may be, in contrast, publicly condemned or praised for the same actions. This private/public dialectic interacts with the ideals and realities of communicating in friendship.

The Dialectic of the Ideal and the Real

This dialectic formulates the interplay between the abstract ideals and expectations often associated with friendship and the nettlesome realities or unexpected rewards of actual communication between friends. Indeed, refined and idealized images and forms of friendship develop in the public domain at given historical junctures and are culturally transmitted. Therefore, despite its marginal status vis-à-vis other social roles, people are socialized into normative expectations regarding certain ideal conceptions and practices of friendship (Sampson, 1977; Brown, 1981).

For instance, Naegele (1958), maintaining that a dialectical relationship between "norms of personal and impersonal conduct" produces a given epoch's guidelines for both types of interpersonal activity, observes, "Indeed, ideals of impersonal relations are necessary for the elaboration of our kind of ideals of personal relations" (p. 236). If a given era encourages less reserve with relative strangers, heightened strategies for revealing oneself to another may be endorsed to distinguish friends. When people are encouraged to be *friendly* with everybody, certain practices become necessary for indicating *friendship*. In contrast, if the norms of impersonal communication promote distance and considerable politeness, more personalized dyads may deviate from rigid stylized expectations without exposing significantly private thoughts and feelings. As mentioned earlier, these practices will receive differential endorsement in terms of a particular cultural epoch's valuations of the public and private spheres, and the appropriate communicative strategies for linking them (Rawlins, 1985).

In addition, Liebow (1976) argues that the public and private realities impinging on the tenuous nature of friendship as a cultural double agent result in its frequent idealization. He states:

> Lacking depth in both past and present, friendship is easily uprooted by the tug of economic or psychological self-interest or by external forces acting against it.
>
> The recognition of this weakness, coupled with the importance of friendship as a source of security and self-esteem, is surely a principal source of the impulse to romanticize relationships. (pp. 206-207)

In his view, idealized images of friendship derive from, yet serve to mute, concerns about its sometimes harsh situational realities.

Whether it is championed as a vital, idiosyncratic haven from a humdrum, bureaucratized social order or simply endorsed as a humanizing complement to a complacent conventional society, the notion of friendship retains idealistic overtones. The Western conception of this bond, Van Vlissingen (1970) maintains, reflects a constant from ancient Greek thought, "In order for a friendship to last it must be permeated with ethical concerns" (p. 230). As a cultural ideal, friendship appears to be a categorical repository for the hope of a mutually edifying moral covenant voluntarily negotiated between people.

The discursive practices of friendship both manage and regenerate the tensions between its ideal and real forms. According to Bloch (1971), the terminology of relationships can pivot between "moral and tactical meanings." The moral meaning of friendship terms indexes its idealistic connotations in our cultural system of values. Describing someone as a friend or speaking in the name of friendship draws upon cherished categorical notions. In contrast, the tactical meaning of friendship labels uses their moral associations in the interest of transforming social situations and strategically defining certain types of relationships. As a result, the specific meanings of these friendship terms derive from how they are operationalized in given cases.

Actual discourse within and about friendships appears to blend moral and tactical meanings in constituting a range of relationships that run the gamut from private to public in scope and responsibility, and from idealistic to realistic in primary impulse. Thus the word *friend* itself has multiple meanings, including moral ones, and can be employed tactically to reflect changing social circumstances and various definitions of self and others. For example, the term may be used to acknowledge someone who has fulfilled various expectations personally or culturally associated with friendship, to recognize an affectionate and loyal other, or to ingratiate oneself to another person. The word may be withdrawn under contrasting conditions to emphasize social distance (Jacobson, 1976). Maines (1981) states that the unspecified use of the word *friend* renders it "a catchall term which is conventionally understood and recognized as having no fixed referent outside of the situation itself" (p. 172).

However, the prevalence of distinctions between "real friends" versus "casual acquaintances" and the preoccupation with determining gradations of friendship register the problematic aspects of managing friendships in the face of such situational definitions and the persistence of and need for moral meanings of the term. A variety of expressions and nicknames are typically developed to indicate degrees of intimacy and the communicative aspects of relationships (Knapp, Ellis, & Williams, 1980). People reflect cultural values in developing core conceptions of what they variously term "best" or "real" friendship and then identify and rank other relationships according to their achievement of its defining attributes (Rawlins & Holl, 1987; Rawlins, Leibowitz, & Bochner, 1986). Investigators have shown that these categories are rather resilient and are preserved by certain strategies. For example, a person who actually achieves a "best" friendship typically will view it as continuing even without identifiable rewards or interaction (Allan, 1979; Rose & Serafica, 1986). Yet, should a best friendship unequivocally end, persons can decide that it could not really have been a best friendship in the first place. In both cases, one revises the perception of a given friendship while maintaining the ideals of friendship (Allan, 1979; Rose & Serafica, 1986).

Consequently, although friendship persists as an enduring cultural ideal, its purer forms are frequently experienced as elusive personal realities. There may be great disparity between its cultural connotations and its meanings deriving from the concrete interaction of particular friends. This situation recurs, Paine (1969) argues, because "the highest ideals of friendship are (a) proclaimed as realizable and (b) not protected institutionally" (p. 521). As a result, aspiring to an ideal friendship comprises an ongoing challenge for specific individuals across constantly changing personal and social circumstances. To complicate matters, measures taken to preserve certain vaunted aspects of friendship may subvert other cherished values. For example, a person may strategically breach the code of honesty between friends in order to protect the other's sensitivity about an issue (Rawlins, 1983b). Paine (1969) observes, "The ideals of friendship are likely to be spoiled without such protection. Of course, the fact that the protection is necessary suggests that the ideals are, in some measure, factitious values" (p. 521).

A dialectical conception maintains that any social formation is revealed through and constituted by the endless interweaving of idealistic and realistic factors (Ball, 1979). Such a view regards the ideals of friendship not as "factitious values" in light of concrete limitations but as guiding principles shaping and shaped by the actual practices of friends. Communicating within friendship is an active process; it is praxis occurring between specific people at a given time and place. Friends may attempt to communicate in ways that conform with the ideals of their era, but in doing so, they create and encounter real constraints and contradictions. The manner in which they handle these exigencies may revise or ratify the original ideals. Indeed, a culturally patterned set of expectations is associated with friendship. These patterns, however, are produced and reproduced through a dialectical interplay of ideal conceptions and real constraints across a continuum of private and public discursive realms in the actual communication of a variety of types of friends. Let us examine some dialectical patterns of interaction identified within friendships.

Interactional Dialectics

Perhaps the most ubiquitous concern for communication scholars is codification, the relationships among self's and others' behaviors and the meanings self and others assign to those behaviors. This practice comprises a vital concern in negotiating friendships as well. Friendships are potentially fraught with ambiguity, both in the friends' attempts to interpret each other's words and actions and the significance assigned to their behavior by third parties and/or society at large.

Ambiguity in friendship is often compounded by ambivalence (Brain, 1976; Harre, 1977). The intermittent delights or disruptions of fulfilling or disappointing an array of publicly and/or privately produced ideals and realities within a given friendship can threaten stable interpretations of even the most straightforward actions. An important challenge to friends, therefore, is to behave and to interpret behaviors in a manner that preserves an assumption of benevolent as opposed to malevolent intentions underpinning each other's actions. To perceive good intentions constitutes an "insurance policy" for the relationship when contradictory conditions may result in ostensibly negative behavior by one's friend. Accordingly, communicating within friendship involves a constant interaction between interpretive and behavioral practices to maintain a mutual definition of the relationship as friendship.

In what follows, I will consider four dialectical principles that organize, yet compose, ongoing challenges and antagonistic choices in the practical management of communication sustaining friendships. These coherences have been identified in participants' descriptions of their relational practices and supplemented by reports of other scholars of friendship. As such, they constitute conceptual and interactional structures informing what ideally/typically occurs in friendships. Though these principles may or may not consciously inform the actual behavior of friends, they are useful as interpretive tools for understanding the communicative predicaments of friendship. They include the dialectic of the freedom to be independent and the freedom to be dependent, the dialectic of affection and instrumentality, the dialectic of judgment and acceptance, and the dialectic of expressiveness and protectiveness.

The Dialectic of the Freedom to Be Independent and the Freedom to Be Dependent

As we have stressed, in American culture free choice and voluntary action are definitive qualities of friendship; people remain friends because both individuals choose to do so. The dialectic of the freedom to be independent and the freedom to be dependent conceptualizes the patterns of availability and copresence negotiated in light of this voluntary essence of friendship (Rawlins, 1983a).

Basically, in forming a friendship, each friend grants the other a pair of contradictory prerogatives. The freedom to be independent is the liberty to pursue one's life and individual interests without the friend's interference or help. In contrast, the freedom to be dependent is the privilege of calling upon or relying on one's friend in times of need. Both liberties engender choices for self and other. Yet, exercising individual options of independent or dependent behavior poses de facto contingencies restricting the other's choices. For example, if self innocently plans a vacation at a time when other requests assistance, their options collide. Ironically, the issue may become, who has more freedom to be constrained by the other's choice?

Clearly, in granting each other these freedoms, friends cocreate relational patterns of interaction that may foster or curtail their individual liberties. Of course, each friendship emphasizes different aspects of this dialectic which organize the relationship in particular ways (Rawlins, 1983a). Some pairs value their privilege of depending upon each other to the extent that either person's independent behavior is infrequent and resented. Conversely, other friendships are characterized by a pattern of such mutual independence that dependence is primarily ritually enacted by "touching base" or is actualized only when there is serious need.

Despite typical and predictable practices established in a given friendship, the contradictory nature of these freedoms can make it difficult to know for certain whether a given pattern is affirming or weakening the friendship. A primarily dependent relationship may unwittingly destroy the individuals' capacities for independent action that give friendship its liberating quality. Choosing dependence may become a conscription. Further, independent friends must renew contact to be sure that they are still involved in a friendship. Perhaps one of them has changed careers or fundamental values and views encounters with the other as too limiting and/or undesirable. However, the freedoms are based on mutually contingent choices by both parties that allow for multiple functional arrangements as well as corruptions. Elsewhere, I have detailed possible modes of prohibiting or obligating independent or dependent behavior in friendship in the role of either granting or receiving these liberties (Rawlins, 1983a).

To summarize, the ongoing negotiation and enactment of both contradictory freedoms is necessary to preserve friendship though it is difficult to specify their precise functional interrelationship. I have termed them *conjunctive freedoms* for two related reasons. First, each freedom is valued in friendship only if negotiated in connection with the other. Independence from a friend is appreciated only if one retains the option of depending on him or her. Likewise, the privilege of depending on someone is prized only if one's autonomy is also preserved. Second, sharing these two freedoms in combination serves to connect friends. Complete independence means no relationship at all, and total dependence constrains both persons by subverting their individual integrity. The ongoing mutual enactment of some composite of these freedoms is essential to maintain a bond of friendship.

The Dialectic of Affection and Instrumentality

This principle formulates the interpenetrated nature of caring for a friend as an end-in-itself and/or as a means-to-an-end. Various communicative quandaries revolve around qualifying one's expressions of need for a friend within the tensions produced by this dialectic.

Few people would question the importance of affection in friendship, and several authors include it as one of the defining characteristics of such bonds (Paine, 1969; Kurth, 1970; Brain, 1976; Rawlins, 1982). Empirical research also attests to its significance across the course of friendships. After surveying a variety of behavioral and attitudinal indices in a longitudinal study of friendship development and maintenance, Hays (1984) concludes, "It may be affection behavior which is primarily responsible for both stimulating the initial formation of a friendship . . . and maintaining that friendship despite environmental constraints and periods of non-interaction" (p. 94). A primary basis for distinguishing between "real friendship" and "casual acquaintance" in Williams's (1959) investigation of suburban friendships involves the extent of "affective involvement" and "norms of affectivity rather than neutrality" (p. 7). Finally, affection figures significantly in Rose and Serafica's (1986) examination of hypothetical and actual strategies for maintaining and ending a variety of friendships and for discriminating "best" and "close" from "casual" ones. Such findings reinforce notions of friendship dating back to Aristotle's (1980) friendships of virtue that stress noninstrumental "person-qua-person" caring for one's friend (Suttles, 1970).

Instrumentality, using one's friend to benefit self, receives far less endorsement as an attribute of friendship. In fact, as readily as affection is associated with "true" friendships, instrumentality tends to connote "false" ones. Aristotle (1980) argues that utilitarian bonds are inferior and less constant, stating, "Those who are friends for the sake of utility part when the advantage is at an end; for they were lovers not of each other but of profit" (p. 198). From this perspective a primarily useful conception of friends defines friendship in a highly specialized and somewhat tainted way.

In actuality, drawing a sharp boundary between friendships based on affection and on instrumentality comprises a false dichotomy (Paine, 1970). Persons derive utilitarian rewards from friendships regardless of their original purposes for engaging in them. Even Aristotle (1980) admits that pleasure and utility could be byproducts of a friendship of virtue. Moreover, Paine (1969) suggests that recognizing a useful relationship as an "instrumental friendship" implies that expressive and emotional factors are also involved. What other considerations operate, then, in preserving or undermining the polar conceptions of friendship as either a true one based on affection or a false one premised on instrumentality, and how do they function in the communicative management of this dialectical pair?

An array of contradictory tensions influences how *both* affection and instrumentality are manifested and experienced within friendships. Expressions of affection may be spontaneously and generously offered or communicated largely to receive displays of caring and/or instrumental aid in return. Likewise, one may help a friend unselfishly or to obtain increased affection or instrumental gains from him or her. Whether a spirit of generosity or reciprocity motivates or is perceived to inspire caring or helpful behaviors affects the ethos of such actions between friends.

Indeed, many authors extol the generous, altruistic impulse in friendship (Paine, 1969; Rake; 1970; Dubois, 1974). One could argue, however, against drawing such a clear line between selfishness and altruism. This view recognizes selflessness as an ideal pursuit but maintains that self-referent agency is an unavoidable reality, even in the best of friendships (Annas, 1977; Wright, 1984). People may derive self-oriented pleasure from their affection for a friend or the opportunity to help him or her. In a sense, one's selfishness draws one toward a friend and one's generosity attracts that friend to one.

Closely associated with attributions of unselfish or selfish inclinations, an instance of affection or help may be perceived as voluntary or obligatory. Ironically for the interpretation of behavior by friends, there is a dialectical relationship between these bases for action. Voluntary services or spontaneous displays of affection can make a friend feel obligated to engage in similar behaviors. Consequently, tacit contracts often develop that are experienced as particularly forceful because they are voluntarily undertaken (Kurth, 1970; Wiseman, 1986). Paradoxically, it is important for friends to fulfill voluntarily binding obligations that they have freely developed. If one feels or makes the other feel that his or her concern or aid in a given instance is obligatory, it sours the more edifying interpretations of the gesture. Repeated occurrences render the friendship barely distinguishable from more mundane partnerships.

Underlying this delicate traffic in sentiment and assistance are fears of inadvertent exploitation and/or indebtedness. Accordingly, within friendships, various models of exchange develop, designed to circumvent such risks without exhibiting rigorous or overtly economic practices. Friends take care to recognize that they share a variety of "things," both tangible and intangible (Hays, 1984). Thus friends will strive to maintain approximately equivalent exchange, realizing that the assets of friendship are difficult to specify, especially by outsiders (Paine, 1969; Szwed, 1969). Sometimes an overall pattern of equitable exchange may ameliorate a constant concern with ledgers. Even so, La Gaipa (1981) suggests, "Short-term 'balancing of accounts' is discouraged because of the economic overtones, but long-term imbalance generally leads to the termination of the relationship" (p. 80). Yet whether one is an observer or an actual participant, Paine (1969) argues, economic conceptions of friendship may be inadequate because the nature of the equivalency may vary greatly in specific circumstances.

The dispersal of benefits within the friendship can be recast in terms of mutuality instead of exchange or economics. Paine (1969) asserts that the notion of a bargain takes on a different meaning between friends. He states, "Expressed as a bargain, A, in his concern with *his own side* of a bargain with B, is, in friendship, *also concerned with B's,* and vice versa" (p. 512). Such conceptions acknowledge individuals' selfish concerns but view them as necessarily supplemented and fundamentally altered by the mutuality and communality of friendship (Mills & Clark, 1982; Wright, 1984).

Even within mutual friendships, however, dynamic tensions persist among generosity versus reciprocity and spontaneity versus obligation. How friends experience each other's affectionate and instrumental behaviors derives from their ongoing management of both the actualities and symbolic qualities of these contradictory facets of friendship. Szwed (1969) warns, "All that can be known of a partner's motives in a contract is his willingness to continue the alliance.... Beyond this fact, individual motivations and goals remain veiled" (p. 108). Thus the meaning and value of particular actions depend upon interpretive frames established and maintained between the friends. Optimally, the interplay of routinely benevolent actions and the favorable codification of self's and other's intentions comprises and reflects the self-reinforcing orientation, "The relationship is experienced as a whole and for its own sake" (Peters & Kennedy, 1970, p. 450). Problematically, self-sustaining negative spirals may also occur and suspicious or cynical attributions then prevail.

The particular stance that develops is a function of both specific events and the patterns emerging over the course of the relationship. Frequent or poignant communication of disinterested affection can qualify a friend's experience of instrumental obligations. Yuan (1973) found that sufficient affect is necessary within friendship to allow for unquestioned altruism and to "remove the burden of strict reciprocity" (p. 12). Conversely, instrumental acts confirm a friend's affection. La Gaipa (1981) notes the convincing quality of expressing one's caring through instrumental assistance, "those actions which speak plainer than words" (p. 80).

Indeed, the interweaving of the contradictory dimensions of affection and instrumentality appears to distinguish various types of friends. For example, we found that best friendships were viewed as more intimate *as well as* more useful than were other friendship types (Rawlins et al., 1986). However, various friends' practices may blend these dimensions to constitute relationships ranging from apparently less caring but highly useful forms to tender bonds studiously avoiding utilitarian exchange. Some friendships begin with patently instrumental purposes and become quite affectionate as well, or instead; opposite trajectories can also occur. Ultimately, the friends determine the actual combination of affection and instrumentality characterizing their relationship and the particular enactment and interpretation of these aspects.

The Dialectic of Judgment and Acceptance

This dialectic articulates the interrelationship between these two interpersonal practices in shaping the communication of friends. Interaction with a friend is widely and duly celebrated for its potential to validate one's self-concept and enhance one's self-esteem (Sullivan, 1953). People are at ease with their friends because they feel liked and accepted by someone familiar with both their strengths and their weaknesses, their charming and irritating qualities. Yet, as considered in the foregoing, this legacy of acceptance masks a variety of antagonistic tendencies and negotiated practices inherent in friendships whose ongoing management subverts any permanently placid picture.

Laing (1971) stipulates that all interpersonal messages are implicitly evaluative. Even the most accepting response from another person implies an appraisal of one's self or one's actions as worthy of support. Laing (1971) further indicates that criticizing one's behavior can also be confirming since it communicates that a person is important enough to judge. It is difficult to experience another person's reactions to self as neutral. People tend to perceive positive and/or negative intentions in others' responses to them (Rawlins & Holl, 1988). Of course, individuals often intentionally formulate critical messages as negative feedback designed to curtail another's behaviors. Likewise, people purposefully indicate acceptance or encouragement of another by responding positively.

Evaluation requires criteria. One friend invokes certain standards by communicating either judgmental or accepting messages to another. Because of the nature of friendship, these messages may reflect appraisals of the friend informed by private codes developed within the friendship or by public norms. Comments may regard specific actions, ideas or feelings, the person's comportment as a friend in private or public circumstances, and/or his or her overall worth as a person. Ironically, the sanctioned friend may in turn criticize or accept the appropriateness of these remarks and/or the criteria applied.

Lack of clarity or disagreement about the source of evaluative standards for appraising the behavior of friends, and how or whether the resultant judgments should be communicated, poses continuous quandaries within friendships. For example, one friend may sharply distinguish between public and private contexts in assessing proper behavior, while the other insists that the friendship transcends such arbitrary boundaries. Moreover, some individuals or pairs of friends hold such idealistic expectations of friendship that there is the constant potential for criticism expressed over inevitable shortfalls unless, of course, their ideals preclude the friends from criticizing each other. To complicate matters, guidelines for appropriate behavior between friends change over the course of friendships and across the individuals' life cycles.

How much friends are perceived to care about each other mediates the dialectical relationship between judgment and acceptance (Rawlins & Holl, 1988). Frequently, friends will not criticize one another's failings or lapses because they care enough about each other to "look the other way." Bensman and Lilienfeld (1979) state, "Tolerance, turning a blind eye, is thus a basic requirement of intimacy" (p. 103). In contrast, we have studied adolescents who maintained that criticism could also indicate a person's concern. They felt their friends could easily accept actions that their parents criticized because their friends did not seem to care as much about them as their parents did (Rawlins & Holl, 1988). Accordingly, the boundaries shift between others' responses perceived as judicious and those viewed as judgmental. Perceptions of differential caring temper the experience of judgment and acceptance.

Acceptance remains a vital aspect of communication between friends. But it functions in a dialectical relationship with the friends' judgments. People value a friend's acceptance, especially when they know the other takes their ideas, thoughts, and actions seriously. They also appreciate judgment and criticism from a person who primarily accepts and cares about them. Particular friendships thus develop specific criteria and practices to communicate in light of this dialectical pair.

The Dialectic of Expressiveness and Protectiveness

This final principle delineates the contradictory impulses to be open and expressive and to be strategic and protective of self and/or of another while communicating in friendship (Rawlins, 1983b). Though open and trusting communicative practices often constitute a desired outcome of becoming friends, they are also the primary means for their own achievement. Thus the apt management of this dialectical principle constitutes a reflexive challenge.

Developing and maintaining a friendship conversationally involves revealing personal thoughts and feelings and commenting on the messages and actions of one's friend, in short, expressiveness. Typically, as relationships become more personal, the participants are more relaxed and expressive with each other (Bochner, 1984). However, when friends communicate more openly, they create the necessary conditions for closedness (Rawlins, 1983b). Disclosing private concerns reveals areas of personal vulnerability, and unrestrained comments on the friend's ideas or actions may uncover areas of great sensitivity.

To avoid hurting each other, friends develop protective communicative practices. Each friend tries to curb self-disclosures that render him or her too vulnerable, preserve the other's confidences and exercise restraint in commenting on topics tender to the other. Trust develops within friendships to the extent that the dialectic of expressiveness and protectiveness is appropriately managed. That is, self limits self's own vulnerability and strives to protect other's sensitivities while still expressing thoughts and feelings (Rawlins, 1983b).

Establishing and preserving trust comprises a continuous discursive challenge within the contradictory responsibilities of this dialectic. Friends expect and want to trust in the honesty of each other's remarks. However, they also trust their friends not to hurt them by candid comments on personally vulnerable issues about which only a close friend is likely to know. Self might reveal a sensitive concern to other, expecting a restrained reaction. A discreet response would reinforce self's trust in him or her. But what if the friend wants to elicit self's trust in his or her candor and, in honestly addressing the issue, hurts self? Both friends' efforts to enhance trust achieve conflicting results because contradictory assumptions inform their actions. Eventually, friends must negotiate the areas of their discourse in which exercising *restraint* furthers trust and the topics for which *candor* affirms it (Rawlins, 1983b).

No universal recommendations can specify what communicative practices will preserve trust in ongoing friendships. Throughout their relationship, friends continually confront the antagonistic tendencies of unrestrained and expressive versus strategic and protective communication.

Summary of Contextual and Interactional Dialectics

The preceding discussion of contextual and interactional dialectics exaggerates the clarity of the dilemmas and choices facing friends. These dialectics actually interweave in numerous ways. For example, the pattern of two friends' mutual independence and/or dependence will shape and reflect the nature and extent of their affection for and/or use of each other. Further, one may utilize a friend for critical appraisals, or like a friend for exercising judiciousness. Finally, the very act of revealing to or concealing from a friend implies an evaluation of the person as able or unable to handle that information.

Particular configurations of enacting these dialectical principles characterize specific friendships and types of friendships. Certain contradictions, such as publicness versus privacy and affection versus instrumentality, may be of principal significance in constituting given relationship, while other dialectics comprise secondary oppositions. Moreover, some of these friendships may be enervated by continuous tensions that result from managing the boundaries between private and public concerns and the functional expressions of affection and instrumentality. In contrast, other bonds may be negotiated or situated such that polar aspects of these dialectics are so pronounced that the friendships persist in encapsulated forms as primarily public and instrumental or private and affectionate in composition.

Significantly, then, these dialectical features of managing friendships configure and function differently according to a variety of factors. First, specific individuals will negotiate particular practices within given friendships at various stages in the development of the relationship and in light of each participant's qualities (such as gender). Second, influenced by the foregoing factors, distinct configurations of these dialectical principles develop that characterize certain types of friendships. Third, particular friendship types will exhibit different enactments of these contradictions at various stages in the friends' life cycles. Finally, the typical patterning of all of these factors will reflect the prevailing cultural practices of the moment.

These considerations emphasize the contextual and mutable nature of communication within friendships. In the next section I will employ the dialectical perspective and the contextual and interactional dialectics as critical tools for analyzing the research literature regarding young adults' friendships.

THE DEPLOYMENT OF YOUNG ADULT FRIENDSHIP: ARTICULATING SELVES, TIME, AND VALUES

Young adulthood, generally encompassing ages 20 to 30, comprises a pivotal stage for determining the role that friendships will play in one's adult life, constrained by the demands of work, love relationships, and/or family. Meanwhile, friends may provide crucial input regarding one's self-conceptions, mate selection, career options, and recreational activities. This section will sketch some praxic features of young adult friendships—how communicative and behavioral choices made within and without such dyads shape and are shaped by one's sense of self, values, and social nexus. In particular, I shall briefly examine research findings regarding the relationships among friendship, gender, marriage, and work during this period in light of previously discussed dialectical issues. Space limits a systematic analysis of cross-sex friendship here, though an initial attempt has been made elsewhere (Rawlins, 1982).

Gender and Interactional Dialectics Within Same-Sex Friendships

As ideal-types constructed from extant research, female and male friendships exhibit distinctive patterns of enacting the interactional dialectics. Overall, in managing the contradictions between independence and dependence, young adults maintain friendships because of volition, not obligation (Shulman, 1975). Moreover, they report more contact with friends than at any other adult stage except for the elderly (Williams, 1958; Verbrugge, 1983).

Although Caldwell and Peplau (1982) identified no gender differences in quantitative indicators, such as the number of intimate, good, or casual friends or the amount of time spent with friends, there is evidence that young men and women experience their similar ostensive management of the dialectic of conjunctive freedoms differently. Wright (1982) found that women typically associate the satisfactions of friendship with greater interdependence, whereas men do not. Despite quantitative similarities, men and women report qualitatively different interactions and activities with friends, implying greater interconnection of lives and dependence in women's friendships than in men's (Caldwell & Peplau, 1982; Aries & Johnson, 1983).

More dramatic distinctions are demonstrated in males' and females' management of the dialectic of affection and instrumentality. Women's friendships appear charged by ongoing tensions between the interwoven demands of caring and utility. Research reveals not only emotional sharing (Caldwell & Peplau, 1982), affective generosity (Fox, Gibbs, & Auerbach, 1985), and greater intimacy than men's bonds (Fischer & Narus, 1981) as characterizing female friendships, but also high expectations for assistance (Margolies, 1985) and "getting as well as giving" (Davidson & Packard, 1981, p. 506). How female friends manage these contradictory aspects in particular contexts can compose relationships ranging from uplifting and functional to emotionally draining and burdensome (Margolies, 1985). Constant motion and transformational potential derive from these antagonistic tendencies in women's friendships.

In contrast, male friendships are typically encapsulated by their instrumental emphasis. Consistently, males report doing things, shared activities, and instrumentality as fundamental properties of their friendships (Caldwell & Peplau, 1982; Fox et al., 1985). Men also exhibit less intimacy and affection in their friendships than women do (Williams, 1985; Fischer & Narus, 1981; Hays, 1984): what Fox et al. (1985) term a "lack of emotional involvement in friendship" (p. 499). With instrumentality clearly dominating this dialectical pair, the composition of male friendships evidences a static quality.

The differences in female versus male enactments of the dialectic of judgment and acceptance reflect prior divergences. For females a highly charged dialectical relationship between these two practices persists because women seem to care more and be more involved with their friends (Fischer, 1981). Wright (1982) indicates that women tend to identify and confront problematic practices and sources of discord in their friendships. Moreover, they are likely to withdraw gradually from the relationship if they cannot resolve the issue. Fox et al. (1985) also remark on the fragility of women's friendships that results from this propensity for addressing disturbing issues. Wright (1982) notes, however, that women who elect to accept their friends and not to confront areas of disagreement try to preserve the friendship, presumably because of their affection for the friend.

A weak opposition between these evaluative tendencies typifies men's friendships; unconcerned acceptance that results from less involvement prevails. Thus males do not criticize their friends much, but neither do they communicate robust acceptance. Wright (1982) describes how males sidestep problematic facets and emphasize the more serene areas of their friendships. Echoing this finding, Fox et al. (1985) depict men as "reluctant to confront friends about bothersome attitudes or behaviors" (p. 493). This apparent tendency to accept friends' foibles can be interpreted positively, but these practices seem to derive more from a superficial judgment of the friend's value and minimal caring. In contrast to women, Wright (1982) observes the nearly even chances that "a man who decides against confronting such strain will eventually terminate the friendship without ever bringing up the troublesome issue" (p. 14).

The patterns of expressiveness and protectiveness identified in women's and men's friendships have been extensively documented and closely parallel those of judgment and acceptance. Female friendships manifest considerable expressiveness; male friendships exhibit much more protectiveness. As considered in the foregoing, women tend to confront their friends even at the risk of severing the bond, whereas men are inclined to skirt threatening issues. In addition, women share more emotional concerns, personal feelings and values (Davidson & Packard, 1981; Tokuno, 1983; Aries & Johnson, 1983). On the contrary, men limit their vulnerability by revealing less about themselves to their friends, avoiding the discussion of feelings or personal issues and focusing more on activities and objective issues such as sports or politics (Davidson & Packard, 1981; Davidson & Duberman, 1982; Tokuno, 1983; Aries & Johnson, 1983).

Indeed, a degree of concern, affection, or involvement appears necessary to animate the contradictions of judgment and acceptance and expressiveness and protectiveness. A given relationship may be too superficial for these antagonistic tendencies to compose its practices significantly. Yet, every interaction within a more interlaced bond may bristle with critical versus accepting overtones and expressive versus protective dilemmas. The potential for two friends' practices to transform their relationship from one type to another always exists.

Thus far I have examined gender-linked patterns in managing the interactional dialectics abstracted from empirical research. The actual configurations of these practices within a specific friendship and their functional or dysfunctional implications derive from and contribute to its place within the two individuals' social matrix of relationships, which include marriage and work affiliations.

Marriage and Young Adult Friendship

As young adulthood unfolds, the typical middle-class American encounters important developmental tasks that include entering the adult world of work, developing personal relationships of varying degrees of intimacy and commitment, and consolidating one's identity (Tokuno, 1986). Critical incidents in any of these processes have ramifications throughout the others. Without commitments to a career or spouse, and with diminished contact with kin, the young single adult has time to spend with other friends in similar circumstances (Shulman, 1975). Through shared activities and interaction, this network of friends helps them shape each other's values and self-conceptions and influences choices of career paths and spouses (Shulman, 1975; Tokuno, 1983).

A friend's marriage sponsors the most sweeping changes in singles' friendship practices (Brown, 1981). Accordingly, there is ambivalent interplay among friendship, courtship, and marriage. Friends aid in mate selection and are frequently involved in a couple's original meeting (Ryder, Kafka, & Olson,

1971). However, when a friend is perceived as too involved with someone, efforts at sabotaging the courtship often occur, including highlighting the prospective mate's faults and siding with the friend in quarrels (Ryder et al., 1971). Yet when a marital commitment is announced, friends will shift from criticism to acceptance; instead of expressing misgivings, they will practice self-restraint to protect the engaged friend's images of self and his or her prospective mate (Mayer, 1957).

Later courtship and early marriage strikingly constrict friendship networks. Each spouse's contact with peripheral friends disappears and gradually diminishes with close friends (Milardo, Johnson, & Huston, 1983). Following marriage, both males and females confide less in all of their friends (Booth & Hess, 1974). Within the marriage, problems develop regarding the blending of spouses' individual friendship networks, concerns about acceptance by the partner's friend and each spouse's freedom to see his or her own friends (Dickson-Markman & Markman, in press; Ryder et al., 1971). To deal with conflicts generated by opposing choices of individual friends, married pairs often develop "couple friendships" (Ryder et al., 1971; Hess, 1972). This practice thoroughly constrains the identity-building possibilities of self-chosen dyadic friendships in the interests of marital stability (Askham, 1976). As time passes, married partners repeatedly face the desire for and challenge of selecting and maintaining both couple and individual friendships that can survive both spouses' scrutiny and fit into increasingly restricted schedules.

Work and Young Adult Friendship

Rivaling marriage in its eventual impact on young adults' friendships, values, and self-conceptions is the career choice. Almost imperceptible in their omnipresence, the demands of a serious commitment to work redefine an individual's world view and practical management of everyday living. Henry (1971, pp 127, 131) observes:

> Man [*sic*] at work *is* at work—working through on a daily basis, his views of himself, the tasks set by his work environment, his hopes for future relationship and rewards.... The world of work takes our time, molds our daily interactions, structures our beliefs and values.

Initially, friendships with coworkers are uncommon for single young adults, possibly reflecting their attempts to preserve previously existing and more encompassing relationships (Verbrugge, 1979). However, having already commenced rearranging their friendship networks and realizing the limited time for independent bonds, married young adults are more likely to mention coworker friends (Verbrugge, 1979). Other factors influence the likelihood of friendship at work. Fine (1986) cites the physical setting, specific type of job, and organizational culture as either facilitating or subverting employees' autonomy and/or willingness to engage coworkers. Further, most organizational norms limit friendships to people with equal status, except for mentoring (Kurth, 1970; Fine, 1986). The ideologies of certain types of work also affect friendship possibilities. For example, Parker (1964) discovered that people in service professions evidenced a much greater probability of close friends in similar or related work than business executives did. Finally, individuals so deeply involved with their work that they have few contacts outside of it tend to become friends with coworkers (Parker, 1964; Verbrugge, 1979).

Though developed under the rubric of friendship, work affiliations range from patently "friendly relations" to more involved bonds transcending the work setting (Kurth, 1970). The former may compose a "friendly career" in which friendships are primarily cultivated and strategically employed to further one's job advancement (Maines, 1981). Friendly networks premised on members' status and instrumental capabilities (Bensman & Lilienfeld, 1979; Fine, 1986) often replace the friendship networks based on a blend of caring, utility, and personal characteristics that predated work preoccupations. These networks persist only to the extent that they are successfully used (Bensman & Lilienfeld, 1979). The shifting sands of promotion and demotion render some friends expendable.

Involvement with a work friend risks the complexities of personal versus professional appraisals and obligations, and activates the contradictions of private versus public enactments of the relationship, and idealized versus realized blends of affection and instrumentality and judgment and acceptance. Suppose one friend has access to resources or information that could help the other but is restricted by corporate policy. This person may feel respected professionally if the friend does not ask him or her to compromise public rules but may also be insulted personally, especially if it would provide an important opportunity to be of service. Even so, too frequent or extensive requests may also be offensive (Bensman & Lilienfeld, 1979). Both one's influence at work and the friendship's definition are tested by how and whether demands are made and the nature and interpretation of the privileged friend's response. Not asking a friend may suggest limited openness between the friends, and refusal to accept constraints on the friend's freedom to help could be seen as lacking trust in his or her good intentions (Bensman & Lilienfeld, 1979).

Moreover, how will other employees view the assisting friend? Perceived favoritism could damage both friends' credibility in the organization (Davis & Todd, 1982). Davis and Todd (1982) remark, "A person valuing loyalty over appearance may favor friends and punish enemies within the organization. A person valuing fairness and impartiality above all may be evenhanded to the point of coldness in dealing with friends within the organizations" (p. 85). But what if the two persons in this quotation are parties to the same friendship? How are such predicaments realistically managed in light of contradictory public and private interpretations of the ideal friend or professional? Eisenstadt (1974, p. 142) synoptically observes:

> It is because of this emphasis on pure symbolic relations—which at the same time cannot escape the problems of struggle over power and resources—that these relationships are potentially both very brittle and heavily laden emotionally. Only when they shade off into mere "acquaintance" can these tensions disappear, to erupt once again if either party tries to transform the relationship into one of more "basic" or "real" friendship.

The prevailing practices of male friendship conform well with the ambivalent friendship ethic of the working world. To the extent that a man is accustomed to friendships emphasizing independence, instrumentality, withheld personal judgments, token acceptance, and carefully measured expressiveness, managing work relationships is easier. In fact, these friendships function to cement the sense of self and personal values accompanying a thorough commitment to the values of an organization (Whyte, 1965).

In contrast, to the degree that a woman engages in friendships stressing interdependence, a vital interpenetration of affection and instrumentality, caring criticisms and heartfelt acceptance, and extensive confidence and candor, the glib "hail-fellow-well-met" style of working world friendships may seem alien and/or unethical. Adjusting to these practices may prove difficult and ultimately situational if she attempts to form her customary brand of friendships with female and/or male colleagues.

Frequently, both men and women become more adept at "the structured use of personal associates" (Feld, 1984). Careful distinctions are made between relationships of "convenience" and "commitment" to correspond with the segmented quality of adult life (Feld, 1984). Yet research suggests that an individual's pattern of discriminating friends may say as much about the chooser as the chosen. Snyder and Smith's (1986) synthesis of self-monitoring research reports that high self-monitors tend to develop situation-specific, activity-oriented, instrumental friendships allowing them to exhibit multiple identities across various contexts; and their close friends are higher self-monitors than are their casual friends. By comparison, low self-monitors negotiate personal disposition-oriented, affective, emotional friendships that permit them to enact a consistent, principled self across contexts; and their close friends are lower self-monitors than are their acquaintances (Snyder & Smith, 1986).

Snyder and Smith (1986) may be identifying people with clear yet different evaluative standards for selecting and appraising close friendships. High self-monitors are sensitive to public appearances and objective expectations for excellence in specific activities, whereas low self-monitors are more concerned with private dictates and subjective codes regarding adherence to personal standards, regardless of setting. Interestingly, Snyder and Smith

(1986) found no reliable gender differences, implying that self-monitoring research may tap underlying "orientations to friendship" (p. 66) missed by other studies. Despite many dissimilarities, Wright (1982) argues that women's and men's best and most longstanding friendships transcend gender-associated divergencies.

Middle-class young adulthood begins with considerable time for friends and multiple options for ways of life and identity consolidation. Ironically, the praxic functions of friendships at this stage involve helping each other make decisions regarding self, marriage, and career, which ultimately constrict the valuation of and opportunities for involvement with friends.

CONCLUSION

This monograph demonstrates the utility and richness of viewing interpersonal communication in relationships from a dialectical perspective, including totality, contradiction, motion, and praxis as its basic elements. Analyzed as a totality, communicating in friendships inherently involves the interconnection and reciprocal influence of multiple factors. The contextual dialectics of private and public domains, and ideal and real attributes give meaning to and derive significance from the various configurations of interactional dialectics that friends negotiate and articulate through their actual communicative practices in everyday situations. How friends manage the interactional dialectics of conjunctive freedoms, affection and instrumentality, judgment and acceptance, and expressiveness and protectiveness reflects each friend's gender, life course stage, and personal circumstances, as well as the stage of the relationship's development and currently favored cultural practices. The parties' mutual enactment and management of these interlayered facets constitute their friendship as a dynamic totality.

Contradictions are central features of a dialectical perspective. These antagonistic yet interdependent aspects of communication between friends comprise the bases for the routine as well as the volatile and transitional moments of such dyads; they form their pulse. Individuals and social relationships continually alter and develop through internally generated oppositions, contradictions between individual and relational functioning, and disjunctions between particular relationships and their cultural context.

A dialectical perspective views motion as constant in social domains. The present state of any relationship is considered an incessant achievement. Configurations of constitutive and emergent contradictions produce the potential for the transformational or encapsulating motion characterizing various friendships. Accordingly, I underscore the importance of deciphering principal and secondary contradictions and aspects of contradictions, and the intensity of their interplay for understanding how enacting countervailing tendencies within friendships generates differential possibilities for significant changes in relational practices or slightly altered editions of the status quo.

The concept of praxis delineates the human communicator as the ongoing producer and product of his or her own choices. Throughout this analysis, individuals are depicted as conscious, active selectors of possible choices from a field that is partially conceived by them, partially negotiated with others, and partially determined by social and natural factors outside of their purview. In any case, the choices a person makes simultaneously engender and restrict options. Because of the contradictory and interrelated nature of interaction within friendship, there are unanticipated consequences of interacting in particular ways to which the communicators must then adapt.

I employed these principles to examine the interconnections among gender, marriage, and work in composing the practices of young adult friendship. Studying friendship reveals the seams of the multiple social systems in which we live. Young adult life becomes increasingly compartmentalized and friendships are conditional (Lopata, 1981). A dialectical perspective emphasizes that these exigencies affecting friendship in given cases are not abstract trends, but the ongoing products of active human choices.

Time and energy are finite. Individual and negotiated choices regarding marriage, children, career, civic involvement, and leisure reflect and influence self-conceptions and begin to articulate networks of human relationships within which one's values and priorities are continuously enacted. Simultaneously, these pursuits also generate constraints typically patterning the forms and functions of one's friendships at any juncture, owing to their marginal status and total reliance on voluntary effort for continued existence.

Consequently, the ways in which friendships are managed, the bases for distinctions among friends, and the overall significance of friendship in a given adult's existential milieu are strongly indicative of his or her self-defining values. Discriminating among people in developing friendships and managing dialectical contingencies produce modes of interaction which shape and are shaped by certain modes of being a person. Individuals' self-conceptions and conceptions of personal relationships are continually devised and revised as friendships are negotiated within various social systems exhibiting diverse public and private exigencies and evaluative standards.

REFERENCES

Allan, G. A. (1979). *A sociology of friendship and kinship*. London: Allen & Unwin.

Altman, I., Vinsel, A., & Brown, B. B. (1981). Dialectic conceptions in social psychology: An application to social penetration and privacy regulation. In L. Berkowitz (Ed.), *Advances in experimental social psychology* (Vol. 14, pp. 107-160). London: Academic Press.

Annas, J. (1977). Plato and Aristotle on friendship and altruism. *Mind, 86*, 532-554.

Aries, E. J., & Johnson, F. L. (1983). Close friendship in adulthood: Conversational content between same-sex friends. *Sex Roles, 9*, 1183-1196.

Aristotle. (1980). *The Nichomachean ethics.* (D. Ross, Trans.). Oxford: Oxford University Press.
Askham, J. (1976). Identity and stability within the marriage relationship. *Journal of Marriage and the Family, 38,* 535-547.
Ball, R. A. (1979). The dialectical method: Its application to social theory. *Social Forces, 57,* 785-798.
Bellah, R. N., Madsen, R., Sullivan, W. M., Swidler, A., & Tipton, S. M. (1985). *Habits of the heart: Individualism and commitment in American life.* Berkeley: University of California Press.
Benjamin, J. (1983). The Greek concept of dialectic. *The Southern Speech Communication Journal, 48,* 356-367.
Bensman, J., & Lilienfeld, R. (1979). *Between public and private: The lost boundaries of the self.* New York: Free Press.
Benson, J. K. (1973). The analysis of bureaucratic-professional conflict: Functional versus dialectical approaches. *The Sociological Quarterly, 14,* 376-394.
Berger, R., & Luckman, T. (1966). *The social construction of reality.* Garden City, NY: Doubleday.
Bloch, M. (1971). The moral and tactical meaning of kinship terms. *Man, 6,* 79-87.
Bochner, A. (1984). Functions of communication in interpersonal bonding. In C. Arnold & J. Bowers (Eds.), *Handbook of rhetoric and communication theory* (pp. 544-621). Boston: Allyn & Bacon.
Booth, A., & Hess, E. (1974). Cross-sex friendship. *Journal of Marriage and the Family, 36,* 38-47.
Bopp, M. J., & Weeks, G. R. (1984). Dialectical metatheory in family therapy. *Family Process, 23,* 49-61.
Brain, R. (1976). *Friends and lovers.* New York: Basic Books.
Brown, B. B. (1981). A life-span approach to friendship: Age-related dimensions of an ageless relationship. In H. Z. Lopata & D. Maines (Eds.), *Research in the interweave of social roles: Friendship* (Vol. 2, pp. 23-50). Greenwich, CT: JAI.
Caldwell, M. A., & Peplau, L. A. (1982). Sex differences in same-sex friendship. *Sex Roles, 8,* 721-732.
Davidson, L. R., & Duberman, L. (1982). Friendship: Communication and interactional patterns in same-sex dyads. *Sex Roles, 8,* 809-826.
Davidson, S., & Packard, T. (1981). The therapeutic value of friendship between women. *Psychology of Women Quarterly, 5,* 495-510.
Davis, K. E., & Todd, M. J. (1982). Friendship and love relationships. In K. E. Davis & T. Mitchell (Eds.), *Advances in descriptive psychology* (Vol. 2, pp. 79-122). Greenwich, CT: JAI.
Dickson-Markman, F., & Markman, H. J. (In press). The effects of others on marriage: Do they help or hurt? In P. Noller & M. A. Fitzpatrick (Eds.), *Perspectives on marital interaction.* Philadelphia: Multilingual Matters.
DuBois, C. (1974). The gratuitous act: An introduction to the comparative study of friendship patterns. In E. Leyton (Ed.), *The compact: Selected dimensions of friendship* (pp. 117-137). St. John's: Institute of Social and Economic Research.
Eisenstadt, S. N. (1974). Friendship and the structure of trust and solidarity in society. In E. Leyton (Ed.), *The compact: Selected dimensions of friendship* (pp. 138-145). St. John's: Institute of Social and Economic Research.
Feld, N. (1984). The structured use of personal associates. *Social Forces, 62,* 640-652.
Fine, G. A. (1986). Friendships in the work place. In V. J. Derlega & B. A. Winstead (Eds.), *Friendship and social interaction* (pp. 185-206). New York: Springer-Verlag.
Fischer, J. L. (1981). Transitions in relationship style from adolescence to young adulthood. *Journal of Youth and Adolescence, 10,* 11-23.
Fischer, J. L., & Narus, L. R., Jr. (1981). Sex roles and intimacy in same sex and other sex relationships. *Psychology of Women Quarterly, 5,* 444-455.

Fox, M., Gibbs, M., & Auerbach, D. (1985). Age and gender dimensions of friendship. *Psychology of Women Quarterly, 9,* 489-502.

Handelman, D. (1984). Inside-out, outside in: Concealment and revelation in Newfoundland Christmas mumming. In E. M. Bruner (Ed.), *Text, play, and story: The construction and reconstruction of self and society: 1983 proceedings of the American Ethnological Society* (pp. 247-277). Washington, DC: American Ethnological Society.

Harre, R. (1977). Friendship as an accomplishment: An ethogenic approach to social relationships. In S. Duck (Ed.), *Theory and practice in interpersonal attraction* (pp. 339-354). London: Academic Press.

Hays, R. B. (1984). The development and maintenance of friendship. *Journal of Social and Personal Relationships, 1,* 75-98.

Hegel, G.W.F. (1966). *The phenomenology of mind.* London: Allen & Unwin.

Henry, W. E. (1971). The role of work in structuring the life cycle. *Human Development, 14,* 125-131.

Hess, B. (1972). Friendship. In M. W. Riley, M. Johnson, & A. Foner (Eds.), *Aging and society: A sociology of age stratification* (Vol. 3, pp. 357-393). New York: Russell Sage.

Israel, J. (1979). *The language of dialectics and the dialectics of language.* Brighton, Great Britain: Harvester.

Jacobson, D. (1976). Fair weather friend: Label and context in middle-class friendships. In W. Arens & S. P. Montague (Eds.), *The American dimension* (pp. 149-160). New York: Alfred.

Kieve, R. A. (1983). The Hegelian inversion: On the possibility of a Marxist dialectic. *Science and Society, 47,* 37-65.

Knapp, M. L., Ellis, D. G., and Williams, B. A. (1980). Perceptions of communication behavior associated with relationship terms. *Communication Monographs 47,* 262-278.

Kurth, S. B. (1970). Friendships and friendly relations: In G. J. McCall (Ed.), *Social relationships* (pp. 136-170). Chicago: Aldine.

La Gaipa, J. J. (1981). Children's friendships. In S. Duck & R. Gilmour (Eds.), *Personal relationships: Developing personal relations* (Vol. 2, pp. 161-185). New York: Academic Press.

Laing, R. D. (1971). *Self and others.* Middlesex: Penguin.

Liebow, E. (1967). *Tally's corner.* Boston: Little & Brown.

Lopata, H. Z. (1981). Friendship: Historical and theoretical introduction. In H. Z. Lopata & D. Maines (Eds.), *Research in the interweave of social roles: Friendship* (Vol. 2, pp. 1-19). Greenwich, CT: JAI.

Maines, D. R. (1981). The organizational and career contexts of friendship among postdoctoral students. In H. Z. Lopata & D. Maines (Eds.), *Research in the interweave of social roles: Friendship* (Vol. 2, pp. 171-195). Greenwich, CT: JAI.

Mao Tse-Tung (1966). *Four essays on philosophy.* Peking: Foreign Language Press.

Marcuse, H. (1964). *Reason and revolution.* Boston: Beacon Press.

Margolies, E. (1985). *The best of friends, the worst of enemies.* Garden City: Doubleday.

Marquit, E. (1981). Contradictions in dialectics and formal logic. *Science and Society, 45,* 306-323.

Mayer, J. E. (1957). The self-restraint of friends: A mechanism in family transition. *Social Forces, 35,* 230-238.

Milardo, R. M., Johnson, M. P., & Huston, T. L. (1983). Developing close relationships: Changing patterns of interaction between pair members and social networks. *Journal of Personality and Social Psychology, 44,* 964-976.

Mills, J., & Clark, M. S. (1982). Exchange and communal relationships. In L. Wheeler (Ed.), *Review of personality and social psychology* (Vol. 3, pp. 121-144). Beverly Hills, CA: Sage.

Mirkovic, D. (1980). *Dialectic and sociological thought.* St. Catharines, Ontario: Diliton.

Naegele, K. D. (1958). Friendship and acquaintances: An exploration of some social distinctions. *Harvard Educational Review, 28,* 232-252.

Paine, R. (1969). In search of friendship: An exploratory analysis in "middle-class" culture. *Man, 4,* 505-524.
Paine, R. (1970). Anthropological approaches to friendship. *Humanitas, 6,* 139-159.
Parker, S. R. (1964). Type of work, friendship patterns, and leisure. *Human Relations, 17,* 215-220.
Parsons, E. C. (1915). Friendship, a social category. *American Journal of Sociology, 21,* 230-233.
Peters, G. R., & Kennedy, C. A. (1970). Close friendships in the college community. *The Journal of College Student Personnel, 11,* 449-456.
Rake, J. M. (1970). Friendship: A fundamental description of its subjective dimension. *Humanitas, 6,* 161-176.
Rawlins, W. K. (1982). Cross-sex friendship and the communicative management of sex-role expectations. *Communication Quarterly, 30,* 343-352.
Rawlins, W. K. (1983a). Negotiating close friendship: The dialectic of conjunctive freedoms. *Human Communication Research, 9,* 255-266.
Rawlins, W. K. (1983b). Openness as problematic in ongoing friendships: Two conversational dilemmas. *Communication Monographs, 50,* 1-13.
Rawlins, W. K. (1985). Stalking interpersonal communication effectiveness: Social, individual or situational integration? In T. W. Benson (Ed.) *Speech communication in the twentieth century* (pp. 109-129). Carbondale: Southern Illinois University Press.
Rawlins, W. K., & Holl, M. (1987). The communicative achievement of friendship during adolescence: Predicaments of trust and violation. *Western Journal of Speech Communication, 51,* 345-363.
Rawlins, W. K., & Holl, M. (1988). Adolescents' interactions with parents and friends: Dialectics of temporal perspective and evaluation. *Journal of Social and Personal Relationships, 5,* 27-46.
Rawlins, W. K., Leibowitz, K., & Bochner, A. P. (1986). Affective and instrumental dimensions of best, equal, and unequal friendships. *Central States Speech Journal, 37,* 90-101.
Riegel, K. F. (1976). The dialectics of human development. *American Psychologist, 31,* 689-700.
Rose, S., & Serafica, F. C. (1986). Keeping and ending casual, close and best friendships. *Journal of Social and Personal Relationships, 3,* 275-288.
Rossi, I. (1983). *From the sociology of symbols to the sociology of signs.* New York: Columbia University Press.
Ryder, R. G., Kafka, J. S., & Olson, D. H. (1971). Separating and joining influences in courtship and early marriage. *American Journal of Orthopsychiatry, 41,* 450-464.
Sampson, E. E. (1977). Psychology and the American ideal. *Journal of Personality and Social Psychology, 35,* 767-782.
Sayers, S. (1982). Contradiction and dialectic in the development of science. *Science and Society, 45,* 409-436.
Sennett, R. (1978). *The fall of the public man.* New York: Vintage.
Shulman, N. (1975). Life-cycle variations in patterns of close relationships. *Journal of Marriage and the Family, 37,* 813-820.
Snyder, M., & Smith, D. (1986). Personality and friendship: The friendship worlds of self-monitoring. In V. J. Derlega & B. A. Winstead (Eds.), *Friendship and social interaction* (pp. 63-80). New York: Springer-Verlag.
Sullivan, H. S. (1953). *Interpersonal theory of psychiatry.* New York: Norton.
Suttles, G. D. (1970). Friendship as a social institution. In G. J. McCall (Ed.), *Social relationships* (pp. 95-135). Chicago: Aldine.
Szwed, J. F. (1969). The mask of friendship: Mumming as a ritual of social relations. In H. Halpert & G. M. Story (Eds.), *Christmas mumming in Newfoundland* (pp. 105-118). Toronto: University of Toronto Press.
Tokuno, K. A. (1983). Friendship and transition in early adulthood. *The Journal of Genetic Psychology, 143,* 207-216.

Tokuno, K. A. (1986). The early adult transition and friendships: Mechanisms of support. *Adolescence, 21,* 593-606.

Van Vlissingen, J. F. (1970). Friendship in history. *Humanitas, 6,* 225-238.

Verbrugge, L. M. (1977). The structure of adult friendship choices. *Social Forces, 56,* 576-597.

Verbrugge, L. M. (1979). Multiplexity in adult friendships. *Social Forces, 57,* 1286-1309.

Verbrugge, L. M. (1983). A research note on adult friendship contact: A dyadic perspective. *Social Forces, 62,* 78-83.

Wells, S. (1985). *The dialectics of representation.* Baltimore: Johns Hopkins University Press.

Whyte, W. H., Jr. (1965). *The organization man.* New York: Simon & Schuster.

Williams, D. G. (1985). Gender, masculinity-femininity, and emotional intimacy in same-sex friendship. *Sex Roles, 12,* 587-600.

Williams, J. H. (1958). Close friendship relations of housewives residing in an urban community. *Social Forces, 36,* 358-362.

Williams, R. M., Jr. (1959). Friendship and social values in a suburban community: An exploratory study. *The Pacific Sociological Review, 2,* 3-10.

Wiseman, J. P. (1986). Friendship: Bonds and binds in a voluntary relationship. *Journal of Social and Personal Relationships, 3,* 191-211.

Wozniak, R. H. (1975). Dialecticism and structuralism: The philosophical foundation of Soviet psychology and Piagetian cognitive developmental theory. In K. F. Riegel & G. C. Rosenwald (Eds.), *Structure and transformation: Developmental and historical aspects* (pp. 25-45). New York: John Wiley.

Wright, P. H. (1982). Men's friendships, women's friendships, and the alleged inferiority of the latter. *Sex Roles, 8,* 1-20.

Wright, P. H. (1984). Self-referent motivation and the intrinsic quality of friendship. *Journal of Social and Personal Relationships, 1,* 115-130.

Yuan, Y. (1973, September). *Affectivity and instrumentality in friendship: An examination of friendship patterns among American women.* Paper presented at the Ninth International Congress of Anthropological and Ethnological Sciences.

Further Dialectics: Strangers, Friends, and Historical Transformations

DAVID R. MAINES
Pennsylvania State University

IF scholars in the humanities and social sciences reason honestly enough, they will eventually find themselves faced with inevitable, but I hope not paralyzing, uncertainties. This inevitability has always unsettled the hegemony of rationalism which has manifestly driven Western societies during the past four centuries. Formal rationalism, ultimately the legacy of Greek geometry and Western dualistic philosophy, presses its major influence now in the form of computerized thought. As everyone knows, however, such thought cannot map human thought. Nor can computerized language map human natural language. The situation facing such efforts, and indeed facing the entire rationalistic thrust, is that humans are incorrigibly ambiguous. That ambiguity, inherent in human communicative conduct, resists and grinds against the rationalistic disposition toward ever-increasing theoretical and metric precision, which rests at the center of contemporary logico-deductive research (Levine, 1985). Honest, careful thinking would recognize this fact.

Of course, there are many sources of human ambiguity and uncertainty, the vast majority of which are related to the evolutionary release of humans from the dictates of instincts and the emergence of symbolic communication so characteristic of our species. In the course of that evolution, humans have invented countless things, and among those "things" are three extremely complex and consequential processes: reflexive time, symbol systems, and

AUTHOR'S NOTE: Discussions with Elaine Bass Jenks, Sandy Rawlins, Bill Rawlins, and Norman Denzin helped to sharpen several of the points made in this essay.

Correspondence and requests for reprints: David R. Maines, Department of Sociology, 206 Oswald Tower, Pennsylvania State University, University Park, PA 16802.

Communication Yearbook 12, pp. 190-202

social contexts. These three processes and their structural arrangements intersect and interpenetrate in profound ways to provide much of what we call human society. Humans communicate about time and within time; they temporally organize their communication and discourse; they create the circumstances and situations within which and about which they communicatively act; they build up communication and temporal structures and technologies that then constrain and shape the conduct they form (Blumer, 1962; Brown, 1987; Duncan, 1968; Innis, 1951; Bateson, 1972). In other words, given their evolutionary heritage, human beings and their societies have become inherently dialectical in character. The various ontologies and metaphors proposed as basic human nature—purposeful, profit-driven, mechanistic, antagonistic, playful, and so on—must therefore bow to the basic proposition that humans transform themselves and their environments through communication and then respond to those transformations (see Stone and Farberman, 1970).

It seems to me that Professor Rawlins profoundly understands that proposition and thus is freed from the struggle of recognizing the problem of ambiguity. He assumes from the outset that human experience is never totally unambiguous and that human conduct is inherently emergent. In its most general expression, the analytical situation immediately presented by that recognition is the relation between continuity and discontinuity, and the most general expression of that relation is given in dialectical analysis. As Mead (1929; 1932) brilliantly showed, continuity and discontinuity constitute one another. They depend on one another for their existence: "The continuity is always of some quality, but as present passes into present there is always some break in the continuity—within the continuity, not of the continuity. The break reveals the continuity, while the continuity is the background for the novelty" (Mead, 1929, p. 239; see also Maines, Sugrue, & Katovich, 1983). The dialectic of the predictable and unpredictable, of social structure, and the episodic, of boredom and chaos, thus constitute the enduring circumstance of our evolutionary loss of instincts. It is within these dialectics that the problem of meaning and interpretation rests. And, as I have reflected on Rawlins's analysis of friendship, it is within the dialectical nature of human existence—of continuity and discontinuity—that he has very honestly and powerfully located a conceptual scheme that systematically, but without the pretensions of scientific precision, reveals the dialectics of friendship.

Accordingly, my response to Rawlins's analysis will take the form of an extension of his ideas. In doing so, I will first present a brief analytical summary of his argument that will serve to frame other dialectical processes that have an important bearing on understanding friendship relations. Next I will discuss the historical transformation of (1) strangers and friends and (2) the ecology of friendship. I will conclude by offering a critical assessment of selected aspects of contemporary work on friendship that will be related to what I see Rawlins attempting to accomplish.

RAWLINS'S DIALECTICAL PERSPECTIVE

Friendship is a form of relatedness (in Simmel's, 1950, sense of the word) that contains several elements. The most important element, emphasized by Rawlins and others (e.g., Matthews, 1986), is that it is a noninstitutionalized relationship. Friendship begins and ends with the participants; it is maintained and sustained by them; it is transformed by them; its existence depends minimally upon dyadic existence. This is not the case with institutionalized relations, such as a marriage. Marital relationships are created and terminated by legal and religious institutions rather than by those who become married. People must be legally, and in some cases religiously, qualified to invoke or avail themselves of a set of rules that then create the relationship. By the same token, it is a set of rules that is activated by those who qualify that ends the marriage. Thus husbands and wives, who out of choice have not communicated for years, who choose to live in different parts of the country, and who have no plans whatsoever to have anything ever to do with one another, still have a marital relationship. They cannot terminate the relationship simply by ceasing to act in the capacity of husband or wife. Yet, that is all it takes to terminate a friendship. There are no rules, few criteria, and no public forum that regulates the flow into and out of friendships. It is the epitome of a self-regulated relationship.

It is this element that gives special warrant to Rawlins's focus on tensions and strategic choice in friendships. But such tensions are not merely hassles or bad feelings or role strain; neither are choices merely linear decision-making processes. These tensions and choices are points of inseparability between personal selves and cultural forms (see Maines, 1984). They are struggles with authenticity (see Denzin, 1984, ch. 5), which are informed by cultural contradictions and channeled through communicative contradictions. Friendship is a process as well as a form of creation and the creation and recreation of a form. It is a pattern of participation that cannot be separated from other patterns of participation (Rawlins's totality dimension), it is a continuous interpretive process that is shaped in part by built-in incompatibilities (the contradiction dimension); it is temporal (the motion dimension); and it is reflexive (the praxis dimension). In this perspective, ambiguity and uncertainty are lodged in movement and the multiple contexts of friendship formation and maintenance. Together ambiguity and uncertainty generate an ongoing interpretive problematic. The dimensions of the dialectical perspective Rawlins discusses allow the analyst to chart that interpretive problematic insofar as "configurations of contradictions compose and organize friendships through an ongoing process of change" (p. 164). That charting, though, can be done only in terms of viewing participants as enacting those dialectics (p. 163). The dialectics of public versus private, of affection versus instrumentalism, of ideal versus the real, of independence versus dependence, and so on, represent issues and concerns that enter into the relationship and that the participants in some way must take into account, whether through negotiation, avoidance, conflict, compromise, or some other mode.

Friendships in Rawlins's analysis thus centrally involve the *configuring* of relationships, which is a view similar to other conceptualizations such as Glaser and Strauss's (1968) concept of structural process, Giddens's (1984) notion of structuration, and Goffman's (1967) treatment of enacted ritual. Young adulthood, as Rawlins shows, contains a number of configuring factors: gender is a primary element that organizes friendships into different patterns, and the "role pile-up" (Hill et al., 1970) of young adulthood entails the simultaneous demands and management of work, education, and marital decisions. The configuring factors of young adulthood reach into the selves of friends as they attempt to form lives with meaning (Maines & Hardesty, 1987) and outward to the large-scale organization of labor force demands, gender stratification systems, and educational timetables. The configurations of contradictions that organize friendships thus collapse the micro and macro orders into meso orders (see Maines, 1982) of ongoing interpretive processes and multiple overlapping contextualizations.

Rawlins appropriately and explicitly takes the position that "dialectical inquiries are intrinsically historical investigations concerned with the developmental and historical specificity of the process in question" (p. 164). I draw two central concepts from this position—context and temporality—that can be added to a third—communication—which is what Rawlins's analysis is about. Though Rawlins focuses most sharply and clearly on interpersonal relations, there is nothing in his perspective that inhibits the analysis of larger scale dialectics of friendships. Indeed, his perspective invites such analysis. Having completed my analytical summary, I therefore turn to my next area of concern that pertains to two historical transformations of the contexts of friendship.

TRANSFORMATION AND CONTEXTS

Rawlins legitimately locates his analysis in the context of contemporary Western society. These societies are urbanized, highly mobile, tourist-inhabited, compartmentalized, secular, and dominated by the electronic media. His dialectics speak to such societal arrangements, and the friendships of his analysis seek authenticity and meaning in terms of those arrangements. As I have indicated, however, his perspective is invitingly rich with suggestions of other aspects of friendship. It is in the spirit of interest and acceptance of that invitation that I take up the following issues that pertain to other contexts and processes relevant to the dialectics of friendship.

Strangers and friends. To most, there is nothing unusual about living among persons one does not know. We live in a world of strangers, as Lyn Lofland (1973) says. Indeed, much of our current terminology regarding friendship is premised on the existence of large numbers of strangers in our social environments—Milgram's "familiar strangers," Kurth's (1970) "friendly relations," Burns's (1953) "fictional friends," and so forth, to include buddies, soul brothers, best friends, acquaintances, life partners, confidants, cliques, old friends, family friends, pals, sidekicks, and main squeezes. That we have so many terms that differentiate types of relationships and basically only one term designating nonrelationships—*strangers*—makes sense in our world. After all, these various terms signify relational meaning to the participants. But I think the numerous terms for friendship and intimate relations signify something else as well, namely that such relations are significantly more problematic in our times than are the anonymous relations with strangers. Modern society struggles with intimacy. It is almost axiomatic in our culture, for example, to acknowledge the paradox of intimacy; that it involves deeply satisfying shared experiences and nurturance as well as enormous vulnerability and risk. Date rape, family violence, murder, marital deception, and the guarded trust of associates common to friendly relations testifies to intimacy and friendship as a cultural problematic. Such problematics, moreover, can be seen as good for the gross national product insofar as they generate (or are generated by) countless service sector occupations, such as counseling centers, self-help groups, therapists of all varieties, how-to books, hot lines, and, less directly, diet plans and exercise programs. The paradox of intimacy is embedded not only in our cultural values, as Rawlins discusses, but in our social structure.

By comparison, strangers are not nearly as problematic as close relationships. The members of modern societies have accommodated their large populations by becoming competent at the ritual exchanges and mechanisms of mutual avoidance between strangers (Goffman, 1963). And such relations are not nearly as dangerous as those between intimates or acquaintances. True, we are more likely to be mugged by a stranger than by a friend, but our friends are more likely than strangers to rape or murder or assault us. The paradox of close relations rests on paradoxes of emotionality: the tenuous separation of love and hate and of pride and jealousy speak to the paradoxes of emotionality. The risk of being nurtured in our society is given in depending on nurturance, and when the nurturing other fails us, we can find ourselves carried from acts of closeness to acts of violence (Denzin, 1987). The social context about which Rawlins writes—the historical specificity, as he puts it—is thus one in which friendships and intimacies are seen and experienced as problematics, and relations with strangers are seen and experienced as relatively nonproblematic. At the heart of that difference, I believe, rests a historical dialectic that might be expressed in the proposition that an increase in strangers generates differentiation among types of close relationships and renders those relationships as interpretive problematics.

Interestingly, and I assume as everyone knows, the routine world of strangers has not always been with us. Indeed, throughout most of human history and certainly in human prehistory, humans existed in small and isolated communities (Lofland, 1973, p.4). People lived out their lives in these communities surrounded almost exclusively by people they knew and who knew them (Redfield, 1953; Childe, 1942). In that kind of context, strangers meant something very different than they mean today. Strangers then rarely appeared in the tiny clusters of huts scattered throughout the forests of Europe of the Dark Ages, for instance, but when they did, they were as likely to be a maurader as a monk, both of whom were feared (Burke, 1985, p. 22-23). The arrival of strangers generally interrupted routine life in preindustrial small communities, with the meaning of such interruptions depending upon the degree of the group's isolation, previous experiences with strangers, belief systems, and so forth. If sufficiently isolated, a group may even think of itself as the only humans on earth; thus, strangers were by definition nonhuman. In such cases, as was true among the Tiwi, it was thought entirely appropriate to simply kill the intruding stranger (Hart & Pilling, 1966). Among other groups, strangers may be met with apprehension, protective rituals, fainting, astonishment, and always suspicion. Throughout most of human history, therefore, it has been strangers who have been problematic rather than those one knew and with whom bonds were formed.[1]

Obviously, population increases and urbanization are processes that have recontextualized the relative problematics of strangers and friends. The historical creation of anonymous relations involved several structural limitations: By virtue of simple population density, such relations became common, which meant that it was impossible to know everyone by social differentiation, such that some people lived more restrictive lives than others and had fewer opportunities to form friendships, and by temporal reorganization, in which larger settlements attracted itinerants who were just passing through. With these changes came changes in modal ways of knowing. Lofland (1973, pp. 15-17) distinguishes categoric knowing (information about another's status) from personal knowing (information about another's biography), which is similar to the distinction Stone (1962) makes between structural and interpersonal identities.

The crucial point here is that increasing population and urbanization themselves were not responsible for the creation of worlds of strangers we have today. Rather, it was the transformation of modal ways of knowing others based on the social organization of information. Anonymous relations are characterized by categorical knowing; friendships are characterized by both categorical and pesonal knowing. Strangers, therefore, are those who are visually available to another, but unreferenced in the viewing person's pool of personal knowledge. Given this conceptualization, the historical transformation of the locus of relational problematics, from that of strangers to that of intimates and friends, centrally involved the transformation in the routine grounds for coding information about others' identities. The critical question raised is who is the other in relation to me?

In the small preindustrial communities, continual copresence without personal knowing was for all practical purposes impossible. There were no structural or relational reasons for anonymous relations to persist. With the press of population density, however, the transformation of all strangers into personally known others was no longer important or viable. Relations now were ordered by categoric codes, and dwellers of urban areas quickly acquired experience with such relations and became competent at them. Out of this transformation emerged a kind of codified fuzziness—a fuzziness we now routinely acknowledge in the use of terms such as *acquaintance.* Twilight is real, as my colleague Carl Couch is fond of saying, but I would add that it is more real in contemporary times than it was in times of the past. With the reality of twilight comes the problem of interpretation and the inherent ambiguities underlying the dialectics of friendship Rawlins analyzes.

The ecology of friendship.[2] The transformation of strangers to intimates and friends as problematic, as I have stated, took place within the context of urbanization, which is the context that also generated the routinization of accommodative relations among strangers. Urbanization, as well, entailed changes in the social organization of information that routinized categorical knowing and identity placement. I wish to focus now on an aspect of urbanization that, at least during the past three centuries, has had a profound effect on the nature of friendship. That aspect pertains to urban space; more precisely, to the ecology of friendship. Space, as scholars such as Edward Hall (1966) and Robert Sommer (1969) have shown, is a kind of semiotic. Urban ecological arrangements presume everyday life theories of the character of those persons who are being arranged, and the use of space symbolizes larger social processes (Lofland, 1988). Moreover, place implies identity; that is, *who* we are is interconnected with *where* we are (Ball, 1973). Urban ecology and the nature of social relations, as Park (1926) so clearly demonstrated, are thus part and parcel of the same thing, and to treat them otherwise violates the proposition that ecological patterns and social relations dialectically constitute one another. Humans confer an enormous variety of meanings on space and place, thus creating a social ecology, and that ecology then becomes a circumstance that facilitates or militates against the various forms of relations humans form. It is the question of the dialectic of place and friendship to which I now turn, focusing primarily on urban public gathering places.

Urban personalization was "discovered" by social researchers only a few decades ago. The early depictions of urban life emphasized superficial and depersonalized relations (Simmel, 1950; Wirth, 1938) in which intimacy and friendship were lacking. Ethnic diversity, occupational segregation, population density, and contractual relations all were seen as forces that denied meaningful personal ties among urban dwellers. Research by Stone (1954) on types of consumer relations, however, uncovered shoppers who personalize their relations with store personnel. Subsequent investigations, such as those by Gans (1962), Suttles (1968) and Leibow (1967), also revealed tightly and elaborately established networks of primary, face-to-face relationships. It appears, therefore, that turn-of-the-century urban scholarship vastly under represented the extent of personalization in urban areas.

A significant element in urban growth that manifestly influenced such personalization was the development of public places designed for informal gatherings. We know from current research (e.g., Fischer, 1982) that "pools of acquaintances" are the primary source of friendships and that such pools are formed to a significant degree on an ecological basis. By and large, our friends are those with whom we have worked, attended school, lived near, and so forth. Public places served much the same function in the early industrial cities. They brought strangers together into a neutral ground and provided a setting in which friendships and friendly relations could be formed. These public places also were contexts in which comfort zones could be established. Schopenhauer's parable of the porcupine comes to mind, in which the animals, in order to keep warm on a cold day, would huddle together only to end up pricking one another with their quills, thus prompting greater distance. The urban public place as neutral ground was therefore a context for people to reduce their sense of isolation through associational ties and, simultaneously, afford sufficient distance to minimize irritation and discomfort.

Community identification was facilitated in the early industrial cities through the availability of these neutral grounds that were close to residential neighborhoods. The bistros of the towns of France, the beer gardens of Germany, and the coffeehouses of Austria all contributed to a sense of community in large urban areas. These were occasions of friendship—places where sociability was interwoven into everyday life. The seventeenth-century London coffeehouses, that spanned two centuries from the mid-1600s to the mid-1800s, are fascinating cases in point (Ellis, 1956). With the introduction of coffee into London came the rapid development of such coffeehouses. These establishments mobilized new forms of appropriate relations, which the British class system had kept separate, representing new freedoms to the customer.

In addition to the coffeehouse as a setting that facilitated class-blind relations, the owners, partly out of business concerns, instituted rules of interaction to ensure a civil and democratic atmosphere. A set of rules was posted in establishments that resulted in customer parity. The rules were fairly simple. Everyone was welcome, people could sit anywhere they pleased and were free to share their company with whomever they chose, each was required to respond in a civil way to anyone who initiated conversations, there were no privileged seating sections, gambling bets were limited to five shillings, and anyone who started an argument had to treat those who were offended. Because women were automatically prohibited, these coffeehouses became institutionalized settings that promoted democratic, noninstitutionalized friendship relations among their male patrons. Favorite coffeehouses were visited by individuals several times a day, which testifies to the significance of the personalization and sociability they occasioned. Such enjoyment took hold as well in the nineteenth-century continental cafe in France. Aries (1965) observes that the spread of sidewalk cafes in Paris were discourse sites that brought strangers together, provided a communication center for the poor and homeless, and served as an informal support system for their participants. Most importantly to Aries, however, the cafes facilitated the meeting of strangers and thus their assimilation into urban community life.

The German beer gardens, which were an ecological feature functioning much like the British coffeehouses and French cafes, were imported to America in the mid-nineteenth century by middle-class Germans. These establishments brought together German speakers of all classes interested in singing or informal conversation. This form of neutral ground eventually disappeared from U.S. cities, however, as Germans "disappeared" through ethnic assimilation (O'Conner, 1968). It is retained now primarily in the form of neighborhood bars, with their "regulars," who indeed do constitute tight-knit friendship circles (Katovich & Reese, 1987; Gusfield, Kotarba, & Rasmussen, 1981).

The neutral ground quality of the public gathering place, to bring myself to the analytical point I want to make, provided a context that facilitated the handling of relations among strangers who populated early urban areas. The democratic zeitgeist and official rules of the house facilitated the transformation of categorical knowing to personal knowing (see also Goffman, 1963, p. 24). By intervening in the traditional status orders, which were based on social distance and the etiquette of hierarchy, these ecological features of cities were significant in the creation of modern sociability and friendship relations containing the element of voluntarism. We see traces of these relations in contemporary neighborhood bars in which membership is defined in terms of biographical knowledge. Regulars become narrators of other people's lives and their membership is secured when their lives become the stories other people tell. Categorical knowledge in these processes becomes much less significant as the identity relations become constructed on the grounds of personal knowledge. The ecology of friendship in this sense is the ecology of knowing.

But contemporary urban life, even with its neighborhood bars and crowded public places, has also become more private. Suburbanization represents a countertrend to the neutral grounds of urban living, and such ecological spread has had the effect of segregating people in single-dwelling private households. One consequence of this process, as Gordon (1976) has shown, is that suburban housewives as a group are among the loneliest in the country. Yearning for the friendly contact missing in their daily lives, they nonetheless resist making their homes available to others on a regular basis. The ecological creation of public sociability a few centuries ago now grinds like sandpaper against the current ecological creation of privacy. The dialectic of the ecology of sociability versus the ecology of privacy reflects Rawlins's dialectic of the public versus the private (pp. 165-167). In his interpersonal perspective, the public marginality of friendship confronts friendship's private morality in a potential clash of accountability and obligation. Friends configure their relationship in terms of its meaning to themselves and its probable lack of meaning to others they encounter, for instance, in the institutionalized relations of work. Those configuring processes, however, occur in complex ecological arrangements in which the nature of the relationship is often revealed by where friends meet. Close friends, assuming they live within reasonable proximity, usually have few spatial limitations to their relationship, whereas friendly relations are typically enacted at the sites of formal role performance. The "need to be alone," which true friends are expected to respect, is often an expression of the ecology of privacy, whereas the "need to go out," which true friends also respect, expresses the ecology of public sociability. Once again, we can see Rawlins's dialectic of friendship in terms of an ecological correlate—this time his dialectic of dependence versus independence.

These suggested parallels and correlates are simply ways of exploring the historical and contextual dialectics Rawlins invites us to ponder. With such pondering at least temporarily satisfied, I will now move on to a few other points that I offer as a set of concluding observations.

CONCLUDING REMARKS

I have spent quite a bit of time in the past decade trying to convince fellow sociologists that the phenomena their theories and concepts reference are communicative and temporal in nature (see Maines, 1977; 1982; 1984; Maines & Couch, 1988). Assuming that *Communication Yearbook* readers need no such lecture from me, I am correspondingly relieved from grinding that particular ax. However, in concluding my remarks, I do have an issue I want to raise regarding research on friendship.

The point I want to address regarding research on friendship is partly expressed in Goffman's (1963) assertion that "a loose speculative approach to a fundamental area of conduct is better than a rigorous blindness to it" (p. 4). The reason I borrow only part of his message is that researchers certainly have options available to them other than speculation or blindness. But Goffman makes a point that the bulk of empirically minded investigators ought to take very seriously. We have become so enamored with our research technologies, our abilities at modeling, our affection for quantophrenic procedures, and our seduction by inappropriate conceptions of precision that we are in danger of pulverizing, in the name of science and rigor, the very phenomena about which we are interested.[3]

Now here is the point of all this carping. Rawlins has produced a dialectical analysis of friendship and he has identified a number of specific dialectics expressed as dichotomies—real versus ideal, public versus private, and so forth, although he explicitly states they are in fact continua. It would be a complete distortion of his analysis, in my opinion, to regard these dichotomies as variables that can be scaled and measured and handled with log-linear analysis. But I can easily imagine someone attempting to undertake such a task. It would not be terribly difficult to come up with a dependence scale, for example, and along with other scales collect a sample of young adults and "test" hypotheses derived from Rawlins's perspective. But to do so would completely miss the heart of his perspective, which is given in the process of participants configuring their relationships as these dialectics become issues and interpretive problematics in ongoing communicative conduct. The latest versions of sophisticated measuring techniques and data analysis have been constructed on the basis of ontologies and epistemologies that run counter to dialectical processes and principles. Thus contemporary social research faces a very profound dilemma: to persist in distorting the phenomena of interest in the name of precision and rigor or to put some real effort into an alternative conception of science that is suitable for the phenomena under scrutiny. This dilemma holds true for the fields of both sociology and communication (Maines & Couch, 1988).

Perhaps without intending to do so, I think that Rawlins's analysis forces honest and thoughtful scholars to face that dilemma in a serious and concerted manner. Far from a "loose speculative approach," he has offered a sophisticated yet flexible framework that attempts to keep the integrity of the phenomena in place. Rawlins's analysis takes very seriously what we know to be true of human conduct: that it is relational, untidy, and ultimately quite specious. Rawlins's perspective attempts to incorporate these truths and represent them in a form suitable for scholarly dialogue and discourse.

In making a few observations on historical transformations and contexts, I have attempted to respond to the merit of the perspective on friendship he has developed. That merit, I am convinced, cannot be tapped by the univocality of contemporary rationalism and logico-deductive reasoning. Scholars, however, who accept the fact that human ambiguity and the reality of twilight constitute both limits and possibilities for their work, are certain to find their imaginations stimulated and their reasoning sharpened by intellectually engaging Rawlins's dialectical perspective on friendship.

NOTES

1. Norman Denzin has reminded me of a point of clarification here. My argument pertains to the translocation of problematics, not the exclusive province of them. To say that strangers used to represent problematics is not to say that socially bonded relationships were unproblematic. That is a different issue that pertains to the dialectics of strangers and friends within that historical context.

2. I appreciate Professor Ray Oldenberg's kind permission to draw from his unpublished manuscript, "The Ecological Variable in Friendship and Sociability" for my analysis of parts of

this section. For a more detailed presentation of Oldenberg's points of view, see his forthcoming *The Great Good Place* (New York: Pergamon).

3. Space limitations prohibit appropriate documentation of this characterization. I would direct readers' attention to two fairly well-known articles on friendship, however, and invite their consideration of how the accepted principles of homophily and proximity (see Lazarsfeld & Merton, 1954) have been tautologically reified in the name of advanced research methods. Blau (1961) sought to show how age and gender homophily structures friendship relations using data from two surveys of friendships among the elderly. The three survey items used for her measures (1961, p. 430), however, had the properties of homophily and opportunity built into them. This produced a tautology insofar as if homophily and proximity are mechanisms of friendship formation, they already had produced the "close friends" specified in her interview questions. Such rigorous blindness also is exemplified in Verbugge's (1977) analysis of adult friendship choices. She used a very up-to-date odds ratio analysis from two large data sets to draw her major conclusion that "social and spatial proximity are strong and pervasive factors in adult friendship choices" (1977, p. 592). The data used to test the proximity principle, however, were based on the question "who are your closest friends and whom do you see most often? (1977, p. 594), thus revealing the tautology. The Blau and Verbugge research, then, exemplify how state-of-the-art data analytic procedures can mask underlying ontological questions and thereby side step fundamental issues of precision. Competence at technical precision, in other words, is proffered as competence at ontological precision.

REFERENCES

Aries, P. (1965). *Centuries of childhood.* NY: Random House.

Ball, D. (1973). *Micro-ecology.* Indianapolis: Bobbs-Merrill.

Bateson, G. (1972). *Steps to an ecology of mind,* NY: Ballantine.

Blau, Z. (1961). Structural constraints on friendship in old age, *American Sociological Review, 26,* 429-439.

Blumer, H. (1962). Society as symbolic interaction. In Arnold Rose (Ed.), *Human behavior and social processes* (pp. 174-192). Boston: Houghton Mifflin.

Brown, R. (1987). *Society as text.* Chicago: University of Chicago Press.

Burke, J. (1985). *The day the universe changed.* Boston: Little, Brown.

Burns, T. (1953). Friends, enemies, and the polite fiction. *American Sociological Review, 18,* 654-662.

Childe, V. G. (1942). *What happened in history.* Harmondsworth, Middlesex: Penguin.

Denzin, N. (1984). *Understanding emotion.* San Francisco: Jossey-Bass.

Denzin, N. (1987). *The alcoholic self.* Newbury Park, CA: Sage.

Duncan, H. (1968). *Symbols in society.* NY: Oxford University Press.

Ellis, A. (1956). *The penny university.* London: Secker & Warburg.

Fischer, C. (1982). *To dwell among friends.* Chicago: University of Chicago Press.

Gans, H. (1962). *The urban villagers.* New York: Free Press.

Giddens, A. (1984). *The constitution of society.* Berkeley: University of California Press.

Glaser, B., & Strauss A. (1968). *Time for dying.* Chicago: Aldine.

Goffman, E. (1963). *Behavior in public places.* New York: Free Press.

Goffman, E. (1967). *Interaction ritual.* New York: Doubleday.

Gordon, S. (1976). *Lonely in America.* New York: Simon & Schuster.

Gusfield, J., Kotarba, J., & Rasmussen, P. (1981). The public society of intimates: Friends, wives, lovers, and others in the drinking-drama. In H. Lopata & D. Maines (Eds.), *Research in the interweave of social roles: Friendship* (pp. 237-257). Greenwich, CT: JAI.

Hall, E. T. (1966). *The hidden dimension.* Garden City, NY: Doubleday.

Hart, C.W.M., & Pilling, A. (1966). *The Tiwi of North Australia*. New York: Holt, Rinehart & Winston.
Hill, R., Foote, N., Aldous, J., Carlson, R., & McDonald R. (1970). *Family development in three generations*. New York: Schenkman.
Innis, H. (1951). *The bias of communication*. Toronto: University of Toronto Press.
Katovich, M., & Reese, W. (1987). The regular: Full-time identities and memberships in an urban bar. *Journal of Contemporary Ethnography, 16*, 308-343.
Kurth, S. (1970). Friendship and friendly relations. In G. McCall et al. (Eds.), *Social Relationships* (pp. 136-170). Chicago: Aldine.
Lazarsfeld, P., & Merton R. (1954). Friendship as a social process: A substantive and methodological analysis. In M. Berger, T. Abel, & C. Page (Eds.), *Freedom and control in modern society* (pp. 18-66). New York: Van Nostrand.
Leibow, E. (1967). *Tally's corner*. Boston: Little, Brown.
Levine, D. (1985). *Flight from ambiguity*. Chicago: University of Chicago Press.
Lofland, L. (1973). *A world of strangers*. New York: Basic Books.
Lofland, L. (1988). Communication and construction: The built environment as message and medium. In D. Maines & C. Couch (Eds.), *Communication and Social Structure* (pp. 307-322). Springfield, IL: Charles C Thomas.
Maines, D. (1977). Social organization and social structure in symbolic interactionist thought. *Annual Review of Sociology 3*, 235-259.
Maines, D. (1982). In search of mesostructure: Studies in the negotiated order. *Urban Life, 11*, 267-279.
Maines, D. (1984). Suggestions for a symbolic interactionist conception of culture. *Communication and Cognition, 17*, 205-217.
Maines, D., & Couch, C. (1988). On the indispensability of communication for understanding social relationships and social structure. In D. Maines & C. Couch (Eds.), *Communication and Social Structure* (pp. 3-18). Springfield, IL: Charles C Thomas.
Maines, D., & Hardesty, M. (1987). Temporality and gender: Young adults' career and family plans. *Social Forces, 66*, 102-120.
Maines, D., Sugrue, N., & Katovich, M. (1983). The sociological import of G.H. Mead's theory of the past. *American Sociological Review, 48*, 151-173.
Matthews, S. (1986). Friendship in old age: Biography and circumstance. In V. Marshall (Ed.), *Later life* (pp. 232-268). Beverly Hills: Sage.
Mead, G. H. (1929). The nature of the past. In J. Coss (Ed.), *Essays in honor of John Dewey* (pp. 235-242). New York: Henry Holt.
Mead, G. H. (1932). *The philosophy of the present*. LaSalle, IL: Open Court.
O'Conner, R. (1968). *The German-Americans: An informal history*. Boston: Little, Brown.
Park, R. (1926). The urban community as a spatial pattern and a moral order. Reprinted in R. Turner (Ed.), *Robert Park on social control and collective behavior* (pp. 55-68). Chicago: University of Chicago Press, 1967.
Redfield, R. (1953). *The primitive world and its transformations*. Ithaca, NY: Cornell University Press.
Simmel, G. (1950). The metropolis and the mental life. In K. Wolff (Ed.), *The Sociology of Georg Simmel* (pp. 400-427). New York: Free Press.
Sommer, R. (1969). *Personal space*. Englewood Cliffs, NJ: Prentice-Hall.
Stone, G., & Farberman, H. (Eds.). (1970). *Social psychology through symbolic interaction*. Waltham, MA: Xerox.
Stone, G. P. (1954). City shoppers and urban identification: Observations in the social psychology of city life. *American Journal of Sociology, 60*, 276-284.
Stone, G. P. (1962). Appearance and the self. In A. Rose (Ed.), *Human behavior and social processes* (pp. 86-118). Boston: Houghton Mifflin.
Suttles, G. (1968). *The social order of the slum*. Chicago: University of Chicago Press.
Verbugge, L. (1977). The structure of adult friendship choices. *Social Forces, 56*, 576-597
Wirth, L. (1938). Urbanism as a way of life. *American Journal of Sociology, 44*, 1-24.

What Is Friendship? A Hermeneutical Quibble

ALLEN SCULT
Drake University

I hope the reader will bear with some introductory self-referencing by way of putting my comments in appropriate perspective. I am a rhetorician with a strong interest in hermeneutics. This explains my concern in the pages that follow with the nature of the discourse in which Professor Rawlins chooses to embody his ideas. Not only is my experience with the theoretical and methodological controversies among empiricists rather limited, but my rhetorical interest constantly diverts my attention to the drama of ideas struggling to be expressed in the discourse. My interest in hermeneutics further prompts me to wonder whether a given discourse is indeed the best one for trying to understand a particular phenomenon.

As I read the essay, I was struck by the richness of the notion of "dialectical tensions" for considering strategic challenges involved in managing friendships. Friendships are, after all, extremely delicate and complex attempts at human bonding that, as Rawlins observes, are not defined by any agreed-upon set of institutional rules or conventions. Because they stand at the margins of institutional life, our attempts to develop and maintain these relationships are beset by a panoply of psychological and social forces, constantly running into one another. The intensity of this interplay is especially severe in times of crisis in the friendship in which the lack of institutional framework for resolving (or even understanding) the problem is strikingly evident. We are "on our own," turned in on ourselves, to negotiate our way through the different dynamics governing our relationship. Rawlins's conceptualization of these complex negotiations as the working through of the central dialectical tensions of friendship is most promising.

But my rhetorical and hermeneutical instincts lead me to wonder if the empirical discourse in which Rawlins chooses to pursue his theme is in fact best suited to it. Rawlins might respond that empirical discourse provides an

Correspondence and requests for reprints: Allen Scult, Department of Speech Communication, Drake University, Des Moines, IA 50311.

Communication Yearbook 12, pp. 203-212

ample and clear frame for the development of his theme: Here is what people do. Here is a conceptual frame for examining what people do. And finally, here are some things that can be said about what people do from the perspective of that conceptual frame. I think this sort of progression is perfectly adequate for discussing easily definable institutional or contractual relationships such as those in families and organizations.

But as we have noted, friendship has no normative or institutional status. This characteristic makes it difficult for me to identify what it is we are talking about when we speak of friendship. In hermeneutical terms, there is no clear "object of investigation," and therefore nothing to focus on as we work our way around the hermeneutical circle. I might be accused here of nitpicking, but I find that in relation to friendship, we are lacking what Gadamer (1975) calls a "common language" for our discussion. The common language would give our discussion a beginning point that also presages its end and thus lends to the hermeneutical circle its logical underpinning. We would either begin with an agreement about something known that we want to learn more about, or something unknown that we wish to identify because such an identification can help us solve some problem. When the common language is of the more specific sort, empirical discourse would be rhetorically appropriate and hermeneutically useful. When it is more general, an investigative pursuit conducted through the medium of empirical discourse might well lack coherence and direction. Rather than a conceptual frame for empirical reportage, the hermeneutical starting point in such cases involves a vision of something sought after to fill a problematical space in the moral universe. The "premonition" of what that thing might be in the form of a hypothesized name which then serves as a basis to investigate the nature of the thing and to discern its moral function. The discourse appropriate to such an open ended inquiry is, of course, philosophy.

Not surprisingly, then, the discussion about friendship in our own tradition has been a philosophical one, begun by the Greeks, especially Aristotle, and joined by (among others) Cicero, Vico, Bacon, and, more contemporaneously, Gadamer. The philosophical discourse on friendship that has taken place at the crossroads of moral philosophy and metaphysics can be seen as a reflexive investigation of a process of naming. It is the very giving of the name followed by the attempt to justify it that constitutes the inquiry. The progression goes something like this: First the name itself is suggested, rather in the nature of a "philosophical hypothesis." Then the implications, especially the moral implications (for naming lends to something a moral character), are examined to see if the name is appropriate. We are presented with a picture of what the world would be like with such a named thing as a significant constituent part. Philosophical naming of this sort is in the nature of "world building" or perhaps "world improving." In any case, the directionality of the hermeneutical circle, the grounds for judging the argument presented, are clear: Does this vision of friendship comport with the evolving moral world view of our philosophical community? In other words, is it justifiable in philosophical terms that we, as a community, can accept?

I propose to respond to Professor Rawlins's essay from the philosophical perspective by first outlining the naming process as it has gone on in the tradition, mainly in Aristotle. The essential questions here are, "What is the nature of the thing our philosophical tradition has chosen to call friendship and why is it of concern to us?" Especially important will be our attempt to identify the moral issues implicit in this evolving notion of friendship, since it will give us an indication of the directionality of the inquiry. I will then examine Rawlins's dialectical theorizing about friendship to try to identify its implicit contributions to this ongoing discussion of the moral place of friendship in the world.

If this way of going about a response seems rather presumptuous on my part, I offer two justifications: First, because I was unable to discern a clear frame of reference for Rawlins's discussion of friendship, I needed to supply one as a basis for my response. Given our common roots in the rhetorical tradition, Aristotle seemed a most appropriate and fruitful source for framing my response. The other justification is simply a rhetorician's conceit: that I was able to discern Rawlins's "true theme" and was able to trace the dialectical drama of its alternate disclosure and concealment through the essay. I will suggest therefore, that Rawlins was engaged in an investigation of a moral vision of friendship, which he holds to quite passionately; but each time he came close to making the nature of this pursuit explicit, the decorum of empirical discourse forced him to retreat, and conceal the progression of his insights in theoretical glosses on neutral reportage. In such cases, perhaps one of the tasks of a commentator-friend might be to recover what the author's sectarian decorum required him to keep hidden. We begin the archaeological portion of this task with Aristotle.

ARISTOTLE'S VIEW

The empiricist in Aristotle recognizes three species of friendship, but Aristotle, the philosopher, focuses on one of these as occupying a central place in the moral universe. The other two are spoken of as derivative of this more central sort of friendship—the one with "real existence." Aristotle further emphasizes its primacy by identifying it as one of the virtues. Friendship of this sort, based on a "recognition of moral goodness," of character in another person, takes the form of a "mutual well-wishing and well-doing out of concern for one another" (Cooper, 1980; p. 302).

Aristotle's exemplar for this kind of friendship—friendship as a virtue grounded in character—is, of course, civic or political friendship. It is in the political arena that friendship assumes its quintessential moral function—a function basic to leading the good life. Aristotle gives the name *homonoia*, "thinking in harmony," to the friendship among citizens that makes political community possible (Beiner, 1983; p. 80).

It is important to note, first of all, that this most primary idea of friendship is not seen by Aristotle as a relationship for itself, for "mere companionship" as he puts it. Rather it "exists for the sake of noble actions" (Ross, 1927; p. 306). The noble actions Aristotle has in mind here depend upon discourse of the right sort among citizens—the kind of deliberation that will eventuate in good judgment. Friendship, then, is seen as the ideal relationship for framing the sort of discourse that leads to good judgment. Thus Aristotle's notion of friendship is definitively instrumental, its purpose being to provide the relational frame for the sort of discourse that produces good judgment. It is the central political virtue, enabling citizens to engage with one another in a process of deliberation and judgment that leads to noble action, thus making the good life possible.

Friendship is able to provide a context for good judgment, because it is a relationship based on essential ideas held in common. As Beiner (1983) observes, "What friends hold in common is a common view of what is just, and it is to this extent that friendship is a form of community" (p. 80). This statement gives us an idea of the moral significance of friendship for Aristotle. Science does not provide us with any method of reaching a clear and certain notion of what is right and wrong, good and bad. That is the task of judgment, and judgment is a capacity we hold in common with others who share our basic values. We need friends to "make our judgments *with*,"—to help us make the sorts of decisions that are essential to living out our lives as moral beings.

This notion of friendship as a relational context for judgment extends beyond politics to the moral dimension of other significant relationships as well. It can be applied to marriage, colleagiality—any institutional or quasi-institutional relationship that requires judgment. The institutional base of the relationship provides us with the occasions for judgment. But in order to be "good" in some moral sense, our judgments need to be made within a broader perspective—a perspective that goes beyond the specific case and brings a communal sense of what is right and wrong to bear on our decision. The requirements for producing the sort of discourse that brings out this *sensus communis* are not satisfied by mere institutional rules and conventions. Those involved in producing this discourse must be committed to realizing a relational ideal together. It is this commitment, this urge to raise their relationship to the highest moral level through discourse, that gives friends the impetus they need to uncover and make use of the tacit knowledge they hold in common. The philosophical process of investigating the nature of that relationship is often conducted by friends in the course of their attempt to realize the ideal (witness, especially, Plato's *Phaedrus,* or more recently, Simons, 1985).

Beiner's (1983) reading of Aristotle further suggests the central moral issue with which this ideal of friendship is concerned: the intrusion of *eros*. "*Eros* collapses the space of friendship, the space that, by enforcing the distinct identity of each, sustains the mutual integrity of friends" (p. 121). The compulsive need of human beings for affiliation leads us to pursue one another in order to form some sort of intimate bond—to establish a source of *companionship* (to use Aristotle's term) we can depend upon. This pursuit is in need of some constraining moral framework. In other words, relationships must develop, at least in part, as instruments in service of some moral end, lest the erotic impulse be its sole motivating force. Friendship, considered as a moral instrumentality, simultaneously enables us to pursue two interrelated objectives: protecting our individual integrity and, at the same time, forming the sort of community that makes good judgment possible. It accomplishes the first by giving us the means to manage our erotic urge for companionship lest we be led to compromise our own principles in order to protect the relationship. A friendship, firmly based in important ideas held in common, gives us a common point of view to guide our discourse, thus introducing a necessary distance in our struggle to achieve dependable and satisfying companionship. Without that distance, we might not only sacrifice our own position, but are also prone to making unreasonable demands on the other person. Our expectation seems to be that unless they think, feel, and act as we do, or at least act as we think they should in their situation, they don't really love us.

Beiner (1983) finds a poignant example of this tension between eros and friendship in the relationship between Hannah Arendt and Gershom Scholem in the aftermath of the Eichmann case (pp. 119-125). In her book, *The Banality of Evil*, Hannah Arendt had tried to understand and judge Adolph Eichmann as a human being who gave into very extreme versions of impulses that plague us all. This effort Beiner sees as an example of the discourse of friendship among intellectuals in the Jewish Community. Arendt did not act simply on the emotional need to be accepted by her fellow Jews, but on an understanding of the deeper ideas that bind the Jewish community together. On the other hand, Scholem, as her longtime friend and fellow Jewish intellectual, reacted emotionally and saw this attempt to understand the actions of one of the generally accepted villains of the holocaust as a denial of Arendt's primary allegiance to her fellow Jews: to love them unequivocally.

In his exploration of the ideal human relationship, Martin Buber (1970) reflects a similar distrust of feelings as the basis of friendship: "A living reciprocal relationship includes feelings but is not derived from them" (p. 94). He goes on to speak of "community" of a "living, active center" as the basis of a true relationship. Again, friends need something beyond themselves, a broader frame that they can understand together but cannot control, to guide the discourse and judgments that constitute the moral dimension of the relationship.

In addition to preserving the integrity of the individual, friendship, as noted here, also enables us to form a community within which the sort of discourse leading to good judgment becomes possible. Again, friendship is able to accomplish this community essentially through the management of *eros*. Gadamer (1975) provides us with the primary contemporary application of this aspect of Aristotle's view of friendship. It occurs in his discussion of the ideal relationship within which to realize "genuine conversation"—that discourse that eventuates in *understanding*, Gadamer's term for good judgment. The relevant portion of that discussion deals with the crucial distinction between understanding the other *individual* as opposed to understanding what the other individual *says* (p. 347). For Gadamer, the pursuit of understanding requires a rigorous focusing and refocusing on the object of understanding, not the other person. Gadamer seems very much aware of the erotic impulses that would divert our attention from the object and move us to err in our discourse in order to further the development of our relationship with the other person. His development of the ideal relationship within which genuine conversation might take place leads him to steer us consistently away from *eros* in order to take those relational steps that will enable us to constitute a community of understanding. The main issue is here again for the friends to manage their discourse with the proper distance so their "give and take" preserves the communal space within which good judgment or understanding, takes place. Hence Gadamer insists that the discourse partners maintain their focus on the object and let the conversation emanating from that focus "conduct them," rather than the other way around.

To summarize our interpretation of Aristotle's notion of *homonoia*, friendship in a political community—it is, first of all, an ideal relationship, a vision to which we might aspire. It is not a relationship that exists for the sake of satisfying our yearning for companionship. It is an ideal to guide us in developing the moral dimension of already existing institutional and quasi-institutional relationships. It is thus instrumental, functioning to bring out the communal sensibilities that exist between individuals in order for them to engage in the sort of discourse that protects their individual integrity and eventuates in good judgment.

It would seem that the logical next step in developing Aristotle's contribution to the philosophical investigation of friendship on the way to applying it to Rawlins's essay would be a generalizing one—to extrapolate the main ingredients of political friendship in order to formulate a more general notion of interpersonal friendship. (The concept seems irresistibly to have begun to move in this direction in the previous pages.) Aristotle, himself, moves his discussion of friendship in the *Ethics* along similar lines and so will continue to provide much of the basis for the ideas that follow. Our discussion will also assume a more narrative form with a focus on how interpersonal friendships begin, develop, reach a crisis point, and resolve the crisis. By providing a medium for discussing the unfolding progression of interpersonal friendship, narrative would seem to be an appropriate discourse for mediating between Aristotle's philosophical discussion and Rawlins's empirical one. Indeed, we find both Aristotle and Rawlins lapsing into narrative by way of exemplifying their claims.

The narrative of interpersonal friendship begins, naturally enough, with some sort of attraction between two people, some perceived characteristic that impels one person to choose to make a friend of another. In Aristotle's moral view of friendship, the source of attraction is obviously not erotic. Rather, the attraction is to the other's perceived virtue that makes him or her a good candidate with whom to engage in those moral pursuits, such as good judgment, that are appropriate to the relationship. As Aristotle puts it, the attraction is that the other is "good and alike in virtue" (Cooper, 1980; p. 304). This perceived similarity of character creates the opportunity to imagine that the ideal vision of the relationship being pursued is shared.

Using our own scholarly community as an example, it would seem that this reading of Aristotle provides a plausible characterization of the choice we make in calling a colleague "friend": It suggests that we see in that colleague the kind of virtuous character that makes him or her a likely possibility with whom to pursue our vision of an ideal relationship between scholars. Because, as is the case with so many relationships, that ideal is enacted through discourse, it becomes essential that the virtues we perceive in the person be similar to our own. Discourse is the epitome of a "transaction," requiring us to be in close and subtle collaboration with one another as we use our discourse to construct a relationship in accordance with a shared ideal. Both the perceived similarity of virtues that makes collaborative discourse possible and the shared ideal vision of the relationship that gives the discourse its direction are firmly grounded in the values of our community. Thus community provides a moral frame for the relationship that goes beyond the feelings people might have for one another. This configuration fits nicely with Aristotle's view of friendship as community.

Within the context of this narrative of friendship as beginning with a judgment of moral character that one finds attractive because of the possibilities it opens up to pursue an ideal vision of the relationship, the moral crisis point in a friendship becomes apparent: What do we do when our friends fail to live up to the virtuous character we judged them to have? Such an event assumes crisis proportions because this moral falling short on their part makes impossible the ideal vision of the relationship we imagined ourselves to be enacting together. We feel betrayed by our friends—betrayed not only because they have failed to live up to who we thought them to be, but perhaps, more importantly, because we took our judgment of their character to be an implicit moral contract that committed them to a vision of the relationship we assumed was shared.

As is often the case with betrayal, here it covers a deeper sense of grief, of loss. The loss is not only a personal one: "You are not the person I thought you were," which is tantamount to saying, "I have lost the friend I thought I had." It is also the loss of an imagined world: The ideal relationship we thought was, or would be ours together, disappears from the horizon.

The fact that the "moral contract" remained unspoken, and indeed that our assumed shared vision of the relationship and our judgment of their character might have been sheer projection does not mitigate this sense of betrayal. Aristotle recognizes this same dilemma as the central crisis point in a friendship: What do we do, he asks, "if we accept another man as good and he turns out badly and is seen to do so, must one still love him" (Aristotle, 1983; p. 225)?

RAWLINS'S VIEW

I see Professor Rawlins as essentially sharing this Aristotelian view of friendship and as having some important contributions to make to the philosophical discussion based on it. However, because he chooses to conduct his inquiry (or at least to record it) primarily in empirical rather than in philosophical or narrative discourse, his contribution must be pieced together from different portions of his essay. The decorum of empiricism required him to submerge his own questions about friendship and his developing response to those questions beneath the pose of neutral reportage. He especially could not let his own moral vision of what friendship might be assume a central thematic role guiding the development of the essay. That is the way of philosophy.

Because of this constraint on his discourse, Rawlins's articulation of what I read as his vision of friendship—the true starting point of the essay—does not appear until page 167. This vision of friendship appears in the midst of his discussion of what he posits as just one of the "contextual dialectics": the dialectic of the ideal and the real. He first observes, in total concert with our own reading of the Aristotelian view, that long-lasting friendships "must be permeated with ethical concerns." (It is interesting to note that he quotes Vlissingen in expressing this thought. Another characteristic of empirical discourse that can inhibit one from developing one's own thought would seem to be that one must forever be quoting someone else in order to make general or theoretical claims.) Then comes his definition of friendship—an eloquent version of Aristotle's "friendship as virtue": "As a cultural ideal, friendship appears to be a categorical repository for the hope of a mutually edifying moral covenant voluntarily negotiated between people."

Providing the appropriate context for the enactment of this view of friendship takes us back to the beginning portion of Rawlins's essay, where again, it is hidden among the four elements in the dialectical view: "The notion of praxis focuses attention on the active choices friends make in the face of objective constraints existing in their temporally and spatially specific social circumstances" (p. 162). Leading us to the crisis point, Rawlins beautifully reflects the interdependence of one's own view of oneself and the actions one takes with another in the formation of significant relationships: "They [individualized persons] are constituted through interaction in their active management of, and communication within, relationships as their actual, lived histories affect and inform their present actions." The actual circumstances occurring in the life of a given relationship provide the inevitable praxic opportunities wherein our initial judgment and subsequent actions based on that judgment are tested.

This focus on praxis leads us to the next step in this "narratization" of Rawlins's essay: his view of the moral crisis point in the life of a friendship. In this case, it is one of the interactional dialectics identified by Rawlins, namely acceptance-judgment, which is the locus at which the crisis appears. Rawlins's characterization of the dialectical tension between acceptance and judgment (pp. 175-176) elegantly describes the contours of the alternative courses of action in response to the moral crisis of friendship as we have identified it: What does one do when a friend fails to live up to one's initial judgment of his or her character?

To oversimplify somewhat, the options appear to be as follows: Do we accept the person's failings (difficult!), or do we express our judgment, criticizing them in the hope of changing them (unlikely!)? Aristotle seems to come down on the side of acceptance with a diminished view of the other person's moral potential and therefore for the possibilities of the relationship: "Surely he should keep a remembrance of their former intimacy, and as we think we ought to oblige friends rather than strangers, so to those who have been our friends we ought to make some allowance for our former friendship, when the breach has not been due to an excess of wickedness" (Aristotle, 1983, p. 226-227).

I read this as a recommendation to resign ourselves to the loss and reconcile ourselves to preserving whatever we can of the relationship "for old time's sake."

Rawlins appears to take a more upbeat strategic view. The only chance one has of bringing the friend back into line with one's original judgment is to first support the friend with acceptance: "They also appreciate judgment and criticism [only] from a person who primarily accepts and cares about them" (p. 176). In thinking through Rawlins's strategic advice, it occurred to me that his recommendation is instructively paradoxical. Our only chance of helping friends become the persons we think they should be is to accept them as they are. Further consideration of this paradox was stimulated again by Rawlins's elaboration of it as a "dialectical tension," and has led me to the realization that accepting the limitations of a cherished friend with whom one wishes to maintain a relationship ultimately means recognizing and coming to terms with one's own limitations. As I ponder this realization, I am moved to thank Professor Rawlins for the "dialectical theorizing" that led me to it and for the philosophical subtext that I presumptuously think I uncovered in his more overt and also useful empirical discourse on friendship.

REFERENCES

Aristotle (1983). *The Nicomachean ethics.* (D. Ross, Trans.). Oxford: Oxford University Press.
Beiner, R. (1983). *Political judgment.* Chicago: University of Chicago Press.
Buber, M. (1970). *I and thou.* (W. Kaufmann, Trans.). New York: Scribner's.
Cooper, J. M. (1980). Aristotle on friendship. In A. Rorty (Ed.), *Essays on Aristotle's ethics* (pp. 301-340). Los Angeles: University Of California Press.
Gadamer, H. G. (1975). *Truth and method* (J.C.B. Mohr, Trans.). New York: Continuum.
Ross, W. D. (Ed.) (1927). *Aristotle selections.* New York: Scribner's.
Simons, H.W. (1985) Chronicle and critique of a conference. *Quarterly Journal of Speech,* 71, 52-64.

4 Second-Guessing Theory: Review and Extension

DEAN E. HEWES
University of Minnesota

MAUDIE L. GRAHAM
University of Wisconsin—Milwaukee

Messages are often biased. Whether these messages are produced by acquaintances, coworkers, governments, or the mass media, social actors believe they can identify biases in them. Not only do they feel they can identify distortions, but they also believe they can correct those distortions, arriving at a more accurate understanding of the messages' referents than if they relied on the messages unreflectively. Hewes and Planalp (1982) called this process of correcting for biases "second-guessing." This chapter describes this process and its implications for communication theory. In addition, it presents a theory of second-guessing that specifies its antecedents and consequences. Included is a review of the relevant literature, suggesting facets of the theory that need further testing and new areas of application.

MESSAGES often carry an inaccurate picture of their referents. People deceive others intentionally and unintentionally. Governments, corporations, the mass media and individuals try to conceal their mistakes or present themselves to others in an unduly positive light. They often hold unwarranted beliefs that they unknowingly inflict on others. Eyewitnesses may remember more than they saw or may remember it incorrectly (Loftus, 1979). Patients undergoing therapy may explain their lives in terms of their own limited, and potentially inaccurate, views of themselves (e.g., Labov & Fanshell, 1977). Virtually every day we encounter people who misrepresent events they have observed, or the attributes of others they have met, as a result of unintended errors in human judgment (see Kahneman, Slovic, & Tversky, 1982).

Whether messages are distorted intentionally or not, receivers of those messages sometimes fail to accept them at face value. In fact, receivers often go to great lengths to see behind the literal or the intended meanings of messages in order to understand what is "really going on." For instance, they

Correspondence and requests for reprints: Dean E. Hewes, Department of Speech Communication, 317 Folwell Hall, University of Minnesota, Minneapolis, MN 55455.

Communication Yearbook 12, pp. 213-248

not only attempt to identify deception (even though, objectively, they do so inaccurately), but they may also attempt to identify the truth behind the lie (Zuckerman, DePaulo, & Rosenthal, 1981). Jurors do not accept eyewitness testimony as sacrosanct; they can specify how such testimony may go awry both intentionally and unintentionally (Loftus, 1979). Counselors question their clients' accounts of their lives and try to construct more viable explanations of those lives, based on their knowledge of the human mind (Cheshire, 1975). And people in everyday life attempt to winnow the truth from messages that they feel are biased (Hewes & Planalp, 1982).

In each of these cases, social actors are engaged in what Hewes and Planalp (1982) have labeled "second-guessing." Second-guessing is a cognitive process by which social actors, upon identifying what they believe to be a biased message, attempt to correct for the bias by means of specialized forms of social knowledge. Thus social actors consciously attempt to "debias" messages in order to identify what they hope to be a "truer" account of the topics discussed therein. Second-guessing is undertaken in reaction to a perceived bias only when there is some threshold need for accurate information (Hewes, Graham, Doelger, & Pavitt, 1985; Hewes, Graham, Monsour, & Doelger, 1988). Moreover, the reinterpretations of those messages that result from second-guessing are assumed theoretically to be approximately "normatively adequate" (Hewes et al., 1985, p. 305). The theory assumes that the belief that many social actors have that they have arrived at a "truer" account of the topic covered in a message is, in fact, approximately accurate when compared to more objective assessments based on socially sanctioned methods of gathering and evaluating evidence.

To make this thumbnail sketch of second-guessing more concrete, consider two commonplace examples. A friend (the source) comes to you upset over a conflict he has just had with his wife (the target). He tells you that his wife is an uncaring and abusive person who will never change. He sees no hope for the relationship (message). Since you (the receiver) wish to offer your friend good counsel, you reflect on his message critically, hoping to gain a better, "truer," understanding of the situation that he faces than he can manage at this moment. In other words, you need more accurate information.

There are several claims in this message that you might second-guess. For instance, in the simplest case, you might have reason to doubt that his wife is either an uncaring or an abusive person based on your prior experiences with her, leading you to reject you friend's claim. Alternatively, you might reinterpret the same claim based on your knowledge that people tend to see others as more consistent and unchangeable than they really are. Thus you may reason that what is really going on here is that your friend is blaming his wife for being an abusive and uncaring person when she is only reacting to the immediate difficulties she faces in the relationship. You might go further, questioning your friend's imputation of her personality as the cause of the conflict. You know him to be a demanding, insecure person who may provoke others to keep their distance from him and who responds angrily when he is asked for too much. Consequently, you may feel that the message is really a reflection of his own insecurity and that he is really the cause of the conflict.

One may also second-guess about concrete experiences, not merely general attributions of character or causality. To illustrate, your sister (the source) tells you that she saw your dating partner flirt with members of the desired sex at a bar last night (the message). Your first reaction is jealousy, but you want be sure that there is reason to feel this way since jealously can damage a relationship. You might second-guess the message based on your knowledge of your dating partner's typical behavior (he or she is innocently flirtatious), the state of your relationship (secure), or your sister's ability to identify flirtation when she sees it (she sees sexual implications in everything). In short, you may use information about source or target to reconstruct what "really" happened last night.

These two examples help to illustrate certain general properties of second-guessing. First, messages that trigger it are salient to the receiver. They may be salient either because they have serious consequences for the receiver's goals ("I want to advise my friend well"; "If I act jealously I could damage this relationship"). Although not illustrated here, they may also simply be striking in their own right (Doelger, Hewes, & Graham, 1986), as in the case of a rumor of a scandal or a presidential address on a politically awkward topic. Second, the messages themselves make synthetic, as opposed to analytic (definitional), truth claims. These claims concern existence ("she flirted"), attributes of person or events ("he is insecure"), the causes of, or reasons for, states of affairs ("she is abusive because . . . "), emotional states ("I love you"), or evaluations of persons or events ("*American Ninja* is a great film"). They may be more or less concrete and may or may not be practically verifiable by the receiver, or even a researcher.[1] Third, something about the message—its form (manifestations of unusual levels of tension) or, as in these examples, its content—gives the receiver reason to question the state of affairs described in the message. Fourth, and finally, prior knowledge, either general ("people generally blame others more than themselves for conflicts"), or specific to the target ("my sister sees sexual connotations in everything"), is brought to bear in the process of reinterpreting the message in order to construct a more satisfying and useful interpretation. Once a reinterpretation is made, it then may be checked by the receiver to determine its veracity.

This thumbnail sketch of second-guessing only hints at its generative mechanism. In this review, we address this issue while undertaking three tasks. First, we identify the contributions that the theory of second-guessing can make to communication theory generally. We argue briefly that an understanding of the process of second-guessing has implications beyond those for the phenomenon itself, implications that challenge specific, simplifying assumptions and limiting foci endemic to modern communication theory. Second, we offer a much expanded version of second-guessing theory that encompasses such previously unaddressed problems as (1) the effects of need for accurate information on cue identification and (2) the relationship between second-guessing and the choice of strategies to assess the subjective adequacy of the reinterpretation that results from second-guessing. Finally, we identify directions for extending second-guessing theory through further elaboration of the theory and its applications to several research domains including interpersonal, organizational, and mass communication.

THE RELEVANCE OF SECOND-GUESSING FOR COMMUNICATION THEORY

The phenomenon of second-guessing has important implications for the study of human communication generally. Let us focus briefly on three of those implications—expanding the role of the hearer, emphasizing the role of nontransactional episodes, and elaborating the connection between cognition and human communication.

Expanding the Role of the Hearer

Much of the current work on communication either ignores strategic considerations altogether or carries an implicit focus on the speaker to the exclusion of the hearer. In either case, little consideration is given to the active, construing, strategic listener except, perhaps, in the group polarization (Alderton & Frey, 1986; Seibold & Meyers, 1986) and deception literatures (see Knapp, Cody, & Reardon, 1987; Zuckerman et al., 1981; also Roloff, this volume, for relevant exceptions in persuasion research). Consider two illustrations of this point.

With the publication of Fisher and Hawes's (1971) ground-breaking theory of group communication, coincident trends in the study of marital interaction (see Rausch, 1965, 1972) and small group decision making (Bales, 1950; Scheidel & Crowell, 1964) were unified into a single philosophical and theoretic focus. Fisher and Hawes, in their interact system model, emphasized the temporal interplay of conventionalized communication acts to the exclusion of either the unique properties of communicators or the processes that might make the connection between the initiation of a message (act) and the response to it problematic. Conveyed to the present by small group (for instance, Ellis, 1979; Hirokawa, 1980, 1983) and relational communication researchers (see Millar & Rogers, 1987; VanLear, 1987), this theoretical stance ignores *both* the speaker's *and* the hearer's strategic orientations in favor of an overly conventionalized view of communication (Hewes & Planalp, 1982).

Another dominant strand of research which tends to ignore the strategic listener draws on the heritage of Miller, Boster, Roloff, and Seibold (1977). These authors literally opened the floodgates on studies of the antecedents of speaker strategy choice (see Cody & McLaughlin, 1985; Seibold, Cantrill, &

Meyers, 1986). Researchers within this tradition emphasize the strategic speaker to the exclusion of the active, construing, strategic listener. For example, current research in uncertainty reduction theory (Berger & Calabrese, 1975) examines factors that promote the use of interrogation (Berger & Kellermann, 1983) or relaxation strategies (Kellermann & Berger, 1984). While there is nothing inherently wrong with trying to adduce antecedents of speaker strategy choice, it is limiting—especially if speaker- and hearer-oriented strategies of information gathering interact, as indeed they do (Hewes et al., 1988, and Section II of this chapter).

The study of second-guessing raises serious questions about these limiting foci on communication. By positing that hearers actively reconstrue the meanings of messages under specifiable conditions (Hewes & Planalp, 1982), hearers are accorded a status lost in either of the two traditions just discussed. And whether or not this strategic construal process is normatively adequate, the phenomenon of second-guessing expands our notions of what a theory of communication must encompass. In order to encompass the strategic hearer, we must include all of the following in our theories of human communication; hearers' motivations, the social knowledge that they use in construing messages, the mechanisms that dictate when, and what, knowledge is brought to bear in any given interaction, and how that knowledge affects subsequent communication (Bowers & Bradac, 1982; Hewes & Planalp, 1982; Winograd, 1977).

Emphasizing Indirect and Nontransactional Episodes

In recent years, interpersonal communication researchers have focused primarily on direct communication. That is, they have focused on dyadic, face-to-face exchanges as social actors' primary source of information about themselves, the other in the interaction, or their relationship with the other (Berger, 1987). While information is often acquired directly, too much emphasis on this modal property of social information gathering serves as a barrier to a fuller understanding of communication. As the phenomenon of second-guessing reminds us, much of our information about the social world arises from less direct sources.

Schutz (1967, chaps. 4, 5) recognized that much knowledge of contemporaries is gained indirectly (also see McCall & Simmons, 1978, on "indirect perception"). Social actors hear about their relationships "through the grapevine"; "their reputations precede them"; and they learn about others "over the back fence." This indirectly obtained information can affect their judgments of others (Gilovich, 1987), the development of their relationships (Parks & Adelman, 1983; Parks, Stan, & Eggert, 1983), the survival of those relationships (Planalp & Honeycutt, 1985), and even mass hysteria (Cantril, 1940; Johnson, 1945; Tummin & Feldman, 1955).

Moreover, the dominant ideology in communication also presumes that interpersonal communication involves some form of mutual engagement; an irreducible sharing of experience (see Stewart, 1978), mutual efforts to attain shared meanings (see McHugh, 1968; Schutz & Luckman, 1973), negotiating a definition of a relationship (see Rogers & Farace, 1975; coordinating activities (Cronen, Pearce, & Harris, 1982), or enacting hedonistic exchanges (see Chadwick-Jones, 1976; Roloff, 1987). In other words, interpersonal communication is a mutually involving symbolic activity. And, again, as second-guessing reminds us, even face-to-face interactions are not necessarily fully engaging.

Often social actors interact with others while simultaneously living separate, and often, secret lives. Liars and other strategic speakers may have hidden purposes, but so do hearers. Hearers may feel that they have detected deception but fear confronting the speaker with their impression; the same may be true in many other high-risk situations, such as acquiring information about the disposition of an attractive other before one is ready to reveal one's own disposition to date or form a relationship. In these instances, communication is not truly transactional. The hearer gathers and interprets social information without making those interpretations part of the communicative process. Too much emphasis on engagement in social interaction draws us away from understanding these essentially nontransactional episodes.

Elaborating the Connection Between Cognition and Communication

A growing core of communication researchers have recognized the importance of cognitive mechanisms such as memory, attention, judgment, message production, and the like for explaining human communication (see Berger & Chaffee, 1987; Hewes & Planalp, 1987; Wartella & Reeves, 1987). They argue that communication theory, unaugmented by knowledge of cognitive representations and processes, is inherently flawed and incomplete. On the other hand, many social psychologists have come to understand that cognitive theory without connections to social processes is distorted and narrow (see Forgas, 1981; Sampson, 1981).

Participants in both theoretical endeavors recognize these limitations and have striven to overcome them. Thus we find theorists in cognition demanding the study of memory in natural contexts (Neisser, 1978) and a growing demand for research into the connection between cognition and behavior (Fiske & Taylor, 1984; Nisbett & Ross, 1980), particularly communicative behavior (as in Kelley et al., 1983). Similar demands have been expressed in the literature in communication theory (Craig, 1979; Greene, 1984; Planalp & Hewes, 1982; Roloff & Berger, 1982).

While responses to these calls have been forthcoming in both theoretical domains, the nature of the connection between cognition and communication is still far from clear. For example, the locus of cognitive research has virtually always been on biases in interpretation (Markus & Zajonc, 1985; Nisbett & Ross, 1980; Sherman & Corty, 1984; Fiske & Taylor, 1984) or on the consequences of those biases in the inappropriate use of social information-gathering strategies (see Snyder, 1984; Fiske & Taylor, 1984; see also, Isen, Means, Patrick, & Nowicki, 1982; Trope & Bassok, 1982). Both these research traditions err in failing to account for the fact that we can successfully coordinate social action despite the existence of all these biases. Somehow social actors compensate for enough distortions to engage in complex organized activity. How do they do so? As Hewes and Planalp (1982) assert and second-guessing theory implies, social actors possess corrective mechanisms that make the effects of those biases less pernicious. A fuller understanding of the complex connection between cognition and communication must reflect this understanding, while further recognizing that cognitive processes take place in social settings in which self-reflection and feedback can correct for cognitive errors.

Because second-guessing is a process of debiasing messages, it serves as an anodyne to the current focus on the biasing effects of cognition (Hewes et al., 1985). By demonstrating the conditions under which biased messages may be reinterpreted accurately (i.e., with "normative adequacy"), second-guessing theory expands the role of cognition in communication, giving it not only a necessary role but a positive role as well. In addition, recent developments in the theory of second-guessing previewed here trace the effects of a message from its initial interpretation through its debiasing reinterpretation to its effects on the selection of specific social tactics that might serve to clarify the hearer's understanding of the "truth" behind the message. In this way, the theory of second-guessing offers a preliminary, though necessarily limited, model of how communication theorists can more fully integrate cognition into the study of human communication without becoming "lost in the head" (Hewes et al., 1988).

SECOND-GUESSING THEORY: REVIEW AND EXTENSIONS

To this point, we have sought to provide a conceptual introduction to second-guessing and to offer some hint of its worth to the field of communication. In this section, we present a model of the process of second-guessing. We then proffer the causal and choice mechanisms that explain what happens at each of the four stages of the process and the status of support for those explanations.

A Model of the Process of Second-Guessing

Our model of the processes of second-guessing combines the reinterpretive aspects of second-guessing discussed in previous studies (Doelger et al., 1986; Hewes et al., 1985; Hewes & Planalp, 1982) with new components in the areas of reinterpretation assessment and, briefly, social information-gathering tactic selection. In describing this model, we will, of necessity, present it in strictly linear terms as it might operate if a social actor were evaluating only one message claim, rather than a set of partially unrelated claims. In this latter case, a social actor might be operating simultaneously at a number of different stages in the process—and be faced with all the difficulties this management might entail. Given this one proviso, we believe the model operates as follows (see Figure 4.1). In the *vigilance* phase, a message is received from some source in a particular context. It is given an initial interpretation that involves accepting the meaning of the message at face value. Then, depending on the cues contained in the message and/or context *and* the importance of obtaining accurate information, some degree of doubt may be generated concerning the veracity of the initial interpretation of the message (Doelger et al., 1986). If there is insufficient reason to doubt, the initial interpretation of the message is accepted at face value. If there is reason to doubt that interpretation, but the importance of accuracy is not sufficiently high, no effort is made to extract the "true" state of affairs behind the message, though it might be recalled to analysis if its importance became greater. If there are cues, however, that raise questions about the veracity of the initial interpretation of the message, and accuracy is important, the social actor enters what Doelger et al. (1986) refer to as "the strategy deployment phase" (p. 328). In this phase, the social actor decides how best to cope with this biased message. A receiver may decide to employ second-guessing, some social information-gathering strategy (e.g., Berger, 1979; Berger & Kellermann, 1983; Kellermann & Berger, 1984), or some combination of both to debias the message depending on his or her perception of social costs and the likely effectiveness of these various strategies.

Since Doelger et al. (1986) described the strategy deployment phase, the complexity of this phase has forced us to abandon it in favor of a series of three-ordered phases that better represent the interrelationships between second-guessing and social information-gathering strategies (Hewes et al., 1988). Our second, third, and fourth phases are now labeled the *Reinterpretation, Reinterpretation Assessment*, and *Social Tactic Choice* phases, respectively. In the *Reinterpretation* phase (Doelger et al., 1986; Hewes et al., 1985), the social actor engages in the reflective, "mindful" process of reinterpreting the message, a process called second-guessing.[2] The outcome of this reinterpretive process is one or more interpretations of the "truth" behind the message, each of which is assigned some level of confidence and each of which may provide a more or less detailed explanation of the subjectively "true" state of affairs behind the message (level of clarity). We assume that the results of this reinterpretive process are approximately "normatively adequate." That is, the reinterpretations are assumed to be closer to the truth about the target than the initial face-value interpretation of the message (Hewes et al., 1985), though

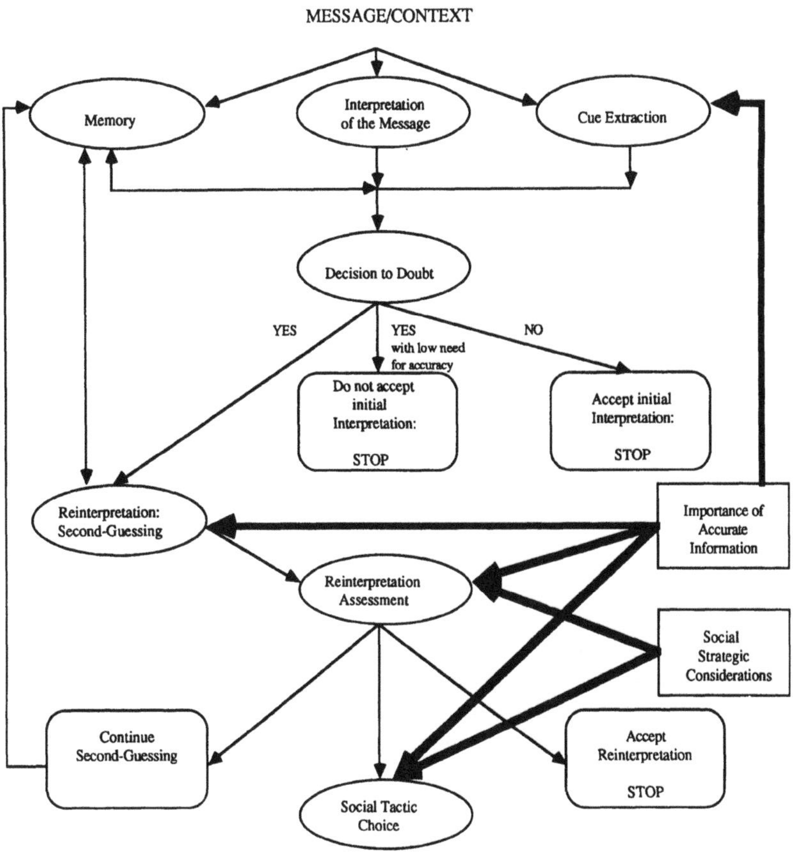

Figure 4.1 A pictorial model of second-guessing. The ellipses represent cognitive processes. Narrow arrows initiating in these processes carry the results of each process to the next stage in processing or to some exit point represented by the rounded rectangles. The standard rectangles represent causal variables, with the wide arrows indicating the causal influence of those variables on some cognitive process. Upon choosing and deploying some social tactic (see Social Tactic Choice at bottom of figure), receivers may be faced with another message/context that reinitiates the whole process described in the figure.

it is still possible that upon reflection in the *Reinterpretation Assessment* phase a social actor will return to the original interpretation.

At this point, the social actor enters the third phase—*Reinterpretation Assessment* (Hewes et al., 1988). Depending on the importance of accurate information, the mental difficulty (cognitive load) involved in assessing the reinterpretations, and certain socially strategic considerations (the social effort needed to gain better information and the social constraints that may prevent one from doing so), the social actors may adopt one or more alternative strategies for assessing the adequacy of each reinterpretation as judged against the original interpretation and other reinterpretations of the same claim. The social actor may decide to accept the best, or only, reinterpretation (or even the original interpretation, although this occurs infrequently in our experience) and stop further analysis of the message. Alternatively, he or she may opt to continue second-guessing by returning to the message and context as stored in memory. Finally, she or he may decide to employ some social tactic designed to test the logical consistency of the reinterpretations or to provide new information that will generate more confidence and/or clarity in one of the reinterpretations, or both. If the social actor desires to seek new information in the social realm, the fourth phase is entered—*Social Tactic Choice* (Graham, Hewes, Doelger, & Monsour, unpublished). In this phase, the choice of some social tactic is guided by the importance of accurate information and social strategic considerations (concerns for conserving social effort). Having sketched the process of second-guessing, we consider in greater detail how each phase functions theoretically and what evidence there is to support these claims.

Phase 1: Vigilance

Most research on second-guessing has focused on the phases of *Vigilance* and *Reinterpretation*. To expedite our discussion, we have subdivided the Vigilance Phase into two parts—the preconditions necessary for the existence of this phase and the theoretical linkages among the variables and cognitive processes functioning at this phase.

Preconditions

Cognitive processes do not arise in a vacuum (Hewes et al., 1985). Rather, some cognitive processes—such as memory, attention, integration, and so on (see Planalp & Hewes, 1982)—probably arise through biological evolution as a function of the press between human survival needs on the one hand and the demands of the physical environment on the other. Other cognitive processes, probably better identified as "skills" (as in Anderson, 1981; Greene, 1984), are acquired through socialization, individual experience, or formal training and are built out of basic, evolution-endowed cognitive processes. For instance, mathematical reasoning, problem-solving, and comprehension of discourse are skills in this sense.

The whole process of second-guessing, including the *vigilance* phase, is also a skill. Viewed in this light, this skill, like any other, results from the press between personal needs and the demands of the environment—in this case not only physical but social demands as well (Hewes et al., 1985; Simon, 1960). Because a skill is not innate, certain preconditions must exist to foster and sustain its development—preconditions both environmental and personal. If these preconditions are met, the existence of the skill is plausible and its etiology understandable. Of course, in order to demonstrate that the skill actually exists one must directly test it in use.

Motivating the development of second-guessing is the basic human need to reduce uncertainty (Berger & Calabrese, 1975; Kagan, 1972). The need to reduce uncertainty about another's intentions, goals, and behaviors arises from simple human curiosity, the desire for a sense of control over one's life (Jones, 1979; also see Tetlock & Levi, 1982 on the motivational bases for attributional biases), and the need to have information necessary to pursue successfully other personal needs (Hewes & Planalp, 1982).

Social actors can meet the first two facets of the need to reduce uncertainty, at least temporarily, without obtaining *accurate* information. Curiosity and the desire for a sense of control can be satisfied by any relevant source of information, at least until the environment demonstrates the inaccuracy of that information—something that may not happen rapidly (Fiske & Taylor, 1984). All that is necessary is that the information must be *perceived* as accurate (Jones, 1979; Tetlock & Levi, 1982). Presumably, the effective pursuit of other personal goals, and especially concrete goals with short-run payoffs, requires a more critical stance toward information—information must be at least approximately accurate in some objective sense (and, of course, relevant to the goals) in order to pursue those goals effectively (Hewes et al., 1988; Hewes & Planalp, 1982). The theory of second-guessing concerns the need to reduce uncertainty by means of *accurate* information.

Do social actors have a desire for accurate information? What stands behind this desire? Social actors express this need freely in both open-ended and close-ended survey formats, yielding substantial evidence of convergent validity when the two operationalizations are correlated ($r = 0.57$, $N = 118$, $p < 0.001$: Hewes et al., 1988). Ample, though indirect, evidence for the existence of a need for accurate information can be found in its power as a predictor of reinterpretation assessment strategy choice (Hewes et al., 1988) and social tactic choice (Graham, Hewes, Doelger, & Monsour, unpublished). Thus we feel justified in making the need for accurate information one of the cornerstones of the theory of second-guessing (see Figure 4.1), although we leave to empirical testing the ability of social actors to gather such information or to recognize it when they have it.

What stands behind the need for accurate information? Here we have little direct evidence (but see Roloff, this volume). We do know that there is an extremely large positive correlation between social actors' perceived need for accurate information and their desire to take social action based on that information ($r = 0.90$, $N = 109$, $p < .001$: Graham et al., unpublished). This finding suggests that the need for accurate information is salient in those situations demanding social action, possibly because it is precisely in those situations in which social actors face real consequences for acting without a firm evidentiary base. Kruglanski and Ajzen (1984) and Kruglanski and

Freund (1983) also suggest that social actors adopt a more critical stance toward the implications of information when their judgments are open to scrutiny by those they believe are in a better position to know the "truth," experts or those who have access to "inside" information, for instance.

In addition, stable differences across individuals may serve as predictors of a need for accurate information. Consider, for example, "self-monitoring" (Snyder, 1987). Self-monitoring correlates with almost anything of interest to communication researchers—or so it seems, reading reviews of self-monitoring (see Roloff, 1987; Snyder, 1987). In the case of need for accurate information, there are good reasons to expect such a correlation. Low self-monitors engage in self-presentation to a minimal degree. Thus whether through lack of skill, lack of motivation, or a counter-motivation to be true to themselves, they do not use contextual information to define who they are to others. On the other hand, high self-monitors are very conscious of the demands of social situations, and through the use of motivated, skillful performances, adapt their presented image to the mandates of certain identifiable contexts (Snyder, 1987).

Characteristic of contexts that are seen as attractive by high self-monitors, but not by lows, are those in which the goals and the goal-path linkages are easily discernible (Mill, 1984; Snyder & Harkness, 1984). Moreover, high, but not low, self-monitors will attempt to transform contexts to make their goals and goal-path linkages manifest (Snyder & Gangestad, 1982). Given this grounding, we anticipate that high self-monitors should have higher needs for accurate information than should low self-monitors in contexts in which goals and goal-path linkages are clear, but that that difference should decrease in contexts characterized by higher levels of goal clarity.

Since high self-monitors have a higher need for information with which to transform their situated identities, they should be more motivated than should low self-monitors to seek the requisite information. And, indeed, some evidence indicates their willingness to do so (Berger & Douglas, 1981; Bercheid, Graziano, Monson, & Dermer, 1976; Elliot, 1979; Jones & Baumeister, 1976; Tomarelli & Graziano, 1981). Thus self-monitoring offers one promising direction to extend second-guessing theory through the inclusion of individual-difference variables. In any event, an understanding of the antecedents of the need for accurate information, both personal and contextual, is crucial to the theory of second-guessing since these antecedents trigger the process of second-guessing and may affect it at subsequent phases in the process.

Unfortunately, understanding the antecedents of the need for accurate information is logically insufficient in itself to explain the development of second-guessing. If we lived in a world with no lies, no misjudgment, and no constraints on the flow of information, we would need but to listen or to ask to satisfy our need. Only when the need for accurate information faces barriers to its satisfaction does a skill for second-guessing develop. What might these barriers be? We can provide part of the answer (Hewes et al., 1985). Social actors must believe that they need to know about persons and/or events outside their direct experience, that such information is available through other people (sources), and that such information is not irredeemably tainted.

Direct and strong evidence supporting the existence of all three of these beliefs was obtained in two distinct populations—college students and subjects in formal organizational settings (Hewes et al., 1985). The only substantial difference between the two samples was that those subjects in organizational settings, who reported using second-guessing, were more inclined to report using interactive information-gathering strategies and less inclined to use hearer-oriented information-gathering strategies than were those who did not report using second-guessing. The college sample did not manifest this pattern (Hewes et al., 1985). Regardless of this apparent anomaly (addressed in the last section), we have good support for the claim that the preconditions necessary to foster the development of the skill of second-guessing exist in the press between a need for accurate information and perceived environmental barriers to the flow of accurate information. However, establishing that there is a perceived need for a skill, and environmental barriers to overcome with it, does not guarantee that a skill has actually developed.

What must be shown is that social actors actually have the necessary skills to engage in second-guessing. Within the *vigilance* phase, according to our sketch of second-guessing, the component of that skill that must be examined empirically is the ability to identify potentially biased messages. In order to do so, social actors must have a set of cues that permit them to discriminate subjectively between the presence and absence of potentially biased messages.

Doelger et al. (1986) undertook the process of identifying these cues. Key to that effort is our conception of what cues are and what they are not. Cues are elements of the message content, form, and context conjointly through which a social actor privileges certain interpretations of the message. Hence, a cue is not simply an objective property of message, but arises from a receiver's interpretation of the message content, form, and such contextual factors as the immediate definition of the situation and background knowledge, relational history, and any implicit goals attributed to the participants in the exchange. Thus cues that promote second-guessing, or any other inference-making process, are interpretations, not simple "objective" linguistic, para-linguistic, or behavioral events (see Ostrom, 1984). These cues arise from an interaction between the objective speech and visual signals and some interpretive process. The process by which these interpretations are made is labeled *cue extraction* in Figure 4.1.

Cue extraction has not been the focus of second-guessing research. The result is that tests of our theory have circumvented a crucial step in any communication theory—the connection between the objective speech and visual signals and the construal of those signals as cues. By permitting cue extraction to function as a "ghost process" in our theory, we have failed to consider what objective properties of messages are feeding the process of second-guessing. In order for a theory of communication to take up its full burden, these objective properties must become part of the theory. Otherwise the communicative connection between speaker and hearer cannot truly be studied. Still, to identify interpretations, as we do by specifying cues to second-guessing, does count as progress, since they provide the foundation against which the process of cue extraction can be anchored.

Evidence supporting the existence of cues to potential bias is provided primarily by Doelger et al. (1986). Table 4.1 summarizes the current list of 18 cues, refined and expanded from Doelger et al.'s 16-cue typology, based on as yet unreported data from a sample used in Hewes et al. (1988) and Graham et al. (unpublished). Following Doelger et al. (1986), four sets of cues are presented—cues attributable to the person or event, to the source, to message form or content, and to the receiver. Updated average coding reliability figures are provided for each category.

Independent support for the existence of some of these cues is available in Hewes et al. (1985). There we demonstrated that subjects had clear, conscious knowledge of the biasing effects of informational cues 2.4a-2.4c as described in Table 4.1. What is most surprising about the support garnered for these cues is that each of them—cues to the availability heuristic (2.4a), cues to the representativeness heuristic (2.4b), and cues to the fundamental attribution error (2.4c)—are, in the bulk of the human judgment literature, supposed to be reflectively inaccessible to social actors under normal circumstances (see Nisbett & Ross, 1980; Fiske & Taylor, 1984; but there are isolated counterexamples as in Isen et al., 1982, on the representativeness heuristic, and Kruglanski, Hamel, Maides, & Schwartz, 1978, on the fundamental attribution error). Overall, then, we have good support for the existence of cues that prompt second-guessing, even cues that should not be accessible given current theory on human judgment.

Theoretical Linkages

Having shown that the preconditions exist for the development of the cognitive skill of second-guessing, we turn to the theoretical linkages posited in the *vigilance* phase. In this section, we examine two such linkages; that between the need for accurate information and cue extraction and that between cue extraction and the decision to doubt.

Second-guessing theory implies that the higher the need for accuracy, the more vigilant social actors should be in identifying sources of biased information that might prevent them from taking appropriate action to attain their goals; however, increased vigilance does not necessarily have the obvious effect of increasing a social actor's sensitivity to the occurrence of cues. Increasing the need for accuracy can have the result of decreasing the detection rate for cues. After all, increasing accuracy can be accomplished in

TABLE 4.1
Coding Scheme for Second-Guessing Cues:
Category Descriptions and Reliability Estimates

	Category Descriptions	Average Percentage Agreement	
(1)	Target Cues		
(1.1)	Inconsistency (specific to target): Message from the source is inconsistent with prior knowledge of the target. (This includes baseline probabilities on events as related to the target as an individual.)	.88	.83
(1.2)	Inconsistency (general): Message from the source is inconsistent with prior knowledge of the target. (This includes baseline probabilities on events as related to norms or information concerning events and/or people like the target.)	n.a.	.83
(2)	Source Cues		
(2.1)	Motivational Cues		
(2.1a)	Source distorts for his or her own benefit.	.85	.73
(2.1b)	Source distorts for altruistic reasons: for example, to avoid embarrassing the target or some other person.	.98	1.00
(2.1c)	Consistency bias: Distortion resorts from source's attempts to keep his/her attitudes and/or beliefs consistent.	1.00	.93
(2.2)	Dispositional Cues		
(2.2a)	Rigid use of knowledge structures: Source always sees things in a particular way (e.g., from a constructivist, Marxist, right wing, or religious perspective) even when such a perspective is inappropriate. Could be the implied result of the source's group membership.	.96	.98
(2.2b)	Dispositional distortions: Source is a habitual liar, exaggerator, distorter, and so on. [Or source has distorted information in similar contents previously.]	.90	.80
(2.2c)	Personal preferences: Not necessarily implying bias or distortion, but acknowledging the role of personal tastes. Source holds different judgmental criteria when evaluating the target. Therefore, he or she cannot provide accurate information for me.	.94	.95
(2.2d)	Diagnosticity: Source is not skilled in identifying or using discriminal clues to reach a conclusion.	.93	.98
(2.3)	Consistency Cues		
(2.3a)	Behavioral consistency: Source's typical behavior patterns are deviated from (would not be a cue for anyone though: These are deviations particular to this source's typical behavior). [Uses *this* source's typical behavior as a baseline, not a baseline of all human behavior (for the latter, see 4.1b).]	.88	.95
(2.4)	Informational Cues		
(2.4a)	Availability heuristic: Source's account of the target was influenced by the availability of objects or events, for example, their accessibility in the processes of perception, memory, or recall; not their actual occurrence. Specific type: Egocentric bias—One's own efforts and actions may be disproportionately available and their frequency compared to those of others may be overestimated ("I helped the group more than they did.")	.95	1.00

(continued)

Table 4.1 Continued

(2.4b)	Representativeness heuristic: Application of simple resemblance or goodness of fit criteria to problems of categorization. Deals with the degree to which salient features of the object are representative of, or similar to features presumed to be characteristic of the category. Source has not considered the relevant base-rate information in drawing conclusions about the target.	.98	1.00
(2.4c)	Fundamental attribution error: Source's comment on the target reflects his or her view that behavior is caused by enduring dispositions of the actor rather than characteristics of the situation.	.99	.98
(2.4d)	Data sufficiency: Source does not have sufficient data to reach the stated conclusion about the target. (This includes the area of expertise normally associated with source credibility.)	.92	.98
(3) Receiver Cues			
(3.1)	Dispositional traits: Receiver makes a global self-attribution concerning his or her own tendencies to question the face interpretations of messages, for example, "I just distrust people."	.92	1.00
(3.2)	Specific tendencies: Receiver makes a specific self-attribution concerning her or his tendency to question messages of a specific kind or messages received in a specific context: "I don't accept flattery well." Excluded from this category are attributions made about others, for example, "Salesmen are untrustworthy."	n.a.	.95
(4) Message Cues			
(4.1)	Message is internally inconsistent: Components of the message are contradictory. Anyone could hear the inconsistency; not based on prior knowledge of the specific source or target. (May also include inconsistencies between claims or between data and claims for specific types of messages.)	.83	.85
(4.2)	Message deviates from expected form: Represents clues that would be evident if provided by *any* source, for example, the delivery was too smooth, too confident, too hesitant, and so on.	.91	.93

SOURCE: The first column of agreement figures is derived from Doelger et al., 1986; the second column from Hewes et al., 1988.
NOTE: Two categories were not used in the study by Doelger et al., 1986, but were in the study by Hewes et al., 1988. Those two categories—1.2 and 3.2—obviously have no reliability estimates in the first column, as indicated by n.a. (not available) designation.

two ways—by increasing the social actors' awareness of cues otherwise undetected, that is, increasing *sensitivity*, or by decreasing the *ambiguity* of cues used in judgments, that is, by discounting normally observed but ambiguous cues.

Social actors tend to prefer the latter alternative. The reporting rate of cue detection for very simple objective cues decreases as motivation to identify those cues increases (Davenport, 1968, 1969; Levine, 1966). The explanation for these findings seems to be that under task conditions in which (1) the task is open-ended and (2) rewarding in its own right, increases in motivation will lead social actors to report more conservatively having detected cues, thus avoiding errors (Eysenck, 1982; McGraw, 1978). It seems reasonable to assume that conditions (1) and (2) are typically met in most second-guessing situations. Second-guessing is certainly open-ended, and it can be rewarding in its own right both as an intellectual exercise and as a means of satisfying curiosity. Thus we predicted that as the need for accurate information increases, the number of cues for second-guessing identified decreases.

Although no experimental studies of this prediction have been conducted to date, preliminary nonexperimental evidence obtained by Hewes, Monsour, and Rutherford, in an unpublished manuscript, provide a test. Drawing on subjects' accounts of their most recent incident of second-guessing, we obtained the predicted significant, negative correlation between need for accurate information and the number of cues identified ($r = -0.16$, $N = 111$, $p < 0.05$). We also regressed the need for accurate information on the number of the 18 cues, described in Table 4.1, occurring in each instance of second-guessing in order to determine if an increase in the need for accurate information resulted in a decrease in the number of cues identified by social actors. We found a marginally significant multiple R^2 of 0.28 ($F = 1.98$, $df = 18, 92$, $p = 0.05$) for the whole model. Of the 18 cues, only two—background consistency cues specific to the target (1.1) and diagnosticity (2.2.d)—were positively associated with need for accurate information, and only one of those two—background consistency cues—had an unstandardized regression coefficient significantly greater than zero (*standardized beta* = 0.22, $t = 2.15$, $df = 110$, $p < 0.05$). Thus as the need for accurate information increases, the number of cues to second-guessing generally decreases—with one exception. In high need situations, social actors shift their focus away from other cues in favor of cues to background inconsistency related to the specific target under consideration.

Obviously, experimental tests of these conclusions must be forthcoming. Experimental tests would greatly aid us in eliminating one troubling alternative interpretation of these results. If we assume that the causal direction between number of cues detected and need for accurate information is reversed, we could quite sensibly assert that as the number of cues increases, social actors become more certain about the persons and/or events described in the message, thus decreasing their need for accuracy. By manipulating the need for accuracy, we can determine if this plausible alternative hypothesis is correct. Even if our original interpretation of this evidence is correct, the normative adequacy of these results must be considered and tested: Does the general decline in cue identification decrease the likelihood of detecting messages that warrant second-guessing? Is the increased reliance on background inconsistency cues in high need situations warranted? As of now, we do not know.

Second-guessing theory also posits that the presence of cues to second-guessing will produce more doubt in the minds of social actors than will the absence of such cues. Direct support for this claim appears in Doelger et al. (1986). In this study, we manipulated three cues—cues to the presence of self-serving motivational biases in the source's message, background cues in which the receiver's knowledge of the target could lead to a different interpretation than the source's, and cues to the presence of the availability heuristic. We contrasted the effects of these three cues with a "no cue" condition over four widely differing contexts, including reactions to a difficult test, a roommate's reactions to his or her partner's impending romantic break-up, a job interview situation, and a blind date. The gender of the receiver was also included in the design. We found that subjects, when asked to evaluate the reasonableness of the face value of a message, reported significantly more reason to doubt it in all the cued than in the "no cue" conditions ($\alpha = 0.05$). No significant effects, either main-effects or interactions, were obtained for sex or context.

The strengths and weaknesses of this study are both clear. On the one hand, there is strong evidence linking cues to second-guessing to the reason to doubt; on the other, only three of the posited 18 cues (see Table 4.1) have been used to test this relationship. Further, testing some of these other cues may prove very difficult. For example, cues to the fundamental attribution error can lead to functionally equivalent but substantively different accounts for bias. Theorists have argued that the source of this error arises from either motivational, or unintended cognitive, factors (Tetlock & Levi, 1982). Assignment of blame is clearly different for each factor; yet, each factor leads to the same functionally equivalent conclusion that social actors inflate the significance of the situational causes of their own behavior while deflating the significance of the situational causes of other actors' behaviors (Kelley, 1967; Ross, 1977). Unfortunately two sets of cues, motivational (2.1 in Table 4.1) and cognitive (2.3), could lead the social actor to the same conclusion. Problems of this type must be solved before independent manipulation of some of these cues is possible. Regardless, extensions of Doelger et al. (1986) to other cues is essential in order to fully test the claims of second-guessing theory.

To conclude, there is good preliminary support for the hypothesized variables and linkages posited in the *Vigilance* phase, although much needs to be done before a detailed picture of this part of second-guessing theory emerges. Aside from those gaps already highlighted, the linkages between memory and both cue extraction and the preliminary interpretation of the message should be explored. Because memory is an active, constructive process (Bartlett, 1932; Hastie, Park, & Weber, 1984) rather than a dustbin filled with the past, it can be expected to both affect and be affected by cue extraction and interpretation (see van Dijk & Kintsch, 1983). Although we have not worked out implications of this view of memory for the process of second-guessing, those implications will undoubtedly be important to future extensions of our theory.

Phase 2: Reinterpretation

During the *Reinterpretation* phase, two theoretical linkages are posited. The first is a choice inspired by the reason to doubt and the need for accurate information (see Figure 4.1). The social actor, faced with sufficient reason to doubt the face value of the message and a sufficient need for accurate information, will attempt to reinterpret the message so as to winnow the truth from behind the message. If there is reason to doubt but insufficient need for accurate information, the social actor will ignore the message and make no attempt to reinterpret it, or at least not until the perceived bias becomes important. Should there be insufficient reason to doubt and an insufficient need for accurate information, the social actor will accept the message at face value. Thus we anticipate an interaction between doubt and need for accurate information in predicting the choice among three reactions to the message (Hewes et al., 1985; Hewes & Planalp, 1982, but see Note 1).[3] No direct tests of this prediction have been performed; however, some indirect supporting evidence appears in Langer's (1978) early work on "mindlessness."

Mindlessness is the complement of second-guessing. Mindlessness is a nonreflective state in which messages are accepted and acted upon without conscious processing of their meaning. Conversely, second-guessing is a mindful state in which the content of messages are examined critically with an eye to reinterpretation (Doelger et al., 1986). Langer demonstrates that compliance-gaining messages with unusual form or content trigger more critical processing and less compliance than do more typical messages (Langer & Abelson, 1972; Langer, Blank, & Chanowitz, 1978). Her results are entirely in line with the notion that doubt and reinterpretation are triggered by the distinctive properties of messages (see cues 1.1, 1.2, 2.3, 4.1, and 4.2 in Table 4.1 and generally in Doelger et al., 1986, p. 304); however, as Doelger et al. note, "although mindfulness is a necessary precondition for second-guessing, it is by no means a sufficient one. Social actors do not attribute bias to all messages while in a mindful state" (p. 304). Thus Langer's evidence is only partially relevant to our predictions concerning the relationship of both the need for accuracy and cue extraction to the reinterpretation of the message; she neither measured need for accuracy nor explored the critical processes that result in a reinterpretation of a message.

More data are available on a second theoretical linkage in the *Reinterpretation* phase. Second-guessing theory predicts that "when confronted with a message displaying cues to both potential cognitive and motivational biases on the part of some source, receivers will adjust their inferences about the target in the normatively correct fashion" (Hewes et al., 1985, p. 306-307). Here we suggest that not only will social actors attempt to reinterpret messages in a way that seems more accurate to them (else why bother), but also their reinterpretations will be closer to the "truth" than will those of persons who do not second-guess, when "truth" is defined by external observers employing both the methods and well-established results of careful inquiry to examine critically the social actors' reinterpretations. In other words, to employ a common distinction in epistemology, whereas social actors base the acceptability of their reinterpretations on "subjective" or "internalist" standards, we wish to employ "externalist" standards for truth so that we as researchers may serve as critics of human cognition (Goldman, 1986; Nisbett & Ross, 1980).

This is no easy row to hoe. Even the claim that there is a truth in some testable sense is controversial, let alone the claim that there are privileged methods of identifying it (see Leplin, 1984; Mehan & Wood, 1975; Suppe, 1974, to name but a few). But we need not go so far as to claim that research can apprehend Metaphysical Truth to demonstrate commonsensical grounds for exploring the normative adequacy of one form of human interpretation. To do so, we offer two criteria which should indicate whether or not social actors' reinterpretations of a message are more normatively adequate than are their initial interpretations.

First, if social actors' reinterpretations are normatively adequate, they should adjust their own judgments about the true state of the affairs referred to in the message so as to reflect an understanding of scientifically validated sources of biases in human judgment. Hewes et al. (1985) undertook to address this criterion for determining the normative adequacy of second-guessing. We manipulate four versions of three cues to biases in human judgment, biases whose effects have been well-documented in the research literature. To ensure that the cues were representative of those particular biases, only cues that had been unanimously accepted by four researchers, three involved in the project and one not, all of whom were familiar with the literature on biases, were incorporated into the design. Those cues were to background inconsistencies (1.1 in Table 4.1), self-serving motivational biases (2.1a), and availability heuristic biases (2.4a). Reinterpretations of messages containing one of these three types of cues were each contrasted to a no-cue condition. Each of the cue types were embedded in four different contexts. The sex of the subject was also included in the design as an independent variable.

The dependent variable in this study was the subjects' assessment of the likelihood that the source's impression of the target was correct. To reflect the normative adequacy of their reinterpretations, subjects needed to respond to cues to bias by judging that the source's impression of the target was less likely than in the no-cue situation. This response apparently happened for all three cues (maximum $p = 0.05$). No significant effects for context or sex were obtained, nor were there any significant interactions among the independent variables (minimum $p < 0.10$).

These results, though supportive of the normative adequacy of second-guessing, are not without their limitations. Beyond the obvious criticism that they relate only to three out of 18 cues that are supposed to trigger and aid in reinterpretation, there lurks a much more serious potential problem. These same results might reflect only a certain cynicism toward the source's conclusions about the target (i.e., lowered source credibility) without implying that the target can correct for different biases in ways consistent with the particular distortions associated with each kind of bias. However, if one could demonstrate that the content of the social actors' reinterpretations reflected specific knowledge of cues being manipulated in each context and the implications of those cues for bias, then there would be stronger support for claims for the normative adequacy of those reinterpretations.

This tack is taken by Doelger et al. (1986). There we demonstrated that subjects' reasons for reinterpreting sources' messages were consistent with the manipulations of the message cues conducted in the aforementioned design. For example, although subjects mentioned background inconsistency as an explanation for reinterpreting the message in all four cue conditions (background inconsistency cues, availability heuristic cues, self-serving motivational bias cues, and the no-cue condition), they almost doubled the percentage of times they mentioned it in the background consistency cue condition (44.9% in this condition versus 25.6% in the no-cue condition). Even more striking, 24.6% of the subjects explained the concept of the availability heuristic in nontechnical terms in their accounts of why they reinterpreted the message in the availability heuristic cue condition, but only 2.3% mentioned it in the no-cue condition. In addition, we found no effects of sex on the identification of cues or in the accuracy with which cues were integrated into accounts of the reinterpretation.

We did find that certain contexts provoked the use of some kinds of explanations more than others regardless of the cues that were manipulated. Although we have developed no theoretical explanation for this finding, it seems likely that social actors have some notions about which biases are more likely in particular interpersonal contexts. To illustrate, in highly emotion-laden interpersonal situations, recall of other situations in which similar emotions dominated should be greater than recall for emotionally different situations (Forgas, Bower, & Krantz, 1984; Isen, 1984; Martins, 1982). Recalling these easily remembered instances should influence one's judgment even when they are not truly relevant to the issue at hand. This is an occasion ripe for the availability heuristic bias (Nisbett & Ross, 1980). If social actors understand this bias, they may view such interpersonal situations as likely to produce this bias regardless of the cues contained in a message. And, in fact, post hoc analyses of Doelger et al.'s data revealed just such a pattern.

Regardless, these results lend credence to the normative adequacy thesis that plays such a major part in second-guessing theory, especially in the *Reinterpretation* phase. Subjects in our studies displayed a range and depth of understanding of biasing strategies that cannot be explained either by conventional theories of human judgment (see Nisbett & Ross, 1980; Sherman & Corty, 1984; Fiske & Taylor, 1984) or by source credibility (see Cronkhite & Liska, 1980; Delia, 1976; McCroskey, 1966). Still, the evidence could be stronger. If we could show that social actors are highly selective in which portion of a complex message they choose to reinterpret, based on the presence of cues to bias, or that qualitative changes in the reinterpretation of the same message arise out of different combinations of multiple cues to bias, the evidence for normative adequacy would be more persuasive. Nevertheless, when one combines the direct evidence for normative adequacy reported here with the evidence from the *Vigilance* phase knowledge of cues and the relationship between cues and reasons to doubt the message, normative adequacy is a very plausible hypothesis.

Phase 3: Reinterpretation Assessment

Early work on second-guessing focused exclusively on the hearer-oriented cognitive process for information acquisition contained in the *Vigilance* and *Reinterpretation* phases (Doelger et al., 1986; Hewes et al., 1985). More recent work has explored the connection between hearer- and speaker-oriented strategies, recognizing the interconnectedness of all facets of uncertainty reduction (as in Berger, 1987). In order to connect cognitive and social sources of uncertainty reduction in the theory of second-guessing, it has proven necessary to posit the existence of a *Reinterpretation Assessment* phase. During this phase, the need for accurate information both directly and indirectly affects the ways in which social actors choose to determine if their reinterpretations of a message are subjectively adequate to their needs. Two other factors—cognitive load and social strategic considerations—also influence this assessment (Hewes et al., 1988).

As Figure 4.1 and our sketch of second-guessing theory indicate, the first theoretical link to be tested in this phase is the connection between need for accurate information and cognitive load. Hewes et al. (1988) hypothesized that the greater the need for accurate information, the more alternative reinterpretations social actors will consider, the less confidence will they express in their reinterpretations, and the less clear will they think their reinterpretations to be. The number of reinterpretations, the confidence with which they are held, and their clarity are all indices of cognitive load during the *Reinterpretation Assessment* phase. For example, if social actors hold two or more incompatible reinterpretations of a message, they must choose among them, a more demanding cognitive task than if there were only one reinterpretation.[4] Similarly, greater reflection is required to reach an acceptable reinterpretation if it is held with little confidence or if its implications are unclear. As the need for accurate information increases, more demands are placed on social actors' cognitive systems. These demands are reflected in the tendency of social actors to see more possible reinterpretations of a message, to question the confidence with which those reinterpretations are held, and to view those reinterpretations as having less clear implications for social action.

Support for this prediction was obtained by Hewes et al. (1988) in a nonexperimental study of 118 undergraduate students who were asked to describe their most recent instance of second-guessing. Using both open- and Likert-type closed-ended response formats, subjects provided assessments of their need for accurate information, descriptions of their reinterpretation(s) of messages, and their confidence in and the clarity of each reinterpretation. Correlations of the predicted sign between an index of need for accurate information (created by pooling the two operationalizations) and each of the cognitive load variables were obtained. One of those correlations, between need for accurate information and confidence, approached significance ($p = 0.07$); the rest were significant at the 0.05 level. Given the small magnitude of the correlations obtained in this study and the high reliability of each of the variables, cognitive load probably has other antecedents beyond the need for accurate information. In all likelihood, these factors, as yet unexplored, included the ambiguity of the message, available cognitive capacity, and the social actor's skill at second-guessing.

The *Reinterpretation Assessment* phase contains another theoretical link, this one directed toward the social actors' subjective (as opposed to "normative") evaluations of their reinterpretation(s). Social actors, according to the theory (see Hewes et al., 1988), must choose among three options to assess the subjective adequacy of their reinterpretation(s): (1) to stop reinterpreting the message and accept the results of the *Reinterpretation* phase, (2) to continue to reinterpret the message relying on information already available to the social actor, or (3) to seek new information from others by selecting and implementing a social information-gathering tactic. Considered in this choice are the need for accurate information, the cognitive load under which the social actor is operating, and, finally, social strategic considerations affecting the accessibility or accuracy of new information. These three considerations are reflected in three theoretically interrelated predictions posited by Hewes et al. (1988).[5]

First, the greater the need for accurate information, the more likely are social actors to engage in social information-gathering. The less the need for accurate information, the more likely will actors stop or continue second-guessing; however, social actors will continue to second-guess in preference to stopping. Results of a nonexperimental test of this hypothesis were supportive, although caution must be exercised in the interpretation of predictions concerning the decision to stop second-guessing—only 9% of the sample reported employing this assessment strategy (Hewes et al., 1988).

Why these results? According to the theory, in the ideal case in which social strategic considerations and cognitive limitations play no part in social actors' decisions, new, relevant information is always desirable, its gathering limited only by the motivation to obtain it. Even when that motivation is low, social actors should prefer to continue second-guessing to stopping since some initially unnoticed information can, at least potentially, be obtained in the performance of the former. (See Hewes et al., 1988, for a more complete rationale for this and the other two predictions for this phase.)

Naturally, the choice of assessment strategies does not always take place under ideal conditions. Social actors are limited in the cognitive capacity that they can devote to any task (Fiske & Taylor, 1984; Mischel, 1981; Navon &

Gopher, 1979; Planalp & Hewes, 1982), including the reinterpretation assessment. Whatever the level of motivation, social actors must shepherd their limited cognitive capacities carefully, lest those capacities become overloaded, resulting in decrements in performance (Eysenck, 1982). Thus we anticipated that the greater the cognitive load, the more likely will social actors be to conserve cognitive effort. As a consequence, the greater the number of reinterpretations, the less confident social actors are in their reinterpretations. The less clear those reinterpretations, the more likely will social actors be to stop second-guessing and the less likely will they be to engage in social information-gathering or continued second-guessing (Hewes et al., 1988).

Partial support for this prediction was obtained in a nonexperimental study based on social actors' descriptions of their most recent second-guessing experiences. The number of reinterpretations did not discriminate among assessment strategy choice, a result we attributed to operational problems with this independent variable (see Hewes et al., 1988, p. 30). Social actors' confidence in their own reinterpretations did discriminate significantly. The perceived clarity of those reinterpretations also discriminated significantly with one anomalous finding. At the lowest levels of clarity, social actors preferred to employ social information-gathering tactics, suggesting that even though cognitive load is an important factor in second-guessing, it may be overridden by the need for accurate information.

According to second-guessing theory, one other factor affects assessment strategy choice—social strategic considerations. Social strategic considerations concern those costs and constraints that affect the availability or usefulness of information obtained in the social realm. For example, the time or effort needed to gather assessment information are costs, whereas the social appropriateness of turning to a particular source on a given topic, the credibility, or the accessibility of that source all represent constraints on either the availability or the usefulness of assessment information.

These costs and constraints taken together are social strategic considerations that affect the amount of social effort needed to evaluate social actors' reinterpretations. Because social actors are thought to work on a principle of conservation of social effort (Boden, 1972; Hewes, 1986: Hewes et al., 1988; McDougall, 1911) that parallels the conservation of cognitive effort discussed previously, we anticipated that the less the social effort to be expended in assessing the adequacy of the results of second-guessing, the more inclined will social actors be to employ social information-gathering tactics and the less inclined will they be to continue to second-guess or to accept the results of second-guessing (Hewes et al., 1988).

Again, the results of the aforementioned nonexperimental study offer partial support for this prediction. Although neither time nor credibility predicted reinterpretation assessment strategy choice—probably a result of high multicolinearity with other independent variables—effort, social appropriateness, and accessibility did. We obtained one unanticipated finding for which we have no explanation. Social actors appear to have a slight preference for using social information-gathering tactics rather than continuing to second-guess in socially effortful situations.

Overall, second-guessing theory has obtained good support in Phase 3. Although our results must be replicated experimentally and observed as they happen in everyday life, still they are highly suggestive of the theory. Furthermore, they imply an expanded role for second-guessing in the study of social information-gathering. Typically, second-guessing has been treated as an alternative to speaker-oriented information-gathering strategies such as strategic self-disclosure, relaxation strategies, and interrogation (see Doelger et al., 1986). Here we have found that second-guessing serves as an antecedent to these speaker-oriented strategies. In fact, in every case examined in Hewes et al.'s, (1988) data, reinterpretation of the meaning of the message preceded the use of social information-gathering tactics. In all but one case, social actors reported having relatively well-formulated reinterpretations in mind before engaging in the interactive quest for new data. Even granting the general tendency of subjects to make themselves look good in the eyes of the researcher, these results are simply too forceful to ignore. Social actors must be seen as potentially thoughtful, naive scientists who use theories of bias, not unlike scientific theories, to explore the social world (see Hewes & Planalp, 1982).

Phase 4: Social Tactic Choice

We know very little about the *Social Tactic Choice* phase. In very general terms, we theorize that if social actors choose to assess their reinterpretations by means of new information gained from the social world, they must choose and implement tactics for doing so. This choice may or may not be conscious. All that is required is that the choice be derived from the activation of a goal to obtain accurate information and that it serve social actors in their reflective examination of a message (see Graham et al., unpublished; see Greene, 1984, and Norman, 1981, on goals and the activation of cognitive processes). Moreover, as both Figure 4.1 and our sketch of second-guessing theory indicate, second-guessing need not stop with the application of social information-gathering tactics. Those tactics may provoke messages that are themselves subject to second-guessing. For instance, in investigating some minor vandalism to your property, you might come to suspect a neighbor's child, over her protestations to the contrary. You might test your suspicions by talking to her parents. Here again, you might find yourself questioning their assertion that their daughter was home the evening of the vandalism after later hearing from a neighbor that the girl's parents were at a party at the time. You might even reinterpret your neighbor's information if he had only second-hand information concerning the party and a motivation to put the girl's parents in a bind.

This pattern of interlocking cycles of second-guessing is not merely a possibility. We have some intriguing qualitative data suggesting that social actors engage in this kind of detective work in everyday life. How often it occurs, what conditions facilitate it, how it affects both cognitive and social factors, and how normatively adequate it is are questions as yet unanswered. For those interested in understanding the interpretative capacities of social actors, the phenomenon of interlocking second-guessing cycles deserves more attention than we have yet been able to give it. However, we will be able to address more mundane issues relevant to Phase 4 soon. In Graham et al. (unpublished) we report the development of a category system to describe social information-gathering tactics. In addition, we are in the process of testing hypotheses concerning the connection between those tactics and their antecedents as characterized in Figure 4.1. The result should be a more complete picture of the connection between the reinterpretive process of second-guessing and its social implications.

CONCLUSIONS AND NEW DIRECTIONS

What can we say about the status of second-guessing theory? Certainly the evidence we have obtained has generally been supportive. Still, both replication of these results and testing of as yet unexplored facets of the theory must be immediate priorities. In particular, efforts should be lent to addressing three key issues. First, we need a more complete understanding of the process of cue extraction. To achieve the requisite understanding at least four questions must be answered: (1) What are the objective properties of messages that interact with the context and interpretive frames of social actors to initiate the process of second-guessing? (2) What psychological differences among individuals, including both temporary states (such as the need for accurate information) and dispositions (such as self-monitoring), affect the identification of cues that trigger second-guessing? (3) To what extent is cue extraction normatively adequate? (4) What factors, if any, moderate the normative adequacy of cue extraction?

Of the four questions, we have addressed briefly the last three in our presentation of the *Vigilance* phase, as has Roloff (this volume) in even greater detail elsewhere. We have made few inroads into answering the first. Preliminary attempts to do so should involve a closer look at two bodies of literature, that on persuasion (covered by Roloff, this volume) and that on deception (see Knapp et al., 1987; Zuckerman et al., 1981). Research efforts to locate objective properties of messages that identify, or are believed by receivers to identify, liars have a direct, though limited, bearing on the *Vigilance* phase of second-guessing.[6] Such research should expand and illuminate our discussion of message (4.1, 4.2) and consistency (2.3a) cues described in Table 4.1, an understanding of which involves, in part, further exploration of the implications of internal inconsistencies in messages as well as nonverbal and paralinguistic cues to arousal for triggering second-guessing. In addition, some research suggests that familiarity with source, based either on the duration of a relationship or repeated exposure to the individual in a laboratory setting, increases the accuracy of deception detection (see Brandt, Miller, & Hocking, 1982; Comadena, 1982; but see Stiff & Miller, 1986). This research not only supports our identification of source cues to second-guessing (2.1a-2.2.d in Table 4.1) but, more importantly, points to mechanisms that make the use of those cues feasible. Finally, the failure of deception researchers to identify objective properties of the communication behavior that indicate deception accurately across situations (Ekman, 1985) provides a challenge for second-guessing theory. This failure is consistent with our notion that cues to bias are not to be found in the objective properties of messages per se. Rather cues to bias result from filtering of the objective properties of behavior through interpretive frameworks—our naive theories of bias. Second-guessing theory may offer a rich source of new cues to deception, especially in descriptions of disposition (2.2), consistency (2.3), informational (2.4), and receiver cues (3.1, 3.2 in Table 4.1). Thus deception research may benefit from the insights of second-guessing theory, just as second-guessing theory will undoubtedly benefit from the insights of deception research.

A second major issue in second-guessing theory that needs more reflection and research relates to Phase 2, the *Reinterpretation* phase. Perhaps the most risky claim made in second-guessing theory, and definitely the most striking, is that social actors' reinterpretations of messages are normatively adequate. This claim is made controversial by the results of the deception literature. The case for accurate reinterpretation of biased messages is weakened by two findings; the low success rates social actors achieve in attempting to detect deception, and the marginal overlap between those properties of messages apparently used by social actors to detect deceit and those properties actually known to do so (see Knapp et al., 1987; Zuckerman et al., 1981). In contradiction, second-guessing research demonstrates that social actors can not only detect bias, they also seem able to correct it. The tension between the claims of these two research traditions commends us to resolve it. Is deception detection a qualitatively different phenomenon than second-guessing because social actors shy away from ascribing deceit, or is the accurate ascription of deceit simply more difficult than the reinterpretation of more mundane message distortions? Are our results supporting normative adequacy of second-guessing insufficiently well-documented, or are there problems in the research paradigms used in the deception research? Both these questions deserve to be addressed. The latter probably deserves more immediate attention since a negative answer removes the tension between claims concerning the interpretive prowess of social actors.

Although replication of existing research and its extension to different contexts and types of cues would test claims to normative adequacy more rigorously, new paradigms of research should be conducted as well. In order to demonstrate further the normative adequacy of reinterpretations, studies should be conducted in which biases are induced experimentally in sources whose messages are then passed on to receivers for reinterpretation. Studies of this type, by improving experimental control over the existence of a particular bias, would put to the test claims that biases in sources' judgments do affect message production and can be detected accurately by receivers. In addition, important evidence on normative adequacy could be garnered if messages containing cues theoretically leading to contradictory reinterpretations could be shown to be more difficult to process and to lead to more tentative reinterpretations than either messages containing no manipulated cues or those containing cues that are theoretically reinforcing.

A third major issue in second-guessing theory that should be explored concerns its implications beyond the confines of interpersonal communication. For instance, Berger (1987) has speculated on the relevance of second-guessing to mass communication research. He suggests, in the spirit of recent conceptions of viewers as active shapers of their own media use (see Katz, 1980), that critical viewers in an "active audience" (Blumler, 1979) may reinterpret the mediated messages in much the same way as social actors in the kinds of interpersonal exchanges discussed here. Thus concerns with "media skepticism" (Cozzens & Contractor, 1987) or the credibility of public figures (see Erickson, 1985) might be more fruitfully cast in terms of second-guessing.

His suggestion seems plausible since we obtained evidence in Hewes et al. (1985) that the media are included by social actors as sources of information to be second-guessed. Given popular concerns over bias in media coverage of political issues (see Lipton, 1988), it seems likely that social actors do more with mediated messages than simply reject or devalue them. Of course, according to second-guessing theory, one can expect social actors to actively reinterpret messages *only* when their need for accurate information is high and when cues to bias are present in the message. Second-guessing theory offers an explanation of the conditions that may foster critical viewership as well as a description of the complex reinterpretive routines that social actors may bring to bear on mediated messages.

Second-guessing theory may also have relevance for the study of informal social networks in organizations. Second-guessing, as originally conceived, was supposed to take place in social networks as a means to explain why the plethora of identified biases in human judgment had so little apparent impact on organized social action (Hewes & Planalp, 1982). Organizations are, after all, rife with information obtained from "the grapevine" or "the rumor mill" (Davis, 1953; 1972; Hellweg, 1983), as much as 50% of which is biased (Freidman, 1981). We know from Hewes et al. (1985) that second-guessing is very common in organizational settings. From the same study we also know that social actors in these settings are more likely to employ social information-gathering tactics than are undergraduates when faced with indirect information of questionable accuracy. Why might this be?

There are at least two explanations, both demonstrating the relevance of second-guessing to the study of organizational communication. First, managers may be concerned about the amount of disinformation flowing through informal channels in an organization, as indeed they should be, given the inaccuracy of much of it. Thus if they doubt the capacity of others to second-guess accurately, they might produce policies designed to discourage second-guessing or, more likely, to discourage purely cognitive, as opposed to social, reinterpretation assessment strategies (Hewes et al., 1988; Pacanowsky, personal communication, provided us with this insight drawn from an actual organizational setting). Second-guessing theory identifies which antecedents of reinterpretation would, or ought to, be brought under policy control. For example, social strategies for reinterpretation assessment directed toward administrative sources might be encouraged as a means of dampening inaccurate gossip. Theoretically, this assessment could be accomplished by institutionalizing opportunities for bottom-up communication or by decreasing the social costs (time and effort) and constraints (accessibility, believability, social appropriateness) to obtaining this information. In addition, use of social reinterpretation assessment strategies directed toward administrative sources might be encouraged by decreasing the need for accurate information through timely, complete, top-down communication, while simultaneously decreasing receivers' cognitive loads by reducing the number of competing interpretations generated by idle speculation.

In the near future, second-guessing theory may also identify which aspects of the need for information, cognitive load, and / or social strategic considerations can be, or are being, manipulated to encourage a preference for social tactics—and, most particularly, to encourage direct communication with the source or target that would minimize idle speculation. This latter function of second-guessing theory is dependent upon the successful conclusion of Graham et al.'s (unpublished) research, since it is there that second-guessing theory is connected to the choice of specific social information-gathering tactics. Thus second-guessing theory offers both a potential explanation of why members of an established informal social network show a preference for social, as opposed to cognitive, reinterpretation assessment strategies while simultaneously providing prescriptions for managers who wish to encourage the use of those same strategies.

There may be a second reason why social actors in organizational settings tend to engage relatively more frequently in social information-gathering tactics. Because the employees of the modest-sized organizations we explored probably had networks that were more durable than those in our student sample, it may have been that the employees had a greater opportunity to reticulate networks in order to meet their informational needs. If so, the antecedents of second-guessing and the feedback from second-guessing may predict the formation and change of informal social networks, making the structuring of networks a proactive social information-gathering tactic. In other words, informal social networks may be formed not only on the basis of such factors as liking, task demands, political power, or organizational prescription (see Corman, 1986; Monge & Eisenberg, 1987), but also a general motivation to reduce uncertainty (as in Albrecht, Adelman, & Associates, 1987) may be satisfied via second-guessing. In this view, we value not only those co-workers who provide us directly with accurate, relevant information, but also those who can be second-guessed accurately or who join us in "plausibility testing" (Hewes et al., 1988) to generate accurate reinterpretations.

Second-guessing theory faces a number of challenges in the future. Some, like these just discussed, involve finding new areas of application. Others require that the deficiencies in extant research identified in this chapter be remedied. We look forward to these challenges. They are the lifeblood of any research program. Moreover, we hope to have offered challenges to modern communication theory. Even though second-guessing is only one of a number of communicative phenomena that must be investigated, even though it is by no means the most common of those phenomena, we believe that it can serve as a catalyst for the reformulation of important aspects of communication theory. Second-guessing theory underscores the importance of viewing hearers as strategic interpreters of messages, both emphasizing the role of interpretation in communication and providing a necessary counterbalance to the current focus on strategic speakers. Second-guessing theory reminds us that "communication" is not synonymous with "face-to-face" or "transactive" communication. Second-guessing theory offers hope that the insights of cognitive research can be incorporated in a theory that extends from message interpretation to message production and beyond. These implications of second-guessing theory for communication theory generally, coupled with the substantive contributions of second-guessing research, commend it for further exploration and extension.

NOTES

1. The normative adequacy of second-guessing can be tested only in those cases in which the truth-value of a claim is amenable to rigorous evaluation. This limitation leaves open the possibility that some classes of claims may not be testable, limiting the generalizability of attributions of normative adequacy.

2. Earlier discussions of second-guessing implied that there is an essentially dichotomous reaction to doubts about the truth of a message (see Doelger et al., 1986; Hewes et al., 1985). That is, since social actors could be in only one of two states—reflective ("mindful") or nonreflective ("mindless")—with respect to the message, either they accepted the message at face value or second-guessed it. We have concluded that there is a third possibility; social actors may have doubts about the veridicality of a message, and thus be in a "mindful" state, but may conclude that

discovering the truth behind the message is not important enough to warrant the effort of engaging in second-guessing.

3. This trichotomous option to respond to an initial interpretation of a message is an important theoretical move. We know from Hewes et al. (1985) that social actors use at least four strategies when faced with a reason to doubt the face-value interpretation of a message: (a) They may discount the message, as in a court of law when evidence or testimony is disallowed; (b) They may weight it differentially in comparison with other messages in which they have more confidence; (c) They may try to reinterpret it, as in second-guessing; (d) They may employ some social tactic to seek out clarifying information (Hewes et al, 1985). Source credibility (Andersen & Clevenger, 1963; McCroskey, 1966), a variable that is encompassed and superseded by second-guessing (Hewes & Planalp, 1982), serves as an antecedent to doubt only for those instances in which the source's good will (2.1a, perhaps 2.1c, or 2.2a-c in Table 4.1), or expertise (2.4d) (McCroskey & Young, 1981) is questioned. Moreover, the conceptualization of source credibility contains no mechanism to discriminate between the four strategies social actors use when faced with a reason to doubt a message—second-guessing does make this discrimination (see Hewes et al., 1988). For other distinctions between second-guessing and source credibility, see Hewes and Planalp (1982, pp. 136-137).

4. Even two compatible reinterpretations increase cognitive load, since their compatibility must be assessed, then they may be combined into an additional reinterpretation in need of subsequent assessment.

5. Hewes et al. (1988) note that because of the nature of the relationships contained in their three predictions, all three must be tested simultaneously. The results reported here were obtained from just such a simultaneous test.

6. Note that second-guessing includes both intentional and unintentional sources of bias. Thus deception research, which focuses on only the most extreme forms of intentional distortion—namely, lying—includes only a subset of the domain of second-guessing situations. Missing are unintended biases such as those produced by cognitive processes as well as the less severe forms of intentional biases—mild forms of self-presentation, face-protection for another, ingratiation, or expressions of generally pessimistic or optimistic attitudes—that would not be judged by members of this society to be lies.

REFERENCES

Albrecht, T. L., Adelman, M. B., & Associates (1987). *Communicating social support.* Newbury Park, CA: Sage.

Alderton, S. M., & Frey, L. R. (1986). Argumentation in small group decision making. In R. Y. Hirokawa & M. S. Poole (Eds.), *Communication and group decision making.* Beverly Hills, CA: Sage.

Andersen, K., & Clevenger, T., Jr. (1963). A summary of experimental research in ethos. *Speech Monographs, 30,* 59-78.

Anderson, J. R. (1981). Concepts, propositions, and schemata: What are the cognitive units? In J. Flowers (Ed.), *Nebraska symposium on motivation, 1980* (Vol. 28). Lincoln: University of Nebraska Press.

Bales, R. F. (1950). *Interaction process analysis.* Chicago: University of Chicago Press.

Bartlett, F. C. (1932). *Remembering.* Cambridge: Cambridge University Press.

Bercheid, E., Graziano, W. G., Monson, T., & Dermer, M. (1976). Outcome dependency: Attention, attribution, and attraction. *Journal of Personality and Social Psychology, 34,* 978-989.

Berger, C. R. (1979). Beyond initial interaction: Uncertainty, understanding, and the development of interpersonal relationships. In H. Giles & R. St. Clair (Eds.), *Language and social psychology.* Baltimore: University Park Press.

Berger, C. R. (1987). Communicating under uncertainty. In M. R. Roloff & G. R. Miller (Eds.), *Interpersonal processes*. Newbury Park, CA: Sage.

Berger, C. R., & Calabrese, R. (1975). Some explorations in initial interaction and beyond: Toward a developmental theory of interpersonal communication. *Human Communication Research, 1*, 99-112.

Berger, C. R., & Douglas, W. (1981). Studies in interpersonal epistemology: III. Anticipated interaction, self-monitoring, and observational context selection. *Communication Monographs, 48*, 183-196.

Berger, C. R., & Kellermann, K. A. (1983). To ask or not to ask: Is that a question? In R. N. Bostrom (Ed.), *Communication yearbook* (Vol. 7). Beverly Hills: Sage.

Blumler, J. G. (1979). The role of theory in uses and gratifications studies. *Communication Research, 6*, 9-35.

Boden, M. A. (1972). *Purposive explanation in psychology*. Cambridge, MA: Harvard University Press.

Bowers, J. W., & Bradac, J. J. (1982). Issues in communication theory: A metatheoretical analysis. In M. Burgoon (Ed.), *Communication yearbook* (Vol. 5). New Brunswick, NJ: Transaction Books.

Brandt, D. R., Miller, G. R., & Hocking, J. E. (1982). Familiarity and lie detection: A replication and extension. *Western Journal of Speech Communication, 46*, 276-290.

Cantril, H. (1940). *The invasion from Mars, a study in the psychology of panic*. New York: Harper & Row.

Chadwick-Jones, J. K. (1976). *Social exchange theory: Its structure and influence in social psychology*. New York: Academic Press.

Cheshire, N. M. (1975). *The nature of psychodynamic interpretation*. New York: John Wiley.

Cody, M. J., & McLaughlin, M. L. (1985). The situation as a construct in interpersonal communication research. In M. L. Knapp & G. R. Miller (Eds.), *Handbook of Interpersonal Communication*. Beverly Hills, CA: Sage.

Comadena, M. E. (1982). Accuracy in detecting deception: Intimate and friendship relationships. In M. Burgoon (Ed.), *Communication Yearbook* (Vol. 5). Beverly Hills, CA: Sage.

Corman, S. R. (1986). *Toward a generative theory of network relationships*. Paper presented to the annual convention of the Speech Communication Association, Chicago.

Cozzens, M. D., & Contractor, N. S. (1987). The effects of conflicting information on media skepticism. *Communication Research, 14*, 437-451.

Craig, R. T. (1979). Information systems theory and research: An overview of individual information processing. In D. I. Nimmo (Ed.), *Communication Yearbook* (Vol. 3). New Brunswick, NJ: Transaction.

Cronen, V. E., Pearce, W. B., & Harris, L. M. (1982). The coordinated management of meaning: A theory of communication. In F.E.X. Dance (Ed.), *Human communication theory*. New York: Harper & Row.

Cronkhite, G., & Liska, J. R. (1980). The judgment of communicant acceptability. In M. E. Roloff & G. R. Miller (Eds.), *Persuasion: New directions in theory and research*. Beverly Hills, CA: Sage.

Davenport, W. G. (1968). Auditory vigilance: The effects of costs and values on signals. *Australian Journal of Psychology, 20*, 213-218.

Davenport, W. G. (1969). Vibrotactile vigilance: The effects of costs and values on signals. *Perception and Psychophysiology, 5*, 25-28.

Davis, K. (1953). Management communication and the grapevine. *Harvard Business Review, 31*, 43-49.

Davis, K. (1972). *Human behavior at work*. New York: McGraw-Hill.

Delia, J. G. (1976). A constructivist analysis of the concept of credibility. *Quarterly Journal of Speech, 62*, 361-375.

Doelger, J. A., Hewes, D. E., & Graham, M. L. (1986). Knowing when to "second-guess": The mindful analysis of messages. *Human Communication Research, 12*, 301-338.

Ekman, P. (1985). *Telling lies.* New York: Norton.

Elliot, G. C. (1979). Some effects of deception and level of self-monitoring on planning and reacting to a self-presentation. *Journal of Personality and Social Psychology, 37,* 1282-1292.

Ellis, D. G. (1979). Relational control in two group systems. *Communication Monographs, 46,* 153-166.

Erickson, P. T. (1985). *Reagan speaks.* New York: New York University Press.

Eysenck, M. W. (1982). *Attention and arousal.* Berlin: Springer-Verlag.

Fisher, B. A., & Hawes, L. C. (1971). An interact system model: Generating a grounded theory of small groups. *Quarterly Journal of Speech, 57,* 444-453.

Fiske, S. T., & Taylor, S. E. (1984). *Social cognition.* Reading, MA: Addison-Wesley.

Forgas, J. P. (Ed.). (1981). *Social cognition.* New York: Academic Press.

Forgas, J. P., Bower, G. H., & Krantz, S. E. (1984). The influence of mood on perceptions of social interactions. *Journal of Experimental Social Psychology, 20,* 497-513.

Freidman, S. (1981). Where employees go for information: Some surprises! *Administrative Management, 42,* 72-73.

Gilovich, T. (1987). Second-hand information and social judgment. *Journal of Experimental Social Psychology, 23,* 59-74.

Goldman, A. I. (1986). *Epistemology and cognition.* Cambridge, MA: Harvard University Press.

Graham, M., Hewes, D. E., Doelger, J., & Monsour, M. (unpublished manuscript). *From cognition to social information-gathering: II. Social Tactic Choice.* Manuscript available from the second author, Department of Speech Communication, University of Illinois, Urbana-Champaign.

Greene, J. O. (1984). A cognitive approach to human communication: An action assembly theory. *Communication Monographs, 51,* 289-306.

Hastie, R., Park, B., & Weber, R. (1984). Social memory. In R. S. Wyer, Jr., & T. K. Srull (Eds.), *Handbook of social cognition* (Vol. 2). Hillsdale, NJ: Lawrence Erlbaum.

Heider, F. (1958). *The psychology of interpersonal relations.* New York: John Wiley.

Hellweg, S. (1983). *Organizational grapevines: A state of the art review.* Paper presented at the annual meeting of the International Communication Association, Dallas.

Hewes, D. E. (1986). A socio-egocentric model of group decision-making. In R. Y. Hirokawa and M. S. Poole (Eds.), *Communication and group decision-making* (pp. 265-292). Beverly Hills: Sage.

Hewes, D. E., Graham, M. L., Doelger, J., & Pavitt, C. (1985). "Second-guessing": Message interpretation in social networks. *Human Communication Research, II,* 299-334.

Hewes, D. E., Graham, M. L., Monsour, M., & Doelger, J. A. (1988). *From cognition to social information-getting tactics: I. Re-interpretation assessment in second-guessing.* Paper presented to the annual meeting of the International Communication Association, New Orleans.

Hewes, D. E., Monsour, M., & Rutherford, D. K. (unpublished manuscript). *Second-guessing: The effects of need for accuracy on cue extraction, doubt, and normative adequacy.*

Hewes, D. E., & Planalp, S. (1982). There is nothing as useful as a good theory . . . : The influence of social knowledge on interpersonal communication. In M. E. Roloff & C. R. Berger (Eds.), *Social cognition and communication.* Beverly Hills, CA: Sage.

Hirokawa, R. Y. (1980). A comparative analysis of communicative patterns within effective and ineffective decision-making groups. *Communication Monograph, 47,* 312-321.

Hirokawa, R. Y. (1983). Communication and problem-solving effectiveness: An investigation of group phases. *Human Communication Research, 9,* 291-305.

Isen, A. M. (1984). Toward understanding the role of affect in cognition. In R. S. Wyer, Jr., & T. K. Srull (Eds.), *Handbook of social cognition* (Vol. 3.) Hillsdale, NJ: Lawrence Erlbaum.

Isen, A. M., Means, B., Patrick R., & Nowicki, G. (1982). Some factors influencing decision-making strategy and risk-taking. In M. S. Clark & S. T. Fisk (Eds.), *Affect and cognition.* Hillsdale, NJ: Lawrence Erlbaum.

Johnson, D. M. (1945). "The phantom anesthetist" of Matoon: a field study of mass hysteria. *Journal of Abnormal and Social Psychology, 40,* 175-186.
Jones, E. E. (1979). The rocky road from acts to dispositions. *American Psychologist, 34,* 107-117.
Jones, E. E., & Baumeister, R. (1976). The self-monitor looks at the ingratiator. *Journal of Personality, 44,* 654-674.
Jungermann, H. (1986). Two camps on rationality. In H. R. Arkes & K. R. Hammond (Eds.), *Judgment and decision-making.* Cambridge: Cambridge University Press.
Kagan. J. (1972). Motives and development. *Journal of Personality and Social Psychology, 22,* 51-66.
Kahneman. D., Slovic, P., & Tversky, A. (Eds.). (1982). *Judgment under uncertainty.* Cambridge: Cambridge University Press.
Katz, E. (1980). On conceptualizing media effects. In T. McCormack (Ed.), *Studies in communication.* Greenwich, CT: JAI.
Kellermann, K. A., & Berger, C. R. (1984). Affect and social information acquisition: Sit back, relax, and tell me about yourself. In R. Bostrom (Ed.), *Communication yearbook* (Vol. 8). Beverly Hills, CA: Sage.
Kelley, H. H. (1967). Attribution Theory in social psychology. In D. Levine (Ed.), *Nebraska symposium on motivation.* Lincoln: University of Nebraska Press.
Kelley, H. H., Berscheid, E., Christensen, A., Harvey, J. H., Huston, T. L., Levinger, G., McClintock, E., Peplau, L. A., & Peterson, D. R. (1983). Analyzing close relationships. In H. H. Kelley, E. Berscheid, A. Christensen, J. H. Harvey, T. L. Huston, G, Levinger, E. McClintock, L. A. Peplau, & D. R. Peterson (Eds.), *Close relationships.* New York: W. H. Freeman.
Kelly, G. A. (1955). *A theory of personality.* New York: Norton.
Knapp, M. L., Cody, M. J., & Reardon, K. K. (1987). Nonverbal signals. In C. R. Berger & S. H. Chaffee (Eds.), *Handbook of communication science.* Newbury Park, CA: Sage.
Kruglanski, A. W., & Freund, T. (1983). The freezing and unfreezing of lay-inferences: Effects on impressional primacy, ethnic stereotyping, and numerical anchoring. *Journal of Experimental Social Psychology, 19,* 448-468.
Kruglanski, A. W., Hamel, I. A., Maides, S. A., & Schwartz, J. M. (1978). Attribution theory as a special case of lay epistemology. In J. H. Harvey, W. Ickes, & R. F. Kidd (Eds.), *New directions in attribution research* (Vol. 2). Hillsdale, NJ: Lawrence Erlbaum.
Labov, W., & Fanshel, D. (1977). *Therapeutic discourse.* New York: Academic.
Langer, E. J. (1978). Rethinking the role of thought in social interaction. In J. Harvey, W. Ickes, & R. Kidd (Eds.), *New directions in attribution research* (Vol. 2). Hillsdale, NJ: Lawrence Erlbaum.
Langer, E. J., & Abelson, R. P. (1972). The semantics of asking a favor: How to succeed in getting help without really dying. *Journal of Personality and Social Psychology, 24,* 26-32.
Langer, E. J., Blank, A., & Chanowitz, B. (1978). The mindlessness of ostensibly thoughtful action: The role of "placebic" information in interpersonal interaction. *Journal of Personality and Social Psychology, 36,* 635-642.
Leplin, J. (Ed.). (1984). *Scientific realism.* Berkeley, CA: University of California Press.
Levine, J. M. (1966). The effects of values and costs in the detection and identification of signals in auditory vigilance. *Human Factors, 8,* 525-537.
Lipton, M. A. (1988, January 23). Campaign '88 and TV: America speaks out. *TV Guide,* 2-7.
Loftus, E. E. (1979). *Eyewitness testimony.* Cambridge, MA: Harvard University Press.
Markus, H., & Zajonc, R. B. (1985). The cognitive perspective in social psychology. In G. Lindzey & E. Aronson (Eds.), *Handbook of social psychology* (Vol. 1, 3rd ed.). Hillsdale, NJ: Lawrence Erlbaum.
Martins, D. (1982). Influence of affect on comprehension of a text. *Text, 2,* 141-154.
McCall, G. J., & Simmons, J. L. (1978). *Identities and interactions* (2nd ed.). New York: Free Press.

McCroskey, J. C. (1966). Scales for the measurement of ethos. *Speech Monographs, 33,* 65-72.
McCroskey, J., & Young, T. (1981). Ethos and credibility: The construct and its measurement after three decades. *Central States Speech Journal, 32,* 24-34.
McDougall, W. (1911). *Body and mind: A history and a defense of animism.* London: Methuen.
McGraw, K. O. (1978). The detrimental effects of reward on performance: A literature review and a prediction model. In M. R. Lepper & D. Greene (Eds.), *The hidden costs of reward.* Hillsdale, NJ: Lawrence Erlbaum.
McHugh, P. (1968). *Defining the situation.* Indianapolis: Bobbs-Merrill.
Mehan. H., & Wood, H. (1975). *The reality of ethnomethodology.* New York: John Wiley.
Mill, J. (1984). High and low self-monitoring individuals: Their decoding skills and emphatic expression. *Journal of Personality 52,* 372-388.
Millar, F. E., & Rogers, L. E. (1987). Relational dimensions of interpersonal dynamics. In M. E. Roloff & G. R. Miller (Eds.), *Interpersonal processes.* Newbury Park CA: Sage.
Miller, G., Boster, F., Roloff, M., & Seibold, D. (1977). Compliance-gaining message strategies: A typology and some findings concerning effects of situational differences. *Communication Monographs, 44,* 37-51.
Mischel, W. (1981). Personality and cognition: Something borrowed, something new? In N. Cantor & J. F. Kihlstrom (Eds.), *Personality, cognition, and social interaction.* Hillsdale, NJ: Lawrence Erlbaum.
Monge, P. R., & Eisenberg, E. M. (1987). Emergent communication networks. In F. M. Jablin, L. L. Putnam, K. H. Roberts, & L. W. Porter (Eds.), *Handbook of organizational communication.* Newbury Park, CA: Sage.
Navon, D., & Gopher, D. (1979). On the economy of the human processing system. *Psychological Review, 86,* 214-255.
Neisser, U. (1978). Memory: What are the important questions? In M. M. Gruneberg, P. E. Morris, & R. N. Sykes (Eds.), *Practical aspects of memory.* London: Academic Press.
Nisbett, R., & Ross, L. (1980). *Human inference.* Englewood Cliffs, NJ: Prentice-Hall.
Norman, D. A. (1981). Categorization of action slips. *Psychological Review, 88,* 1-15.
Ostrom, T. M. (1984). The sovereignty of social cognition. In R. S. Wyer, Jr., & T. K. Srull (Eds.), *Handbook of social cognition* (Vol. 1). Hillsdale NJ: Lawrence Erlbaum.
Parks, M. R., & Adelman, M. B. (1983). Communication networks and the development of romantic relationships. *Human Communication Research, 1,* 55-79.
Parks, M. R., Stan, D. M., & Eggert, L. L. (1983). Romantic involvement and social network involvement. *Social Psychology Quarterly, 46,* 116-131.
Planalp, S., & Hewes, D. E. (1982). A cognitive approach to communication theory: *Cogito Ergo Dico?* In M. Burgoon (Ed.), *Communication yearbook* (Vol 5). New Brunswick, NJ: Transaction-International Communication Association.
Planalp, S., & Honeycutt, J. M. (1985). Events that increase uncertainty in interpersonal relationships. *Human Communication Research, 11,* 593-604.
Rausch, H. (1965). Interaction sequences. *Journal of Personality and Social Psychology, 2*(4), 487-499.
Rausch, H. (1972). Process and change—A Markov model for interaction. *Family Process, 11,* 275-298.
Rogers, L. E., & Farace, R. V. (1975). An analysis of relational communication in dyads: New measurement procedures. *Human Communication Research, 1,* 222-239.
Roloff, M. E. (1987). Communication and reciprocity within intimate relationships. In M. E. Roloff & G. R. Miller (Eds.), *Interpersonal processes.* Newbury Park CA: Sage.
Roloff, M. E., & Berger, C. R. (Eds.). (1982). *Social cognition and communication.* Beverly Hills: Sage.
Ross, L. (1977). The intuitive scientist and his shortcoming: Distortions in the attributional process. In L. Berkowitz (Ed.), *Advances in experimental social psychology* (Vol. 10). New York: Academic.
Sampson, E. E. (1981). Cognitive psychology as ideology. *American Psychologist, 36,* 730-743.

Scheidel, T., & Crowell, L. (1964). Idea development in small discussion groups. *Quarterly Journal of Speech, 50,* 140-145.

Schutz, A. (1967). *The phenomenology of the social world,* (G. Walsh & F. Lehnert, Trans.). Evanston, IL: Northwestern University Press.

Schutz, A., & Luckmann, T. (1973). *The structures of the life-world* (R. M. Zaner & H. T. Engelhardt, Jr., Trans.). Evanston, IL: Northwestern University Press.

Seibold, D. R., Cantrill, J. G., & Meyers, R. A. (1985). Communication and interpersonal influence. In M. L. Knapp & G. R. Miller (Eds.), *Handbook of interpersonal communication.* Beverly Hills: Sage.

Seibold, D. R., & Meyers, R. A. (1986). Communication and influence in group decision-making. In R. Y. Hirokawa & M. S. Poole (Eds.), *Communication and group decision making.* Beverly Hills, CA: Sage.

Sherman, S. J., & Corty, E. (1984). Cognitive heuristics. In R. S. Wyer & T. K. Srull (Eds.), *Handbook of social cognition.* Hillsdale, NJ: Lawrence Erlbaum.

Simon, H. A. (1960). *The sciences of the artificial.* Cambridge: MIT Press.

Snyder, M. (1984). When belief creates reality. In L. Berkowitz (Ed.), *Advances in experimental social psychology* (Vol. 18). New York: Academic Press, 247-305.

Snyder, M. (1987). *Public appearances/private realities.* New York: Freeman.

Snyder, M., & Gangestad, S. (1982). Choosing social situations: Two investigations of self-monitoring processes. *Journal of Personality and Social Psychology, 43,* 123-135.

Snyder, M., & Harkness, A. R. (1984). *E=f(p): The impact of personality on choice of situation.* Paper presented at the annual meeting of the Midwestern Psychological Association, Chicago.

Stewart, J. (1978). Foundations of dialogic communication. *Quarterly Journal of Speech, 64,* 183-201.

Stiff, J. B., & Miller, G. R. (1986). "Come to think of it . . .: Interrogative probes, deceptive communication, and deception detection. *Human Communication Research, 12,* 30-338.

Suppe, F. (Ed.). (1974). *The structure of scientific theories.* Urbana: University of Illinois Press.

Tetlock, P. E., & Levi, A. (1982). Attributional bias: On the inconclusiveness of the cognition-motivation debate. *Journal of Experimental Social Psychology, 18,* 68-88.

Tomarelli, M. M., & Graziano, W. G. (1981). *When opposites attract: Self-monitoring and dating relationships.* Paper presented at the annual meeting of the Southeastern Psychological Association, Atlanta.

Trope, Y., & Bassock, M. (1982). Confirmatory and diagnosing strategies in social information gathering. *Journal of Personality and Social Psychology, 43,* 22-34.

Tummin, M. M. & Feldman, A. S. (1955). The miracle at Sabana Grande. *Public Opinion Quarterly, 19,* 124-139.

van Dijk, T. A., & Kintsch, W. (1983). *Strategies of discourse comprehension.* New York: Academic Press.

Vanlear, C. A., Jr. (1987). The formation of social relationships: A longitudinal study of social penetration. *Human Communication Research, 13,* 299-322.

Wartella, E., & Reeves, B. (1987). Communication and children. In C. R. Berger & S. H. Chaffee (Eds.), *Handbook of Communication Science.* Newbury Park CA: Sage.

Winograd, T. (1977). A framework for understanding discourse. In M. A. Just & P. Carpenter (Eds.), *Cognitive processes in comprehension.* New York: John Wiley.

Zuckerman, M., DePaulo, B. M., & Rosenthal, R. (1981). Verbal and nonverbal communication of deception. In L. Berkowitz (Ed.), *Advances in experimental social psychology* (Vol. 14). New York: Academic Press.

On Second-Guessing the Theory of Second-Guessing: A Comment

MICHAEL E. ROLOFF
Northwestern University

> To question all things—never to turn away from any difficulty; to accept no doctrine either from ourselves or from other people without a rigid scrutiny by negative criticism; letting no fallacy, or incoherence, or confusion of thought step by unperceived; above all, to insist upon having the meaning of a word clearly understood before using it, and the meaning of a proposition before assenting to it—these are the lessons we learn from the ancient dialecticians.
>
> —John Stuart Mill
> (Inaugural Address as Rector,
> University of St. Andrews, 1867)

Given the results of current research focused on human decision making, the quoted lessons are as valuable now as they were in the nineteenth century. Scholars have identified an impressive list of biases that affect human judgment (Fiske & Taylor, 1984; Nisbett & Ross, 1980; Ross, 1977; 1979). The existence of these factors make data received from others somewhat unreliable and possibly invalid. Since people are unable to observe directly all phenomena about which they need information, individuals must discern the biases contained within the accounts of others and overcome them or their ability to understand, predict, and control events could be seriously impaired.

This process of scrutinizing and debiasing messages is the focus of the theory of second-guessing. Hewes and Graham argue that when needing accurate information and believing that available data are tainted, individuals are capable of vigorously applying their social knowledge about decision

AUTHOR'S NOTE: The author gratefully acknowledges bibliographic assistance from Professor Peter V. Miller.

Correspondence and requests for reprints: Michael E. Roloff, Northwestern University, Department of Communication Studies, 1815 Chicago Avenue, Evanston, IL 60201.

Communication Yearbook 12, pp. 249-265

making biases to incoming information and to revise those messages so as to correct partially for the perceived biases.

Their perspective has many positive traits. Hewes and Graham have posited a theoretical orientation that is more complete, specific, and data-based than many. Moreover, their cautious analysis of relevant research is commendable.

Given my positive orientation toward their framework, my commentary is aimed at integrating their approach with similar conceptualizations and attempting to fill in gaps in their perspective rather than debunking their analysis. In pursuit of these goals, my commentary is divided into two sections: (1) perspectives on active message processing and (2) factors biasing the use of second-guessing.

PERSPECTIVES ON ACTIVE MESSAGE PROCESSING

Hewes and Graham argue that

> much current work on communication either ignores strategic considerations altogether or carries an implicit focus on the speaker to the exclusion of the hearer. In either case, little consideration is given to the active, construing strategic listener except, perhaps, in the group polarization literature. (p. 216)

Given that their review of research is focused strictly upon interaction analyses and source strategy selection, they are correct. However, within social psychology (and to a lesser extent communication), there are perspectives that conceptualize information processing in a similar but not identical fashion to the second-guessing framework.

Specifically, several perspectives used to study attitude change have hypothesized the existence of active and critical information processing. When confronting a belief-discrepant message, Festinger and Maccoby (1964) described the receiver this way:

> Certainly such a listener is not passive. Indeed it is most likely that . . . he [*sic*] is very actively, inside his own mind, counterarguing, derogating the point the communicator makes, and derogating the communicator himself. In other words, we can imagine that there is really dialogue going on, one side being vocal and the other subvocal. (p. 360)

This orientation is manifested in three current perspectives on attitude change: the cognitive response approach, the elaboration likelihood model, and the attributional analysis of opinion change. I will briefly explicate each perspective and identify similarities with second-guessing, then indicate how as a group they differ from the second-guessing perspective.

The Cognitive Response Approach

The cognitive response approach has played an important role in understanding a variety of persuasive phenomena (see, Greenwald, 1968; Perloff & Brock, 1980; Petty, Ostrom, & Brock, 1981). Perloff and Brock (1980) describe its assumptions this way:

> In essence, the cognitive response perspective maintains that individuals are active participants in the persuasion process who attempt to relate message elements to their existing repertories of information. In so doing, these individuals may consider material that are not actually contained in the persuasive message. These self-generated cognitions may agree with the position advocated by the source or they may disagree. Insofar as the communication elicits favorable cognitive responses, attitudes should change in the direction advocated by the source. To the extent that the message evokes unfavorable mental reactions, attitude change in the direction advocated by the source should be inhibited. (p. 69)

Thus, when confronting a belief-discrepant message, the receiver evaluates its worth by relating it to prior knowledge, and depending upon the valence of resulting cognitions, accepts or rejects the message. While not mentioning judgments of bias, it seems likely that measures of cognitive responses may contain some indicators of second-guessing activity. Cacioppo, Harkins, and Petty (1981) posit that "cognitive responses are the results of information-processing and information-structuring activity and thus consist of responses such as recognitions, associations, elaborations, ideas, and images" (p. 37). Of particular importance to second-guessing are the elaborations, for they include the evaluative assessments of the message. Responses can be favorable (pro arguments), unfavorable (counterarguments), or neutral toward the advocated position and aimed at the message arguments and/or source.[1]

Unfortunately, I have found no research that coded the content of cognitive responses (especially counterarguments) for allegations of bias toward the source. However, if the necessary conditions for creating second-guessing are met, such activity should be manifest in these reactions. The receiver counterargues against the advocated position by identifying the biases contained in the reasoning/evidence proffered as justifications for message acceptance and/or by identifying source characteristics that suggest bias. If such biases are perceived, confidence in the veracity of the supporting data is reduced, alternative interpretations posited, and persuasion is unlikely.

The Elaboration Likelihood Model

The ELM is a variant of the cognitive response approach. Of its various postulates, two are important for our analysis. First, "people are motivated to hold correct attitudes" (Petty & Cacioppo, 1986, p. 127). The theorists assume that all people want to have accurate evaluations of self, others, behaviors, and events so as to avoid negative consequences that result from misperception. Although not stated, presumably this desire for accuracy extends to the evaluation of incoming information relevant to attitudes. Hence when data are deemed relevant, they should be scrutinized for bias as described by the theory of second-guessing.

Second, "although people want to hold correct attitudes, the amount and nature of issue-relevant elaboration in which people are willing or able to engage to evaluate a message vary with individual and situational factors" (Petty & Cacioppo, 1986, p. 128). In essence, when receivers are sufficiently motivated and able, they will focus and expand the amount of cognitive processing related to interpreting a persuasive message.

Two variables having implications for second-guessing appear to influence the motivation and/or ability to engage in issue-elaboration. First, the degree of personal relevance/involvement attached to an issue has been hypothesized to increase the scrutiny applied to incoming information. Presumably, individuals who see an issue as highly involving are more *motivated* to scrutinize relevant messages since the issue has potential consequences for their lives (Petty & Cacioppo, 1986). Moreover, because such receivers often have a greater store of knowledge about an issue, they are better *able* to evaluate incoming information (Petty & Cacioppo, 1986).

Although it is untested in persuasion research, I would argue that individuals have a higher need for accurate information about topics they define to be personally relevant/involving. Accurate information helps them understand, predict, and control these phenomena that have an impact on their lives (Katz, 1960). Although not a direct test of this speculation, information seeking about a phenomenon is positively related to interest in it (see, Atkin, 1973) and its importance to the individual (Lanzetta & Driscoll, 1968).

Research indicates that personal relevance/involvement produces effects similar to second-guessing activity. Receivers who define a topic as personally involving, generate more unfavorable thoughts and fewer positive thoughts when processing counterattitudinal rather than proattitudinal messages (Howard-Pitney, Borgida, & Omoto, 1986; Petty & Cacioppo, 1979, Study 1). The amount of these cognitive responses made by low-involved receivers did not vary significantly across message type. This finding does not mean that highly involved receivers are universally skeptical of counterattitudinal messages. Individuals who are personally involved generate fewer unfavorable cognitive responses and more favorable ones when processing strong rather than weak counterattitudinal arguments (Benoit, 1987; Petty & Cacioppo, 1979, Study 2; Petty & Cacioppo, 1984). Low-involved receivers are less able to make such discriminations. Hence personal relevance/involvement may identify when individuals are better able to discriminate the presence or absence of bias.

The second variable is need for cognition. Cohen, Stotland, and Wolfe (1955) define the need for cognition as "a need to structure relevant situations in meaningful, integrated ways. It is a need to understand and make reasonable the experiential world" (p. 291). Research indicates that individuals who have a high need for cognition engage in greater information seeking from print media (Buss, 1967). Moreover, people high in this trait are hypothesized to be *motivated* to "think about the issue that they confront" (Cacioppo & Petty, 1982, p. 130). Although they do not evidence greater *ability* to scrutinize, such as verbal or abstract reasoning skills (Cacioppo, Petty, & Morris, 1983), their heightened motivation should be sufficient to prompt detailed processing of information. Indeed, receivers high in the need for cognition report expending significantly greater cognitive effort when processing a persuasive message than do their counterparts having a lower need (Cacioppo, Petty, Kao, & Rodriguez, 1986, Study 1; Cacioppo, Petty, & Morris, 1983).

Their greater cognitive effort appears to pay dividends. Individuals high in the need for cognition are better able to evaluate differentially the effectiveness of strong and weak counterattitudinal arguments (Cacioppo et al. 1986, Study 1, Cacioppo, Petty, & Morris, 1983) and generate more unfavorable cognitive responses to weak rather than strong counterattitudinal arguments (Cacioppo et al., 1986, Study 1). This relationship may indicate that persons high in the need for cognition are better able to identify when bias is present.

Although none of the aforementioned studies specifically measured second-guessing activity, they do suggest similar processes. Some topics or some individuals are associated with elaborated scrutiny of incoming information. In essence, they produce vigilance. Hence, both personal relevance/involvement and need for cognition could be related to the need for accurate information and subsequent second-guessing.

The Attributional Analysis of Opinion Change

The attributional approach is focused on the perceived basis for a source's position on a topic. Wood and Eagly (1981) argue that individuals have a store of knowledge about human traits and external pressures that cause communicators to advocate particular positions with regard to an issue. Receivers have conceptions about why a source has a particular "axe to grind."

This information is applied to communicators in order to determine if they are biased or not. Two biases are identified: knowledge bias and reporting bias. The former refers to the belief that a source has a limited or selective knowledge base upon which to draw. For example, persons who did not serve in the Vietnam War may have a different store of information upon which to justify their attitudes about the conflict than would individuals who did serve.

That difference in knowledge may imply that each will be perceived to be biased with regard to their stance on that issue. The reporting bias stems from the perception that the source may be unwilling to present an accurate view of reality. As another example, one might be suspicious of compliments received from a person known to be extremely polite, manipulative, or who needs something we possess. Consistent with this reasoning, Eagly, Wood, and Chaiken (1978) found that receivers perceived a communicator to be less biased when the communicator advocated a position inconsistent with his or her background (knowledge bias) and/or promoted a position that significantly diverged from that held by most of his or her other audience (reporting bias).

In subsequent research, Wood and Eagly (1981) argue that this search for bias occurs through three postmessage stages. After decoding a message, receivers initially attempt to determine whether the source advocated the position based upon personal characteristics, situational forces, or factual evidence. At the second stage, message recipients attribute bias to the message if it is perceived to be the result of personal characteristics or situational forces. If the message is perceived to have resulted from factual evidence, less bias is attributed to the communicator. If the source is perceived to be biased, then the message should be closely scrutinized and its arguments recalled. On the other hand, the relative absence of bias should not require much scrutiny, and argument comprehension should be low. The final stage is the decision to accept or reject the message.

In general, this analysis was supported by their data. When a source advocated a position inconsistent with his or her background, he or she was perceived to have advanced it more so because of factual information and, to a lesser extent, personal background. Moreover, the source was judged to be less biased, and stimulated lower argument comprehension than when his or her advocated position was consistent with his or her prior history. Only when the source advocated an inconsistent position did the perceived absence of bias reduce message comprehension which in turn was positively related to opinion change.

This perspective is similar to the theory of second-guessing in that receivers are perceived to apply prior knowledge about bias to the sources of incoming messages. When such bias is perceived, greater scrutiny of incoming information occurs (at least as evidenced by greater postmessage comprehension) and rejection of the advocated position results.

Differences Among the Perspectives

At this juncture, one might perceive that the theory of second-guessing is redundant with the three persuasion approaches. That perception is inaccurate; at least six differences between the perspectives exist.

First, the theory of second-guessing describes a *strategic* hearer, whereas the persuasion approaches characterize the receiver as merely *active*. The theory of second-guessing posits that the hearer is not only mindfully considering the message, but may apply particular techniques so as to correct for perceived bias. Because not all mindful hearers are able or motivated to use such correcting techniques, active cognitive responding or issue-elaboration is a necessary but not sufficient condition for second-guessing. The attributional analysis comes closer to the concept of the strategic hearer because it posits that prior knowledge is used to deduce bias. However, it does not focus on techniques used to counter such distortions.

Second, the theory of second-guessing identifies both cognitive and behavioral reactions to perceived bias, whereas the persuasion approaches are primarily focused on cognitive processes. Hewes and Graham argue that individuals may employ social information-gathering strategies to supplement and evaluate the results of cognitive, second-guessing activity. Although research associated with the three persuasion perspectives has investigated a variety of dimensions contained in cognitive responses (see Cacioppo, Harkins, & Petty, 1981), few studies have examined the relationships between cognitive responses and behavioral reactions (see Cacioppo & Petty, 1979a, and Cacioppo et al., 1986, as exceptions).

Third, the theory of second-guessing describes a process that is less temporally bounded than that posited by the persuasion approaches. Hewes and Graham hypothesize that second-guessing activity and social information-gathering may continue beyond initial reception of the message. Individuals may continue second-guessing and information seeking as long as the need for accurate information remains high, and cognitive load is not excessive. The persuasion approaches focus on information processing just prior to message reception, during message reception, or immediately after receiving the message. Whether or not processing continues beyond the encounter is ignored.[2]

Fourth, the theory of second-guessing is not bounded by any particular type of communication context, whereas the persuasion approaches are primarily focused on persuasive contexts. Hence, a receiver may engage in second-guessing even if a message is not perceived to be sent with persuasive intent. Although cognitive responses and issue-elaboration could also occur in nonpersuasive contexts, the persuasion approaches do not focus upon them.

Fifth, the theory of second-guessing posits that reinterpretation processes are driven by uncertainty reduction, whereas the persuasion approaches are not entirely specific about the underlying variable guiding their approach. The cognitive response approach must rely upon other persuasion perspectives (e.g., psychological reactance, cognitive dissonance) to predict when cognitive responding will occur and the basis of its relationship to persuasion (Eagly & Himmelfarb, 1978; Petty & Cacioppo, 1981). The elaboration likelihood model is clearer in specifying that individuals want to hold correct attitudes, but this postulate is not directly tied to subsequent tests of the theory. The attributional analysis makes no mention of its fundamental process.[3] This is not to say that uncertainty reduction might not be applied to the three persuasion approaches. Koslin, Pargament, and Suedfeld (1971) argued that induced uncertainty and attempts at its reduction may play a pivotal role in persuasion. However, the three perspectives do not explicitly consider the possibility.

Sixth, the theory of second-guessing is focused exclusively upon the process of identifying bias and reinterpreting biased messages, whereas the persuasion approaches extend such processes to other domains. Obviously, the persuasion approaches are intended to describe processes leading to attitude change. The theory of second-guessing stops short of specifying implications for other variables.

Though different, the theory of second-guessing and the persuasion approaches may offer insights into each of their respective processes. The theory of second-guessing offers a more specific analysis of what receivers may do when encountering persuasive messages. It provides an expanded list of biases that might be discovered and specifies activities used to correct for them. It also extends the analysis beyond the immediate situation in which the message is received. By focusing only on short-term cognitive responding, persuasion researchers have ignored mulling processes that may lead to continued attitude modification. While it is clear that recalling the initial cognitive responses will predict persistence of attitude change (Love & Greenwald, 1978; Petty, 1977), subsequent second-guessing activity may provide insight into what determines the recollection of initial cognitive responses and may be a better predictor of later attitudes.

The persuasion approaches may provide insight into antecedents and consequences of second-guessing. Hewes and Graham argue that it is important to identify the antecedents of the need for accurate information and, though unstated, it is equally crucial to discover variables that cause a receiver to doubt the veracity of incoming information. The ELM specified two potential correlates of the need for accurate information: personal relevance/involvement and need for cognition. The attribution analysis implies that when a person's background is consistent with his or her advocated position, doubt increases about the accuracy of his or her views. All of these variables may play significant roles in stimulating the second-guessing process.

On the consequence side, the theory of second-guessing has not been extended to potential effects. It might be useful to explore the effect of second-guessing in other domains. If second-guessing results in less confidence in the stated opinion and a revision that corrects for the perceived bias, will the receiver hold more accurate attitudes and be better able to predict and control the environment? More importantly, what might prevent people from achieving these advantages? The latter question is the one I will address in the second part of the commentary.

FACTORS BIASING THE USE OF SECOND-GUESSING

Research cited by Hewes and Graham indicates that receivers have an adequate store of information about the kinds of biases affecting information providers and that they are able to apply their knowledge appropriately when cues of bias are present. This claim implies that receivers have the *potential* to debias information.

However, certain factors may reduce the likelihood that individuals will be able to fulfill their potential. I would argue that these variables exert influence at the vigilance stage of the model and reduce the likelihood that second-guessing will be appropriately activated. Two sets of factors may cause second-guessing to be less effective: general suspiciousness and selective application of second-guessing.

There is evidence that people vary in the degree to which they trust others. For example, Christie and Geis (1970) argue that high Machiavellians have generally cynical and negative views of other people and such a dimension has been identified within one of their scales (Hunter, Gerbing, & Boster, 1982). This outlook is evidenced by the negative correlation between Machiavellianism scores and trait measures of trust in other people (Lamden & Lorr, 1975; Wrightsman, 1964).

Although no research has directly investigated this possibility, individuals who are either very trusting or suspicious may inappropriately engage in second-guessing activity. After reviewing research, Christie and Geis (1970) concluded that low Machiavellians seem to be "soft touches. They are more likely to do or accept what another wants simply because he [*sic*] wants it" (p. 295). On the other hand, high Machiavellians appear to be "suspicious of experimenters' and others' explanations" (p. 298).[4]

If so, when needing accurate information, low Machiavellians may engage in *less* second-guessing and high Machiavellians *more* second-guessing than is warranted by cues in the situation. Although not tied to Machiavellianism, Doelger, Hewes, and Graham (1986) similarly noted, "Clearly, social actors who second-guess all the time, and those who never do, are unable to gain an accurate picture of the world. The former are likely to be labeled as paranoid, whereas the latter would be considered gullible and/or excessively naive" (p. 303).

Unfortunately, research has not investigated whether Machiavellianism, trust, or any other relevant orientation makes individuals over- or undersensitive to cues of bias. However, it is clear that some individuals do perceive bias in message contexts containing no *explicit* indicators. Doelger, Hewes, and Graham (1986, p. 325) found that 25% of their respondents perceived background inconsistency and 23% found self-serving motivational bias in contexts containing no such cues. While the observation of such bias was significantly higher in contexts actually containing appropriate cues, the aforementioned proportions suggest that some individuals are actively (and perhaps, inappropriately) applying social knowledge to low information or ambiguous contexts.

While general suspiciousness or trust may prove to be a problem, *selective vigilance* may be of greater concern. Rather than generally distrusting information, individuals may be selective about when they bring to bear their cognitive skills. Only when screening cues activate uncertainty will receivers employ their social knowledge to identify and correct bias. If those cues are not present, an individual may be insufficiently attentive and less able to identify cues of bias that are present. There may be two fundamental criteria that affect the initiation of second-guessing: attitudinal agreement and source characteristics.

Petty and Cacioppo (1986) speculated that in some circumstances, issue-elaboration "is more biased and may be guided mostly by the person's initial attitude" (p. 128). In essence, we may second-guess the veracity of attitudinally discrepant messages to a greater extent than we do those with which there is agreement.

A variety of studies indirectly support this analysis. Receivers of counter-attitudinal messages generate more unfavorable thoughts than those receiving proattitudinal ones (Cacioppo & Petty, 1979a, Study 2; Cacioppo & Petty, 1979b, Petty & Cacioppo, 1979, Study 1). My own research discovered this pattern even though pretesting indicated that the arguments contained in the counterattitudinal and proattitudinal messages were of equal strength (Roloff, in press). This effect occurs primarily when a receiver is personally involved in the issue (Petty & Cacioppo, 1979, Study 1; Howard-Pitney, Borgida, & Omoto, 1986) and has a great deal of behavioral experience with the topic (Wood, 1982). Moreover, premessage attitudes are positively correlated with generating negative cognitive responses to a counterattitudinal message (Greenwald, 1968; Love & Greenwald, 1978; Roloff, in press).

Attitudinal agreement may also cause receivers to overlook or forgive moderate bias. Sternthal, Dholakia, and Leavitt (1978) focused on reactions to a proattitudinal message attributed to either a competent and unbiased (advocated a position inconsistent with background) source or to a communicator having no expertise and potential bias (job aspirations are consistent with the advocated position). They found no difference in counterargumentation and greater *proarguing* with the inexpert, biased source. Rather than reject the information from the less credible source, they seemed to bolster it with their own. Similar bolstering has been observed when individuals recall information contained in the political advertisements of a candidate they favor (Donohue, 1973-74). While this effect does not generalize to sources of extremely low credibility (see Tan, 1975), it does suggest that attitudinal agreement may reduce second-guessing.

Beyond experimental evidence, there is survey data indicating that attitudes may determine perceived bias. Some media critics have argued that news reporting reflects a liberal bias (Corry, 1986; Efron, 1971) while others have posited a bias toward the status quo (Miliband, 1969; Lauderdale & Estep, 1980). Such diverse opinion as to the direction of news bias is also reflected in public opinion polls wherein segments of the population are convinced that news reporting is biased in either a liberal or conservative direction (Stevenson & Greene, 1980). However, if one uses balanced reporting (i.e., roughly equal coverage of all sides of an issue) as a criterion of bias, content analyses of news content have not demonstrated significant bias (e.g., Pride & Wamsley, 1972; Pride & Richards, 1974; Hallin, 1984).[5] Why then do some believe it exists? Stevenson and Greene (1980) have argued that perceived bias is affected by the attitudes of the media user. To the extent that information is inconsistent with a media user's attitudes, then that message will be viewed as biased. Indeed, Swindel (1987) found that liberals thought that groups reflecting their own political orientation were treated less favorably by the media than were those groups that are conservative and moderate. Conservatives held the opposite perceptions. Perhaps individuals are overly sensitive to any information that implies criticism of their attitudes and readily attribute bias to such a source.[6]

Research directly related to the *ability* to evaluate information critically is also supportive of the biasing effects of attitudes. Lord, Ross, and Lepper (1979) discovered that attitudes affected the decision to accept at face value the results of a belief-confirming or belief-contradicting study. Individuals on different sides of an issue read the results and then methodological critiques of two studies: one that supported their side and another that contradicted it. Instead of reducing confidence in the results, criticism of the studies was interpreted in such a manner so as to support the receiver's initial attitude, and attitude polarization resulted.

The biasing effects of attitudes may also be exacerbated by personality. Rokeach (1960) argued that highly dogmatic individuals evidence a greater rejection of alternative belief systems than do low dogmatics. Hence, Robbins (1975) found that high dogmatics expressed greater liking for another whose opinions agreed with their own than one whose opinions were discrepant. Given this orientation, high dogmatics may question the accuracy of counterattitudinal information and accept the validity of proattitudinal data regardless of actual flaws contained therein.[7] Indeed, Bettinghaus, Miller, and Steinfatt (1970) found that low dogmatics were better able to identify the accuracy of valid, belief-discrepant syllogisms than were high dogmatics. Low dogmatics evidenced the same advantage when evaluating belief-congruent, invalid syllogisms.

The final criterion influencing vigilance is related to the source of the message. Receivers may be more skeptical of some sources than are others, even when all of them send identical message content. There is evidence that receivers begin counterarguing against certain sources *prior* to receiving any information from them (e.g., Baron & Miller, 1969). If so, then premessage assessments of bias may influence the degree of scrutiny applied to subsequent information. If the source is thought to be generally unbiased, then less scrutiny is required (see Hass, 1981). For example, Gillig and Greenwald (1974) found that priming receivers with counterarguments *prior* to message reception only increased counterarguing *during* decoding for messages from a low credible source. In essence, those receiving a persuasive message from a high credible source did not use the counterarguments they had. Also, research indicates that withholding the identification of a high credible source until *after* message processing does not increase message acceptance (Mills & Harvey, 1972; Ward & McGinnies, 1974). Thus, if the source is unknown, information may be processed and evaluated differently than if a citation is included.

The potentially debilitating effect of attitudes toward the source is especially evident in highly dogmatic individuals. Rokeach (1960) argued that high dogmatics are easily influenced by authority figures. Hence, they do not differentiate between their evaluation of the source of the message and the validity of the message (Powell, 1962). This binding implies that high dogmatics are less able to identify bias in the reasoning of certain sources. Indeed, low dogmatics are better able to evaluate the logical accuracy of invalid syllogisms attributed to high credible sources and valid syllogisms advanced by low credible sources (Bettinghaus, Miller, & Steinfatt, 1970).

Thus Hewes and Graham are correct when arguing that individuals have the necessary skills to second-guess. The problem of not second-guessing may stem from the lack of motivation to do so. When confronting attitudinally consistent information or a credible source, the potential for second-guessing is low. Only when individuals are forced to consider actively the opposite of what they are processing may second-guessing of such information occur (Lord, Lepper, & Preston, 1984).

SUMMARY

At the outset, I professed my positive regard for the theory of second-guessing. The reader will note that none of my comments challenge the essential nature of the theory. Instead, I tried to integrate the theory with other perspectives and suggest clarifications. In doing so, I noted that the research I cited was not designed to test the theory. Hence it does not include many measures that are directly related to the framework. However, I believe that the concepts may be useful and the relationships can and should be empirically evaluated.

One irony is worthy of note. Hewes and Graham provide evidence that individuals have a store of knowledge about actual biases that affect human observation and that they can use that information to correct for such bias in the accounts of others. Because all information users are also information providers, one might wonder why we find data derived from our direct observation of events to be more useful and generally preferable to those garnered from the observations of others (Hewes, Graham, Doelger, & Pavitt, 1985). Do we suffer from an "ownness bias" whereby we believe that our perceptions are more original and untainted than those of others (Perloff & Brock, 1980)? Perhaps, people are engaging in a form of what Davison (1983) calls the "third person effect." We believe that biases affect others to a greater extent than they do ourselves. In any case, individuals who believe that data received from others are inherently more tainted than those derived from their own senses may be as "out of touch" as persons who hold the opposite view.

NOTES

1. Cognitive responses might also be coded so as to access the alternative explanations and reinterpretations that might result from second-guessing. For example, Greenwald (1968) coded cognitive responses into three categories: externally originated (those thoughts related to the persuasive message), recipient-modified (those thoughts in which the receiver illustrated, qualified, and reacted to the persuasive message), and recipient-generated (thoughts not directly related to the persuasive message). The latter two categories might include indicators of second-guessing. Two of his results are of interest. The majority of thoughts were recipient-generated and only recipient-generated thoughts were significantly and positively related to opinion change.

2. This focus on cognitive responses occurring concomitantly with message reception is reflected in the operations used to elicit them. Miller and Baron (1973) urge researchers to employ a restrictive time limit for listing cognitive responses (as little as 45 seconds) so as to preclude the elicitation of postmessage thoughts and less relevant cognitions that occurred during processing. Much research employs a limit of three minutes (see Petty & Cacioppo, 1986).

3. Since the attribution analysis was stimulated by work focused on inference-making about plausible causes of a person's behavior (see Eagly & Chaiken, 1984), one might assume that uncertainty reduction plays a role in the perspective. However, an explicit link is not made.

4. These conclusions are problematic given that Hunter, Gerbing, and Boster (1982) found that the cynicism dimension of Machiavellianism was significantly correlated with dogmatism (Rokeach, 1960). However, since Rokeach (1960) found that high dogmatics are "blindly loyal" to even irrational instructions from experimenters, it is doubtful that the general suspicion (also aimed at experimenters) observed by Christie and Geiss reflects dogmatism. But, it is unclear as to which of the other dimensions of Machiavellianism might be related to suspicion.

5. Not all scholars would agree that balance is the only content measure of media bias. Groups may receive equal coverage, but one may be labeled in such a fashion that it is treated unfairly. For example, Shoemaker (1984) found that groups perceived to be deviant by the editors of large, metropolitan newspapers were portrayed in newspaper stories as more negative, less legitimate, and less viable than groups perceived to be less deviant. One problem with such a measure of bias is that one cannot discern whether such groups are being portrayed unfairly or actually possess such characteristics. In Shoemaker's study, groups perceived to be highly deviant included the Moral Majority, Jewish Defense League, communists, the Ku Klux Klan, and the American Nazis.

6. It should be noted that research on media bias may be cast at a broader level than is applicable to the theory of second-guessing. Generally, perceived media bias is not aimed at a specific message and, at most, only compares judgments about several media (e.g., Swindel, 1987). In the only study I found focused on specific media messages, Stevenson and Greene (1980) discovered that readers of newspaper accounts they judged to be biased stopped reading more frequently to disagree, question, and agree with the author than did readers of unbiased stories.

Even though the stories were focused on political candidates, the researchers did not relate political preference or attitudes to perceived bias or cognitive reactions. Hence we cannot tell if stopping to disagree or question a biased passage occurred primarily when one's own candidate was attacked or if stopping to agree with a biased passage occurred when the opposition candidate was defamed.

7. Donohew and Palmgreen (1971) provide indirect evidence of this relationship. They discovered that low dogmatics experienced greater stress when exposed to attitudinally discrepant, important information than did high dogmatics. The researchers interpreted this pattern as reflecting a tendency for high dogmatics to reject "out of hand" any belief-discrepant information, whereas low dogmatics attach potential plausibility to the data. Hence, high dogmatics might be prone to second-guess belief-discrepant information and low dogmatics to second-guess their own beliefs and suffer uncertainty. The greater uncertainty is evidenced by their greater stress. Unfortunately, no cognitive measures were included in the study. Therefore, the speculation cannot be evaluated.

REFERENCES

Atkin, C. (1973). Instrumental utilities and information seeking. In P. Clarke (Ed.), *New models for communication research* (pp. 205-242). Beverly Hills, CA: Sage.

Baron, R. S. & Miller, N. (1969). Credibility, distraction, and counterargument in a forewarning situation. *Proceedings of the 77th Annual Convention of the American Psychological Association, 4*, 411-412.

Benoit, W. L. (1987). Argument and credibility appeals in persuasion. *Southern Speech Communication Journal, 52*, 181-197.

Bettinghaus, E., Miller, G. R., & Steinfatt, R. (1970). Source evaluation, syllogistic content, and judgments of logical validity by high- and low-dogmatic persons. *Journal of Personality and Social Psychology, 16*, 238-244.

Buss, L. J. (1967). Motivational variables and information seeking in the mass media. *Journalism Quarterly, 44*, 130-133.

Cacioppo, J. T., Harkins, S. G., & Petty, R. E. (1981). The nature of attitudes and cognitive responses and their relationships to behavior. In R. E. Petty, T. M. Ostrom, & T. C. Brock (Eds.), *Cognitive responses in persuasion* (pp. 31-54). Hillsdale, NJ: Lawrence Erlbaum.

Cacioppo, J. T., & Petty, R. E. (1979a). Attitudes and cognitive responses: An electrophysiological approach. *Journal of Personality and Social Psychology, 37*, 2181-2199.

Cacioppo, J. T., & Petty, R. E. (1979b). Effects of message repetition and position on cognitive responses, recall, and persuasion. *Journal of Personality and Social Psychology, 37*, 97-109.

Cacioppo, J. T., & Petty, R. E. (1982). The need for cognition. *Journal of Personality and Social Psychology, 42*, 116-131.

Cacioppo, J. T., Petty, R. E., Kao, C. F., & Rodriguez, R. (1986). Central and peripheral routes to persuasion: An individual difference perspective. *Journal of Personality and Social Psychology, 51*, 1032-1043.

Cacioppo, J. T., Petty, R. E., & Morris, K. (1983). Effects of need for cognition on message evaluation, recall, and persuasion. *Journal of Personality and Social Psychology, 45*, 805-818.

Christie, R., & Geis, F. C. (1970). *Studies in Machiavellianism*. New York: Academic Press.

Cohen, A., Stotland, E., & Wolfe, D. (1955). An experimental investigation of need for cognition. *Journal of Abnormal and Social Psychology, 51*, 291-294.

Corry, J. (1986). *TV news and the dominant culture*. Washington: Media Institute.

Davison, W. P. (1983). The third-person effect in communication. *Public Opinion Quarterly, 47*, 1-15.

Doelger, J. A., Hewes, D. E., & Graham, M. L. (1986). Knowing when to "second-guess": The mindful analysis of messages. *Human Communication Research, 12*, 301-338.

Donohew, L., & Palmgreen, P. (1971). An investigation of "mechanisms" of information selection. *Journalism Quarterly, 48*, 627-639.
Donohue, T. R. (1973-74). Impact of viewer predisposition on political TV commercials. *Journal of Broadcasting, 18*, 3-15.
Eagly, A. H., & Chaiken, S. (1984). Cognitive theories of persuasion. In L. Berkowitz (Ed.), *Advances in experimental social psychology* (Vol. 17, pp. 268-361). New York: Academic Press.
Eagly, A. H., & Himmelfarb, S. (1978). Attitudes and opinions. *Annual Review of Psychology, 29*, 517-554.
Eagly, A. H., Wood, W., & Chaiken, S. (1978). Causal inferences about communicators and their effect on opinion change. *Journal of Personality and Social Psychology, 36*, 424-435.
Efron, E. (1971). *The news twisters.* New York: Manor Books.
Festinger, L., & Maccoby, N. (1964). On resistance to persuasive communications. *Journal of Abnormal and Social Psychology, 68*, 359-366.
Fiske, S. T., & Taylor, S. E. (1984). *Social cognition.* Reading, MA: Addison-Wesley.
Gillig, P. M., & Greenwald, A. G. (1974). Is it time to lay the sleeper effect to rest? *Journal of Personality and Social Psychology, 29*, 132-139.
Greenwald, A. G. (1968). Cognitive learning, cognitive response to persuasion, and attitude change. In A. G. Greenwald, T. C. Brock, & T. M. Ostrom (Eds.), *Psychological foundations of attitudes* (pp. 147-170). New York: Academic Press.
Hallin, D. C. (1984). The media, the war in Vietnam and political support: A critique of the thesis of an oppositional media. *Journal of Politics, 46*, 2-24.
Hass, R. G. (1981). Effects of source characteristics on cognitive responses and persuasion. In R. E. Petty, T. M. Ostrom, & T. C. Brock (Eds.), *Cognitive responses in persuasion* (pp. 141-172). Hillsdale, NJ: Lawrence Erlbaum.
Hewes, D. R., Graham, M. L., Doelger, J., & Pavitt, C. (1985). "Second-guessing": Message interpretation in social networks. *Human Communication Research, 11*, 299-334.
Howard-Pitney, B., Borgida, E., & Omoto, A. M. (1986). Personal involvement: An examination of processing differences. *Social Cognition, 4*, 39-57.
Hunter, J. E., Gerbing, D. W., & Boster, F. J. (1982). Machiavellian beliefs and personality: Construct invalidity of the Machiavellianism dimension. *Journal of Personality and Social Psychology, 43*, 1293-1305.
Katz, D. (1960). The functional approach to the study of attitudes. *Public Opinion Quarterly, 24*, 163-204.
Koslin, B. L., Pargament, R., & Suedfeld, P. (1971). An uncertainty model of attitude change. In P. Suedfeld (Ed.), *Attitude change: The competing views* (pp. 234-245). Chicago: Aldine-Atherton.
Lamden, S., & Lorr, M. (1975). Untangling the structure of Machiavellianism. *Journal of Clinical Psychology, 2*, 301-302.
Lanzetta, J. T., & Driscoll, J. M. (1968). Effects of uncertainty and importance on information search in decision making. *Journal of Personality and Social Psychology, 4*, 479-486.
Lauderdale, P. & Estep, R. E. (1980). The bicentennial protest: An examination of hegemony in the definition of deviant political activity. In P. Lauderdale (Ed.), *A political analysis of deviance.* Minneapolis: University of Minnesota Press.
Lord, C. G., Lepper, M. R., & Preston, E. (1984). Considering the opposite: A corrective strategy for social judgment. *Journal of Personality and Social Psychology, 47*, 1231-1243.
Lord, C. G., Ross, L., & Lepper, M. R. (1979). Biased assimilation and attitude polarization: The effects of prior theories on subsequently considered evidence. *Journal of Personality and Social Psychology, 37*, 2098-2109.
Love, R. E., & Greenwald, A. G. (1978). Cognitive responses to persuasion as mediators of opinion change. *Journal of Social Psychology, 104*, 231-241.
Miliband, R. (1969). *The state of capitalist society.* London: Weidenfield & Nicolson.

Mills, J., & Harvey, J. (1972). Opinion change as a function of when information about the communicator is received and whether he is attractive or expert. *Journal of Personality and Social Psychology, 21*, 52-55.

Nisbett, R. E., & Ross, L. (1980). *Human inference: Strategies and shortcomings of social judgment*. Engelwood Cliffs, N J: Prentice-Hall.

Perloff, R. M., & Brock, T. C. (1980). ". . . And thinking makes it so": Cognitive responses to persuasion. In M. E. Roloff & G. R. Miller (Eds.), *Persuasion: New directions in theory and research* (pp. 67-100). Beverly Hills, CA: Sage

Petty, R. E. (1977). *A cognitive response analysis of the temporal persistence of attitude changes induced by persuasive communications*. Unpublished doctoral dissertation, Ohio State University, Columbus.

Petty, R. E., & Cacioppo, J. T. (1979). Issue involvement can increase or decrease persuasion by enhancing message-relevant cognitive processes. *Journal of Personality and Social Psychology, 37*, 1915-1926.

Petty, R. E., & Cacioppo, J. T. (1981). *Attitudes and persuasion: Classic and contemporary approaches*. Dubuque, IA: William C. Brown.

Petty, R. E., & Cacioppo, J. T. (1984). The effects of involvement on responses to argument quantity and quality: Central and peripheral routes to persuasion. *Journal of Personality and Social Psychology, 46*, 69-81.

Petty, R. E., & Cacioppo, J. T. (1986). The elaboration likelihood model of persuasion. In L. Berkowitz (Ed.), *Advances in experimental social psychology* (Vol. 19, pp. 123-205). New York: Academic Press.

Petty, R. E., & Cacioppo, J. T., & Goldman, R. (1981). Personal involvement as a determinant of argument-based persuasion. *Journal of Personality and Social Psychology, 41*, 847-855.

Petty, R. E., Ostrom, T. M., & Brock, T. C. (Eds.). (1981). *Cognitive responses in persuasion*. Hillsdale, NJ: Lawrence Erlbaum.

Powell, F. A. (1962). Open- and closed-mindedness and the ability to differentiate source and message. *Journal of Personality and Social Psychology, 65*, 61-64.

Pride, R. A., & Richards, B. (1974). Denigration of authority? Television news coverage of the student movement. *Journal of Politics, 36*, 637-660.

Pride, R. A., & Wamsley, G. L. (1972). Symbol analysis of network coverage of Laos incursion. *Journalism Quarterly, 49*, 635-640.

Robbins, G. E. (1975). Dogmatism and information gathering in personality impression formation. *Journal of Research in Personality, 9*, 74-84.

Rokeach, M. (1960). *The open and closed mind*. New York: Basic Books.

Roloff, M. E. (in press). Issue schema and mindless processing of persuasive messages: Much ado about nothing? In C. Roberts & K. Watson (Eds.), *Intrapersonal communication*. New Orleans: Spectra.

Ross, L. (1977). The intuitive psychologist and his shortcomings: Distortions in the attribution process. In L. Berkowitz (Ed.), *Advances in experimental social psychology* (Vol. 10, pp. 173-220). New York: Academic Press.

Ross, L. (1979). Some afterthoughts on the intuitive psychologist. In L. Berkowitz (Ed.), *Cognitive theories in social psychology* (pp. 385-400). New York: Academic Press.

Shoemaker, P. J. (1984). Media treatment of deviant political groups. *Journalism Quarterly, 61*, 66-75.

Sternthal, B. Dholakia, R., & Leavitt, C. (1978). The persuasive effect of source credibility: Test of cognitive response. *Journal of Consumer Research, 4*, 252-260.

Stevenson, R. L., & Greene, M. T. (1980). A reconsideration of bias in the news. *Journalism Quarterly, 57*, 115-121.

Swindel, S. H. (1987). *Spatial considerations for the study of perceived bias in the news: The role of political ideology*. Paper presented at the annual meeting of the Midwest Association for Public Opinion Research, Chicago, IL.

Tan, A. S. (1975). Exposure to discrepant information and effect of three coping modes. *Journalism Quarterly, 52*, 678-684.

Ward, C. D., & McGinnies, E. (1974). Persuasive effect of early and late mention of credible and non-credible sources. *Journal of Psychology, 86*, 17-23.

Wood, W. (1982). Retrieval of attitude-relevant information from memory: Effects on susceptibility to persuasion and on intrinsic motivation. *Journal of Personality and Social Psychology, 42*, 798-810.

Wood, W., & Eagly, A. H. (1981). Stages in the analysis of persuasive messages: The role of causal attributions and message comprehension. *Journal of Personality and Social Psychology, 40*, 246-259.

Wrightsman, L. S., Jr. (1964). Measurement of philosophies of human nature. *Psychological Reports, 14*, 743-751.

Second-Guessing Second-Guessing: Yet Another Comment

GERALD R. MILLER
Michigan State University

Neither a borrower nor a lender be.

—William Shakespeare

Though Shakespeare's familiar caveat counsels that both borrowing and lending are social taboos, most people, including the Bard himself, would doubtless opt for the latter practice over the former. To be cast in the role of lender implies possession of some economic, social, or intellectual resource deemed sufficiently valuable to be coveted by others not fortunate enough to possess it in adequate supply. By contrast, borrowing is a humbling activity, for borrowers are forced to concede that through the vagaries of either fate or chance or because of some character or performance flaw, they have failed to amass a sufficient store of the valued resource.

THE HISTORICAL SETTING

Throughout much of its relatively brief history, communication has suffered the scholarly and professional indignities of being dismissed as a "borrower" discipline. During the 1950s and the 1960s, the theoretical postures and conceptual schemata guiding the work of most communication scholars were appropriated from such related disciplines as psychology, sociology, political science, and the various offshoots of linguistics. Although these frequent trips to the academic loan department caused periodic attacks of cognitive dissonance (to use one oft-borrowed concept from social psychology) typically signaled by yet another essay advocating the develop-

Correspondence and requests for reprints: Gerald R. Miller, Department of Communication, CAS 472, Michigan State University, East Lansing, MI 48824.

Communication Yearbook 12, pp. 266-275

ment of "communication theories," few actual partly or fully developed theories emerged. Thus I can recall squirming in my convention-audience seat as recently as the early 1970s while listening to a prominent researcher from a related discipline dismiss communication as a "derivative field." Though the precise meaning of the label escaped me, it was clear from verbal context and the accompanying paralinguistic cues that being a member of a "derivative field" implied a borrowing posture not to be crowed about.

Fortunately, the 1970s and the 1980s have witnessed a rebalancing of the scales such that in 1988, the discipline of communication has accumulated some valuable theoretical and conceptual resources of its own. It seems fair to say our scientific pockets are no longer empty, and while some may contend that we still suffer from a deficit in the disciplinary balance of payments, few would question our increasing potential to shed the pervasive onus of borrowers and to don the more rewarding mantle of intellectual lenders. One significant resource, prominently mentioned by Hewes and Graham, is the uncertainty reduction theory developed by Berger and his colleagues (e.g., Berger & Calabrese, 1975; Berger & Kellermann, 1983), as well as its more primitive, less fully developed manifestations, such as the developmental conceptualization of interpersonal communication sketched by Steinberg and myself (Miller, 1975; Miller & Steinberg, 1975). Similarly, the constructivist position developed by Delia and his colleagues (e.g., Delia, 1977; Delia, O'Keefe, & O'Keefe, 1982) has broken important theoretical and conceptual ground, as has the rules-oriented work on the coordinated management of meaning carried out by Pearce and his associates (e.g., Pearce & Cronen, 1980; Cronen, Pearce, & Harris, 1982). And as a final specific example, the violation of expectations perspective reflected in the work of Judee Burgoon and others on nonverbal communication (e.g., Burgoon & Jones, 1976), as well as a recent chapter by Michael Burgoon and myself (Burgoon & Miller, 1985) outlining a theory of persuasive effects, offers a relatively original theoretical vantage point for generating future communication research and for synthesizing and reinterpreting the findings of a large body of prior persuasion studies grounded in a variety of theoretical positions.

THE IMPORTANCE OF SECOND-GUESSING THEORY

This brief historical backdrop, while admittedly far from a comprehensive chronicle of recent conceptual and theoretical advances in the field, provides a context for my comments about the work of Hewes and his associates on second-guessing theory and, particularly, the description and current evaluation of the theory detailed in the Hewes and Graham *Communication Yearbook* chapter. I agree with both these authors and with my fellow commentator, Professor Roloff, that second-guessing theory represents a shiny, new theoretical resource crafted by communication scholars. Moreover, upon pondering present research trends in the field, I conclude that the three implications of the theory for communication research identified by Hewes and Graham constitute a generally sound argumentative foundation for the theory's utility. Despite my general agreement with this foundation, however, I do want to nitpick a point or two: First, because I think it will reveal several distinctions worth making; second, because nitpicking is the academic's order of the day when insufficient insight and/or absence of ideological fervor dictate concurrence with the major substantive thrust of a position.

Hewes and Graham contend that the first virtue of second-guessing theory is its central concern with an "active, construing, strategic listener" (p. 216), a concern largely absent in the current work of communication scholars. If attention is directed solely at empirical, data-driven scholarship, this charge, given the occasional exceptions noted by both Hewes and Graham and by Roloff, has much to recommend it. Ironically, however, even the most cursory examination of the way that scholars in our field have written about and conceptualized the communication process reveals a quite different picture. Berlo's (1960) *The Process of Communication*—a book that exerted great influence in shaping our field, even though it seems simple, elemental, and dated in 1988—consistently stresses the centrality of active, construing receivers, placing emphasis on such notions as perceptual relativity, a subjective conception of reality, and the now commonplace saw, "Meanings are in people." To be sure, Berlo's discussion of these concepts largely bypasses the *strategic* dimension envisioned by Hewes and Graham; indeed, when taken at face value, one could easily conclude that the activating forces operating on receivers predispose them to respond thoughtlessly or irrationally and that the strategic trick of communication lies in pinpointing the right message and channel choices to capitalize on this thoughtlessness or irrationality. I will later comment briefly on some questions raised by what I perceive to be Hewes and Graham's staunch commitment to the importance of classical conceptions of the rational message recipient; my point here is not that earlier writers such as Berlo totally anticipated the cognitive and affective picture of listeners painted by Hewes and Graham, but to indicate the longstanding tendency to pay at least hearty conceptual lip service to the active receiver as a crucial element of the communication process.

A second signpost of the considerable discrepancy between the way we have talked about communication conceptually and the approaches we have used to study it empirically can be found in the almost universal assent to view communication as a process—a stubborn habit exemplified by my own use of the phrase "communication process" twice in the preceding paragraph. As I understand it, commitment to a process view mandates that communication is most richly construed as *an interactive phenomenon involving two or more active, construing, and (perhaps) strategic communicators*. Thus, though I concur heartily with Hewes and Graham's point that Miller, Boster, Roloff, and Seibold (1977) "opened the floodgates" for a deluge of monadic, unidirectional research focusing on an active, construing, strategic persuader practicing her or his wiles on inert, cognitively invisible persuadees, I am confident that, if pressed, all of the involved researchers, including the four manning the floodgates, would quickly profess belief in the indispensable role of active, construing, and strategic persuadees if persuasive exchanges and outcomes are to be described accurately. In fact, it is perhaps worth noting that second-guessing theory itself exhibits the same unidirectional bias, focusing entirely on the activities of listeners while largely ignoring the ongoing cognitive and symbolic activities of speakers. To say this certainly does not negate the force of Hewes and Graham's argument that message recipients are not afforded fair and equitable empirical treatment in our research. Rather, what I have sought to do is to place their argument in a disciplinary context that has consistently manifested a substantial void between our metatheoretical and theoretical commitments and our research practices.

Hewes and Graham next contend that second-guessing theory has the virtue of emphasizing indirect, nontransactional episodes, rather than focusing on direct, transactional, symbolic exchange. For those mindful of an era when the commonplace criticism was that communication theory and research suffered from too much of the former and too little of the latter, this virtue will rightly be interpreted as a modest pendulum swing, not as a dramatic harbinger of a new research outlook. As such, evaluation of their argument hinges on a personal reading of whether such a swing is apt to be fruitful given the current state of the scholarly Zeitgeist. My own reading places me solidly in their corner. Just as I believe that the recent trend toward transactionalism, documented by Hewes and Graham, has represented a useful avenue for research practices, I fear it has also signaled an inordinate disinterest in the ways individuals process and "make sense" of incoming messages. And lest I be accused of blatant inconsistency with my earlier comments, I hasten to add my position does not represent allegiance to a monadic conception of communication, but endorsement of the view that individual cognitive activities and affective states are crucial ingredients of a scientific understanding of the total communicative process.

The preceding assertion captures my substantial agreement with the third virtue of second-guessing theory claimed by Hewes and Graham: That the theory centers on the important and, perhaps, overly neglected task of elaborating connections between cognition and communication. My reading of Hewes and Graham suggests that they have stated the argument too loosely and generally, for I interpret second-guessing theory as being primarily concerned with only a certain genre of cognitive processes, namely, those processes culminating in cognitive and behavioral responses that conform with a set of established and, to some extent, prescriptive norms or standards for rational social reasoning. This preoccupation with *rational thought* (in a classical, humanistic sense of the term) posed some initial problems for me in grasping the content and scope of the theory, and indeed, as I will shortly consider, in understanding their meaning for the term *second-guessing.* Furthermore, though Hewes and Graham may question my interpretation, this concern with the rational processing of messages sometimes seems to transcend boundaries of scientific concern to embrace an ideological commitment to the personal desirability and social utility of such processing. Such a commitment, if indeed it exists, is at least partially rooted in assumptions about communication that have traditionally influenced the theorizing and research of most communication scholars including myself. Because I have become increasingly skeptical about the validity of these assumptions, I will consider them later in conjunction with an assessment of possible social limitations of the theory. Notwithstanding the preceding demurrals and reservations, I still am in accord with Hewes and Graham in their positive assessment of the theory's emphasis on the connection between cognition and communication.

TWO QUESTIONS ABOUT SECOND-GUESSING THEORY

Having commented on the claims made to justify the scientific import of second-guessing theory, my remaining remarks will center on two considerations relating to the theory itself. Both have already been previewed: First, I will share some ambiguity and uncertainty I experienced in coming to grips with the meaning and scope of the theory's central concept, "second-guessing;" second, I will examine some questions that occurred to me regarding the theory's possible social limitations. It bears repeating that my primary urges are to tinker with the theory and to tease out one or two of its potential implications and limitations, because my overall judgment of the theoretical contributions of Hewes and his colleagues is overwhelmingly positive.

A Concept by Another Name Might Be Less Confusing

If queried, I would describe myself as an inveterate second-guesser. When asked by a colleague on Monday to air my opinion of MSU's Saturday football performance, I am never hesitant to point out a crucial moment in the game when the coach should have punted instead of running on fourth and one from midfield (the familiar "Monday morning quarterback" syndrome). Similarly, no poker game goes by that I do not chastise myself, either subvocally or vocally, for choosing to break up a four-flush or an open-end straight to draw three to a pair. In short, I am one of countless living testimonies to the wisdom of the tired cliché, "Hindsight is better than foresight."

This self-descriptive vignette captures what I presume to be the ordinary, widely held meaning for the term *second-guessing:* criticizing the prior decisions of oneself or others, given the benefit of knowledge about the outcomes resulting from the original decisions. When viewed in this light, second-guessing is primarily a communicative activity (an episode of verbal behavior) rather than a cognitive process. As long as one is capable of recalling the original alternatives involved in the decision and the outcome(s) accruing from the chosen alternative, any previous decision is fair game for second-guessing messages.

Upon encountering the label "second-guessing theory," then, I initially assumed that the theory was primarily concerned with certain types of messages, as well as the variables influencing production of such messages. As I began to examine the theory, of course, I was quickly disabused of this assumption; clearly Hewes and Graham are focusing on cognitive processes not symbolic behaviors. Nevertheless, I encountered another semantic roadblock when I mistakenly concluded that " second-guessing" referred to the general cognitive process of reinterpreting messages that listeners perceive as biased. In other words, I found myself thinking of second-guessing as encompassing *any situation* in which a reader or listener reinterprets a message either because of doubts about the source's ability to communicate accurately (the *expertise* dimension of credibility) or questions about the source's integrity or motives (the *trustworthiness* dimension). Of central import to this interpretation of "second-guessing" is the possibility that because of attitudinal and perceptual biases of their own, message recipients may err in their judgments of source attributes and/or message content: Instead of "debiasing" the message, they may, to use a term first suggested to me by Dailey (1988), "rebias" it.

Subsequent readings of second-guessing theory revealed that it is not concerned with such a general cognitive process, but instead, a more limited domain of message reinterpretation. Specifically, as Hewes and Graham indicate, second-guessing is of interest to them only when a message is reinterpreted in a manner that conforms more closely with appropriate norms of social reasoning. The authors indicate that second-guessing produces a "truer" account of the message topic. Here, "true" (and in fairness to Hewes and Graham, I should note that they consistently use quotation marks around words such as "true" or "truer" in their chapter) does not refer to the degree to which the message conforms with some objective state of affairs (e.g., the used car salesperson tells the customer the speedometer has not been altered, and, in fact, it has not been), but to the application of sound social reasoning criteria to the reinterpretation. Thus, as used in second-guessing theory, the term *second-guessing* refers to the *cognitive skill* of debiasing messages that fall short on certain yardsticks of social reasoning.

To be sure, Hewes and Graham say most, if not all, of this in their chapter. Nevertheless, considerable "noise" could have been eliminated, at least in my reading of the theory, by simply substituting a label such as "message debiasing" for the more fuzzy "second-guessing." The perils involved in appropriating ordinary language for use in social scientific writing have been underscored by numerous writers, and these perils are heightened if casual, idiomatic language is employed. Despite the fact that Hewes and Graham are free to choose any concept label they wish and despite the fact that they provide a definition of the concept as it is used in their theory, the label "second-guessing" strikes me as having so much excess semantic baggage that it obfuscates rather than informs. Moreover, it deflects attention from the major issues addressed by the theory and causes readers (or, at least, this particular reader) to get bogged down in psuedo problems and definitional confusions.

A second reason for substituting a term such as *message debiasing* relates to the potential scope of second-guessing theory as it is presently formulated. Hewes and Graham are doubtless correct in asserting that people can and do reinterpret messages in line with the predictions of second-guessing theory. Nonetheless, such processing outcomes are but one form of reinterpretation, and at this time, it is anyone's guess as to how frequently they will prevail. My own guess is that "rebiasing" outcomes are more common than "debiasing" outcomes. If my guess is correct, second-guessing theory may be situated at a level of generalizability that severely limits its explanatory and predictive utility. By contrast, a more general theory of message reinterpretation that *includes* message debiasing as one of its cognitive processing alternatives could eventually yield richer scientific returns.

The "All I Want Are the Facts" Bias

By and large, the writings of contemporary scholars are guided by the underlying assumption that effective communication is (or perhaps more accurately, *ideally ought to be*) rooted in thoughtful, "rational" behavior. A more cynical way of putting this claim is to say that academics equate effective communication with the kinds of cognitive activities and message behaviors that largely dominate formal academic discourse.

The first manifestation of this bias appears in the widespread tendency to treat communication as though almost all message exchanges, no matter how mundane or routine, involve considerable conscious cognitive activity—in short, to conceptualize communication as predominantly a highly mindful activity. The claims of second-guessing theorists avoid this potential pitfall, a situation I number as one of the theory's strengths. According to Hewes and Graham, message recipients respond to many messages relatively mindlessly, simply because the messages deal with matters so uninvolving and unimportant as to ensure minimum motivation for careful thought and reflection. Conscious attempts to reinterpret messages (mindful processing activities) are limited to salient messages; that is messages of potentially serious consequence for the recipient's goals or messages that are simply striking in their own right, such as a juicy rumor or a political address on an awkward topic. Thus second-guessing theory makes a useful and reasonably clear distinction between mindful and mindless processing domains.

A second manifestation of the prevailing commitment to a thoughtful, "rational" conception of communication is found in the typically unquestioned belief that effective communication is best fostered by directing mindful processing activities toward the goal of "getting at the *truth* of the message," "acquiring *accurate* information," "finding out what is *really* going on," or some similar phrase: In short, the guiding assumption seems to be that favorable communicative outcomes are most likely to be achieved by realizing an accurate, objective understanding of physical, social, and/or symbolic reality and then responding accordingly.

To be sure, many communicative transactions fall within the purview of this assumption. When purchasing a used car (or making any purchase or investing any money, for that matter), it is clearly in my best interest to acquire an accurate reading of the car's present condition. Moreover, my communication with the salesperson is all but certain to be driven by the knowledge that his or her desired communicative outcome is to sell the car at a profit. Given such potential conflicts of communicative and economic interest, reinterpretation of the salesperson's messages, both by my own message debiasing and by my seeking relevant social information—for example, "Is the dealership and the salesperson reputable?"—is the only prudent course of action.

In other instances, however, the eventual utility of dispassionate, objective cognitive processing and consequent symbolic response is much more problematic. Consider Hewes and Graham's example of counseling a friend suffering the throes of a marital conflict. Throughout this example, they assume that the desired outcomes of both the counselor and the person being counseled are best served by the former's accurate, "true" interpretation of what is actually poisoning the relationship *and* by communicating advice consistent with this interpretation. Thus their suggested counseling options are largely a litany of the friend's relational and personal shortcomings: blaming the spouse unjustly, demanding too much from the spouse, reacting to personal insecurities, and so forth.

This rather simplistic approach to the counseling transaction has several interesting features. First, it ignores other outcomes that may be of primary import to the involved parties in favor of stressing the hegemony of a dispassionate, objective account of the reasons and causes of the relational conflict. Perhaps the friend cares not a whit about understanding the "real" causes of the marital conflict, but instead is seeking social support for his position. Perhaps the counselor is most interested in behaving supportively toward the friend, either because of concern for sustaining their relationship or because of reactance occasioned by past supportive actions by the friend. In short, perhaps neither party is motivated primarily by a desire to understand the "true" nature of the marital conflict, but by a host of other personal or relational considerations.

A second, closely related feature is the implicit assumption that the most effective course of action lies in "telling it like it is," or perhaps more accurately, telling it as it is most "rationally" interpreted to be. Such a course of action would be preferable only if both parties' interests were best served by reconstructing the most accurate possible account of the reasons for, or causes of, the conflict. At the risk of being unduly cynical, this move would be more likely to occur in a scholarly article on marital conflict than in a conversation between two friends regarding an actual marital spat. As a result, comments such as, "Yes, your wife is a real shrew," or, "I think you've always given more to your marriage than you've gotten from it," may be totally congruent with desired personal and relational outcomes, even though they are grounded in biased cognitive processing and communicative response.

Hewes and Graham may contend that these comments do not detract seriously from the scientific utility of second-guessing theory. Moreover, they may also argue that the scenario I have painted itself requires message debiasing, because communicators cannot respond supportively and congruently unless they can accurately determine the actual motives and goals of other communicators—motives and goals that themselves may be masked by biased messages. To avoid any misunderstanding, let me say that I would agree with both claims. My major intent is to question what I perceive as Hewes and Graham's tacit acceptance of the unqualified value of a "rational" view of human communication and to second-guess (in the general cognitive process sense explicated earlier) a substantial dash of ideological commitment that underlies their entire description and current evaluation of the theory. Whether my second-guessing has resulted in "debiasing" or "rebiasing" remains an open question best addressed by future research and theoretical refinement. In light of the theory's promise, such future scientific undertakings are a virtual certainty.

REFERENCES

Berger, C. R., & Calabrese, R. J. (1975). Some explorations in initial interaction and beyond: Toward a developmental theory of interpersonal communication. *Human Communication Research, 1*, 99-112.

Berger, C. R., & Kellermann, K. A. (1983). To ask or not to ask: Is that a question? In R. N. Bostrom (Ed.), *Communication yearbook 7* (pp. 342-368). Newbury Park, CA: Sage.

Berlo, D. K. (1960). *The process of communication*. New York: Holt, Rinehart & Winston.

Burgoon, J. K., & Jones, S. B. (1976). Toward a theory of personal space expectations and their violations. *Human Communication Research, 2*, 131-146.

Burgoon, M., & Miller, G. R. (1985). An expectancy interpretation of language and persuasion. In H. Giles & R. N. St. Clair (Eds.), *Recent advances in language, communication, and social psychology* (pp. 199-229). London: Lawrence Erlbaum.

Cronen, V. E., Pearce, W. B., & Harris, L. M. (1982). The coordinated management of meaning: A theory of communication. In F.E.X. Dance (Ed.), *Human communication theory: Comparative essays* (pp. 61-89). New York: Harper & Row.

Dailey, W. O. (1988). *Second-guessing, familiarity, and in-group bias: Do cognitive responses help*? Paper presented at the Annual Conference of the International Communication Association, New Orleans.

Delia, J. G. (1977). Constructivism and the study of human communication. *Quarterly Journal of Speech, 63,* 66-83.

Delia, J. G., O'Keefe, B. J., & O'Keefe, D. J. (1982). The constructivist approach to communication. In F.E.X. Dance (Ed.), *Human communication theory: Comparative essays* (pp. 147-191). New York: Harper & Row.

Miller, G. R. (1975). Interpersonal communication: A conceptual perspective. *Communication, 2,* 93-105.

Miller, G., Boster, F., Roloff, M., & Seibold, D. (1977). Compliance-gaining message strategies: A typology and some findings concerning effects of situational differences. *Communication Monographs, 54,* 37-51.

Miller, G. R., & Steinberg, M. (1975). *Between people: A new analysis of interpersonal communication.* Chicago: Science Research Associates.

Pearce, W. B., & Cronen, V. E. (1980). *Communication, action and meaning: The creation of social realities.* New York: Praeger.

SECTION 2

INTERCULTURAL RELATIONSHIPS AND CULTURAL IDENTITY

5 Intercultural Communication Revisited: Conceptualization, Paradigm Building, and Methodological Approaches

FRED L. CASMIR
Pepperdine University

NOBLEZA C. ASUNCION-LANDE
University of Kansas

Beginning with a review of the intellectual antecedents of intercultural communication, this essay goes on to document its successes, failings, and uncertainties. It then turns to the development of a "third culture" model in which cultural domination and subjugation are rejected but opportunities for mutual development are provided. Central to the model is the realization that it is the human capacity to synthesize that will provide success and not the simple export and import of technology.

INTERCULTURAL communication scholars are concerned with understanding what happens when human beings from different cultures meet, interact, and attempt to resolve problems in various interrelationships. Unfortunately, scholars and practitioners in the field have been unable to agree on a knowledge base that would distinguish intercultural communication from the various disciplines that have provided the original intellectual impetus for the development of this field of study.

To put it another way, intercultural communication has been faced with "intercultural" challenges within itself, because specialists have been unable to adequately adjust the input from other areas of study to their own unique professional concerns and needs. Intercultural communication can, in fact, be seen as a kind of "third culture" (Casmir, 1978), which has been the result of interactions by representatives of older, academic disciplines. To mention only one specific instance, intercultural communication has to deal with challenges resulting from its symbiotic relationship with the academic field of

Correspondence and requests for reprints: Fred L. Casmir, Department of Communication, Pepperdine University, Malibu, CA 90265.

Communication Yearbook 12, pp. 278-309

study known as "communication," seemingly condemned to suffer many of the same problems and experience the same victories common to that discipline.

HISTORICAL ANTECEDENTS

In the 1970s, there began to emerge among communication and speech scholars the realization that if their disciplines were to have any impact upon the ever increasing problems experienced in human interactions, the use of a variety of approaches and methodologies would be necessary (Delia, 1977). Yet even the term *communication* seemed to defy attempts to come up with one commonly accepted definition (Dance, 1970). Finally, it became clear that the development of even *one* communication theory, responsive to all of the insights and needs of scholars in the field, was also not an attainable goal (Littlejohn, 1983). During that period, when the model for scholars and researchers in most of the social sciences was the one provided by physics, it did not seem to occur to anyone that coming up with *a theory of communication* was akin to coming up with *a comprehensive theory of physics*. Such a variety of needs, applications, interests, and approaches had been brought together under the umbrella term of *communication* that it became impossible to develop one single definition or methodological approach. That this confusion of symbolic activity with observable reality or identifiable processes was not understood more quickly was not one of the finest hours of communication scholars in general, or of intercultural communication scholars in particular, as the latter followed the imperfect examples set by their predecessors.

Under these circumstances, intercultural communication was predictably condemned to experience developmental phases, growing pains, and problems very similar to those of its parent discipline. These included questions relating to organizational structure, the use and careful application of a variety of methodologies, and the clear definition of a *unique* role or subject matter. All these problems were not made easier by a lack of willingness to reexamine the *roots* of intercultural communication studies by those now engaged in various activities as they tried to establish themselves in the field. As is true for the rest of the academic world, intercultural communication scholars must carve out their own professionally significant niches, which they hope will result in meaningful contributions, or simply recognition, advancement, and acceptance as equals by other social scientists within the academy. Of course, unwillingness to regularly reexamine roots as a *basis* for future development is not unique to this area—it is a weakness of every field of human study, including the natural sciences. While a growth or development orientation brings its own rewards, it also can lead to the repetition of prior mistakes by those who neither understand their bases nor are willing to learn from them.

At the present time, as is true of communication studies in general, intercultural communication is more involved in describing and defining specific instances than in the development of any general theory. Of course, those methodologies that had been borrowed from prior communication studies, the social sciences, and, in turn, from the physical sciences have not resulted in the discovery of anything comparable to lawlike responses in human actions.

Many early contributors were concerned with the challenges faced in the United States by individuals who had to deal with confrontations between ethnic and racial segments of our population (Blubaugh & Pennington, 1976; Daniel, 1970; Rich, 1973; Smith, 1973). There was, furthermore, an emerging realization that the United States, following World War II, was suddenly and unexpectedly thrust into a world leadership role that resulted in almost daily interactions by individuals representing political, economic, cultural, and trade organizations. These situations required intercultural and language skills that had previously not been part of the training or education offered in the United States. In addition, these arenas of conflict were often far removed from an academic environment in which objectivity and scientific processes, not necessarily related to common, daily human experiences, were seen as ideals.

Much of the past work in intercultural communication has been anecdotal, and it has relied heavily upon situational descriptions. That approach was in no small measure encouraged by the seminal work of individuals like Edward T. Hall (1959, 1966). Hall's earliest approaches to the study of human behavior and interactions across cultural lines of demarcation were attempts to provide *specific* categories and measurements. The result was an impression that we might be able to identify and label "pigeonholes" into which we could easily sort cultural differences. His major contributions to our understanding that human beings use space differently in different settings because of different cultural demands were, nevertheless, flawed by the illusion of specificity or definiteness through the assignment of numerical values and measures. This illusion of precision, and the assumption of generalizability, provided the basis for a great deal of early enthusiastic growth in the available literature, only some of it of lasting value (Doob, 1961; Jules, 1963; Oliver, 1962; Smith, 1966). Once it became clear, however that mere categories or classifications had little necessary relationship to the complex realities faced by individuals concerned with human interactions across cultural lines of separation, the foundations were laid for an evolutionary process that still continues.

An attempt was made by Kohls (1983) to identify some significant milestones in the evaluation of intercultural communication study. He lists some publications, institutions, and events from the 1930s to the 1960s. Among these are: the establishment of the Experiment in International Living in Vermont (1932); The American Institute of Foreign Trade (1946), renamed

The American Graduate School of International Management (1973); the Interagency Roundtable for Intercultural and Area Studies by the Government (1955); and the Area Studies Centers at major universities.

Other events, mostly of post-World War II vintage, that focused on international affairs and cross-cultural understanding also influenced the development of intercultural communication study, including the establishment of the United Nations and its subsidiary agencies and assistance programs; the United States Information Agency, renamed the International Communication Agency; the Fulbright Exchange Programs for academicians, students, and its foreign leader seminars; the Agency for International Development (a Marshall Plan for developing countries); and the Center for Technical and Cultural Interchange between East and West. These activities created a need to understand the interface of communication and culture.

Movements and events in the United States that marked an awareness of cultural differences and human rights concerns include: the "hippie revolution" of the 1960s, the demonstrations for and against the Civil Rights Act of 1964, the Immigration Act of 1965 dealing with immigrant quotas imposed on several countries, the influx of refugees from various parts of the world that continues to the present time, and the technological innovations that opened up more possibilities for cultural interactions in all parts of the world. From these historical happenings, studies about intercultural interactions began to accrue.

Within the fields of communication and speech communication, a number of individuals began to develop international contacts with those who had similar interests, during the period following World War II. At this point, it is instructive to note that out of these early contacts and interests came the conviction held by William S. Howell, among others, to not contribute to the development of a new academic discipline. He argued that it would simply be another level added to the already existing professional structures or another attempt to justify its existence merely by *assuming* significant differences or unique contributions (Howell, 1975). It was argued that the very nature of the intercultural interactions that were being studied suggested that scholars concerned with such efforts should attempt to build new models of *cooperation* between and within already existing disciplines, such as communication, business management, and anthropology. That approach would have enabled scholars in various academic areas to make their contributions more readily available to individuals across academic "cultural" lines of division. To Howell and others, the question of whether or not intercultural communication should be a discipline, a field, or an area of study seemed unimportant. They preferred to deal with it as an emphasis that could be applied to and used in a variety of fields that were already well established and that had to be made more useful in a world of expanding human contacts. At the same time, a certain amount of faddism could be noted. In some cases, unprofessional practitioners in the field of intercultural communication took advantage of existing needs, and attempted to fill the relative vacuum created by the absence of extensive scientific research and recognized publications by providing less than adequate information or questionable techniques.

Following the example of the social sciences, intercultural communication scholars attempted to overcome the negative effects of such faddism and self-serving approaches by employing methodological rigor. As had been tried earlier in the field of communication and in the social sciences, attempts began to abound in the 1970s and early 1980s to give meaning to that which was vague and inadequately understood by careful application of mathematical and statistical models (Gudykunst, 1983a). At the same time, calls for theory development abounded that were similar to those in other areas of communication study (Gudykunst, 1983b). Critics from outside the field noted that nothing significantly new happened if one merely added the word *culture* to communication without demonstrating that such interactions differed significantly from interpersonal, group, or media communication within one culture.

It did not help that in some cases vaguely anthropological settings or anecdotes were used to demand an even vaguer "cultural" *awareness*. To many who were attempting to apply models of physics to human behavior, this seemed more akin to voodoo than to science. Finally, in the 1970s, a variety of books and journals containing research findings were published that began to provide a meaningful corpus of knowledge. This corpus included an early effort by Bystrom, Casmir, Stewart, and Tyler (1971) to understand the explosively developing field, which resulted mainly in the realization of how complex and diverse the already existing information was. Other publications attempted to provide structure by developing encyclopedic formats intended to provide information concerning existing organizations, significant component parts, and divergent communication strategies (Hoopes & Ventura, 1979; Seelye & Tyler, 1977).

In much of this work, the influence of atomistic, reductionist assumptions as to how understanding is produced played a significant role. The ease with which physicists could predict that water could boil under specified circumstances in any environment could, however, never be replicated in intercultural communication studies, or for any other human interactional processes. Interrelationships were found to be complex, and they constantly reminded us of the earlier work by symbolic interactionists who had insisted that the process of socialization and acculturation could not easily be fitted into existing scientific models (Mead, 1934). Understanding universal principles thus proved to be a significant challenge, and the extensive listing of component parts did not produce closure.

Intercultural communication provided opportunities to identify and deal with important human needs, and the framework and controls developed in well established disciplines appeared to provide good bases to overcome disciplinary inadequacies as scholars attempted to apply already accepted standards or formats. This effort is reflected in the early textbooks on intercultural communication that came out in the 1970s. They were published in response to a need for textbooks in courses on intercultural communication, which at the time were proliferating at institutions of higher learning. Among those contributions were books by Harms, 1973; Condon, 1975; Ruhly, 1976; Sitaram, 1976; Dodd, 1977; Prosser, 1978b; and Sarbaugh, 1979.

Significantly, most of these publications were not truly "intercultural." They provided neither interactional opportunities for work with students and scholars in a variety of areas or opportunities for "practitioners" to readily learn or benefit from the work of researchers, theoreticians, and educators. Some of these books became *cultural artifacts*, representing the concerns of specialists in one academic field rather than *intercultural resources* directed to a variety of individuals, institutions, or interests. Publications during the early 1980s often still indicated the lack of a truly *inter*cultural emphasis in communication studies. There also could be noted the absence of a unified effort by practitioners and scholars to reach conclusions based on all, or a significant portion of, the efforts and insights of the past 20 to 25 years. Thus while intercultural communication has become established at American universities and colleges as an identifiable subject matter that can be taken as a major at both the undergraduate and graduate levels, there is still a need for a unifying concept, construct, or theoretical base that would affirm and demonstrate its uniqueness vis-à-vis other areas of communication study.

In the following pages, we will attempt to provide some indication of what we consider to be important developments in contemporary, intercultural communication research that may provide future direction, integration, and identification of the unique contributions that this field of study can make.

CONTEMPORARY CONCEPTS AND RESULTING CHALLENGES

There is, of course, a seeming paradox in intercultural communication. The basic process begins with the perception of differences that suggest that the participants often do not share norms, beliefs, values, and even patterns of thinking and behavior. The focus on the differences that separate the participants in an intercultural encounter is what distinguishes intercultural communication, in part, from the rest of communication studies. Yet there is also an implicit assumption, though less critically examined in this context, that a degree of homogeneity must be present in order for communication to be initiated. All human beings have some understanding of each other. This commonality is recognized in publications in the area of communication theory, but even more so in the work of intercultural communication specialists such as Prosser (1973), Condon and Yousef (1975), Ellingsworth (1977), Sarbaugh (1979), and Dodd (1977).

Nicassio and Saral (1978) offer a different view of the "intercultural paradox." They argue that intercultural communication has ignored the element of "personality" in interpersonal interactions. By examining the impact of individual personality in an interaction, we are introduced to the heterogeneity of individuals, which forces us to recognize that, despite everything human beings have in common, there are also unique features that have impact on the interactions between individuals. Such unique features are indicative of an individual's personality. This view, which is consistent with concepts evolved by Smith (1966), Ellingsworth (1977), and Sarbaugh (1979), among others, holds that *every* communication act includes an element of interculturalness in the sense that there are no two individuals or situations that are identical at any given time or in any given place. This approach may also have significant implications for the determination of what is the domain of intercultural communication, and what contributions the field can make to other areas of study.

Work related to intercultural communication has usually dealt with interpersonal communication in a context of cultural differences. Such diversities can have either a negative or a positive impact on the intercultural encounter. Cultural differences will have a negative effect if they impede the flow of communication between participants. They will have a positive effect if they motivate two individuals to work harder at understanding each other. Thus the crux of the whole process is HOW *cultural* differences are managed by the participants in any act of communication. It is this phenomenon that is used to further distinguish intercultural communication from other forms or contexts of communication.

What we can thus conclude is that early studies of intercultural communication often treated it as a wholly separate field, with its own systemic structure and distinct process. Later investigations, however, indicated that the elements and processes of intercultural communication are not totally different from those that are part and parcel of other types of communication (Asuncion-Lande, 1981; Ellingsworth, 1977; Gudykunst & Kim, 1984; Sarbaugh, 1979).

Much of the contemporary research on intercultural communication has attempted to clarify the interpersonal nature of the process. Various interpersonal constructs have been used to analyze interaction behavior in intercultural contexts (Yum, 1982). Among those constructs that have provided direction and guidance to the study of intercultural communication within the past few years are the "coordinated management of meaning" concept, developed by Pearce and associates (Pearce, 1976); the "rule-governed perspective," developed by Cushman and Whiting (1977); the "constructivist approach," developed by Delia (1977); and attribution theory (Kelley, 1971).

The view that intercultural communication is an extension of the study of interpersonal communication has been based on the "principle of difference" as a prime discriminator between interpersonal communication in intercultural and intracultural contexts. Thus a critical issue has been the specification of the *degree* of difference that would make one communication event intercultural, another intracultural.

The following example should illustrate this problem. A German and an American know that they are from different cultures and that, therefore, problems of intercultural communication are to be expected. But what about communication between an American and a Canadian? Their language and nonverbal codes are quite similar. The American, representative of a dominant political entity, may be inclined to assume that the two also share a common culture. The American may, therefore, be unable to accept the fact that there are cultural differences between them to which he or she must be sensitive, and which the Canadian counterpart may have assumed all along.

Sarbaugh's conceptual scheme of a homogeneity-heterogeneity continuum provided one starting point for the discussion of this definitional problem. He explained heterogeneity and homogeneity as follows: If two circles represent the life experiences of two persons (or groups), and the circles have minimal overlap (indicating minimal similarity of experience), the two persons would be near the heterogeneous end of the continuum. If the circles have maximum overlap, the two persons would be near the homogeneous end of the continuum. Sarbaugh labeled the heterogeneous end of the continuum as "intercultural" and the homogeneous end of the continuum as "intracultural" (Sarbaugh, 1979). He conceded that there are no completely heterogeneous or homogeneous pairs, but he insisted that the heterogeneity of participants in an interpersonal encounter can be plotted through points along the continuum. These points are labeled "levels of interculturalness." Sarbaugh's basic assumption is that communication becomes increasingly difficult and decreasingly efficient as the heterogeneity of the participants increases.

Let us go back to the example of the American and the German. Their life experiences would normally have minimal overlap, and they could easily acknowledge that fact. They are close to the heterogeneous end of Sarbaugh's continuum. Thus their communication could be labeled intercultural. In our second example, that of the American and the Canadian, classification of their communication as intercultural or intracultural depends on their perceptions of the degree of homogeneity or heterogeneity of their experiences and cultural diversity beyond language similarities. Sarbaugh thus attempts to identify "key" variables in which differences between the participants can be expected and a specific "location" on the heterogeneity-homogeneity continuum can be determined. The amount of difference will increase as we move from the most intracultural (homogeneous) to the most intercultural (heterogeneous) acts. The more heterogeneous the participants, the more dissimilar are their perceptions and interpretations. The main strengths of Sarbaugh's proposed scheme are: (1) its attention to the operations of basic communication principles at different levels of intra-/interculturalness, and (2) its classification of events according to the different levels of intercultural communication. What is needed, however, are some empirical efforts to operationalize his categories, and an attempt to consider creative interactions that go beyond the mere "overlapping" of existing components.

Samovar, Porter, and Jain (1981) proposed a model in which differences are measured along a minimum-maximum axis. This model is a refinement of one developed by Porter (Samovar & Porter, 1972). According to them, the amount of difference between two cultural groups can be seen to depend on the relative social uniqueness of the two groups. Although the scale they developed has limitations, it allows them to examine an intercultural communication act and thereby gain an insight into the impact of cultural differences in an encounter. The major problem with this instrument is that it is very subjective in terms of measuring the "amount" of difference, and it fails to consider the myriad of both positive and negative variables that are simultaneously affecting the interaction.

An interesting approach to the conceptual refinement of the process of intercultural communication has been proposed by Gudykunst (Gudykunst & Kim, 1984). The model starts with the premise that communication is a transactional, symbolic activity that involves making predictions and reducing uncertainty. Gudykunst claims that the greatest amount of uncertainty exists when strangers communicate with each other. Strangers are people who are unknown and unfamiliar to us and who exist in an environment that we do not know. Whenever we encounter a stranger, our primary concern is to increase our ability to identify our most suitable behavior, as well as predicting that of the other person. This conceptualization of uncertainty reduction while communicating with strangers is, of course, not original with Gudykunst. Miller and Steinberg (1975) and Berger and Calabrese (1975) used it in their studies on interpersonal communication. But Gudykunst is the first to adopt this notion as a framework for delineating intercultural communication. He observes that in our communication with strangers, we are influenced by our conceptual filters, just as the strangers are influenced by theirs. The conceptual filters that influence our communication are categorized as the cultural, the sociocultural, the psychocultural, and the environmental. Each of these filters influences our interpretation of strangers' messages and our predictions about their behaviors. If we do not understand the strangers' filters, we cannot make accurate predictions or interpretations related to their behaviors. Gudykunst's proposed framework specifies that the process of intercultural communication is not unique, but it is one that reflects the basic processes of human communication. In this, he reinforces Sarbaugh's (1977) and Ellingsworth's (1977) proposition that the variables and the underlying processes that operate in any communicative act are the same. The value of Gudykunst's model lies in the refinement of the conceptual boundaries of intercultural communication. It is another step toward conceptual clarification and simplification. Its apparent limitation is in its failure to explain what is taking place in specific encounters between strangers, and how the limitations imposed by filters can be overcome in interactional efforts.

Theorizing in intercultural communication has been greatly benefited by sojourn, acculturation, and diffusion of innovation studies. Sojourn studies (Austin, 1986; Bochner, 1982; Brislin, 1981; Ellingsworth, 1982) have typically examined face-to-face contact experiences and their outcomes between members of a host society and the visitors, including foreign students. Their analysis of these situations have produced some useful concepts for the examination of intercultural encounters. Included are such concepts as the historical background that would affect the interactants' views of their worlds, individual factors such as personality traits and skills, and group factors that would predispose individuals toward a specific outcome of their interactions. Also considered were situational factors that lead to positive and negative sojourn experiences, task factors that can affect the success or failure of intended goals, organizational factors that would form part of the support systems during the sojourn experience, social problems that sojourners face when moving into different cultures, and coping mechanisms leading to adjustment.

Results of some of these sojourn studies point to two opposing views concerning the outcomes of cross-cultural contacts that have implications for intercultural communication. One point of view holds that cross-cultural contact can lead to development of mutual understanding, tolerance, and respect. This belief is the main justification for the many cross-cultural exchange programs operating throughout the world. It is also one of the principal reasons for the emergence of intercultural communication as a field of study. Another point of view holds that frequent contacts between different cultures leads to increased suspicion, hostility, and even war. This particular consequence of cross-cultural contact has not been dealt with seriously in the study of intercultural communication. However, it is closely related to a factor discussed earlier in this chapter. When cultures increasingly interact in an environment that *requires* the sharing of limited resources and they cannot avoid such contacts, inadequate intercultural communication skills could lead to attempted resolutions by means of violent conflict. Better identification of contact situations that can be systematically related to either improving or destroying intergroup cooperation or harmony should be helpful in predicting or explaining when and why intercultural communication may succeed or fail.

Other studies have focused on acculturation processes and the communicative aspects of such intercultural encounters (J. Kim, 1980; Y. Kim, 1977; Ruben, 1977; Ruben & Kealy, 1979; Yum, 1982). These scholars have found that interpersonal communication between expatriates and members of a host culture, as well as host and expatriate media usage, are important indicators of the degree of acculturation of immigrants into any society's mainstream. Such studies have determined several key factors in the acculturation process. They include the degree of similarity or difference between the original culture and the host culture, degree of familiarity with the host culture, as well as personality characteristics, demographic features, and educational levels that are useful for successful integration. Most of these factors feature an element of communication or are very similar to attributes already found to be associated with successful communication. These scholars have also identified specific verbal and nonverbal communication patterns and they have related them to acculturation processes.

Approaching the subject of intercultural communication from a different orientation, studies dealing with the diffusion of innovations from one culture to another have focused on the role of communication in initiating and influencing social change and development. Some of them found in earlier efforts that communication is an effective instrument for social change (Chu, 1977; Dodd, 1987; Rogers, 1976; Schramm & Lerner, 1976). Others have insisted that communication should not be treated as a simple stimulus for change, but that it is a basic social process that includes complex verbal, nonverbal, and visual behaviors that, in turn, depend upon or change dynamically and concomitantly with various social structures.

The main contribution of diffusion studies to theory building in intercultural communication can be seen in moving the locus of communication research from the United States to various cultures in which communication concepts, structures, styles, and functions are not similar to our own. These insights have expanded the domain and context of intercultural communication studies. They have also sensitized intercultural communication specialists to the fact that conclusions based on culture-specific research may not have universal applicability.

CONCEPTUAL AND METHODOLOGICAL DEVELOPMENT IN INTERCULTURAL COMMUNICATION

Several state-of-the-art surveys of intercultural communication studies have described significant advancements in the field over the last decade (Gudykunst, 1983; Nwanko, 1979; Prosser, 1978b; Saral, 1977). Yet, some critical issues continue to plague contemporary research. Some of these concerns include a more adequate reconceptualization of both culture and communication as bases for intercultural communication studies, of the role of similarity and difference in intercultural communication, and a reassessment of the overall intellectual terrain of intercultural communication studies.

Culture, which has been defined in many different ways by many different people (see, among others, Dodd, 1987; Geertz, 1973; Smith, 1966; Singer, 1987), can initially be identified as a process involving relations between human beings in a given environment for purposes of interaction, adaptation, and survival. Intercultural communication results when two or more human cultures interact as parts of the same environment, and either competition or cooperation is called for in order for the participants in that interaction to continue existing. It is the differences between the cultures or their different survival systems and processes, their different adaptations to the environment, and the fact that the sharing of that environment becomes desirable or necessary that create the bases for intercultural communication. What is *not* intercultural communication is any attempt to enable representatives of one culture to learn, understand, *and adopt* the patterns of the culture. If a human being is trained to be integrated into a different culture, it requires joining one and leaving the other. Under those circumstances, one can speak of cultural integration, not of intercultural communication.

Furthermore, we need to realize that culture is not the same as the artifacts constructed by it. Artifacts are visible evidence of the existence of a culture, but the principles used in *relating* all the component parts and making them into a nurturing, supportive, securing, *interactional pattern* are of central concern to intercultural communication scholars. The mere collection, identification, and categorization of artifacts leads to the establishment of a museum or the writing of a catalogue, but it does very little to help us understand the living, ongoing, ever-changing process of human interaction.

Many of the efforts that have been based upon the concept of understanding culture by understanding its component parts are based on a fundamentally *technological* paradigm. They are based on a kind of "Erector Set model," which is used in an attempt to indicate that culture is inevitably the result of construction patterns that are limited and defined by their component parts. The creative, interactive processes that produce *inter*cultural and *inter*national results, however, require a very different kind of model that produces a very different kind of insight. The mere piling of event upon event, or detail upon detail, is very different from understanding the interactive *process* that is closely interlinked with the *creation* of culture and the production of a new or "third culture." Thus the traditional models of interlinking circles, so often used in earlier communication textbooks (Rich, 1973), are not very helpful. Nontraditional approaches are required to describe the processes involved in culture creation, maintenance, and destruction, all of which are based on communication.

Culture, thus is the product or result of interaction, not merely the result of available parts whose use may have been constrained by earlier settings. Indeed, the very fact that alternatives and new survival patterns have emerged throughout history is an indication that technologically oriented "construction models" are inadequate. What we need for successful intercultural communication is not merely a compromise or an overlap model. We must provide for the possibility of the creation of a third or new culture that does not merely use earlier component parts, but that can create new insights, new goals, new techniques, and new roles, precisely because diversity of experience requires something new without domination by any one of the partners contributing to the process.

Probably one of the greatest tragedies related to the study of human behavior around the world has been the insistence that *Western* models of persuasion, influence, control, domination, and confrontation best describe the evolution of human cultures in an ongoing survival process. That domination is probably one of the most important reasons why contemporary approaches to organizations as "cultures" (Kilmann, 1985; Richardson, 1983) are becoming increasingly unsatisfactory. They appear to assume that an organization can be seen as an autonomous, independent, unresponsive institution that has no particular relationship to, or does not need to be dependent upon, the larger environment and the initial, originating culture that created it. If anthropology's major contribution to our understanding of human beings has been the identification of component parts of culture and the *description* of culture, it is the major contribution of intercultural communication, not yet fully realized, to help us understand what happens when cultures meet or when the *need* for a new culture arises. That engagement is something that is strictly a communication process that can be only imperfectly sensed in traditional anthropological and linguistic emphases because those emphases were not process-oriented. In recent years, attempts have been made to change that. The *interactive* role of symbols, and not merely their creation or their existence, has become of interest to linguists and anthropologists who strive to go beyond the facts of evolution or structure (Comaroff & Roberts, 1981; Kay & Kempton, 1984).

In connection with this emphasis, the earlier discussion of Howell's vision needs to be recalled. That model represented a new approach that could not have been readily robbed of its vitality because it deliberately assisted in the formation of "third cultures," based upon the experience of a variety of academic fields. It was a deliberate attempt to go against the technological "construction patterns" that had dominated other academic disciplines. How strong the latter models are, however, can be seen in that intercultural communication, as a "field," has not been very successful in overcoming their impact. One of the tragic results has been that attempts in such diverse areas as organizational communication and education, which are trying to understand contemporary challenges and difficulties on the basis of a cultural model, have had to be carried out without early input by those who have been identified as intercultural communication scholars. Other academic disciplines had to "discover" culture as a root metaphor on their own, without intercultural communication theorists available to assist them, because of a lack of interchange.

Earlier models of intervention/change or compromise were often carried over, accepted, or unknowingly followed by scholars in the new field of intercultural communication at the same time that they attempted to overcome ethnocentric concepts, cultural domination, cultural imperialism, and a variety of factors that were associated with the American way of doing things. In effect, it took time to realize that even the research methods and logical constructs used by American scholars were not necessarily adequate or even applicable to the study of other cultures and their communication processes (Brislin, 1981).

Intercultural communication scholars may have been dimly aware of the fact that there existed alternatives to Western or Northern models of interaction based on domination or the collapse and replacement of old cultures, according to some evolutionary predispositions. However, the possibility of a creative interaction to bring about *new* survival models suited to our contemporary needs was explored only inadequately. It may be important to recall that not since the "conquest" of Greece by Rome has a subjugated culture in the Western world found a way to play a direct and powerful part in the creation of a new or "third" culture (which in that case was neither entirely Greek nor entirely Roman). Even a moment's consideration of that historic development indicates important implications, but it is unfortunately true that that particular cultural change event has not been studied in any detail by intercultural communication scholars. In fact, we lack basic understanding of what happens when cultures meet and integrate rather than destroy each other (Casmir, 1983a).

As long as contemporary students and scholars do not clearly conceptualize what needs to be or could be done beneficially, we should not wonder that some are consistently drawn into the belief that the struggle is all about methodology or that switching from traditional statistical methods to ethnographic or other recent approaches will make a significant difference (Gudykunst & Kim, 1984). Unfortunately, such simplistic solutions to contemporary challenges do not make a real difference to the field. Furthermore, older practitioners of the art of ethnography have already developed considerably greater skills and more finely honed techniques than those representing the field of intercultural communication. As a result, ethnographers, anthropologists, and others have been rather free, at times, in their criticism of those whom they consider to shoddily apply, or misapply, the techniques originally developed by them.

At a time when Americans are reaching out to others around the world, our efforts seem condemned to be identified as cultural imperialism, electronic colonialism, or hegemony (McPhail, 1987; Schiller, 1976). Not withstanding the fact that many Americans are seeking a better understanding of both other cultures and their own, we do find ourselves increasingly drawn into confrontational encounters with other cultures because of models that appear to have worked so well for us over a long period of time. In other words, we are learning that the exchange of ideas, discussion, understanding, or even adaptation simply are not enough. Members of two cultures who learn to understand each other quite well can simply "pass" each other and end up, as it were, walking in each other's shoes. Thus they can literally subvert the possibilities of a creative *inter*cultural process for bringing about a new situation that is meaningful to *both* of them. To do "other people's things their way" is not intercultural communication. It is simply a matter of adopting somebody else's way that was developed for reasons that may be foreign or strange to us. It is not the creation of a common ground, and will not tend to be conducive to *mutual* satisfaction.

Consider the example of the well-known Trojan horse. Neither horses nor soldiers were unknown to the Trojans. What trapped them was not the component parts, but a basic change in relationship that the Greeks used to subvert Trojan defenses. Separately, the Trojans could have dealt with a wooden horse and with Greek soldiers. In an unknown combination, they became a decisive weapon because of significant misunderstandings. We could conclude that few Trojans would ever have been fooled again by a Grecian horse like the one brought inside their walls. But what about other means of accomplishing the same thing used by other enemies or, heaven forbid, even friends? That example well summarizes our repeated insistence that a mere understanding of the artifacts of culture or of component parts is not enough. It is our understanding of communicative interactions that can make a significant additional contribution. Because it is a human creative activity, culture is able to constantly redefine itself. Technology cannot do so. Its evolution is predictable, based on an understanding of its component parts. It is, in effect, a closed process. Its products will experience entropy in a predictable way, in accordance with the second law of thermodynamics, unless human design intervenes. Culture as an active human definitional process, on the other hand, allows for the creative combination of factors not even previously identified as being interrelated or independent.

The subject matter of intercultural communication thus can be seen as having to do directly with defined versus constructed systems. We need to contrast technological solutions based on the notion of constructed reality, and the open process of intercultural communication between component parts in an environment, whose result is not merely additive or summative. It needs to be remembered that in the Western world, culture defined technology and science and the logical systems supporting both. Yet that technology and science became countercultures that redefined their original purposes of serving their nourishing and foundational culture by defining their own, new values, artifacts, processes, and goals. It is little wonder that in the Western world, in recent decades, proposed solutions to our dilemmas were not the result of cultural definition and redefinition of our survival by participating human beings. Rather, it was assumed that survival of the human race would be based on an evolutionary process of science and technology, in some combination, making available constructed systems that would bring about desirable results. That assumption was basic in such areas of study as the diffusion of innovations (Rogers & Svenning, 1969) that concluded that by simply sharing our technology with other nations, they could *develop* just as well and just as successfully as we had done. Only later did it become clear that technological systems included value systems that required cultural adaptation and change, and that these often resulted in cultural domination. That fact had not even been considered by those who believed that technology and science were neutral or objective. The result was, of course, that *more* communication did not result in better communication, and that *more* intercultural awareness did not result in the resolution of differences. More was not better—a realization that is always accompanied by some shock in individuals who see human endeavors and interactions basically as technological constructions.

A relatively brief statement, concluding a contemporary motion picture titled *Children of a Lesser God*, is startling in this connection. This film explores the difficulties that arise as two human beings, one male and one female, attempt to build a life together, though one of them is deaf and the other is able to hear. The realization that they are living in two different worlds, that they are representatives, as it were, of two different cultures, is expressed in the question the man asks: "Do you think there's a place where we can meet? Not in silence, and not in sound?" That is a good summary statement of the entire point that intercultural communication scholars have to make. Successful "meetings" between cultures must finally take place "someplace" that belongs to neither one or the other of those seeking interaction.

The ability of human beings to think the seemingly "unthinkable," to do the "undoable," and to believe the "unbelievable" has brought about human developments because we were able, through interaction, to transcend that which we had found limiting in our own cultures. It may very well be that a generation in that not-too-distant future will be astonished that we could not understand that it was not our ability to analyze and dichotomize, but our ability to metabolize and synthesize, that was most significant to our survival. Our ability to see not only "either one" but "both" at the same time may, sometime in the near future, be understood as something that makes us truly human. It may be argued by some that understanding and knowing human beings on a technical level is enough. However, culturally we have a need for fulfillment that requires considerably more than a technologically defined purpose as we strive for completion of self and others. Historically, we can demonstrate that there is a place to meet that is neither "sound nor silence," and it has always been created and always will be created by human beings coming from different spheres who see a need for each other and for the new. Just as human beings initially created both "sound" and "silence" as meaningful concepts, they are able to create yet unthought concepts, as long as they communicate on the basis of their intercultural needs for survival.

Intercultural communication is a way of reminding us, in our studies of human behavior, that what "can be" is probably best accomplished by technology, but what "ought to be" is the province of human definition and thus of culture, based on continuity and not mere change. Helping us to understand how third cultures are developed could well be a significant contribution to the human beings on this planet who are having difficulty finding technological answers to their problems.

THIRD CULTURE BUILDING—A CONCEPTUAL PARADIGM

The notion of a third culture (Casmir, 1978; Useem & Useem, 1967) is both intriguing and useful. It helps to clarify the dynamics of communication in an intercultural setting. Though beginning with contrasting perceptions and behaviors, two individuals, through their interaction, create a unique setting for their interaction. In the conjoining of their separate cultures, a third culture, more inclusive than the original ones, is created, which both of them now share. Within that third culture, the two can communicate with each other more effectively. Thus a third culture is not merely the result of the fusion of two or more separate entities, but also the product of the "harmonization" of composite parts into a coherent whole. When viewed in this way, we go beyond the assumption that by studying the original cultures of communications, including their accompanying patterns of communication, we can understand how the whole communication process functions. We also avoid making the unwarranted conclusion that we have uncovered the underlying rules governing all communicative interactions.

A third culture is a situational subculture wherein temporary behavioral adjustments can be made by the interacting persons as they attempt to reach a mutually agreed upon goal(s). In their efforts to adjust to each other, they build upon a commonality experience that can later serve as a starting point for their renewed interactions.

A third culture can develop only through interaction. It develops by necessity when culturally dissimilar persons combine to carry out a mutually agreed-upon task. Finally, a third culture cannot be understood without the backdrop of the participants' original cultures. This grounding is for the purpose of making comparisons, contrasts, and interpretations of behaviors.

Some fundamental assumptions underlying third culture building are as follows: (1) It is open-ended. Not only is it capable of absorbing additional elements, but it also has the potential for instant growth. (2) It is expansive. It can enlarge its contextual boundaries to include individual, organizational, institutional, and mediated communication situations. (3) It is responsive to new demands emerging from constant adjustments and readjustments in order to realign the participants' own perceptions and expectations of each other and of the situation. (4) It is future-oriented in that a third culture marks the beginning instead of the end point of a joint venture that may continue over time. This mood establishes attitudes toward the current situation as the start for increased communication.

A conceptualization of a third culture must include three interrelated levels of integration and analysis: the individual, the organization, and mediated communication. Each level can be viewed as part of a road map for describing, analyzing, and postulating a model of intercultural communication.

At the individual level, there emerges a type of person whose philosophical and psychological outlooks exceed the limits of his or her indigenous culture. This new individual is partly a product of the cultural synergy that characterizes most modern contacts and exchanges, and partly the product of a composite of social, political, economic, and educational interacting of the time. Various new conceptualizations of this phenomenon include "universal communicator" (Gardner, 1962); "universal man" (Walsh, 1973); "mediating person" (Bochner, 1973, 1981); and "multicultural man" (Adler, 1974). They all refer to a person who is oriented toward a third culture, and whose essential identity is grounded in both the universality and diversity of cultural forms and human conditions. Such an individual is committed to the preservation of fundamental differences, but also to the discovery of essential similarities that can enrich his or her interpersonal relationships. Thus the aim is to create a third culture in which the individual can function unfettered by the original cultural constraints and limitations. This type of person has the ability to suspend cultural identity in order to create new forms of reality based on human diversity and the unpredictability of the human condition.

A critical role for this type of individual is to serve as a link, as a facilitator, and as a catalyst for contact and change within and between cultures. These individuals build bridges to connect segments of various cultures. They serve as gatekeepers in the flow of information between cultures. They serve as translators of messages that are sent and the interpreters of messages that are received from other cultures. They possess certain attributes, such as cognitive flexibility, cultural sensitivity, relativism in cultural values and attitudes, empathetic understanding, and innovativeness. These attributes are necessary for effective intercultural communication, and they demonstrate the effects of increased cross-cultural contacts and exchanges.

The concept of a third culture can also be dealt with from the standpoint of institutions and organizational structures used by human beings to ensure ongoing interrelationships and their control over them. At this level, we would use contemporary family structures in the West or North to make our point. A "successful family" does not provide only *immediate* nurture, instructions, safety, and a number of other vital contributions to a child's life as he or she grows up, it also prepares her or him for *future* interactions with other human beings. In contemporary Western societies, that future frequently means a marriage to a partner who comes from a different background, has different expectations, and one who has experienced a different upbringing.

Thus marriage partners can either insist on "doing it the way we did it at home," leading to conflict or be ready to participate in the building of a "third culture family." That "third culture family" certainly will contain initially a large number of component parts borrowed from the original two families. If the new husband and wife, however, have been adequately "culturally" prepared, they will increasingly want to create their own traditions, value systems, ways of operating, interests, and a multitude of other factors that may be based on, but that also can be significantly dissimilar from, the original components they brought into their marriage. That kind of developmental pattern, of course, may also continue with their own children. The reason for such an approach is clear. Increasingly, on a global scale in the West and North, individuals are being faced with both rapid changes in their environment and interactions in that environment with people whom, in days past, they would not have met, or known, or married. Thus the opportunities for "third culture" development are a significant component part of our sociocultural environment.

This basic model, however, does not need to be limited to such primary institutions and organizational structures as the family. In recent years, interest has been shown in "organizations as cultures." Putnam and Pakanovsky (1983) and others (Frost, Moore, Craig, Lundberg, & Martin, 1985) have spent considerable effort in explaining their conceptualizations of organizations as entities that engage in activities and organize behavior quite similar to traditional, "natural" cultures. While their approach has been provocative, it certainly has done little to provide us with answers to serious problems that can arise when two or more organizations have to interact in the same space (geographic, economic, and otherwise) and compete for the same limited resources. In other words, contributions to our understanding of *inter*cultural communication and third culture development resulting from these efforts remain very limited.

As mentioned earlier, culture can be studied from the standpoint of power relationships and the role that trust needs to play in human institutions. These are significant factors in the family, in which the initial power of parents can be counterbalanced over time by experiences leading to trust and interdependence. Similar areas of concern arise in the institutions of business, industry, government, and education, among others. If it is accepted that power in ongoing legitimate interrelationships is not taken but given or granted (Milgram, 1974), then the role of communication in applications of various intercultural aspects of human organizing behavior is significant.

Every system, and every organization that uses members to establish contact with other cultures, faces similar important challenges. While culture shock (Draguns, 1977) and reentry shock (Brislin & Van Buren, 1974), as phenomena related to integration and intercultural communication, have been given considerable attention, other factors significantly related to our understanding of third culture development have not. That lack is not surprising if one remembers that the major concern of cultures and their representatives has always been their own survival and supremacy, even as indicated in contemporary studies of organizations "as cultures." As a result, many approaches to intercultural interaction in the past, sometimes even subconsciously, were based on "us-against-them" models of interaction.

Some 20 years ago, Oliver (1962) wrote about an insight that, at best, was shocking and at worst, very painful, to Americans. It was his contention that the United States and its representatives had for decades engaged in activities that in their own eyes were helpful, sometimes even unselfish, and certainly intended to help the unfortunate nations of our world to improve their status. When those attempts were either rejected or seen as cultural and media imperialism or colonialism (McPhail, 1987), we tended to profess that we neither understood nor could we accept such a lack of gratitude.

In such interactions, well-ingrained concepts of freedom, democracy, and capitalism played a major role, often not because of imperialistic tendencies, but simply because they were what we knew, and represented something that demonstrably had worked for us. Only recently have we dealt with such subjects more carefully and thoughtfully. While some individuals like Schiller (1969), based on his own Marxist orientation, simply see the impact of multinational companies and the use of capitalistic models as wrong and bad, others have dealt with related subjects more thoughtfully (Deetz, 1979; de Sola Pool, 1979). In all cases, the issues of power and trust play a major role as change and the impact of media and Western or Northern economic institutions are discussed. However, discussions of the subject typically have been based on political and state orientations rather than on cultural or national concerns (Olson, 1987). That was the case even though traditional, thus familiar and easily accepted terms such as *culture* and *nationhood* were used by proponents who actually were engaged in building modern states. In other words, they were in reality using models developed following the Peace of Westphalia that were based on technopolitical rather than cultural considerations.

Dealing with issues of power, communication, and state building are, of course, part of the ongoing efforts to understand their interrelationships as well. Innis (1972) attempted to indicate comprehensively the roles communication as well as economic models play in the development of various empires, all based on the use of language and media within a culture. McCluhan (1964, 1970) picked up on these issues developed by his mentor, but became clearly enamored with a technological approach to *resolving* problems of intercultural and international communication. His concept of the "global village," poorly defined and inadequately supported by insights from other fields such as anthropology, as Michaels (1985) points out, clearly skirted the issue of how and why third cultures can and must be built. The underlying hope or expectation in these early efforts was that technological innovations could resolve any difficulties that might exist. Though that approach fits models that have a technological orientation very well, it has been attacked in the recent past by those not sharing that orientation (Benson, 1977; Clegg & Dunkerley, 1980; Giddens, 1979; Hawes, 1974). Ong (1967, 1977) has been among those who took a different approach, as they explored in more detail the relationship of language, specifically orality, literacy, and the "second orality" represented by contemporary electronic media, to cultural and societal changes.

While there continues an optimistic hope that media and technology will bring about something that is conceived of as "one world," some point out that contemporary technological changes in the media tend to result either in "privatization" rather than interaction or in major cultural upheavals. Meyrowitz (1985) makes that point for the United States when he insists that important cultural changes have resulted because the media have torn away the "curtains" between the front of the stage, where we have traditionally observed actors (Goffman, 1971, 1974), and the back of the stage. It used to be true that those who were powerful and influential among us used and hid whatever insights, knowledge, or interrelationships they needed to maintain their power backstage so that the "audience" could not share or observe them. Now, according to Meyrowitz's (1985) culturally oriented book, *No Sense of Place*, we no longer have a clear understanding of what our specific place in time or space is, nor does there seem to be any more "privileged" knowledge. Anyone, regardless of age, sex, or education, can know the same things at the same time, however far removed in space they are, by sitting in front of the same television set. Michaels (1985) makes similar points about changes in primitive or aboriginal societies, in which the impact of modern media drastically changes old power relationships and communication patterns.

What then is the significant difference between such media-induced changes and what we have discussed as third culture building? (Casmir, 1982, 1983b, 1984). Media are quite unidirectional and "opaque" (Jamieson, 1985). They create *illusions* of interaction and more than one-way communication, but they are actually merely suppliers of various input that audience members either accept or reject. In effect, whenever a contemporary media approach is used, there is little chance of interactionally developing a third culture, as happens in traditional cultures or in families. Culturally significant individuals in the media remain hidden behind their own curtains, such as sources protected by the First Amendment or the technical aspects of the media and their organizational structures. In effect, old authorities are thus simply replaced by new ones, without a great deal of information provided as to why they are to be accepted as authorities. The institutions they belong to appear to give them all the rights to their position, as used to be true, for instance, of royal houses. New high priests protecting the "holy First Amendment grail" speak, just as the old ones, of utter destruction of their new culture if we do not protect them from the unwarranted attacks by unprincipled enemies. The list could go on. The point is that the model used by the media, as in the case of industrial organizations, is one of confrontation and replacement, one of destruction of the old culture for the sake of something "better"—which is always determined by the more powerful. Such actions can, of course, easily be interpreted as empire building or imperialistic acts.

As Oliver (1962), Schramm (1964) and Rogers (1969) have pointed out, one can always assume that we are doing a favor only for those over whom we seek control. There remain serious challenges to such oversimplifications, however. The so-called revolution of rising expectations (Nam, 1983) and concerns over the role of Western advertising (Sauvant, 1979) in promoting products representative of an apparently desirable life-style, but that may be threatening to weak economies in the Third World, are only two of them. It also seems that we have learned little from the past, because current debates over information sharing in our so-called information age have a very familiar ring to them. People involved in such confrontations in many instances still appear to be convinced that

(1) technology, in general, will resolve our human and cultural problems;
(2) new technology is just around the corner that will provide exactly the means needed for the resolution of problems not yet resolved or stubbornly "resisting" improvement in the past; and
(3) such new technology *and the information that it carries is* neutral and does not threaten national or cultural values.

These simplistic points of view do depend, as was already discussed, on the illusion that the human interactional problems that cultures and nations have experienced over past centuries can be eliminated by various technical constructs, including the modern state. Such political entities are seen as being capable of welding together many cultural and national entities into a modern institution, in the process making use of contemporary media and technology. Nothing in that approach is significantly different from models of conquest used in the past, even if it seems to be more subtle, and in spite of the fact that different "types" of cultural change control agents have emerged. Excellent examples of the fact that such *replacement* models sidestep the more difficult process of third culture building can be seen, for instance, in India, where Indian bureaucracy is simply British colonial bureaucracy with a vengeance. Much of the heritage of the despised former colonial overlords continues because the English way is the only one that can "tie together" the multiplicity of cultures found in that modern state.

Third World news agencies are another example. In spite of the insistence of various people in developing countries that Western and Northern news agencies have controlled the news flow and that regional institutions should replace them, in most instances the models for news gathering, news distribution, and institutional organization familiar in the West were simply copied by such new Third World organizations. The question is, of course, whether the copying of institutions that were developed in another culture has a cultural impact far beyond what we are willing to acknowledge (Nasser, 1983). The problem is similar to one faced in the United States, where various people are concerned with the redefinition of the traditional cultural roles of men and women. When equality for women is sought, the goal often is "equality with men" based on a system and values originally developed by males. No attempt to build a third culture was stipulated as the beginning point for such a struggle; rather, it was tacitly accepted that what men had built and accomplished represented a desirable value base. No wonder men can continue to feel as if they are "in charge." To put it in very simplistic language, the question has not been whether we ought to develop a third kind of "garment," but whether it is all right for women to wear pants, "just like men." There is little threat here to the existing culture as compared, for instance, to possible female insistence that men wear skirts, "just like them," nor is there any focused attempt to build something new, meaningful, or effective that can be mutually decided upon.

What we have considered then is the fact that cultural integration can be of importance to us as a subject for study. However, it has little to do with the subject of *inter*cultural communication for purposes not of domination and control of another culture, but for the purpose of mutually beneficial control over the environment, development of trust, and the creation of third cultures. Only the latter assists in continued growth with a minimum of confrontation and effort expended on fighting each other rather than on the challenges presented by material, intellectual, and spiritual problems existing among and around us.

To make our point more precisely, let us consider for a moment one specific scenario relating to culture, media, development, and third culture building. Walt Disney and Disney characters are known around the world, as are "The Flintstones." The organizations involved in both cases have developed powerful means for representing cultural values and making statements about human relations. One need be reminded only that both Uncle Scrooge and Fred Flintstone basically are representing the capitalistic, technologically oriented value system of the United States. Because they originated within, and served as parts of U.S. culture, that representation is obviously to be expected. (Whether those value systems and the expectations raised by them are good or bad, we will leave for the moment to people who seem much more certain about such matters than we are.)

We do not wish to overlook the legitimate economic aspirations of organizations involved in the production and dissemination of these cartoon characters, as well as such issues as copyrights. However, the "imperialistic" model based on simply *translating* the *content* of material produced for American audiences and then distributing it to other parts of the world could be replaced and made culturally less threatening and positive. That could be accomplished if the same characters and the same overall artistic format were to be used in each of the countries distributing the material to produce their own version directed to the needs of their own citizens. Such a model is similar to one used by Japanese auto makers opening plants in the United States.

Obviously, as is true of all culturally oriented change, this adaptation is a slower and more difficult process but one that brings its own rewards.

Unfortunately, in a world where desirable change is often seen as instantaneous, only cultural disasters may make us sufficiently aware that we may be violating vital, natural processes because we cannot, at this point, be certain about the implications of *technologically* induced and controlled change. Mao's government in China realized very well that if deep, far-reaching changes were to be brought about, China had to have more than a technological revolution, it needed a cultural one. He technologically orchestrated it, implemented it, and nearly succeeded in ruining thousands of years of human accomplishment. Correct identification of contemporary cultural problems and their relationship to change processes thus requires more than inadequate solutions based on an inapplicable technological model. On the other hand, intercultural communication, and a careful study of third culture building, can make major contributions to human development.

The early efforts of Christian missionaries are one more example of models brought to the situation that were based on inadequate Western or Northern expectations. In the process of sharing a message, one that its adherents considered vital to others as well as to themselves, little or nothing was done to consider the implications of changing life-styles, putting women into unsuitable clothes for hot humid climates, or forcing musical and other cultural patterns on people who copied appearance forms but who had trouble developing a personal, meaningful faith. It should be added that today's missionaries have been in the forefront of efforts to implement interactional patterns that are based on understanding and respect for many of the cultural traditions and value systems they find in countries to which they carry their messages while desiring to implement certain changes (Richardson, 1974).

How badly a third culture approach is needed can be demonstrated by the fact that organizations that spend millions of dollars to send people abroad have developed little or no means of benefiting from those experiences once these sojourners return home (Brislin, 1981). Reentry, as a result, becomes more of a challenge to facilitate the reintegration of sojourners than to the development of new patterns of interaction that involve entire organizations. Third World students sent abroad to learn the ways of people in developed countries often return home finding it impossible to apply their newly gained knowledge. They may, as a result, return to the West or North, and become part of the "brain drain" that hurts developing states (Glaser, 1974).

Another example can be seen in the attempt to use second or third generation American citizens of Japanese ancestry in negotiations with Japanese business concerns in that country, because they were thought to be "natural" intermediaries between the two cultures. Similarly naive assumptions also formed the basis for expectations by American blacks in search of their roots and acceptance in their "homeland," Africa. When such individuals were met with suspicion or downright rejection, because they were seen as "Americans" and not as natives, the shallowness of naive assumptions, based on simple transfer models of cultural exchange or negotiation processes, became more apparent (Gudykunst & Kim, 1984).

Related intercultural communication problems are experienced, for instance, by ethnographers. Their research models require close interaction with the cultures they study in order to gain sufficient understanding. The problem then becomes how one shares such knowledge with members of one's own academic or other culture, since they have not had the same experiences themselves and they have little in their own cultural repertoire to help them understand (Clifford & Marcus, 1986).

In all of these cases, it can be argued, simplistic replacement or integration models cause difficulties because they are inadequate. Millions or even billions of dollars will continue to be wasted unless the basic inadequacy of such models is questioned. Meanwhile, successes and failures of internationally and interculturally active organizations like the Catholic church and the bureaucratic society known as the United Nations (Magee, 1978) in developing third-culture approaches, including those used for the preparation of personnel suited to their purposes, need to be studied to better understand the process and its implications.

CONCLUSIONS: MORE UNANSWERED QUESTIONS IN INTERCULTURAL COMMUNICATION RESEARCH

As the field of intercultural communication continues to develop, there are additional emerging issues that must be confronted. The first issue deals with the ethical aspects of intercultural communication. What is ethically responsible behavior in an intercultural encounter? Should we impose our own standards of communication behavior, even if they are alien to the other participants? Can we, and should we, develop an ethical code that could be used as a guideline for communication between cultures? Toward what ends should the work of scholars in intercultural communication be directed? Finally, on a practical level, how can we deal effectively with the fact that ethical, successful, meaningful intercultural communication depends on *all* participants, not only on representatives, of one of the cultures involved?

The second issue also deals with the development of instructional materials and innovative methods of instruction that will reflect the changing nature of education in an interdependent world. What teaching methods should we develop and use to teach competence in intercultural communication? How do we define *competence* in intercultural communication?

The third issue deals with practical applications of intercultural research. How can researchers make their findings readily available to practitioners? How can we facilitate collaborative efforts between researchers, practitioners, and subjects to achieve desirable ends? How can such cooperation be extended to incorporate other "cultures" in both the academy and the "real world"?

The fourth question specifically deals with the value of research to the subjects and to the cultures that are under study. How can we, as intercultural communication scholars, make our research valuable to the subjects of our study? What types of research should be undertaken that would be useful to other cultures?

Solutions to these questions may not come easily. Obviously, coordinated efforts by intercultural scholars and practitioners from diverse cultures, who hold a variety of viewpoints, will be needed to accomplish that task. A prerequisite for all such efforts will be that intercultural specialists practice what they preach.

Work related to intercultural communication undertaken during the last two decades has led to the formation of some common bases facilitating explanations dealing with the nature of communication in cross-cultural contexts. But, although there have been some significant advances in theory development, notably in the definition, identification, and delineation of the parameters of intercultural communication studies, there is need for improvement in empirical testing, methodological refinement, and the development of conceptual bases. It is clear by now that there is no one approach, no one methodology, that is best suited to *all* intercultural communication research. As a result of continuing, innovative efforts to understand, define, and practice *inter*cultural communication, our effectiveness in understanding, predicting, and modifying human communication in general may be improved.

REFERENCES

Adler, P. (1974). Beyond cultural identity: Reflections on cultural and multi-cultural man. *Topics in Culture Learning, 2*, 23-40.

Asante, M., Newmark, E., & Blake, C. (Eds.). (1978). *A handbook of intercultural communication*. Beverly Hills: Sage.

Asuncion-Lande, N. (Ed.). (1980). *Ethical perspectives and critical issues in intercultural communication*. Annandale, VA: Speech Communication Association.

Asuncion-Lande, N., & Pascasio, E. M. (Eds.). (1981). *Building bridges across cultures*. Manila, Philippines: Solidaridad.

Austin, C. (1986). *Cross-cultural re-entry: A book of readings*. Abilene, TX: Abilene Christian University Press.

Barnlund, D. C. (1975). *Public and private self in Japan and the United States: Communicative styles for two cultures*. Forest Grove, OR: International Scholarly Book Services.

Benson, J. K. (1977). Organizations: A dialectial view in *Administrative Science Quarterly, 22*, 1-21.

Berger, C., & Calabrese, R. (1975). Some explorations in initial interactions and beyond. *Human Communication Research, 1*, 99-112.

Blubaugh, J. A., & Pennington, D. L. (1976). *Crossing difference*. Columbus, OH: Merrill.

Bochner, S. (1973). The mediating man and cultural diversity. *Topics in Culture Learning, 1*, 23-37.

Bochner, S. (1981). *The mediating person: Bridges between cultures.* Cambridge, MA: Schenkman.

Bochner, S. (Ed.). (1982). *Cultures in contact: Studies in cross-cultural interaction.* New York: Pergamon.

Bock, P. (1970). *Culture shock.* New York: Alfred Knopf.

Brislin, R. W. (1981). *Cross-cultural encounters: Face-to-face interaction.* New York: Pergamon.

Brislin, R. W., & Van Buren, H. (1974). Can they go home again? *International Educational and Cultural Exchange, 4*, 19-24.

Bystrom, J., Casmir, F. L., Stewart, E. C., & Tyler, V. L. (1971). Intercultural communication: Development of strategies for closing the gap between the is and the ought-to-be. *International and Intercultural Communication Annual, I*, 152-160.

Casmir, F. (1974, December). *International and Intercultural Communication Annual.* Los Angeles: Speech Communication Association.

Casmir, F. (1978). *Intercultural and international communication.* Washington, DC: University Press of America.

Casmir, F., & Harms, L. S. (1970). *International studies of national speech education systems.* Minneapolis: Burgess.

Casmir, F. L. (1982). Mass communication and the individual: Mutuality vs. dominance as models for human survival. *Journal of Asian-Pacific and World Perspectives, 6, 2*, 3-14.

Casmir, F. L. (1983a). Phenomenology and hermeneutics: Evolving the approaches to the study of international and intercultural communication. *International Journal of Intercultural Relations, 7*, 309-324.

Casmir, F. L. (1983b). U.S. perspectives on the new information order. In Robert & Jonathan Woetzel (Eds.), *The new ethics of international communications.* Los Angeles: United Nations.

Casmir, F. L. (1984). *Communication and development alternatives: Foundation for policy implementation designed to meet development needs of 3rd world nations.* (U.S. Department of State contract, May-November). Washington, DC: U.S. Department of State.

Cherry, C. (1971). *World communication: Threat or promise.* New York: Wiley-Interscience.

Chu, G. (1977). *Radical change through communication in Mao's China.* Honolulu: University of Hawaii Press—East West Center.

Clegg, S., & Dunkerley, D. (1980). *Organization, class, and control.* Boston: Routledge & Kegan Paul.

Clifford, J., & Marcus, G. E., (1986). *Writing culture: The poetics and politics of ethnography.* Berkeley: University of California Press.

Comaroff, J. L., & Roberts, S. (1981). *Rules and processes: The cultural logic of dispute in an African context.* Chicago: University of Chicago Press.

Condon, J. C., & Yousef, F. (1975). *An introduction to intercultural communication.* New York: Bobbs-Merrill.

Condon, J., & Saito, M. (Eds.). (1974). *Intercultural encounters with Japan: Communication, contact and conflict.* Tokyo: Simul.

Condon, J., & Saito, M. (Eds.). (1976). *Communicating across cultures for what?* Tokyo: Simul.

Cushman, D., & Cahn, D. D., Jr. (1984). *Communication in interpersonal relationships.* Albany: State University of New York Press.

Cushman, D., & Whiting, G. (1977). An approach to communication theory: Toward consensus on rules. *Journal of Communication, 22*, 217-238.

Dance, F. (Ed.). (1970). *Comparative human communication.* New York: Harper & Row.

Daniel, J. L. (1970). The facilitation of white-black communication. *Journal of Communication, 20*(2), 134-141.

Davey, W. (1979). *International theory and practice: Proceedings of the 1978 SIETAR conference.* Washington, DC: Society for Intercultural Education, Training and Research.

de Sola Pool, I. (1979). Direct broadcast satellites and the integrity of national cultures. In K. Nordenstreng & H. I. Schiller, *National Sovereignty and International Communication*. Norwood, NJ: Ablex.
Deetz, S. (1979). De-institutionalization, legitimation, and the possibility of mutual problem solving. *Journal of the Communication Association of the Pacific, VII*(2), 13.
Delia, J. (1977). Alternative perspectives for the study of human communication: Critique and response. *Communication Quarterly, 25*, 30-35.
Delia, J., O'Keefe, B. O., & O'Keefe, D. (1984). The constructivist approach to communication. In F. Dance (Ed.), *Comparative Human Communication*. New York: Harper & Row.
Dodd, C. (1977). *Perspectives on cross-cultural communication*. Dubuque, IA: Wm. C. Brown.
Dodd, C. (1987). *Dynamics of intercultural communication*. Dubuque, IA: Wm. C. Brown.
Doob, L. (1961). *Communication in Africa—A search for boundaries*. New Haven, CT: Yale University Press.
Doob, L. (1970). *Resolving conflict in Africa: The Fermeda workshop*. New Haven, CT: Yale University Press.
Dood, C. H. (1977). *Perspectives on cross-cultural communication*. Dubuque, IA: Kendall Hunt.
Dood, C. H. (1981). *Dynamics of intercultural communication*. Dubuque, IA: William C. Brown.
Draguns, J. (1977). Mental health and culture. In D. Hoopes, P. Pedersen, & G. Renwick (Eds.), *Overview of intercultural education, training and research*. Washington, DC: SIETAR.
Ehrenhaus, P. (1982). Attribution theory: Implications for intercultural communication. *Communication yearbook, 6* (pp. 721-734). Beverly Hills: Sage.
Ellingsworth, H. (1977). Conceptualizing intercultural communication. In *Communication yearbook* (Vol. I). New Brunswick, NJ: Transaction Books.
Ellingsworth, H. (1982). The sojourner: Some communication aspects of cultural entry and re-entry. In N. Asuncion-Lande & E. Pascacio (Eds.), *Building bridges across cultures—perspectives on intercultural communication theory and practice* (160-169). Manila, Philippines: Solidaridad.
Feig, J. P., & Blair J. G. (1975). *There is a difference: Twelve intercultural perspectives*. Washington, DC: Meridian House International.
Fisher, G. (1979). *American communication in a global society*. Norwood, NJ: Ablex.
Fisher, H. D., & Merrill, J. C. (Eds.). (1974). *International and intercultural communication* (rev. ed.). New York: Hastings House.
Frost, P. J., Moore, L. F., Louis, M. R., Lundberg, C. C., & Martin, J. (Eds.). (1985). *Organizational culture*. Beverly Hills, CA: Sage.
Furnam, A., & Bochner, S. (1982). Social difficulty in a foreign culture: An empirical analysis of culture shock. In S. Bochner (Ed.), *Cultures in contact*. (161-198). New York: Pergamon.
Gardner, G. (1962). Cross cultural communication. *The Journal of Social Psychology, 58*, 241-256.
Geertz, C. (1973). *The international culture*. New York: Basic Books.
Gerbner, G. (Ed.). (1983). Ferment in the field: Communication scholars address critical issues and research tasks of the discipline. *Journal of Communication, 33*(4).
Giddens, A. (1979). *Central problems in social theory*. Berkeley: University of California Press.
Giles, H. (Ed.). (1977). *Language, ethnicity and intergroup relations*. London: Academic Press.
Glaser, W. (1974). *The migration and return of professionals*. New York: Columbia University, Bureau of Applied Social Science.
Goffman, E. (1971). *Relations in public*. New York: Basic Books.
Goffman, E. (1974). *Frame analysis: An essay on the organization of experience*. Cambridge, MA: Harvard University Press.
Gordon, R. L. (1975). *Living in Latin America*. Skokie, IL: National Textbook.
Gudykunst, W. (1983a). Intercultural communication theory, current perspectives. In W. Gudykunst (Ed.), *International and intercultural communication annual, VII*. Beverly Hills: Sage.

Gudykunst, W. (1983b). Toward a typology of stranger-host relationships. *International Journal of Intercultural Relations, 7,* 401-413.

Gudykunst, W. (1984a). Intercultural research methods. In W. Gudykunst (Ed.), *International and Intercultural Communication Annual VIII.* Beverly Hills, CA: Sage.

Gudykunst, W. (Ed.). (1984b). *Methods for intercultural communication research.* Beverly Hills, CA: Sage.

Gudykunst, W., Stewart, L. P., & Ting-Toomey, S. (1985). *Communication, culture and organizational processes.* Beverly Hills, CA: Sage.

Gudykunst, W., & Kim, Y. Y. (Eds.). (1984). *Communicating with strangers.* Reading, MA: Addison-Wesley.

Hall, E. T. (1959). *The silent language.* Garden City, NY: Doubleday.

Hall, E. T. (1966). *The hidden dimension.* Garden City, NY: Doubleday.

Hall, E. T. (1977). *Beyond culture.* New York: Anchor.

Harms, L. S. (1973). *Intercultural communication.* New York: Harper & Row.

Harris, P. R., & Moran, R. T. (1979). *Managing cultural differences.* Houston, TX: Gulf.

Hawes, L. (1974). Social collectivities as communication: A perspective on organizational behavior. *Quarterly Journal of Speech, 60,* 497-501.

Hofstede, G. (1984). *Culture's consequences.* Beverly Hills, CA: Sage.

Hoggart, R. (1972). *On culture and communication.* New York: Oxford University Press.

Hoopes, D. (Ed.). (1971-1976). *Readings in intercultural communication* (Vols. I, II, III, IV, V). Pittsburgh, PA: Regional Council for International Education, Intercultural Network, and Society for Intercultural Education, Training and Research.

Hoopes, D., Pederson, P., & Renwick, G. (Eds.). (1977). *Overview of intercultural education, training and research* (Vols. I, II, III). Washington, DC: Society for Intercultural Education, Training and Research.

Hoopes, D., & Ventura, P. (Eds.). (1979). *Intercultural sourcebook: Cross-cultural training methodologies.* LaGrange, IL: Intercultural Network.

Howell, W. S. (1975). A model for the study of intercultural communication in colleges and universities in the United States. In F. L. Casmir (Ed.), *International and intercultural communication annual* (II, pp. 98-101). Speech Communication Association.

Howell, W. S. (1982). *The empathic communicator.* Belmont, CA: Wadsworth.

Innis, H. (1972). *Empire and communications.* Toronto: University of Toronto Press.

Isaacs, H. R. (1972). *Images of Asia: American views of China and India.* New York: Harper & Row.

Jamieson, G. H. (1985). *Communication and persuasion.* London: Croom Helm.

Jules, H. (1963). *Culture against man.* Middlesex, England: Penguin.

Kanter, R. M. (1977). Men and women of the corporation. *American Journal of Sociology, 82,* 965-990.

Kapp, R. (Ed.). (1983). *Communicating with China.* Chicago: Intercultural Press.

Kay, P., & Kempton, W. (1984). What is the Sapir-Whorf hypothesis? *American Anthropologist, 86*(1), 65-79.

Kelley, H. (1971). *Attribution in social interaction.* New York: John Wiley.

Kilmann, R. H. (1985). Corporate culture. *Psychology Today, 19,* 62-68.

Kim, J. K. (1980). Explaining acculturation in a communication framework: An empirical test. *Communication Monographs, 47*(3), 155-179.

Kim, Y. Y. (1977). Interethnic and intraethnic communication: A study of Korean immigrants in Chicago. *International and Intercultural Communication Annual, 4,* 53-68.

Kitano, H.N.L. (1976). *Japanese Americans: The evolution of a subculture.* Englewood Cliffs, NJ: Prentice-Hall.

Klopf, D. (1987). *The fundamentals of intercultural communication.* Englewood, CO: Morton.

Kohls, R., & Howard, S. (1983). *Benchmarks in the field of intercultural communication.* Unpublished manuscript.

Kroeber, A., & Kluckhohn, C. (1972). *Culture: A critical review of concepts and definitions.* New York: Vintage.
Kumar, K. (Ed.). (1979). *Bonds without bondage: Explorations in transcultural interactions.* Honolulu: University of Hawaii Press.
Leach, E. (1976). *Culture and communication: The logic by which symbols are connected.* New York: Cambridge University Press.
Littlejohn, S. W. (1983). *Theories of human communication.* Belmont, CA: Wadsworth.
Luhmann, M. (1979). *Trust and power.* Chichester, England: John Wiley.
Magee, J. (1978). Communication in international organizations with special reference to the United Nations and its agencies. In F. L. Casmir (Ed.), *Intercultural and international communication.* Washington, DC: University Press of America.
McCluhan, H. M. (1964). *Understanding media: The extension of man.* New York: New American Library.
McCluhan, H. M. (1970). *Culture is our business.* New York: New American Library.
McPhail, T. L. (1987). *Electronic colonialism.* Newbury Park, CA: Sage.
Mead, G. H. (1934). *Mind, self and society.* Chicago: University of Chicago Press.
Meyrowitz, J. (1985). *No sense of place.* New York: Oxford University Press.
Michaels, E. (1985). Constraints on knowledge in an economy of oral information. *Current Anthropology, 26*(4), 505-510.
Milgram, S. (1974). *Obedience to authority: An experimental view.* New York: Harper & Row.
Miller, G. (in press). Rites, roles, rules and relationships: Putting the person into interpersonal communication. In N. Dahnke, G. Carols, & F. Collado (Eds.), *Communication as a social science: An intermediate survey.* Belmont, CA: Wadsworth.
Miller, G., & Steinberg, M. (1975). *Between people.* Chicago: Science Research Associates.
Moore, C. (Ed.). (1968). *Philosophy and culture: East and West.* Honolulu: University of Hawaii Press.
Nam, S. W. (1983). Media entertainment in the Third World. In L. J. Martin & A. G. Chandhary (Eds.), *Comparative mass media systems.* New York: Longman.
Nasser, M. K. (1983). News values versus ideology: A Third World perspective. In L. J. Martin & A. G. Chandhary (Eds.), *Comparative mass media systems.* New York: Longman.
Nwanko, R. (1979). Intercultural communication: A critical review. *Quarterly Journal of Speech, 65,* 324-346.
Olien, M. D. (1973). *Latin America: Contemporary peoples and their cultural traditions.* New York: Holt, Rinehart & Winston.
Oliver, R. T. (1962). *Culture and communication: The problem of penetrating national and cultural boundaries.* Springfield, IL: Charles C Thomas.
Oliver, R. T. (1971). *Communication and culture in ancient India and China.* Syracuse, NY: Syracuse University Press.
Olson, R. S. (1987). *Development without states: Mass media and revolutionary nationalism.* Unpublished manuscript, International Communication Association National Conference, Montreal, Canada.
Ong, W. J. (1967). *The presence of the word: Some prolegomena for cultural and religious history.* New Haven: Yale University Press.
Ong, W. J. (1977). *Interfaces of the word.* Ithaca: Cornell University Press.
Patai, R. (1976). *The Arab mind.* New York: Scribner's.
Pearce, W. B. (1976). The coordinated management of meaning: A rules-based theory of interpersonal communication. In G. Miller (Ed.), *Exploration in interpersonal communication.* Beverly Hills, CA: Sage.
Prosser, M. H. (1973). *Intercommunication among nations and peoples.* New York: Harper & Row.
Prosser, M. H. (Ed.). (1975). *Syllabi in intercultural communication.* Charlottesville, VA: Department of Speech Communication, University of Virginia.

Prosser, M. H. (1978a). *The cultural dialogue.* Boston: Houghton Mifflin.
Prosser, M. H. (1978b). Intercultural communication theory and research: An overview of major constructs. In B. D. Ruben (Ed.), *Communication yearbook* (Vol. II). New Brunswick, NJ: ICA-Transaction Books.
Putnam, L. L., & Pacanowsky, M. E. (Eds.). (1983). *Communication and organizations: Interpretive approach.* Beverly Hills, CA: Sage.
Reischauer, E. (1979). *The Japanese.* Cambridge, MA: Harvard University Press.
Renwick, G. W. (1976). *Australian and American cultures: Similarities, differences, difficulties* (Intercultural Management Series No. 1). Scottsdale, AZ: Intercultural Network.
Renwick, G. W. (1977). *Malays and Americans: Definite differences, opportunities* (Intercultural Management Series No. 2). Scottsdale, AZ: Intercultural Network.
Rhinesmith, S. (1975). *Bring home the world.* New York: American Management Association.
Rich, A. (1973). *Interracial communication.* New York: Harper & Row.
Richardson, D. K. (1974). *Peace child.* Glendale, CA: G-L Regal.
Richardson, D. K. (1983). Corporate culture. *Vital Speeches, 1*(49), 677-681.
Rogers, E. (Ed.). (1976). *Communication and development—critical perspectives.* Beverly Hills, CA: Sage.
Rogers, E. M., in association with Svenning, L. (1969). *Modernization among peasants: The impact of communication.* New York: Free Press.
Ruben, B. (1977). Human Communication and cross-cultural effectiveness. *International and Intercultural Communication Annual, 4,* 95-105.
Ruben, B. (1983). *Handbook of intercultural skills, 1.* New York: Pergamon.
Ruben, B. (1985). Human communication and cross-cultural effectiveness. In L. Samovar & R. Porter (Eds.), *Intercultural communication: A reader* (pp. 338-346). Belmont, CA: Wadsworth.
Ruben, B., & Kealey, D. (1979). Behavioral assessment of communciation competency and the prediction of cross-cultural adaptation. *International.*
Rucker, M., Raik, D., Rossiter, R., & Uhes, M. (1973). *Improving cross-cultural training and measurement of cross-cultural learning.* Denver: Center for Research and Education.
Ruhly, S. (1976). *Orientations to intercultural communication* (ModCom Series). Chicago: Scientific Research Associates.
Samovar, L., & Porter, R. (Eds.). (1972). *Intercultural communication: A reader.* Belmont, CA: Wadsworth.
Samovar, L. A., & Porter, R. (Eds.). (1985). *Intercultural communication: A reader.* Belmont, CA: Wadsworth.
Samovar, L. A., Porter, R. E., & Jain, N. C. (1981). *Understanding intercultural communication.* Belmont, CA: Wadsworth.
Saral, T. (1977). Intercultural communication theory and research: An overview. In B. D. Ruben (Ed.), *Communication yearbook* (Vol. I, pp. 389-396). New Brunswick, NJ: ICA—Transaction Books.
Sarbaugh, L. (1979). *Intercultural communication.* Rochelle Park, NJ: Hayden.
Sauvant, K. P. (1979). Sociocultural emancipation. In K. Nordenstreng & H. I. Schiller (Eds.), *National sovereignty and international communication.* Norwood, NJ: Ablex.
Schiller, H. I. (1969). *Mass communications and American empire.* New York: Augustus M. Kelley.
Schiller, H. (1976). *Communication and cultural domination.* White Plains, NY: M. E. Sharpe.
Schramm, W. (1964). *Mass media and national development: The role of information in developing countries.* Stanford: Stanford University Press.
Schramm, W., & Lerner, W. D. (Eds.). (1976). *Communication and change in the last ten years—and the next.* Honolulu: University of Hawaii Press—East West Center.
Seelye, N., & Tyler, V. L. (1977). *Intercultural communication resources.* Provo, UT: Brigham Young University.
Singer, M. R. (1987). *Intercultural communication.* Englewood Cliffs, NJ: Prentice-Hall.

Sitaram, K. S., & Cogdell, R. T. (1976). *Foundations of intercultural communication.* Columbus, OH: Charles E. Merrill.

Smith, A. G. (Ed.). (1966). *Communication and culture: Readings in the codes of human interaction.* New York: Holt, Rinehart & Winston.

Smith, A. (1973). *Transracial communication.* Englewood Cliffs, NJ: Prentice-Hall.

Smith, E. C., & Luce, L. F. (Eds.). (1979). *Toward internationalism: Readings in cross-cultural communications.* Rowley, MA: Newbury House.

Stewart, E. (1975). *American cultural patterns: A cross-cultural perspective.* Pittsburgh, PA: University of Pittsburgh Intercultural Communication Network.

Triandis, H. (1972). *The analysis of subjective culture.* New York: John Wiley.

Triandis, H. (1977). Subjective culture and interpersonal relations across cultures. In L. Loeb-Adler (Ed.), Issues in cross-cultural research. Annals of the New York Academy of Sciences (pp. 418-434). *Annals of New York Academy of Sciences, 285,* 418-434.

Useem, J., & Useem, R. (1967). The interface of a binational third culture: A study of the American community in India. *Journal of Social Issues, 23*(1), 130-143.

Walsh, J. (1973). *International education in the community of man.* Honolulu: University of Hawaii Press.

Weeks, W. H., Pedersen, P. B., & Brislin, R. W. (1977). *A manual of structured experiences for cross-cultural learning.* Pittsburgh: Society for Intercultural Education, Training and Research.

Yum, J. (1982). Communication diversity and information acquisition among Korean immigrants in Hawaii. *Human Communication, 8*(2), 154-169.

Ceteris Paribus in the Global Village: A Research Agenda for Intercultural Communication Theory Building

WILLIAM J. STAROSTA
Howard University

> Critics from outside the field noted that nothing significantly new happened if one merely added the word *culture* to communication, without demonstrating that such interactions differed significantly from interpersonal, group, or media communication within the culture.
>
> —Casmir and Asuncion-Lande (this volume)

> It commonly is accepted that cultural variability in peoples' backgrounds influences their communication behavior. This "fact" leads many scholars studying intercultural communication to view it as a unique form of communication differing in kind from other forms of communication (e.g., communication between people from the same culture). This point of view, however, is not widely accepted.
>
> —Gudykunst and Kim (1984, p. 19)

A certain strain of communication researchers finds culture to be an extraneous factor in interpersonal communication theorizing. Theoretic regularities in patterns of human communication can now be validated by means of comparison between persons of theoretically preselected different points on a continuum, a spectrum, an overlapping circle, or a "level" of communication. Such researchers use culture as a source of cross-cultural

Correspondence and requests for reprints: William J. Starosta, School of Communication, Howard University, Washington, DC 20059.

Communication Yearbook 12, pp. 310-314

amplification of psychologically universal laws. The quest for a field-invariant theory of communication need not be slowed by the unfortunate imposition of man-made symbolic structures. These are the *culture discounters.*

A second strain of communication researchers wonders aloud whether communication is possible at all between identical twins, let alone between cultures. But they resign themselves to raising consciousness about particular differences, with relatively little attention to the evolution of relationships that are to be built in spite of such differences. These are the *culture particularists.* To them, discourse is but an afterthought.

A third strain of communication researchers focuses on desired outcomes. They set out an abstract goal such as synergy or cooperation or culture learning, and hope that persons of different cultural traditions will seek higher, transcendent goals, for the good of humankind. These are the *ethicists.*

Fourth come those researchers who seek to know how realities are constructed between persons of culturally diverse experiences. They dwell on matters of perception and attribution, on the phenomenology and hermeneutics of finding "meaning" in intercultural exchange. Their central concern is with perception, and they may be termed Meadian symbolic interactionists, or *attributionists* for short.

A fifth type of researcher deals with the specifics of the ways in which culture manifests itself in the discourse of a people. The result may be a study of sub-Saharan *nommo,* Middle Eastern sermons, or Native American rhetoric. Seldom do the *culture specifiers* explore the nature of a specific culture's interactions with persons of other cultures.

Sixth, certain researchers are enamored with outcomes, the *resolutionists.* They often resemble the culture discounters in their disinterest in the specifics of given cultures, for the most part, as a decisive factor in achieving a desired result. They fear conflict, and seek its avoidance.

Finally come the *culture conceptualizers*, who advance new lexicons to describe the commonplace. Many times, they draw concepts from one or another existing discipline; prospectively, they suggest hybrid conceptualizations that draw their force, a la Casmir and Asuncion-Lande, from numerous disciplines. Casmir and Asuncion-Lande's discussion of a "third-culture perspective" illustrates the culture conceptualizer at work.

The question is posed: Can these disparate approaches to the study of intercultural communication be merged? Otherwise phrased, must a researcher from one strain of research argue for its supremacy over all other approaches? One answer to this question follows that aims to avoid the isolation and finger pointing that has too long stymied efforts-building in intercultural communication.

(1) Spatial metaphors are insufficient to carry the researcher far toward an understanding of intercultural communication. Temporal studies (i.e., interaction over time) are an important step forward in describing how persons of

different cultures come to intercommunicate. Better still, conceptual, mentalistic metaphors that center on subjective culture, "making sense," construction of mutual meanings, and on adjusting perceptions to accommodate the other (Starosta, 1971) lead to deeper insights into interaction than might spatial descriptions of populations of a certain "distance" from each other. Resolutionists could strengthen their approach with greater attention to mental landscapes.

Casmir and Asuncion-Lande extend, in their analysis, a discussion of third cultures begun by Casmir in an earlier forum (Casmir, 1978, pp. 249-250). Their initial premise that culture equals discipline represents a novel definition that soon is abandoned, with good reason, for more traditional uses of the notion of culture: It would seem that one could call for an interdisciplinary perspective on a given matter without seeking to become more intercultural.

But their treatment of third culture creation has a greater significance, a worth that would be enhanced by sharpening definitions. A third culture, it would appear, is any interactive defining of a situation between two entities in a way that avoids imposing the will of either entity, but that respects the worldviews and cultural traditions of both. The attempt to use one and the same framework to discuss individuals, organizations, and nations is at the same moment parsimonious, heuristic, and confusing, because the questions to be posed for the levels are not completely parallel. The writers do not clearly decide, as one example, whether they accept an organization as capable of having one (or more) cultures; but they do allow that interorganizational communication represents potentially third-culture communication.

At the present stage of conceptualization, the greatest value of the Casmir and Asuncion-Lande position on third cultures is hortative: It advocates a value posture for all cultural entities that interact with other such entities. The authors' position should provide a basis for further development of insights in the future.

(2) A third orientation (i.e., the dispassionate observer-quantifier) must make room for the second-person perspective of the participant-observer. Casmir and Asuncion-Lande's example of the Canadian who views the U.S. interactant as a "foreigner" while the U.S. interactant expects no differences of the Canadian would not occur as easily from the second-person perspective as it would in the third person. Culture specifiers, conceptualizers, and attributionists could combine their insights to their mutual benefit in a second-person orientation.

(3) Environment must be understood (Starosta & Merriam, 1986), since it shapes rules, tasks, possible relationships, social hierarchies and male-female expectations for discourse. Culture specifiers are correct in this assertion. But their studies seldom extend to explanations of how environment influences actual interaction within that setting or between settings.

(4) While language is the medium of much exchange across cultures, few studies (Glenn, 1972) take this fact into account in any penetrating sense. For example, will the Spanish medium lead to predictably different patterns of interaction on a given topic than will the English language? Culture classifiers and conceptualizers must begin to answer such questions to make their work interculturally important.

(5) Too seldom is content used as an intercultural communication study variable. Ethnographers have some idea *within* a culture as to which topics may be appropriate for which occasions, but little parallel work can be cited to speak to between-culture choice of topics or to intergender choice of topics across cultures.

(6) Communication across cultures is certainly, in the culture discounter sense, first—communication. But the sole stress on cross-cultural continuities of process speaks more to psychology than to environment, task, or content matters. The discounter tradition must become more cognizant of micro climates within which laws must be altered (Starosta, 1987) and should begin to add footnotes noting exceptions to covering laws for specific intercultural and cultural contexts.

(7) Intercultural communication events have a history or an etiology (Starosta & Coleman, 1987) that must be understood in order to interpret a given interaction. Culture specifiers, ethicists, and resolutionists should more actively cooperate in providing historical facts for understanding and predicting the course of exchange between any two peoples.

(8) Motivation to communicate must certainly influence outcome and affect. Along these lines, conceptualizers and resolutionists have begun to explore attitudes and factors of "intercultural communication competence" that contribute to a better prediction of outcomes in any given instance of intercultural exchange.

(9) Ethicists should pursue more vigorously the way in which ideology, hegemony, cultural imperialism, xenophobia, ethnocentrism, historical isolationism, the absence of language training and area studies programs in schools, to name a few factors, shape mutual perceptions (attributionists) (Starosta, in press) and outcomes (resolutionists) (Starosta, 1984).

(10) In short, a myopic view that sees only its own favored framework does not transcend its own limitations. The view that one perspective gains only by the diminution of another is surely shortsighted. Unless insights are shared, collaboration between traditions is requested, and conceptualizers build on historically-contexted studies of discourse, the "critics" quoted at the onset will chisel an epitaph for the headstone of a stillborn field of study. The view that communication is communication, *ceteris paribus,* just add culture, can lead researchers no further than the boundary of the most accessible mainstream culture. A village that is global is not a village, nor is a *global* theory an *intercultural* one.

REFERENCES

Casmir, F. L. (Ed.). (1978). *International and intercultural communication.* Washington, DC: University Press of America.

Glenn, E. S. (1972). Meaning and behavior: Communication and culture. In L. Samovar & R. Porter (Eds.), *Intercultural communication: A reader* (2nd ed., pp. 170-187). Belmont: Wadsworth.

Gudykunst, W. B., & Kim, Y. (1984). *Communicating with strangers.* Reading, MA: Addison-Wesley.

Starosta, W. J. (1971). United Nations: Agency for semantic consubstantiality. *Southern Speech Journal, 36,* 243-254.

Starosta, W. J. (1984). On intercultural rhetoric. In W. B. Gudykunst (Ed.), *Methods on intercultural communication research* (pp. 229-238). Beverly Hills, CA: Sage.

Starosta, W. J. (1987). A little compulsion with our persuasion? "De facto coercion" in Mrs. Gandhi's family planning communication campaign. *Journal of Political Communication and Persuasion, 4*(2), 123-134.

Starosta, W. J. (in press). A national holiday for Dr. King? A qualitative content analysis of arguments carried in the *Washington Post* and the *New York Times. Journal of Black Studies.*

Starosta, W. J., & Coleman, L. (1987). A study of rhetorical interethnic analysis: Reverend Jackson's "Hymietown" apology. In Y. Kim (Ed.), *Interethnic communication: Current research* (pp. 117-135). Newbury Park, CA: Sage.

Starosta, W. J., & Merriam, A. (1986). Appropriate media technology in peasant societies: The case of India and SITE. *Educational Technology and Communication, 34,* 39-46.

6 Culture and the Development of Interpersonal Relationships

WILLIAM B. GUDYKUNST
Arizona State University

The purpose of this chapter is to examine the influence of culture on communication in interpersonal relationships. Initially, research on social penetration and uncertainty reduction processes in interpersonal relationships across cultures is reviewed. The differences and similarities which emerge then are linked theoretically to communication in interpersonal relationships. This is accomplished by isolating the underlying dimension of cultural variability (e.g., individualism-collectivism) on which the cultures where the studies were conducted differ, thereby allowing culture to be treated as a theoretical variable. The next section focuses on the influence of cultural similarity/dissimilarity on social penetration and uncertainty reduction processes in interpersonal relationships between members of different cultures. The conclusion contains a summary of recent theoretical statements and a discussion of the issues which need to be addressed in future research and elaborations of uncertainty reduction theory.

UNCERTAINTY reduction theory is one of the major theories designed to explain human communication. In the context of the theory, uncertainty refers to the ability to accurately predict others' attitudes, feelings, and how they will behave, and to the ability to explain others' attitudes, feelings, and behavior (Berger & Calabrese, 1975). Uncertainty reduction, therefore, involves the creation of proactive predictions and retroactive explanations about others' feelings, attitudes, and behavior. The major assumption of the theory is that an individual tries to reduce uncertainty about others when they can provide rewards, behave in a deviant fashion, or may be encountered in future interactions (Berger, 1979). Cross-cultural studies suggest that the theory can be generalized to initial interactions

AUTHOR'S NOTE: An earlier version of this chapter benefited from Mark Knapp's comments and suggestions. The research reported herein would not have been possible without the contributions of my coauthors, Tsukasa Nishida, Seung-Mock Yang, Young-Chul Yoon, Mitchell Hammer, Elizabeth Chua, Lori Sodetani, and Hiroki Koike. Michael Bond and Harry Triandis provided valuable feedback on many of the studies reported in this chapter.

Correspondence and requests for reprints: William B. Gudykunst, Department of Communication, Arizona State University, Tempe, AZ 85287.

Communication Yearbook 12, pp. 315-354

(Gudykunst & Nishida, 1984), as well as can communication in developed relationships across cultures (Gudykunst, Yang, & Nishida, 1985). Recent research also reveals that the theory can be extended to elucidate initial interactions between blacks (Gudykunst & Hammer, 1988), account for differences in intra- and interethnic communication (Gudykunst, 1986a), and explain communication between people from different cultures (Gudykunst, 1983a, 1985a, 1985c; Gudykunst, Chua, & Gray, 1987), including the influence of the language spoken (Gudykunst, Nishida, Koike, & Shiino, 1986).

The original focus of uncertainty reduction theory was initial interactions between strangers, but as Berger (1979) argues, "the communicative processes involved in knowledge generation and the development of understanding are central to the development and disintegration of most interpersonal relationships" (p. 123). Recent research has examined uncertainty reduction processes in developed relationships (e.g., Gudykunst, 1985c; Gudykunst, Nishida, & Chua, 1986; Gudykunst, Yang, & Nishida, 1985; Parks & Adelman, 1983). This research, however, does not account for developmental stages of relationship growth. A developmental perspective that is compatible with uncertainty reduction theory is Altman and Taylor's (1973) social penetration theory. This theory hypothesizes that interpersonal exchanges gradually progress from nonintimate to intimate areas of the personalities of the individuals involved in a relationship. Research conducted in the United States (Altman, 1973; Altman & Haythorn, 1965; Hays, 1985; Taylor, 1968), cross-cultural comparisons (Gudykunst & Nishida, 1983, 1986; Won-Doornink, 1979, 1985), and intercultural studies (Gudykunst, 1985b; Gudykunst, Nishida, & Chua, 1987; Sudweeks, Gudykunst, Ting-Toomey, & Nishida, 1988) support predictions derived from the theory. Recent research indicates social penetration and uncertainty reduction processes are associated positively across cultures and at different stages of relationship development (Lu & Gudykunst, 1988).

The purpose of the present chapter is to examine the effect of culture on communication in interpersonal relationships. To accomplish this purpose, cross-cultural studies of social penetration and uncertainty reduction processes are reviewed. The objective of the review is to explain how culture theoretically influences these processes. In addition to cross-cultural variability, differences in social penetration and uncertainty reduction processes in relationships between members of the same culture and members of different cultures are examined. Comparisons of communication in intra- and intercultural relationships allow for the effect of cultural similarity on social penetration and uncertainty reduction processes to be isolated. Prior to examining differences owing to culture or cultural similarity, however, it is necessary to briefly overview social penetration and uncertainty reduction theories.

SOCIAL PENETRATION AND UNCERTAINTY REDUCTION PROCESSES

Social Penetration

Altman and Taylor's (1973) theory of social penetration is based on earlier models of personality and social relationships developed by Lewin (1948) and Simmel (1950). Social penetration theory gives central importance to the concept of self-disclosure, hypothesizing that it gradually progresses from superficial, nonintimate areas to more intimate, central areas of the individuals in a relationship. This process involves increased amounts of interpersonal exchange (breadth of penetration), as well as increasingly intimate levels of exchange (depth of penetration). Altman and Taylor do not view this as a mechanistic process; they make no assumptions to indicate that penetration moves at the same speed for different people, or that it proceeds to the same level for all dyads. In fact, they argue that the level and rate of social penetration varies with the interpersonal cost/reward characteristics of the relationship (e.g., casual acquaintances, role relationships, and close friendships all have different cost/reward characteristics).

Social penetration theory (Altman & Taylor, 1973) posits four stages of relationship development: orientation, exploratory affective exchange, affective exchange, and stable exchange. The orientation stage is characterized by responses that are stereotypical and reflect superficial aspects of the personalities of the individuals involved in a relationship. Exploratory affective exchange involves interaction at the periphery of the personalities of the partners. This stage includes relationships that are friendly and relaxed, but commitments are limited or temporary. The third stage, full affective exchange, involves "loose" and "free-wheeling" interaction and an increase of self-disclosure in central areas of the partner's personalities. Stable exchange, the final stage, emerges when partners have described themselves fully to each other and communication is efficient. This stage, however, is achieved in very few relationships.

Eight broad dimensions of communication behavior are hypothesized to vary with the stage of a relationship (Altman & Taylor, 1973; Knapp, 1978). As relationships become more intimate: (1) communication takes on a more personal focus, (2) depth of interaction increases, (3) breadth of interaction increases, (4) difficulty of interaction decreases, (5) flexibility of interaction increases, (6) spontaneity of interaction increases, (7) smoothness of interaction increases, and (8) evaluation of interaction increases. Changes along these dimensions, however, do not necessarily involve "linear progressions" such that increases on one dimension involve corresponding increases on another dimension (Knapp, Ellis & Williams, 1980; see Altman, Vinsel, & Brown, 1981, for a discussion of social penetration as a "dialectical" process). The changes along each dimension also do not go on forever. Rather, changes occur until both partners feel comfortable with the interaction. While the theory focuses on actual changes that occur in relationships, perceptions of change should covary with actual changes that occur.

Knapp, Ellis, and Williams (1980) examined perceptions of communication along the eight dimensions as a function of type of relationship, sex of respondent, sex of partner, and selected demographic variables. Their data revealed three factors: (1) "personalized communication," which includes items that relate to the intimacy of communication (e.g., "We tell each other personal things about ourselves—things we don't tell most people"); (2) "synchronized communication" involves items that relate to the coordination of communication between partners (e.g., "Due to mutual cooperation, our conversations are generally effortless and smooth flowing"); and (3) "difficult communication" encompasses items that relate to "barriers" to communication (e.g., "It is difficult for us to know when the other person is being serious or sarcastic"). Knapp, Ellis, and Williams (1980) concluded that personalized communication is aligned most closely with Altman and Taylor's (1973) depth dimension, but some aspects of other dimensions (i.e., uniqueness, flexibility, and evaluation) are included. Synchrony, in contrast, was associated most closely with smoothness, but it also includes some statements from spontaneity. Difficulty was aligned most closely with Altman and Taylor's difficulty dimension, but it includes some statements that are the opposite of smoothness (i.e., awkwardness). At least seven of the eight dimensions isolated by Altman and Taylor, therefore, were included in the three factors. "The dimensions of communication which predicted changes in the depth, smoothness and difficulty of interaction with perceived changes in intimacy seem to have centrality around which the other dimensions cluster" (Knapp et al., 1980, pp. 273-274).

Results of Knapp, Ellis, and Williams's (1980) research revealed main effects for relationship type, respondents' sex, as well as an interaction between respondents' sex and partners' sex. Relationships were perceived as more personal as intimacy increased, with intimate relationships being less discrepant from each other than nonintimate. Males also perceived their relationships as less personal and synchronized than did females. Two-way interactions indicated that males perceived relationships with females as more personal than relationships with other males; females also rated relationships with males as more personal than relationships with other females. These results suggest that both type of relationship and dyadic composition (same/opposite sex relationships) influence perceptions of communication.

Uncertainty Reduction

Communication involves "the exchange of messages which may or may not be spoken and linguistic in form" (Berger & Bradac, 1982, p. 52). The primary function of the exchange of messages is the reduction of uncertainty (Berger & Calabrese, 1975). Uncertainty in this context refers to two phenomena: (1)

individuals' inability to predict their own and others' beliefs and attitudes (cognitive uncertainty); and (2) their inability to predict their own and others' behavior in a given situation (behavioral uncertainty). Uncertainty reduction, therefore, involves the creation of proactive predictions and retroactive explanations about our own and others' behavior, beliefs, and attitudes (for a more detailed discussion of current conceptualizations of uncertainty, see Berger & Gudykunst, in press).

When uncertainty is reduced, understanding is possible. Understanding involves perceiving meaning, knowing, comprehending, interpreting, and/or obtaining information. Three levels of understanding can be differentiated: description, prediction, and explanation (Berger, Gardner, Parks, Schulman, & Miller, 1976). Description involves delineating what is observed in terms of physical attributes (i.e., to draw a picture in words). Prediction involves projecting what will happen in a particular situation. Explanation involves stating why something occurred. Understanding, therefore, is the ability to make accurate descriptions, predictions, and/or explanations.

Berger and Calabrese's (1975) theory of initial interactions is presented in seven axioms and 21 theorems that specify the interrelationships among uncertainty, amount of communication, nonverbal affiliative expressiveness, information seeking, intimacy level of communication content, reciprocity, similarity, and liking. The first axiom of the theory posits a reciprocal relationship between amount of communication and uncertainty. This axiom is based on Lalljee and Cook's (1973) research which revealed that speech acts increase and filled-pause rates decrease as interaction between strangers progresses. Axiom 1 also is consistent with research on the desire to obtain information under conditions of uncertainty (Berlyne, 1960, 1965; Weick, 1979). Not only does the amount of communication reduce uncertainty, but information seeking (Axiom 3) and similarity between communicators (Axiom 6) reduces it too. Axiom 3 is derived from Frankfurt's (1965) research that revealed that the number of questions strangers ask each other declines as a function of time. The posited relationship between similarity and uncertainty reduction is supported by extensive research (Clatterbuck, 1979; Prisbell & Anderson, 1980; Parks & Adelman, 1983).

Under high levels of uncertainty, responses to question-seeking information involve low levels of intimacy (Axiom 4), yet high levels of uncertainty tend to decrease interpersonal attraction, and liking tends to increase attributional confidence (Axiom 7). Axiom 4 is consistent with studies on relationship development (Altman & Taylor, 1973). Support for Axiom 7 can be found in Clatterbuck's (1979) research that indicated that there is a positive correlation between several standard measures of attraction and attributional confidence and that people are more confident about their predictions for those they like than for those they do not like.

Berger and Calabrese (1975) also argue that uncertainty produces high rates of reciprocity (Axiom 5). This axiom was generated in part from

Jourard's (1960) research that found evidence for a "dyadic effect" with respect to the intimacy of self-disclosure. Specifically, he discovered that there is an association between what people disclose and what others disclose to them. The notion of self-disclosure reciprocity is consistent with some research (e.g., Feigenbaum, 1977), but other research suggests there is a difference depending upon the sex composition of the dyad (Cline, 1983).

Recent manifestations of uncertainty reduction theory have posited an influence on the process by self-monitoring and self-consciousness (both of which influence uncertainty reduction processes across cultures, Gudykunst, Yang, & Nishida, 1985; and differ systematically across cultures, Gudykunst, Yang, & Nishida, 1987). Snyder (1974) characterized self-monitoring as "self-observation and self-control guided by situational cues to social appropriateness" (p. 526). Snyder's research indicated that high self-monitors, in contrast to low self-monitors, are judged by peers to be better able to discover appropriate behavior in new situations, have more control over emotional expressions, and are better able to create the impressions they wish to. Snyder and Monson (1975) found that high self-monitors modify their behavior to changes in social situations more than do low self-monitors, while Berscheid, Graziano, Monson, and Dermer (1976) reported that high self-monitors make more confident and extreme attributions and recall more information about an anticipated date viewed on video tape. In a related study, Elliott (1979) reported high self-monitors seek more information about others with whom they anticipate interacting than do low self-monitors.

Recent work by Berger and his associates (Berger, 1979; Berger & Douglas, 1981; Berger & Perkins, 1978) suggests that passive uncertainty reduction strategies are influenced by self-monitoring. Berger and Douglas, for example, discovered differences in perception of how informative formal and informal situations are in reducing uncertainty by level of self-monitoring: low self-monitors perceive formal situations as more informative, and high self-monitors see informal situations as more informative. This finding is consistent with Ickes and Barnes (1977) who reported that high self-monitors initiate and regulate conversations more, initiate more conversational sequences, and have a greater need to talk than do low self-monitors. Research by Tardy and Hoseman (1982) revealed that high self-monitors exhibit more self-disclosure flexibility than do low self-monitors, and Gudykunst and Nishida (1984) discovered that self-monitoring has an impact upon two of the interactive strategies: intent to self-disclose and intent to interrogate. Self-monitoring also has been found to be related to the third interactive strategy—deception detection: High self-monitors are more accurate than low self-monitors in detecting deception (Brandt, Miller, & Hocking, 1980a, 1980b; Siegman & Reynolds, 1983).

"The consistent tendency to direct attention inward or outward is the trait of self-consciousness" (Fenigstein, Scheier, & Buss, 1975, p. 522). Three dimensions of self-consciousness have been isolated. Private self-consciousness involves a private, cognitive focus upon the self as an object, while public self-consciousness "emphasizes an awareness and concern over the self as a social stimulus" (p. 525). The final dimension, social anxiety, is similar to conceptions of communication apprehension (McCroskey, 1978), but is more oriented toward social situations than is speaking per se. Research indicates that the three dimensions of self-consciousness have an impact on selected aspects of behavior. Scheier and Carver (1977), for example, found that high private, self-conscious persons react in a more extreme fashion than do persons low on the dimension. Similarly, Scheier, Buss, and Buss (1978) reported that high private self-conscious persons are more attentive and knowledgeable about their own attitudes than are those low in self-consciousness.

CROSS-CULTURAL STUDIES OF SOCIAL PENETRATION AND UNCERTAINTY REDUCTION

Cultural Variability

Interpersonal relations between individuals vary across cultures. At the same time, however, there appears to be general dimensions of interpersonal relations that are "universal" across cultures. *Universal,* as used here, implies that the dimension of social relations exists in all cultures. Triandis (1978) isolated four dimensions of social relations that appear to be universal (see Lonner, 1980, for research supporting this claim): (1) association-dissociation—associative behaviors include being helpful, supportive, or cooperative, while dissociative behaviors involve fighting or avoiding another person; (2) superordination-subordination—superordinate behaviors include criticizing or giving orders, while subordinate behaviors involve asking for help, agreeing, or obeying; (3) intimacy-formality—intimate behaviors include self-disclosure, expressing emotions, or touching, while formal behaviors involve socially sanctioned, public behavior; and (4) overt-covert—overt behaviors are visible to others, while covert behaviors are internal and not visible to others.

While dimensions of social relations may be universal, specific aspects of interpersonal relations vary across cultures. Differences in interpersonal communication and interpersonal relations typically are studied by collecting data in two (or more) cultures selected because of convenience or the researchers' interest in the cultures. Cross-cultural comparisons made in this way do not allow for theoretical statements regarding culture to be generated. Cross-cultural comparisons of social penetration and uncertainty reduction processes, therefore, should treat culture as a theoretical variable. Stated differently, specific differences between particular cultures are not of theoretical interest; specific cultures are of theoretical interest only when they are used to operationalize dimensions of cultural variability. Foschi and Hales

(1979) succinctly outline the issues involved in treating cultural differences as a theoretical variable: "a culture X and a culture Y serve to operationally define a characteristic *a*, which the two cultures exhibit to different degrees" (p. 246). There are several characteristics on which cultures differ (i.e., conceptualizations of cultural variability) that could be used to explain the influence of culture on interpersonal relationships. The focus of research on social penetration and uncertainty reduction processes has been based upon Hall's (1976) and Hofstede's (1980) theories of cultural variability (for a complete discussion of the influence of culture on interpersonal communication, see Gudykunst & Ting-Toomey, in press).

Hall's (1976) low- and high-context schema, for example, has been used to explain cultural differences in uncertainty reduction processes (Gudykunst, 1983b) and differences in conflict styles (Ting-Toomey, 1985). Hall (1976) differentiates cultures on the basis of the communication that predominates in the culture. A high-context (HC) communication or message is one in which more of the information is either in the physical context or internalized in the person, and very little is in the coded, explicit part of the message. A low-context communication is just the opposite; i.e., the mass of information is vested in the explicit code" (Hall, 1976, p. 79). While no culture exists at either end of the low/high-context continuum, the culture of the United States is toward the low end, slightly above the German, Swiss, and Scandinavian cultures. Most Asian cultures (e.g., Japanese, Chinese, and Korean), on the other hand, fall at the high-context end of the continuum.

The level of context influences all other aspects of communication. Context affects language (both written and spoken), legal codes, material culture (e.g., automobiles, houses), patterns of social organization, and business systems, to name only a few. Hall (1976) points out the following:

> High-context cultures make greater distinctions between insiders and outsiders than low-context cultures do. People raised in high-context systems expect more of others than do the participants in low-context systems. When talking about something that they have on their minds, a high-context individual will expect his [or her] interlocutor to know what's bothering him [or her], so that he [or she] doesn't have to be specific. The result is that he [or she] will talk around and around the point, in effect putting all the pieces in place except the crucial one. Placing it properly—this keystone—is the role of his [or her] interlocutor. (p. 98)

Okabe (1983) extends this analysis, arguing that verbal skills are more necessary and prized more highly in low-context cultures than in high context cultures. In high-context cultures verbal skills are considered suspect and confidence is placed in a nonverbal aspect of communication.

An alternative multidimensional schema was developed by Hofstede (1980, 1983). Hofstede isolated four dimensions of culture: uncertainty avoidance, individualism, masculinity, and power distance. Uncertainty avoidance is "the extent to which people feel threatened by ambiguous situations and have created beliefs and institutions that try to avoid these" (Hofstede & Bond, 1984, p. 419). This dimension is related to how people deal with conflict and aggression, how they release energy and use formal rules, and the tolerance they have for ambiguity. Members of high uncertainty avoidance cultures try to avoid uncertainty, but at the same time show their emotions more than members of low uncertainty avoidance cultures do. Differences in the uncertainty avoidance dimension should be related to expression of emotion in relationships; that is, members of cultures high on uncertainty avoidance should express more emotion in relationships than do members of cultures low on the dimension.

Hofstede's (1980) second dimension involves a bipolar continuum between individualism and collectivism. In individualistic cultures, "people are supposed to look after themselves and their immediate family only;" while in collectivistic cultures, "people belong to in-groups or collectivities which are supposed to look after them in exchange for loyalty" (Hofstede & Bond, 1984, p. 419). Triandis (1986) sees the key distinction between individualistic and collectivistic cultures as the focus on the ingroup in collectivistic cultures. Collectivistic cultures emphasize goals, needs, and views of the ingroup over those of the individual; the social norms of the ingroup rather than individual pleasure; shared ingroup beliefs rather than unique individual beliefs; and a value on cooperation with ingroup members rather than maximizing individual outcomes. Triandis goes on to argue that the larger the number of ingroups, the narrower the influence and the less the depth of influence. Since individualistic cultures have many specific ingroups, they exert less influence on individuals than ingroups do in collectivistic cultures in which there are few general ingroups. Triandis also points out that ingroups have different rank orders of importance in collectivistic cultures. Some, for example, put family ahead of all other ingroups while others put their company ahead of other ingroups.

Hofstede's (1980) third dimension is a bipolar continuum, masculinity-femininity. Masculinity predominates in countries where the dominant values "are success, money, and things," while femininity predominates where "caring for others and quality of life" are predominant values (Hofstede & Bond, 1984 pp. 419-420). Cultures high in masculinity differentiate sex roles clearly, while cultures low in masculinity (high in femininity) tend to have fluid sex roles. The rationale for the influence of masculinity-femininity on perceptions of communication behavior associated with relationship terms is straightforward; it should influence how same-sex and opposite-sex relationships are perceived. Specifically, because of differentiated sex roles, members of high masculinity cultures should perceive opposite-sex relationships as less intimate than members of low masculinity cultures.

Power distance, Hofstede's (1980) final dimension, involves the degree to which members of a culture accept the unequal distribution of power in the society. High power distance cultures assume that inequality should exist, that most people should be dependent on others, and that hierarchy results from existential inequality. Lower power distance cultures, in contrast, assume that inequality should be minimized, people should be interdependent, and that hierarchy results from role inequality and roles are established for convenience. This dimension of cultural variability should influence social penetration in those relationships in which there are power differentials (e.q., superior-subordinate). Also some cultures (e.g., Chinese) reconstruct or explain interpersonal relationships in power distance terminology (Forgas & Bond, 1985).

Social Penetration

Variability along Hofstede's (1980) dimensions influences social penetration processes across cultures. Differences in the uncertainty avoidance dimension, for example, are related to expression of emotion in relationships; that is, members of cultures high on uncertainty avoidance should express more emotion in relationships than do members of cultures low on the dimension. Translating this line of argument to Knapp, Ellis, and Williams's (1980) dimensions, members of high uncertainty avoidance cultures perceive their relationships to be more personal than do members of low uncertainty avoidance cultures. The rationale for the influence of masculinity-femininity on communication behavior in relationships is straightforward: It influences how same-sex and opposite-sex relationships are perceived. Specifically, because of differentiated sex roles, members of high masculinity cultures perceive opposite-sex relationships as less intimate than do members of low masculinity cultures. Further, it follows that members of cultures high on masculinity perceive less personalization and synchronization, but more difficulty in opposite-sex relationships than do members of cultures low on masculinity.

Triandis (1986) suggests that members of collectivistic cultures draw sharper distinctions between members of ingroups (e.g., those with whom they go to school or work) and outgroups, and perceive ingroup relationships to be more intimate than do members of individualistic cultures. Ingroup relationships include co-worker and colleague (company ingroup) or classmate (university ingroup), to name only a few. Because of the perceived intimacy of these relationships, members of collectivistic cultures also perceive these same ingroup relationships as involving more personalization and synchronization and less difficulty than do members of individualistic cultures.

Power distance also has a direct influence on selected aspects of relationship development and organizational communication. Cultural variability along this dimension affects the way interpersonal relationships form and develop when differences in "power" are perceived. In high power distance cultures, for example, differences in power are assumed to be natural. "Superiors" and "subordinates" are considered as being of a different kind, and this difference simply reflects an "existential inequality" (Hofstede, 1980). In low power distance cultures, in contrast, people are seen as equal and inequalities in roles are viewed as being established for the sake of convenience. While the impact of this dimension communication between superiors and subordinates in an organization is obvious, other types of relationships also are affected; for example, teacher-student, old person-young person, and parent-child, to name only a few.

Gudykunst and Nishida (1983, 1986b) compared social penetration in Japan and the United States. The first study (1983) examined perceptions of social penetration across 10 topics of conversations isolated by Taylor and Altman (1966). Only three of the 10 analyses, (own marriage and family; love, dating, and sex; emotions and feelings) revealed differences by culture in same-sex close friendships; with North American means being higher than Japanese means on each topic (i.e., North Americans perceived more social penetration on these topics than did Japanese). Overall, the patterns of social penetration in close friendships in Japan and the United States were very similar. The differences that emerged in Gudykunst and Nishida's (1983) study appear to be related to Hofstede's (1980) masculinity dimension. The Japanese have the highest masculinity score of all cultures studied, and the culture of the United States falls in the middle. It, therefore, would be expected that the Japanese would place less emphasis on opposite-sex relationship than would people in the United States.

Gudykunst and Nishida's (1986b) research extended Knapp, Ellis, and Williams's (1980) work in the United States. Specifically they examined the influence of culture (Japan versus the United States), relationship type (stranger, acquaintance, classmate, friend, best friend, and lover), and dyadic composition (same versus opposite sex relationships) on perceptions of the intimacy of relationship terms (Study I) and on perceptions of personalization, synchronization, and difficulty in communication with specific partners (Study II). To illustrate the effect of culture on perceived intimacy of relationship in Japan and the United States, the results of Gudykunst and Nishida's Study I are presented in Table 6.1.

Consistent with Triandis's (1986) description of the focus on ingroup relationships in collectivistic cultures, Gudykunst and Nishida's (1986b) Japanese respondents rated relationship terms associated with two of their major ingroups, people from their university and people with whom they work, as more intimate than did respondents from the United States. The same individuals are members of ingroups for people in the highly individualistic culture of the United States, but relationships with the ingroup are not emphasized or perceived as important in individualistic cultures unless individuals are engaging in intergroup behavior.

Though the score on Hofstede's (1980) masculinity dimension for the United States falls in the middle and Japan's score is high, six of the seven opposite-sex relationships in Gudykunst and Nishida's (1986b) Study I

TABLE 6.1
Means of Intimacy Ratings of Relationship Terms by Culture

Relationship Terms	United States	Japan	p
Cohort (Nakama)	5.40	2.85	.001
Brother (Kyodai)	3.12	3.51	ns
Mother (Hahaoya)	2.35	2.06	ns
Acquaintance (Chijin)	6.79	4.95	.001
Co-worker (Shigato-makama)	5.76	5.27	.05
Aunt (Oba)	4.53	4.99	.05
Employer (Koyosha)	6.39	6.86	.05
Colleague (Doryo)	5.33	4.76	.05
Lover (Koibito)	1.25	2.81	.001
Sister (Shimai)	2.88	3.78	.01
Roommate (Doshukusha)	3.85	4.88	.001
Cousin (Itoko)	4.67	4.66	ns
Grandparent (Sofubo)	3.75	4.15	.05
Fiance (Konyakusha)	1.29	4.32	.001
Classmate (Dokyusei)	5.72	3.84	.001
Best Friend (Ichiban no shinyu)	2.51	1.73	.001
Father (Chichioya)	2.75	2.57	ns
Son (Musuko)	2.59	4.76	.001
Uncle (Oji)	4.55	5.21	.001
Neighbor (Kinjo no hito)	5.72	5.92	.001
Mate (Tsureai)	1.75	4.45	.001
Companion (Tomodachi)	3.08	3.05	ns
Spouse (Haigusha)	1.33	4.32	.001
Boy/Girlfriend (Otoko/onna tomodachi)	1.70	3.32	.001
Daughter (Musume)	2.55	4.87	.001
Date (Detonoaite)	4.02	3.48	.05
Close Friend (Shinyu)	2.85	1.83	.001
Stranger (Shiranai hito)	8.35	7.99	.05
Friend (Tomo)	3.67	3.42	ns
Steady (Kosai shiteiru hito)	2.27	2.92	.01

SOURCE: Gudykunst and Nishida (1986b).
NOTE: Items were rated on a nine-point scale with 1 = intimate and 9 = nonintimate. Japanese translations for each term is given in parentheses following the term in English.

revealed significant differences in the posited direction. Consistent with Hofstede's description, sex roles in high masculinity cultures are differentiated clearly, while sex roles in low masculinity cultures are fluid and a unisex or androgyny ideal predominates. When sex roles are differentiated clearly, relatively little informal interaction occurs between males and females, and when interaction take place, the content of communication tends to be superficial. These relationships, therefore, are perceived as less intimate in highly masculine cultures than in cultures low on the dimension.

The Japanese sample perceived six of the nine family relationship terms as less intimate than the United States sample in Gudykunst and Nishida's

(1986b) first study. Nakane (1974) argues that the company for which a Japanese works is the ingroup with the most influence on individuals' behavior. In cultures in which the company is the most influential, other ingroups (e.g., family) appear to be less important, and relationships with these ingroups are perceived as less intimate. The clear pattern that emerged in the data is consistent with Triandis's (1986) conceptualization of individualism-collectivism; that is, collectivistic cultures that do not rank family as the prime ingroup do not perceive family relationships to be highly intimate (e.g., less intimate than individualistic cultures). The ingroup that is perceived as most important may be related to other dimensions of culture; that is, it is plausible that cultures high in masculinity attribute a larger social role to the organizations for which they work, while cultures low in masculinity attribute larger social roles to other institutions, such as the family.

Gudykunst and Nishida (1986b) examined the cross-cultural generalizability of Knapp, Ellis, and Williams's (1980) analysis of the dimensions of communication behavior hypothesized to vary with intimacy of relationship (see the preceding for the specific dimensions) in their Study II. Using *confirmatory* factor analysis, they compared the factor structure of Knapp, Ellis, and Williams's items in Japan and the United States. Gudykunst and Nishida's data indicated that the same three factors (personalization, synchronization, and difficulty) emerge in both cultures, and Gudykunst, Nishida, and Yoon's (1987) study (discussed in detail next) revealed that the three factors generalize to Korea as well. It appears therefore, that personalization, synchronization, and difficulty are relevant dimensions of communication in interpersonal relations across cultures.

While Gudykunst and Nishida (1986b) found that the dimensions of social penetration were the same in Japan and the United States, their Study II revealed culture by relationship type and culture by dyadic composition interactions. The interaction between culture and relationship term was a result of differences in perceptions of classmate and acquaintance relationships. The Japanese perceived acquaintance relationships as more personalized and synchronized than classmate relationships, while the opposite pattern emerged for North American respondents. The culture by dyadic composition interaction revealed that North American female-male relationships were perceived as the most personalized, followed by male-male, male-female, and female-female dyads. The Japanese, in contrast, perceived the most personalization in male-female dyads, followed by female-female, female-male, and male-male dyads.

Gudykunst and Nishida's (1986b) data displayed patterns predictable from three of Hofstede's (1980) four dimensions: individualism-collectivism, uncertainty avoidance, and masculinity-femininity. Specifically, the masculinity-femininity dimension influences perceptions of communication behavior associated with opposite- versus same-sex relationships and has direct bearing on generalizing theory and research regarding interpersonal relationship development, in general, and the development of romantic relationships in particular. It would be predicted, for example, that oppposite-sex relationships are formed and develop more easily in feminine cultures than in masculine cultures. The uncertainty avoidance dimension influences the expression of emotion in relationships, with more emotion being expressed in high uncertainty avoidance cultures than in low uncertainty avoidance cultures. This dimension also affects the amount of consensus present in a relationship. To illustrate, it would be hypothesized that there is greater consensus within dyads on the nature of their communication in high uncertainty cultures than in low uncertainty avoidance cultures. Results predicted from the individualism-collectivism dimension were somewhat inconclusive to Gudykunst and Nishida's (1986b) study.

The effect of individualism on social penetration processes was also examined in Gudykunst, Yoon, and Nishida's (1987) study of ingroup and outgroup relationships in Japan, Korea, and the United States. This study revealed that the greater the degree of collectivism present in a culture, the greater the amount of personalization and synchronization, but the less the difficulty perceived in communication with classmates (ingroup). These results for communication in ingroup relationships clearly support predictions derived from Triandis's (1986) conceptualization of individualism-collectivism. Members of collectivistic cultures perceive greater social penetration (more personalization and synchronization, but less difficulty) in ingroup relationships than do members of individualistic cultures.

Gudykunst, Yoon, and Nishida's (1987) results for communication with outgroup members were not as clear-cut. The data indicated that there is an inverse linear relationship between perceived personalization of communication with members of outgroups and individualism; that is, the greater the individualism, the less the perceived personalization. This finding is consistent with the prediction derived from previous research in collectivistic cultures (Leung & Bond, 1984; Wetherall, 1982). Specifically, since there are strong situational demands on behavior in collectivistic cultures, the amount of personalization in communication with members of outgroups is specified by the situation, while in individualistic cultures in which situational demands are relatively weak, the amount of personalized communication is determined by the specific individuals involved.

Perceptions of synchronization in communication with outgroup members did not fit the same pattern in Gudykunst, Yoon, and Nishida's (1987) study. Rather, the least synchronization occurred in Japan, while approximately the same amount was perceived in the United States and Korean samples. One potential explanation for this pattern is that Japan and Korea emphasize different forms of collectivism. Japan emphasizes what Triandis (1986) labels "contextual collectivism," in which the ingroup's influence is specific. Korea, in contrast, emphasizes what Triandis calls "simple collectivism," in which, if more than one ingroup influences a person's behavior, the person can balance the views of the various groups and decide how to behave without feeling norm or role conflict. The relevant ingroups with which Korean students use to deal with strangers, therefore, appear to prescribe that relatively the same degree of personalization takes place, but not all prescribe the same degree of synchronization between their behavior and that of strangers. The contextual collectivism of Japanese student ingroups, on the other hand, appears to require both relatively low levels of personalization and synchronization in communication with members of outgroups.

Finally, Gudykunst, Yoon, and Nishida's (1987) results for perceived difficulty in communicating with strangers were consistent with the predicted pattern: The least difficulty was perceived in the United States, and the most was perceived in Japan and Korea, with their mean scores being approximately the same. This finding is consistent with Triandis's (1986) conceptualization of individualism-collectivism.

Won-Doornink (1979, 1985) also has examined aspects of social penetration theory across cultures. She examined reciprocity process over time in Korean dyads (1979) and compared reciprocity over time in dyads in Korea and the United States (1985). The data revealed a linear inverse association between stage of relationship and reciprocity of nonintimate self-disclosure. Her results, therefore, support predictions made from social penetration theory.

Won-Doornink's (1979, 1985) research, in combination with Gudykunst and Nishida's (1983, 1986b; Gudykunst, Yoon, & Nishida, 1987) research suggests that social penetration theory is generalizable across cultures. Research by Hammer and Gudykunst (1987) also suggests that the theory is generalizable across ethnic groups in the United States. They found that even though ethnicity influences perceptions of the amount of social penetration across most of Taylor and Altman's (1966) topics of conversation, ethnicity does not influence the relative agreement between friends on the degree of social penetration in their relationship.

Uncertainty Reduction

Cross-cultural differences in uncertainty reduction processes appear to be related to Hall's (1976) low/high-context distinction and Hofstede's (1980) individualism-collectivism dimension. The conceptual link is clearest to low/high-context, but this dimension appears to be isomorphic with individualism-collectivism (Gudykunst & Ting-Toomey, in press). Specifically, low-context communication predominates in individualistic cultures, and high-context communication is prevalent in collectivistic cultures. While there are no empirical data to support this claim, Hall's description of high-context cultures is consistent with Triandis's (1986) description of collectivistic cultures and virtually all of the low-context cultures Hall discusses are individualistic and all high-context cultures are collectivistic.

Exploratory research by Gudykunst (1983c) with international students in the United States revealed that members of high-context cultures are more cautious in initial interactions with strangers, make more assumptions about strangers based upon their background, and ask more questions about strangers' backgrounds than do members of low-context cultures. His research also suggested that members of low-context cultures engage in more nonverbal affiliative expressiveness than do members of high-context cultures.

Gudykunst and Nishida (1984) found that culture influences self-disclosure, interrogation, nonverbal affiliative expressiveness, and attributional confidence. As would be predicted from Hall's (1976) theory, the Japanese sample displayed a higher level of attributional confidence about strangers' behavior than did the United States sample. Moreover, higher levels of interrogation and self-disclosure were reported in the United States sample than in the Japanese sample. These results are consistent with Nakane (1974), Johnson and Johnson (1975), and Okabe (1983), who point out that people in the United States engage in more verbal communication, including interrogation and self-disclosure, than do Japanese. This finding, however, is inconsistent with Gudykunst (1983c), who reported that members of high-context cultures asked more questions about a stranger's background than did members of low-context cultures. The difference in results of the two studies may be the result of the high-context respondents in Gudykunst's study being international students from Japan, Korea, Hong Kong, and Taiwan studying in the United States, while the high-context respondents in Gudykunst and Nishida's study were Japanese living in Japan. Japanese also were reported as displaying more nonverbal affiliative expressiveness than were the respondents from the United States. This finding is consistent with Johnson and Johnson's (1975) position that there is "a conspicuous focus on the interpretation of nonverbal communication" in Japan (p. 445). Similarly, Okabe (1983) points out that Japanese "use *haragei*, or the 'art of the belly' for the meeting of minds or at least the viscera, without clear verbal interaction" (p.39).

Gudykunst and Nishida (1986a) argue that two types of attributional confidence can be isolated across cultures. These correspond to patterns of communication in low- and high-context cultures and, accordingly, were labeled low- and high-context attributional confidence. As pointed out earlier, high-context cultures emphasize nonverbal forms of communication. Tsujimura (1987), for example, isolates four major characteristics of Japanese communication: (1) *ishin-denshin* ("traditional mental telepathy"), (2) taciturnity, (3) *kuki* (mood or atmosphere), and (4) respect for reverberation (i.e., indirect communication). Yum (1987a) points out that *i-sim jun-sim* (telepathy) is regarded as the highest form of communication in Korea. She also contends that silence and the use of indirect forms of communication are used widely in Korean cultures. Hall (1976) makes a similar observation about communication in the Chinese cultures.

Because of the emphasis on nonverbal communication, members of high-context cultures need to know whether others understand them when they do not verbally express their ideas and feelings and, in addition, whether they can understand others under the same circumstances in order to reduce uncertainty. Although these forms of uncertainty are not totally absent in low-context cultures, they are emphasized less. Not only is it important for members of high-context cultures to know whether others understand them when they don't express themselves, it is also necessary for them to know whether others will make allowances for them. The concept *sassi* in Japan illustrates this claim. Nishida (1977) defines *sassi* as a noun meaning conjecture, surmise, guess, judgment, understanding what a person means, and what a sign means. In its verb form (*sassuru*), its meaning is expanded to include imagine, suppose or empathize with, feel or make allowances for. This concept is so important in Japan that Ishii (1984) used it as the basis for his model of Japanese interpersonal communication.

In low-context cultures, oral (or written) messages require less knowledge of the context in order to be interpreted correctly. Members of low-context cultures, therefore, can gather information about others' attitudes, values, emotions, and past behavior and use it to predict their future behavior (i.e., reduce uncertainty). The type of information gathered is individual specific. Members of high-context cultures, in contrast, seek out social information (e.g., where others went to school, their company). To illustrate, Alexander, Cronen, Kang, Tsou, and Banks (1986) found that Chinese college students infer more about others' intellectual and academic potential based on knowing their high school background than do college students in the United States. Nakane (1974) argues similarly that Japanese ignore an individual whose background is unknown because his or her behavior is unpredictable, and it is unknown whether he or she will follow the norms/conventions appropriate in the context. In order to be able to predict others' behavior their background and relative status must be known. Background information not only tells Japanese whether strangers' behavior is predictable, but it also tells them how to talk with strangers (i.e., it tells them how to address strangers and which form of the language to use). Without this knowledge it is impossible to communicate with strangers in the Japanese language with any degree of comfort. Yum (1987b) makes similar observations about communication in Korea.

Gudykunst and Nishida (1986a) expanded Clatterbuck's (1979) earlier work and developed a two-factor measure of attributional confidence that is consistent with the preceding descriptions of communication in low- and high-context cultures. Each factor emphasizes sources of information that are more important in one type of culture. Members of low-context cultures *focus* on information specific to the individuals with whom they are communicating that increases accuracy in direct forms of communication. Members of high-context cultures, in contrast, *focus* on information that increases accuracy in indirect, nonverbal forms of communication. Both types of culture, however, do attune to the information upon which the other culture focuses. Members of high-context cultures use information on individual's attitudes, values, feelings, and empathy to predict others' behavior, but this information appears to be secondary to the information used to reduce uncertainty resulting from the indirect forms of communication that predominates in the culture. Similarly, people in low-context cultures use information regarding whether or not the others understand their feelings, make allowances for them when they communicate, and the degree to which they understand the other person, but these sources of information appear to be secondary to those isolated by Clatterbuck (1979). This is consistent with Hall's (1976) contention that both low- and high-context communication are used in every culture, but one tends to predominate.

Significant differences in low- and high-context attributional confidence scores emerged by culture and stage of relationship in Gudykunst and Nishida's (1986a) study. As would be expected from research on interpersonal relationship development (Altman & Taylor, 1973), both low- and high-context attributional confidence increased as relationships increased in intimacy. The interaction effect between culture and stage of relationship that emerged suggests that there may be differences in the perceived intimacy of relationships across cultures. At least one of the findings is consistent with previous research. Members of high-context cultures, for example, establish relationships with classmates early in their school careers. These relationships are part of the in-group and last for life (Nakane, 1974; Yum, 1987a, 1987b). It therefore would be expected that members of high-context cultures would have more low- and high-context attributional confidence regarding classmates than acquaintances. Members of low-context cultures, however, do not establish the same type of relationships with classmates. Rather, acquaintance relationships tend to be perceived as more intimate and members of low-context culture are more confident in predicting acquaintances' than classmates' behavior.

Gudykunst and Nishida (1986a) also found that high-context attributional confidence was higher in the low-context culture of the United States than in the high-context culture of Japan, an unexpected finding. On the surface, this finding might suggest that the two dimensions are not conceptually distinct. This, however, does not appear to be the case. When frequency of communication, length of relationship, shared networks, interaction with others' friends, and percentage of free time spent with others were correlated with the two dimensions, different patterns emerged. The only variable to have a significantly different correlation with low-context confidence was frequency of communication. Frequency correlated significantly higher with low-context attributional confidence in the United States sample than in the Japanese sample, suggesting that frequency of communication has less influence in high-context cultures than in low-context cultures. The correlation between frequency of communication and high-context confidence was also significantly higher in the United States sample than in the Japanese sample. Three other variables, in contrast, correlated significantly higher with high-context attributional confidence in the Japanese sample than in the United States sample: overlap in social network, interaction with others' friends, and percentage of free time spent with others.

Gudykunst and Nishida's (1986a) data are consistent with previous work on communication in high-context cultures. Nakane (1974), for example, argues that Japanese differentiate others into three categories—strangers, people whose social backgrounds are known, and members of the ingroup—and that effectiveness of communication varies as a function of others' group membership. Yum (1987b) and Hsu (1981) make similar observations about Korean and Chinese cultures respectively. Shared communication networks, interaction with others' friends, and spending free time with others—the variables correlated with high-context confidence in Japan—are characteristic of in-group relationships, rather than relationships with members of out-groups. This suggests that high-context attributional confidence emerges from in-group relationships, rather than from frequency of communication with the specific other person, in high-context (collectivistic) cultures like that in Japan. High-context attributional confidence, in contrast, appears to be a function of individualistic interaction (i.e., frequency of communication) in low-context (individualistic) cultures like that in the United States.

Finally, recent research by Gudykunst, Nishida, and Schmidt (1988) indicates that individualism-collectivism influences uncertainty reduction processes in ingroup and outgroup relationships. Specifically, this study found differences in ingroup and outgroup relationships (e.g., more attributional confidence in ingroup than in outgroup) in collectivistic cultures, but not in individualistic cultures. This finding is consistent with Triandis's (1986) conceptualization of ingroup and outgroup in individualistic and collectivistic cultures. Gudykunst, Nishida, and Schmidt also observed that there are differences in same- and opposite-sex relationships (e.g., more attributional confidence in same- than in opposite-sex relationships) in masculine cultures that do not appear in feminine cultures, consistent with the prediction derived from Hofstede's (1980) masculinity-femininity dimension of cultural variability.

INTERCULTURAL RESEARCH ON SOCIAL PENETRATION AND UNCERTAINTY REDUCTION

Cultural Similarity

The research just cited focused on cross-cultural comparisons of social penetration and uncertainty reduction processes; what follows focuses on social penetration and uncertainty reduction in intercultural relationships. Relationships between members of different cultures involve perceptions of cultural similarity and dissimilarity. Bishop (1979) argues that "to understand the ways in which the perception of similarity influences interpersonal relations, it is necessary that the problem be approached from the point of view of a wide variety of types of similarity . . . one general type of similarity which could be fruitfully explored is that of cultural similarities"(p. 461).

When cultural dissimilarities exist, communication is, in part, a function of group membership. "Whenever individuals belonging to one group interact collectively or individually, with another group or its members *in terms of their group identifications*, we have an instance of intergroup behavior" (Sherif, 1966, p. 12). Tajfel (1978) argues that behavior can be viewed as varying along a continuum from purely interpersonal to purely intergroup. Recent conceptualizations, however, suggest that a single continuum may oversimplify the analysis. Stephenson (1981) and Gudykunst and Lim (1986), for example, contend that both interpersonal and intergroup factors are salient in every encounter between two individuals and that intergroup salience affects interpersonal processes (and vice versa).

Cultural dissimilarities have a differential effect on relationships at different levels of intimacy. Altman and Taylor (1973) argue that in the affective exchange stage (i.e., close friendships) "the dyad has moved to the point were interaction is relatively free in both peripheral and in more central areas of personality. Cultural stereotypy is broken down in these more intimate areas and there is willingness to move freely in and out of such exchanges" (Altman & Taylor, 1973, pp. 139-140). If cultural stereotypy is broken down, the culture from which a person comes should not be a major factor influencing interaction. This line of reasoning is consistent with Bell's (1981) conceptualization of friendship: "The development of friendship is based on private negotiations and is not imposed through cultural values or norms" (p. 10).

The position just outlined also is compatible with Miller and Steinberg's (1975) "developmental" theory of interpersonal relationships. Specifically, it can be inferred that when communicators move from using cultural and sociological data in making predictions about their partners to the use of psychological data, the culture from which a person comes is no longer a major relevant variable in making predictions about their communication behavior. Given this position, it would be expected that when relationships reach the point of close friendship, and the individuals are basing their predictions about their partners on psychological data, that the degree of social penetration in which people engage should not differ in intracultural and intercultural relationships as a function of culture.

Both Altman and Taylor's (1973) and Miller and Steinberg's (1975) theories support the argument that the influence of culture on interpersonal relationships varies as relationships become more intimate. Initially, cultural dissimilarities have an effect on the relationship and how it develops. As relationships between people from different cultures move through the stages of relationship development, however, the impact of cultural dissimilarities begins to disappear. Once interpersonal relationships between people from different cultures reach the friendship stage (i.e., Altman & Taylor's, 1973, full effective exchange stage), cultural dissimilarities appear to have little impact on the relationship because the majority of interaction in friendships has a personalistic focus. As Wright (1978) observes, "in friendship, each person reacts to the other as a person-qua-person or, more specifically, with respect to his/her genuineness, uniqueness, and irreplaceability in the relationship" (p. 199).

Social Penetration

One study has compared social penetration processes in intracultural and intercultural relationships. Gudykunst (1985b) found a high correlation between perceptions of social penetration across Taylor and Altman's (1966) 13 topical areas in close intra- and intercultural relationships. The canonical coefficients and canonical component loadings had very similar patterns in the intra- and intercultural relationships. Gudykunst's data also revealed a moderate correlation between the amount of perceived similarity in the two types of relationships.

Given results of Gudykunst's (1985b) and Gudykunst and Nishida's (1983, 1986b) research, Gudykunst, Nishida, and Chua (1987) predicted that as relationships increase in intimacy, communication is perceived as more personalized and synchronized, but less difficult. Knapp, Ellis, and Williams's (1980) research and Gudykunst and Nishida's (1986b) study also suggest that the social penetration process is influenced by dyadic composition. Extending their findings, Gudykunst, Nishida, and Chua (1987) argued that opposite-sex relationships are perceived as more personal than are same-sex relationships. Data were collected from both partners in Japanese-North American dyads, and examined using both summation and dispersion scores. Results of this study were consistent with predictions derived from Altman and Taylor's (1973) social penetration theory, as well as with Knapp, Ellis, and Williams's (1980) intracultural research in the United States. Summation scores (i.e., the average of the two partners' responses) for high intimacy dyads revealed that partners perceive more personalized and synchronized communication, but less difficulty in communication than for low intimacy dyads. These results are clearly consistent with social penetration theory. Mixed dyads (i.e., dyads for which the partner defined the relationship as high in intimacy and the other defined it as low in intimacy), however, were between the low and high intimacy dyads with respect to personalized communication and higher than both groups for synchronized communication and difficulty of communication. Relationship type explained 62% of the variance in personalized communication, 20% of synchronized communication, and 15% of difficulty in communication.

The results from the analysis of the dispersion scores (i.e., the difference between the two partners' responses) in Gudykunst, Nishida, and Chua's

(1987) study revealed that mixed dyads had significantly less agreement than did low intimacy dyads on the amount of personalized communication, and less, but not significantly less, agreement than did low intimacy dyads. On the remaining two factors, high intimacy dyads had lower dispersion scores than did low intimacy dyads, but the low intimacy dyads' scores were higher than were the mixed dyads' scores. These findings suggest that there is greater agreement in high intimacy dyads than in low intimacy dyads, but mixed dyads do not fit a specific pattern.

Several noteworthy patterns also emerged in Gudykunst, Nishida, and Chua's (1987) correlational analysis. Perceived synchrony and perceived difficulty of communication, for example, had a high negative correlation, suggesting that as difficulty is reduced synchronization occurs, or vice versa. Furthermore, while perceived personalization and perceived synchronization had a moderate correlation, perceived personalization and perceived difficulty were uncorrelated. These patterns imply that perceived personalization and perceived synchrony covary in intercultural dyads, but perceived personalization and perceived difficulty do not, a finding consistent with Knapp, Ellis, and Williams's (1980) intracultural research. The length of relationship and frequency of communication also were correlated moderately with perceived personalization, but neither correlated with perceived synchronization or perceived difficulty of communication. These findings, in combination with the analysis by relationship type, suggest that relationship type, not length or frequency, influences perceived synchronization and perceived difficulty, consistent with Altman and Taylor (1973). Only the perceived synchronization findings, however, are consistent with Knapp, Ellis, and Williams. This difference may suggest that relationship type has more of an influence on perceived difficulty of communication in intercultural relationships than in intracultural relationships.

Perceived second-language competence correlated moderately and positively with each of the three social penetration variables in Gudykunst, Nishida, and Chua (1987). It therefore appears that the ability to use the partner's native language influences perceptions of social penetration in intercultural dyads, or vice versa. It should be noted, however, that these results may be primarily owing to the Japanese partner's ability to use English rather than the North American partner's ability to use Japanese, or a combination of the two because the ethnolinguistic vitality (see Giles, Bourhis, & Taylor, 1977) of Japanese probably was low. Closely related to second-language competence, clear patterns emerged for perceived intercultural effectiveness. Specifically, perceived effectiveness was related moderately to highly to each of the three social penetration dimensions. The results appear to be consistent with Hammer, Gudykunst, and Wiseman's (1978) conceptualization of intercultural effectiveness. Their research suggests that a large part of intercultural effectiveness is the ability to establish interpersonal relationships with people from other cultures.

Finally, communication satisfaction was correlated positively with each of the dimensions of social penetration in Gudykunst, Nishida, and Chua's (1987) study, with the weakest correlation occurring with perceived personalization. These findings appear to be consistent with Hecht (1984), but his research also suggests that the correlations may vary across type of relationship. He found, for example, that personalness and synchrony were related more strongly to satisfaction in relationships at lower levels of intimacy than in relationships at higher levels of intimacy. The data further revealed a high correlation between satisfaction and perceived effectiveness. This is consistent with Hecht's (1978) argument that "communication satisfaction is one of the outcomes commonly associated with competent communication" (p. 253). Gudykunst, Nishida, and Chua's results, therefore, suggest that this conclusion may be generalizable to intercultural relationships.

Uncertainty Reduction

Simard's (1981) research with Francophones and Anglophones in Canada revealed that both groups "perceive it as more difficult to know how to initiate a conversation, to know what to talk about during the interaction, to be interested in the other person, and to guess in which language they should talk" (p. 179) when communicating with someone culturally different than when communicating with someone culturally similar. Her research also indicated that subjects who formed an acquaintance relationship with a culturally different person perceived this person to be as similar to them as did subjects who formed an acquaintance with a person who was culturally similar.

Other research is consistent with Simard's (1981) findings. Gudykunst (1983a), for example, found that people make more assumptions about strangers, prefer to talk less, ask more questions about strangers' backgrounds, and have less attributional confidence in predicting strangers' behavior in initial intercultural encounters than in initial intracultural encounters. Similarly, in a study of Japanese and North Americans, Gudykunst and Nishida (1984) discovered that cultural similarity/dissimilarity has a multivariate effect on intent to self-disclose, interrogate, display nonverbal affiliative expressiveness, attraction, and attributional confidence.

Similarly, Gudykunst (1985c) found a significant interaction effect between cultural similarity and type of relationship. The univariate analyses revealed significant independent effects on two variables: attributional confidence, and shared communication networks, and interrogation and self-disclosure approached significance. With respect to self-disclosure and attributional confidence the mean scores were higher for dissimilar acquaintances than similar ones, but higher for culturally similar friends than for dissimilar ones. Results for shared communication networks indicated that the mean scores were approximately the same for culturally similar and dissimilar acquaintances, but culturally similar friends shared twice as many networks as did culturally dissimilar friends. Culturally dissimilar friends, however, shared significantly more communication networks than did culturally similar acquaintances. This difference can be explained by Blau and Schwartz's (1984) theory of intergroup relations. Drawing upon Simmel's (1950) analysis of "cross-cutting social circles," they point out that close relations between people who do not share similar ethnic or cultural backgrounds "tend to be the result of their having other social relations in common" (Blau & Schwartz, 1984, p. 88).

Findings from Gudykunst's (1985c) study with respect to the cultural similarity by type of relationship interaction did not display the patterns that might be predicted from Altman and Taylor's (1973) social penetration theory. Using this perspective it would be predicted that there are differences between culturally similar and dissimilar acquaintances, but no significant differences between culturally similar and dissimilar friends. Gudykunst's data revealed only one significant difference between the two types of acquaintances, a higher level of attraction in the cultural dissimilarity condition than in the cultural similarity condition. This finding might suggest that a higher level of attraction is necessary to call someone from another culture an acquaintance than is necessary if the person comes from the same culture. The only differences to emerge between culturally similar and dissimilar friends were on attributional confidence and the percentage of shared networks. The difference in shared communication networks is to be expected since a large percentage of the culturally dissimilar friends' networks of international students in the United States are in their home cultures. The level of attributional confidence in culturally dissimilar friendships was significantly lower than for culturally similar ones, but at the same time it is significantly higher than for culturally dissimilar and culturally similar acquaintances. The difference between the two types of friendships may be a result of differences in the shared communication networks, since the correlations between the two variables are approximately equal in the two conditions. This explanation appears to be consistent with Parks and Adelman's (1983) research on romantic relationships.

The lack of predicted interactions may be related to the nature of the relationships studied in Gudykunst's (1985c) study. Specifically, the acquaintance relationships may have been in the later phases of Altman and Taylor's (1973) exploratory affective exchange stage of relationship development (i.e., close to the affective exchange stage), rather than in earlier phases (i.e., nearer the orientation stage). If this is the case, then the predicted interactions would not be observed. Gudykunst's (1985c) results, therefore, appear to extend Ting-Toomey's (1981) and Gudykunst's (1985a) conclusions that once intercultural relationships become established (i.e., acquaintances or friendships are formed) there are few significant differences attributable to culturally dissimilar backgrounds.

Gudykunst, Chua, and Gray's (1987) research revealed significant interaction effects between dissimilarities on all of Hofstede's (1980) dimensions of cultural variability and stage of relationship development. Specifically, they found that power distance interacted with stage of relationship to influence self-disclosure, attraction, similarity, shared networks, low- and high-context attributional confidence; uncertainty avoidance interacted with stage of relationship to influence self-disclosure, similarity, low- and high-context attributional confidence; individualism interacted with stage of relationship to influence self-disclosure, interrogation, shared networks, low- and high-context attributional confidence; and masculinity interacted with stage of relationship to influence self-disclosure, similarity shared networks, low- and high-context attributional confidence. The data suggest that as relationships become more intimate, cultural dissimilarities have less effect on uncertainty reduction processes.

Gudykunst, Sodetani, and Sonoda's (1987) research supports extensions of ethnolinguistic identity theory (Beebe & Giles, 1984; Giles & Johnson, 1987) to interethnic uncertainty reduction processes. Overall, their data indicated that ethnolinguistic identity influences the set of uncertainty reduction processes examined. Specifically, the data revealed that the stronger the interethnic comparisons, the weaker other group identification, and the less the perceived vitality, the greater the perceived similarity. Gudykunst, Sodetani, and Sonoda's (1987) study also suggested that the greater the perceived vitality, the less the self-disclosure, interrogation, and low-context attributional confidence. Similarly, they found that the stronger the interethnic comparisons, the less the high-context attributional confidence. Finally, their study indicated that the more positive the interethnic comparisons, the more interethnic networks overlap. Findings from Gudykunst, Sodetani, and Sonoda's (1987) research are generally consistent with extensions of Giles and Johnson's (1981) and Giles and Byrne (1982), who hypothesize that the lower the perceived vitality, the higher second-language competence.

Recent work by Gudykunst and Hammer (in press) demonstrated that social identity is related to uncertainty reduction processes in general and that it is related positively to interethnic attributional confidence. While inconsistent with the initial version of Giles's (e.g., Giles & Byrne, 1982) intergroup theory of second-language acquisition, this finding is consistent with a recent revision (Giles, Garrett, & Coupland, 1987). Gudykunst and Hammer's finding also is compatible with Hall and Gudykunst's (1986) results, which indicated that the stronger the ingroup identification, the greater the perceived competence in the outgroup language. Moreover, Gudykunst and Hammer's results are consistent with Lambert, Mermigis, and Taylor's (1986) study, which suggests that the more secure and positive that members of a group feel about their identity, the more tolerant they are of members of other groups. Similar observations emerge from other studies (e.g., Bond & King, 1985; Pak, Dion, & Dion, 1985).

Gudykunst and Hammer's (in press) research further revealed that social identity influences uncertainty reduction processes only when members of the outgroup are perceived as typical of their group. When members of the outgroup are perceived as atypical, social identity does not affect uncertainty reduction processes in interethnic relationships. Gudykunst and Hammer also found that social identity influences uncertainty reduction only when ethnic status is activated.

Gudykunst, Sodetani, and Sonoda (1987) also found that type of relationship influences uncertainty reduction processes. Not only was there a significant multivariate effect by stage of relationship, there was a significant univariate effect for all dependent variables (e.g., self-disclosure, interrogation, attributional confidence, attraction). These findings are consistent with Altman and Taylor's (1973) social penetration theory, as well as with Gudykunst's (1985b) research comparing intracultural and intercultural relationships. Uncertainty reduction processes, therefore, appear to vary systematically as the stage of relationship changes, intraculturally, interculturally, and interethnically.

Gudykunst, Nishida, and Chua's (1986) research revealed that high intimacy dyads have greater self-disclosure, interrogation, shared networks, amount of communication, and low-context attributional confidence than have low intimacy dyads, based on the analysis of summation scores. These findings are consistent with Gudykunst's (1985c) research on intercultural relationships and Gudykunst, Sodetani, and Sonoda's (1987) study of Japanese-Caucasian interethnic communication in Hawaii. The results from the analysis of the dispersion scores revealed that high intimacy dyads are more consistent in the amount of self-disclosure and the degree of high-context attributional confidence they have about each other.

Several noteworthy patterns also emerged in Gudykunst, Nishida, and Chua's (1986) post hoc correlational analysis. The data indicated that self-disclosure, interrogation, amount of communication, length of relationship, and shared networks are correlated with low-context, but not high-context attributional confidence. The associations for amount of communication and self-disclosure supported Axioms 1 and 4 of Berger and Calabrese's (1975) original theory, but the data indicated the axioms cannot be extended to high-context attributional confidence in intercultural dyads. Gudykunst, Sodetani, and Sonoda's (1987) findings suggest this constraint may be the result of differences between the North American and Japanese partners. In their study, amount of communication and high-context confidence were correlated for Caucasians, but not for Japanese-Americans. Similarly, Gudykunst and Nishida's (1986a) research revealed that amount of communication and length of relationship were correlated with both low-context and high-context confidence for North Americans, but only related to low-context confidence for Japanese.

Perceived second-language competence was correlated with self-disclosure, interrogation, low-context attributional confidence, and length of relationship in Gudykunst, Nishida, and Chua's (1986) study. These results are consistent with Gudykunst's (1988) theory of intergroup uncertainty reduction that predicts that second-language competence influences the use of interactive uncertainty reduction strategies (i.e., self-disclosure and interrogation), as well as attributional confidence. Closely related to second-language competence, clear patterns emerged for perceived intercultural effectiveness. Specifically, perceived effectiveness was related to self-disclosure, interrogation, attraction, and similarity, as well as to both low- and high-context attributional confidence. These results appear to be consistent with Hammer, Gudykunst, and Wiseman's (1978) conceptualization of intercultural effectiveness. Finally, communication satisfaction was correlated with self-disclosure, interrogation, attraction, similarity, effectiveness, and low- and high-context attributional confidence. These findings appear to be compatible with Hecht's (1978) conceptualization of communication satisfaction and Hecht's (1984) research.

Current Theoretical Models

While the vast majority of the axioms and theorems of uncertainty reduction theory appear to generalize to intercultural encounters, an uncertainty reduction theory of intercultural/intergroup communication must include additional concepts that are not included in the original theory. I have (Gudykunst 1985a) argued that, minimally, these include cultural/ethnolinguistic identity, culture/group similarity, second-language ability, intercultural/intergroup attitudes and stereotypes (attitudes and stereotypes are incorporated under expectancies in Gudykunst's, 1988, theory). Recent work (Gudykunst, 1988; Gudykunst & Hammer, 1987) also includes intercultural/intergroup anxiety as a critical variable in extending uncertainty reduction theory to explain intercultural/intergroup communication. An initial extension of the theory has been proffered (Gudykunst, 1988), but it has not been tested empirically to date (see Table 6.2 for a summary of the assumptions and axioms in the theory). This theory incorporates aspects of ethnolinguistic identity theory (Giles & Johnson, 1987) and expectation states theory (Berger & Zelditch, 1985). It is designed to be applicable to interpersonal and intergroup/intercultural encounters. My theory explicates the factors that account for the reduction of uncertainty and anxiety. Some variables in the original theory are subsumed under higher level concepts (e.g., nonverbal affiliative expressiveness and intimacy of communication content are subsumed under interpersonal salience) and additional concepts (e.g., expectancies) are incorporated. The theory suggests that interpersonal salience and expectancies may also be able to be combined and thereby to integrate Sunnafrank's (1986) notion of predicted outcome value. Moreover, the theory

TABLE 6.2
Axioms from Gudykunst's Theory of Interpersonal and Intergroup Communication

Assumptions

(1) At least one participant in an intergroup encounter is a stranger vis-à-vis the ingroup being approached.
(2) Strangers' initial experiences with a new ingroup are experienced as a series of crises; that is, strangers are not cognitively sure of how to behave (i.e., cognitive uncertainty) and they experience the feeling of a lack of security (i.e., anxiety).
(3) Uncertainty and anxiety are independent dimensions of intergroup communication.
(4) Strangers' behavior takes place at high levels of awareness.
(5) Both intergroup and interpersonal factors influence intergroup communication.
(6) Strangers overestimate the influence of group membership in explaining members of other group's behavior.

Axioms

(1) An increase in the strength of strangers' ethnolinguistic identities will produce an increase in their attitudinal confidence regarding members of other groups' behavior and an increase in the anxiety they experience when interacting with members of other groups. This axiom holds *only* when members of the outgroup are perceived as "typical" and when ethnic status is activated.
(2) An increase in strangers' positive expectations will produce an increase in their attributional confidence regarding members of other groups' behavior and a decrease in the anxiety they experience when interacting with members of other groups.
(3) An increase in the similarity between strangers' ingroups and other groups will produce an increase in their attributional confidence regarding members of other groups' behavior and a decrease in the anxiety strangers experience when interacting with members of other groups.
(4) An increase in the networks strangers share with members of other groups will produce an increase in their attributional confidence regarding members of other groups' behavior and a decrease in the anxiety strangers experience when interacting with members of other groups.
(5) An increase in the interpersonal salience of the relationship strangers form with members of other groups moderates the effect of group dissimilarities and will produce an increase in their attributional confidence regarding members of other groups' behavior, as well as a decrease in the anxiety strangers experience when interacting with members of other groups.
(6) An increase in strangers' second language competence will produce an increase in their attributional confidence regarding members of other groups' behavior and a decrease in the anxiety experienced when interacting with members of other groups.
(7) An increase in strangers' self-monitoring will produce an increase in their attributional confidence regarding members of other groups' behavior and a decrease in the anxiety experienced when interacting with members of other groups.
(8) An increase in strangers' cognitive complexity will produce an increase in their attributional confidence regarding members of other groups' behavior and a decrease in the anxiety experienced when interacting with members of other groups.
(9) An increase in strangers' tolerance for ambiguity will produce an increase in their attributional confidence regarding members of other groups' behavior and a decrease in the anxiety experienced when interacting with members of other groups.
(10) An increase in strangers' attributional confidence regarding members of other groups' behavior will produce an increase in their intergroups adaptation and effectiveness.

(continued)

Table 6.2 Continued

(11)	A decrease in the anxiety strangers experience when interacting with members of other groups will produce an increase in their intergroup adaptation and effectiveness.
(12)	An increase in collectivism will produce an increase in the differences in attributional confidence between ingroup and outgroup communication.
(13)	An increase in uncertainty avoidance will produce an increase in the anxiety strangers experience when interacting with members of other groups.

SOURCE: Gudykunst (1988).

links uncertainty and anxiety to effectiveness and adaptation, a linkage not specified in any previous version of uncertainty reduction theory.

In addition to formal extensions of uncertainty reduction theory, Gudykunst and Hall (1987) integrated ethnolinguistic identity theory with Berger and Bradac's (1982) work on the relationship between language and uncertainty (see Table 6.3). Berger and Bradac suggest four alternative models regarding the relationship between language and uncertainty reduction that are influenced by ethnolinguistic identity. Model 1 specifies that people use others' language to develop hypotheses about their group affiliations, and on the basis of these hypotheses, judgments of similarity are made. The greater the similarity, the more uncertainty is reduced. Model 2 is similar except that a "judgment of psychological trait or state" replaces the judgment of group membership as the mediator for judging similarity. Model 3 posits that language leads to a judgment of group membership that in turn leads to a judgment of psychological trait or state that then forms the basis of a judgment of similarity. Similarity then leads to uncertainty reduction. Model 4 posits that only a judgment of similarity intervenes between language and uncertainty reduction.

Each of the four models "is probably valid in particular circumstances" (Berger & Bradac, 1982, p. 55), however, Berger and Bradac do not specify under which circumstances each model might be valid. Gudykunst and Lim's (1986) argument that the interpersonal intergroup salience of encounters are orthogonal dimensions provides a way to define the circumstances under which each of Berger and Bradac's models should be valid. Four quadrants can be isolated: (I) high interpersonal and high intergroup salience, (II) high interpersonal and low intergroup salience, (III) low interpersonal and high intergroup salience, (IV) low interpersonal and low intergroup salience. The major generative mechanism for intergroup behavior is ethnolinguistic identity, while the major generative mechanism for interpersonal behavior is personal identity.

Gudykunst and Hall (1987) suggest that when intergroup salience is high and interpersonal salience is low (Quadrant III) and ethnolinguistic identity is a major generative mechanism for behavior, individuals use language to make judgments of group affiliation on which judgments of similarity are made, and

TABLE 6.3
Interpersonal and Intergroup Salience and the Relationship Between Language and Uncertainty Reduction

Model 1 (high intergroup and low interpersonal salience)

language → perceived group membership (social categorization) → similarity → uncertainty reduction

Model 2 (high interpersonal and low intergroup salience)

language → perceived trait (trait attribution) → similarity → uncertainty reduction

Model 3 (low interpersonal and high intergroup salience)

language → perceived group membership (social categorization) → perceived trait (trait attribution) → similarity → uncertainty reduction

Model 4 (low interpersonal and low intergroup salience)

language → similarity → uncertainty reduction

SOURCE: Gudykunst and Hall (1987).

uncertainty is reduced (Model 1). When the intergroup salience is high and interpersonal salience also is high (Quadrant I) and both ethnolinguistic and personal identity are generative mechanisms for behavior, it is plausible that judgments of group membership are used to made judgments of psychological traits that form the basis for the judgment of similarity, which reduces uncertainty (Model 3). When intergroup salience is low and interpersonal salience is high (Quadrant II) and personal, *not* ethnolinguistic identity, is the major generative mechanism for behavior, language should lead directly to judgments of psychological traits that form basis of judgments of similarity that are used to reduce uncertainty (Model 2). Finally, when both interpersonal and intergroup salience are low (Quadrant IV), language may cue only similarity judgment (Model 4) because the interaction is of relatively low importance. Integrating this perspective with my theory cannot be accomplished here, but future work may reveal that scope and boundary conditions are necessary for some of the axioms based upon the interpersonal/intergroup salience of the encounter.

FUTURE DIRECTIONS

The cross-cultural research reviewed suggests that there are systematic variations in social penetration and uncertainty reduction processes across cultures that are explainable by Hofstede's (1980) and Hall's (1976) theories of cultural variability. The intercultural research examined indicates that predictions derived from Altman and Taylor's (1973) social penetration theory are applicable to relationships between people from different cultures. Specifically, cultural dissimilarities influence social penetration and uncertainty reduction processes in early stages of relationship development (i.e., orientation and exploratory affective exchange), but not later stages (i.e., full affective exchange and stable exchange). This conclusion is supported when one person or the dyad is studied. Social penetration and uncertainty reduction theories, therefore, provide a powerful heuristic for integrating the study of intracultural relationships.

There are several issues future work on culture and communication in interpersonal relationships must address. The most critical issue that needs to be addressed is the focus on uncertainty reduction. Planalp and Honeycutt's (1985) intracultural research indicated that an increase in uncertainty has negative consequences for interpersonal relationships. Sodetani and Gudykunst's (in press) intercultural study, in contrast, revealed both positive and negative outcomes for interpersonal relationships between members of different cultures following an increase in uncertainty. While there are potential methodological explanations for the different results of the two studies (e.g., Planalp and Honeycutt gave only negative examples of uncertainty increase, while Sodetani and Gudykunst did not provide examples), another plausible explanation involves differences between intracultural and intercultural relationships. Given the findings of these two studies and Berger's (1987) argument that initial affective responses to observable attributes, such as skin color and age (e.g., cues to group membership), can either impede or propel attempts to reduce uncertainty, it appears advisable for future work on the theory to focus on uncertainty change in general, rather than uncertainty reduction in particular.

Uncertainty change might best be conceived as a dialectical process, with continual shifts from increase to decrease and back to increase occurring throughout a relationship. Altman, Vinsel, and Brown (1981) make a similar argument vis-à-vis social penetration. They contend that openness and closedness shift back and forth as relationships become more intimate and social penetration increases: "We speculate that a period of openness eventually gives way to a degree of closedness—as people seek a change in their mode of dealing with one another, as they try to absorb the results of their interaction, as they experience psychological satiation, or because of other factors. This results, over time, in oscillations of openness-closedness" (Altman et al., 1981, pp. 143-144).

Viewing uncertainty change as a dialectical process might suggest an unpatterned relationship between uncertainty and intimacy of relationships. This, however, is not necessarily the case. Work on "chaos" in the physical and social sciences suggests that while disorder or chaos may appear to lurk under the facade of order, ordered patterns undergird the chaos (see Gleick, 1987, for an introduction to the study of chaos). The study of chaos, therefore, may provide a powerful heuristic for future theoretical development on uncertainty and communication.

Future theorizing also should integrate and/or examine the role of the use of ambiguity in general (Levine, 1985) and strategic ambiguity in particular (Eisenberg, 1984), as well as the role of "second guessing" (Hewes, Graham, Doelger, & Pavitt, 1985; Doelger, Hewes, & Graham, 1986) on uncertainty change. Ambiguity and uncertainty are related constructs. Recent work by Levine and Eisenberg suggests that individuals use ambiguity unconsciously and consciously in their relationships with others. Ambiguity plays a large role in communication in high-context cultures. Given the dialectic between uncertainty reduction and uncertainty increase that exists in social relationships and that ambiguity may or may not lead to an increase in uncertainty, the potential dialectic between certainty and ambiguity also should be investigated in future research.

In addition to focusing on uncertainty change and incorporating ambiguity, future work needs to include affective reactions to intercultural contact. Rose (1981) argues that intergroup (including intercultural) contact is a novel form of interaction for most people. Herman and Schield (1961) point out the following:

> The immediate psychological result of being in a new situation is lack of security. Ignorance of the potentialities inherent in the situation, of the means to reach a goal, and of the probable outcomes of an intended action causes insecurity. (p. 165)

Attempts to adapt to the ambiguity of new situations involves a cyclical pattern of tension reducing and information seeking behaviors (Ball-Rokeach, 1973). Information seeking is directed toward individuals increasing their ability to predict or explain their own and others' behavior in the environment; that is, reducing cognitive uncertainty. Tension reduction, on the other hand, is directed toward reducing the anxiety individuals experience. Stephan and Stephan (1985) argue that "anxiety stems from the anticipation of negative consequences. People appear to fear four types of negative consequences: psychological or behavior consequences for the self, and negative evaluations by members of the outgroup and the ingroup" (p. 159). In order to understand fully intercultural relationships, it is therefore necessary to study the anxiety associated with initial intergroup interactions (see Gudykunst, 1988, for an initial attempt to incorporate anxiety into a theory of intergroup communication).

Another issue that needs to be addressed in future work is the effect of anticipated interaction on uncertainty change. Berger (1979) argued that anticipated future interaction was one of the major conditions under which individuals try to reduce uncertainty. Kellermann's (1986) research, however, indicates that anticipated future interaction does not increase attempts to reduce uncertainty. Honeycutt's (1986) study, in contrast, suggests that situational expectancies (e.g., friendly, unfriendly, or no-expectancy) influences uncertainty. Given that intergroup communication often is associated with unfriendly expectancies (Stephan & Stephan, 1985), the influence of the expected outcome should be examined in future research. This position is consistent with Sunnafrank's (1986) argument that the "predicted outcome value" of a relationship plays a major role in uncertainty reduction processes. More generally, this line of argument suggests that expectation states theory (Berger & Zelditch, 1985) should be integrated with the research examined here. Such an integration should provide a powerful heuristic because expectation states theory focuses on how status characteristics (e.g., group memberships) influence expectations, which in turn affect behavior. As indicated earlier, expectancies are included in Gudykunst's (1988) theory (see Table 6.3). The difference between expectancies and interpersonal salience and the relationship of each (or some higher order concept) to predicted outcome value, however, still needs to be examined.

The environment in which interpersonal relationships form and develop also should be studied in future research. The majority of the research cited examined relationships between college students. All of the intercultural relationships studied were between international students studying in the United States and students at United States universities. These relationships, therefore, were initiated following United States cultural norms to some extent and the language spoken in all likelihood was English, since international students' native languages have low vitality (see Giles, Bourhis, & Taylor, 1977) in the United States. The language spoken and location should influence how interpersonal relationships between members of different cultures form and develop over time. This line of reasoning is consistent with Altman's transactional model (e.g., Altman & Rogoff, 1987). The location (e.g., the culture in which the individuals meet) will influence the temporal flow of relationship development, including the pace and rhythm of the relationship. The location also influences the environment in which the relationships occur. Both the physical environment (e.g., the places where people meet) and the social environment (e.g., with whom it is acceptable to communicate) vary across cultures and influence relationship development processes. The transaction among environment, temporal patterns, and psychological processes in interpersonal relations across cultures and in intercultural relationships, therefore, should be examined in future research.

In addition to the theoretical concerns outlined, there are several methodological issues that need to be taken into consideration in future work. Most cross-cultural studies to date, for example, have examined social penetration or uncertainty reduction processes in only two or three cultures. Although using a small number of cultures allows for the generalizability of the relationships among the variables in the theory to be tested, it does not allow theoretical predictions of the influence of culture on uncertainty reduction processes to be tested adequately. In order to accomplish this testing, studies with multiple (e.g., four or more) cultures need to be conducted. The influence of individualism-collectivism on uncertainty reduction processes in ingroup/out-group communication, for example, should be examined in at least two individualistic and two collectivistic cultures. This design is necessary in order to examine both within- and between-group variance.

With respect to intercultural research, more work needs to be conducted on the effect of cultural similarity/dissimilarity on social penetration and uncertainty reduction processes. Of particular interest is whether or not cultural similarity/dissimilarity has a differential influence across cultures. The influence of social/ethnolinguistic identity on social penetration and uncertainty reduction processes in intercultural/intergroup encounters needs to be investigated in more detail, including research on its affect across cultures.

Future cross-cultural and intercultural research also needs to move beyond the use of self-reports of social penetration and uncertainty reduction processes to examine actual communication behavior. Observations of communication behavior need to be conducted both in controlled laboratory settings and natural environments. While there are numerous "problems" in conducting cross-cultural and intercultural observational studies (see Gudykunst & Ting-Toomey, in press, for an overview), actual communication behavior must be observed for definitive tests of the generalizability of social penetration and uncertainty reduction theories to be conducted.

Finally, research and theorizing on culture and interpersonal relationship development needs to be integrated more completely with a higher-order theoretical perspective. Previous research has focused on culture and cultural similarity as separate concepts/variables. Both, however, can be considered aspects of group membership. By focusing upon group membership, cross-cultural and intercultural research on interpersonal relationship development can be integrated with theories of intergroup behavior (namely, Giles & Johnson, 1987, or Gudykunst, 1985a, 1986b, 1988). Such an integration will begin to address Doise's (1986) call for "articulation" of different levels of analysis in explanations of communication behavior.

REFERENCES

Alexander, A., Cronen, V. E., Kang, K., Tsou, B., & Banks, B. J. (1986). Patterns of topic sequencing and information gain: A comparative study of relationship development in Chinese and American Cultures. *Communication Quarterly, 34,* 66-78.

Altman, I. (1973). Reciprocity of interpersonal exchange. *Journal of the Theory of Social Behavior, 3,* 246-261.

Altman, I., & Haythorn, W. (1965). Interpersonal exchange in isolation. *Sociometry, 28,* 411-426.

Altman, I., & Rogoff, B. (1987). World views on psychology. In D. Stokols & I. Altman (Eds.), *Handbook of environmental psychology*. New York: John Wiley.
Altman, I., & Taylor, D. (1973). *Social penetration: The development of interpersonal relationships*. New York: Holt, Rinehart & Winston.
Altman, I., Vinsel, A., & Brown, B. (1981). Dialectical conceptions in social psychology: An application to social penetration and privacy regulation. In L. Berkowitz (Ed.), *Advances in experimental social psychology* (Vol. 14, pp. 107-160). New York: Academic Press.
Ball-Rokeach, S. J. (1973). From pervasive ambiguity to a definition of the situation. *Sociometry, 36*, 378-389.
Beebe, L. M., & Giles, H. (1984). Speech accommodation theories: A discussion in terms of second-language acquisition. *International Journal of the Sociology of Language, 46*, 5-32.
Bell, R. (1981). *World of friendship*. Beverly Hills, CA: Sage.
Berger, C. R. (1979). Beyond initial interactions. In H. Giles & R. St. Clair (Eds.), *Language and social psychology* (pp. 122-144). Oxford: Basil Blackwell.
Berger, C. R. (1987). Communicating under uncertainty. In M. E. Roloff & G. R. Miller (Eds.), *Interpersonal processes* (pp. 39-62). Newbury Park, CA: Sage.
Berger, C. R., & Bradac, J. J. (1982). *Language and social knowledge: Uncertainty in interpersonal relations*. London: Edward Arnold.
Berger, C. R., & Calabrese, R. (1975). Some explorations in initial interactions and beyond: Toward a developmental theory of interpersonal communication. *Human Communication Research, 1*, 99-112.
Berger, C. R., & Douglas, W. (1981). Studies in interpersonal epistemology III: Anticipated interaction, self-monitoring, and observational context selection. *Communication Monographs, 48*, 183-196.
Berger, C. R., & Gudykunst, W. B. (in press). Uncertainty and communication. In B. Dervin (Ed.), *Progress in communication science* (Vol. 10). Norwood, NJ: Ablex.
Berger, C. R., & Perkins, J. (1978). Studies in interpersonal epistemology I: Situational attributes in observational context selection. In B. Ruben (Ed.), *Communication yearbook* (Vol. 2, pp. 171-184). New Brunswick, NJ: Transaction.
Berger, J., & Zelditch, M. (Eds.). (1985). *Status, rewards, and influence*. San Francisco, Jossey-Bass.
Berlyne, D. (1960). *Conflict, arousal and curiosity*. New York: McGraw-Hill.
Berlyne, D. (1965). *Structure and direction in thinking*. New York: John Wiley.
Berscheid, E., Graziano, W., Monson, T., & Dermer, M. (1976). Outcome dependency: Attention, attribution, and attraction. *Journal of Personality and Social Psychology, 34*, 978-989.
Bishop, G. (1979). Perceived similarity in interracial attitudes and behavior. *Journal of Applied Social Psychology, 9*, 446-465.
Blau, P., & Schwartz, J. (1984). *Cross-cutting social circles: Testing a macro theory of intergroup relations*. New York: Academic Press.
Bond, M. H., & King, A.Y.C. (1985). Coping with the threat of westernization in Hong Kong. *International Journal of Intercultural Relations, 9*, 351-364.
Brandt, D. R., Miller, G. R., & Hocking, J. E. (1980a). Effects of self-monitoring and familiarity on deception detection. *Communication Quarterly, 28*, 3-10.
Brandt, D. R., Miller, G. R., & Hocking, J. E. (1980b). The truth-deception attribution: Effects of familiarity on the ability of observers to detect deception. *Human Communication Research, 6*, 99-110.
Byrne, D. (1971). *The attraction paradigm*. New York: Academic Press.
Clatterbuck, G. W. (1979). Attributional confidence and uncertainty in initial interactions. *Human Communication Research, 5*, 147-157.
Cline, R. J. (1983). The acquaintance process as relational communication. In R. Bostrom (Ed.), *Communication yearbook, 7* (pp. 396-412). Beverly Hills, CA: Sage.

Doelger, J. A., Hewes, D. E., & Graham, M. L. (1986). Knowing when to "second-guess": The mindful analysis of messages. *Human Communication Research, 12,* 301-338.
Doise, W. (1986). *Levels of explanation in social psychology.* Cambridge: Cambridge University Press.
Eisenberg, E. (1984). Ambiguity as a strategy in organizational communication. *Communication Monographs, 51,* 227-242.
Elliott, G. (1979). Some effects of deception and level of self-monitoring on planning and reacting to a self-presentation. *Journal of Personality and Social Psychology, 37,* 1282-1292.
Feigenbaum, W. M. (1977). Reciprocity in self-disclosure within the psychological interview. *Psychological Reports, 40,* 15-26.
Fenigstein, A., Scheier, M., & Buss, A. (1975). Public and private self-consciousness: Assessment and theory. *Journal of Consulting and Clinical Psychology, 43,* 522-527.
Forgas, J. P., & Bond, M. H. (1985). Cultural influences on the perception of interaction episodes. *Personality and Social Psychology Bulletin, 11,* 75-88.
Foschi, M., & Hales, W. H. (1979). The theoretical role of cross-cultural comparisons in experimental social psychology. In L. H. Eckensberger, W. J. Lonner, & Y. H. Poortinga (Eds.), *Cross-cultural contributions to psychology* (pp. 244-254). Lisse, The Netherlands: Swets & Zeitlinger.
Frankfurt, L. P. (1965). *The role of some individual and interpersonal factors in the acquaintance process.* Unpublished Ph.D. thesis, American University.
Gerard, H. G. (1963). Emotional uncertainty and social comparison. *Journal of Abnormal and Social Psychology, 66,* 568-573.
Giles, H., Bourghis, R., & Taylor, D. (1977). Towards a theory of language in ethnic group relations. In H. Giles (Ed.), *Language, ethnicity, and intergroup relations* (pp. 307-347). London: Academic Press.
Giles, H., & Byrne, J. (1982). An intergroup approach to second language acquisition. *Journal of Multilingual and Multicultural Development, 3,* 17-40.
Giles, H., Garrett, P., & Coupland, N. (1987, September). *Language acquisition in the Basque country: Invoking and extending the intergroup model.* Paper presented at the Second World Basque Congress: Basque Language Conference, San Sebastian, Basque Country, Spain.
Giles, H., & Johnson, P. (1981). The role of language in ethnic group relations. In J. Turner & H. Giles (Eds.), *Intergroup behavior* (pp. 199-243). Chicago: University of Chicago Press.
Giles, H., & Johnson, P. (1987). Ethnolinguistic identity theory: A social psychological approach to language maintenance. *International Journal of the Sociology of Language, 68,* 69-99.
Gleick, J. (1987). *Chaos: Making a new science.* New York: Viking.
Gudykunst, W. B. (1983a). Similarities and differences in perceptions of initial intracultural and intercultural encounters. *The Southern Speech Communication Journal, XLIX,* 49-65.
Gudykunst, W. B. (1983b). Uncertainty reduction and predictability of behavior in low- and high-context cultures. *Communication Quarterly, 31,* 49-55.
Gudykunst, W. B. (1985a). A model of uncertainty reduction in intercultural encounters. *Journal of Language and Social Psychology, 4,* 79-98.
Gudykunst, W. B. (1985b). An exploratory comparison of close intracultural and intercultural friendships. *Communication Quarterly, 33,* 270-273.
Gudykunst, W. B. (1985c). The influence of cultural similarity, type of relationship, and self-monitoring on uncertainty reduction process. *Communication Monographs, 52,* 203-217.
Gudykunst, W. B. (1986a). Ethnicity, type of relationship, and intraethnic and interethnic uncertainty reduction. In Y. Kim (Ed.), *Interethnic communication* (pp. 201-224). Beverly Hills, CA: Sage.
Gudykunst, W. B. (1986b). Toward a theory of intergroup communication. In W. Gudykunst (Ed.), *Intergroup communication* (pp. 152-167). London: Edward Arnold.
Gudykunst, W. B. (1988). Uncertainty and anxiety. In Y. Y. Kim & W. B. Gudykunst (Eds.), *Theory in intercultural communication.* Newbury Park, CA: Sage.

Gudykunst, W. B. (in press). *Strangeness and similarity: A theory of interpersonal and intergroup communication.* Clevendon, England: Multilingual Matters.
Gudykunst, W. B., Chua, E., & Gray, A. (1987). Cultural dissimilarities and uncertainty reduction process. In M. McLaughlin (Ed.), *Communication yearbook 10* (pp. 456-469). Beverly Hills, CA: Sage.
Gudykunst, W. B., & Hall, B. J. (1987, July). *Ethnolinguistic identity and uncertainty reduction in interpersonal and intergroup encounters.* Paper presented at the Third International Conference on Language and Social Psychology, Bristol, England.
Gudykunst, W. B., & Hammer, M. R. (1988). The influence of ethnicity, gender, and dyadic composition on uncertainty reduction in initial interactions. *Journal of Black Studies, 18,* 191-214.
Gudykunst, W. B., & Hammer, M. R. (in press). The influence of social identity and intimacy of interethnic relationships on uncertainty reduction processes. *Human Communication Research.*
Gudykunst, W. B., & Lim, T. S. (1986). A perspective for the study of intergroup communication. In W. Gudykunst (Ed.), *Intergroup communication* (pp. 1-9). London: Edward Arnold.
Gudykunst, W., & Nishida, T. (1983). Social penetration in Japanese and North American friendships. In R. Bostrom (Ed.), *Communication yearbook 7* (pp. 592-610). Beverly Hills, CA: Sage.
Gudykunst, W. B., & Nishida, T. (1984). Individual and cultural influences on uncertainty reduction. *Communication Monographs, 51,* 23-36.
Gudykunst, W. B., & Nishida, T. (1986a). Attributional confidence in low- and high-context cultures. *Human Communication Research, 12,* 525-549.
Gudykunst, W. B., & Nishida, T. (1986b). The influence of cultural variability on perceptions of communication behavior associated with relationship terms. *Human Communication Research, 13.* 147-166.
Gudykunst, W. B., Nishida, T., & Chua, E. (1986). Uncertainty reduction in Japanese-North American dyads. *Communication Research Reports, 3,* 39-46.
Gudykunst, W. B., Nishida, T., & Chua, E. (1987). Perceptions of social penetration in Japanese-North American dyads. *International Journal of Intercultural Relations, 51,* 256-278.
Gudykunst, W. B., Nishida, T., Koike, H., & Shiino, N. (1986). The influence of language on uncertainty reduction: An exploratory study of Japanese-Japanese and Japanese-North American interactions. In M. McLaughlin (Ed.), *Communication yearbook 9* (pp. 555-575). Beverly Hills, CA: Sage.
Gudykunst, W. B., Nishida, T., & Schmidt, K. (1988, May). *Cultural, personality, and relational influences on uncertainty reduction in ingroup vs. outgroup and same vs. opposite sex relationships: Japan and the United States.* Paper presented at the International Communication Association Convention, New Orleans.
Gudykunst, W. B., Sodetani, L. L., & Sonoda, K. (1987). Uncertainty reduction in Japanese-American-Caucasian relationships in Hawaii. *Western Journal of Speech Communication, 51,* 256-278.
Gudykunst, W. B., & Ting-Toomey, S., with Chua, E. (in press). *Culture and interpersonal communication.* Newbury Park, CA: Sage.
Gudykunst, W. B., Yang, S. M., & Nishida, T. (1985). A cross-cultural test of uncertainty reduction theory: Comparisons of acquaintance, friend, and dating relationships in Japan, Korea, and the United States. *Human Communication Research, 11,* 407-454.
Gudykunst, W. B., Yang, S. M., & Nishida, T. (1987). Cultural differences in self-consciousness and self-monitoring. *Communication Research, 14,* 7-36.
Gudykunst, W. B., Yoon, Y. C., & Nishida, T. (1987). The influence of individualism-collectivism on perceptions of communication in ingroup and outgroup relationships. *Communication Monographs, 54,* 295-306.
Hall, B. J., & Gudykunst, W. B. (1986). The intergroup theory of second language ability. *Journal of Language and Social Psychology, 5,* 291-302.

Hall, E. T. (1976). *Beyond culture.* New York: Doubleday.
Hammer, M. R., & Gudykunst, W. B. (1987). The influence of ethnicity and sex on social penetration in close friendships. *Journal of Black Studies, 17,* 418-437.
Hammer, M., Gudykunst, W., & Wiseman, R. (1978). Dimensions of intercultural effectiveness. *International Journal of Intercultural Relations, 2,* 382-393.
Hays, R. (1985). A longitudinal study of friendship development. *Journal of Personality and Social Psychology, 48,* 909-924.
Hecht, M. (1978). The conceptualization and measurement of communication satisfaction. *Human Communication Research, 4,* 253-264.
Hecht, M. (1984). Satisfying communication and relationship labels: Intimacy and length of relationship as perceptual frames of naturalistic conversations. *Western Journal of Speech Communication, 48,* 201-216.
Herman, S., & Schield, E. (1961). The stranger group in a cross-cultural situation. *Sociometry, 24,* 165-176.
Hewes, D. E., Graham, M. K., Doelger, J., & Pavitt, C. (1985). "Second-guessing": Message interpretation in social networks. *Human Communication Research, 11,* 299-334.
Hofstede, G. (1980). *Cultures consequences.* Beverly Hills, CA: Sage.
Hofstede, G. (1983). Dimensions of national cultures in fifty countries and three regions. In J. Deregowski, S. Dziurawiec, & R. Annis (Eds.), *Expiscations in cross-cultural psychology* (pp. 335-355). Lisse, The Netherlands: Swets & Zeitlinger.
Hofstede, G., & Bond, M. (1984). Hofstede's culture dimensions: An independent validation using Rokeach's value survey. *Journal of Cross-Cultural Psychology, 15,* 417-433.
Honeycutt, J. M. (1986, May). *Processing information about others and attributional confidence in initial interaction on the basis of expectancies.* Paper presented at the International Communication Association Convention, Chicago.
Hsu, F. L. K. (1981). *American and Chinese* (3rd ed.). Honolulu: University of Hawaii Press.
Ickes, W., & Barnes, R. (1977). The role of sex and self-monitoring on unstructured dyadic interaction. *Journal of Personality and Social Psychology, 35,* 315-330.
Ishii, S. (1984). Enryo-sasshi communication: A key to understanding Japanese interpersonal relations. *Cross-Currents, 11,* 49-58.
Johnson, C., & Johnson, F. (1975). Interaction rules and ethnicity. *Social Forces, 54,* 45[illegible]-4[illegible]
Jourard, S. M. (1960). Knowing, liking, and the "dyadic effect" in men's self-disclosure. *M[illegible]rill Palmer Quarterly of Behavior and Development, 6,* 178-186.
Kellermann, K. (1986). Anticipation of future interaction and information exchange in initial interaction. *Human Communication Research, 13,* 41-75.
Knapp, M. (1978). *Social intercourse: From greetings to goodbye.* Boston: Allyn & Bacon.
Knapp, M., Ellis, D., & Williams, B. (1980). Perceptions of communication behavior associated with relationship terms. *Communication Monographs, 47,* 262-278.
Lalljee, M., & Cook, M. (1973). Uncertainty in first encounters. *Journal of Personality and Social Psychology, 26,* 137-141.
Lambert, W. E., Mermigis, L., & Taylor, D. M. (1986). Greek Canadian's attitudes toward own group and other Canadian ethnic groups: A test of the multiculturalism hypothesis. *Canadian Journal of Behavioural Sciences, 18,* 35-51.
Leung, K., & Bond, M. H. (1984). The impact of cultural collectivism on reward allocation. *Journal of Personality and Social Psychology, 47,* 793-804.
Levine, D. N. (1985). *The flight from ambiguity.* Chicago: University of Chicago Press.
Lewin, K. (1948). *Resolving social conflicts.* New York: Harper & Row.
Lonner, W. (1980). The search for psychological universals. In H. Triandis & W. Lambert (Eds.), *Handbook of cross-cultural psychology* (Vol. 1, pp. 143-203). Boston: Allyn & Bacon.
Lu, H. N., & Gudykunst, W. B. (1988, February). *The relationship between social penetration and uncertainty reduction across relationships and cultures.* Paper presented at the Western Speech Communication Association Convention, San Diego, CA.

McCroskey, J. M. (1978). Validity of the PRCA as an index of oral communication apprehension. *Communication Monographs, 45,* 192-203.
Miller, G. R., & Steinberg, M. (1975). *Between people.* Chicago: Science Research Associates.
Nakane, C. (1974). The social system reflected in interpersonal communication. In J. Condon & M. Saito (Eds.), *Intercultural encounters with Japan* (pp. 124-131). Tokyo: Simul Press.
Nishida, T. (1977). An analysis of a cultural concept affecting Japanese interpersonal communication. *Communication, 6,* 69-80.
Okabe, R. (1983). Cultural assumptions of East and West: Japan and the United States. In W. Gudykunst (Ed.), *Intercultural communication theory: Current perspectives* (pp. 21-44). Beverly Hills, CA: Sage.
Pak, A., Dion, K. L., & Dion, K. K. (1985). Correlates of self-confidence with English among Chinese students in Toronto. *Canadian Journal of Behavioural Sciences, 17,* 369-378.
Parks, M. R., & Adelman, M. B. (1983). Communication networks and the development of romantic relationships: An expansion of uncertainty reduction theory. *Human Communication Research, 10,* 55-80.
Planalp, S., & Honeycutt, J. (1985). Events that increase uncertainty in interpersonal relationships. *Human Communication Research, 11,* 593-604.
Prisbell, M., & Andersen, J. F. (1980). The importance of perceived homophily, level of uncertainty, feeling good, safety, and self-disclosure in interpersonal relationships. *Communication Quarterly, 28,* 22-33.
Rose, T. L. (1981). Cognitive and dyadic processes in intergroup contact. In D. Hamilton (Ed.), *Cognitive processes in stereotyping and intergroup behavior* (pp. 259-302). Hillsdale, NJ: Lawrence Erlbaum.
Scheier, M. F., & Carver, C. S. (1977). Self-focused attention and expression of emotion: Attraction, repulsion, elation, and depression. *Journal of Personality and Social Psychology, 35,* 625-636.
Scheier, M. F., Buss, A. H., & Buss, D. M. (1978). Self-consciousness, self-report of aggressiveness and aggression. *Journal of Research in Personality, 12,* 133-140.
Scheier, M. F., & Carver, C. S. (1982). Self-consciousness, outcome expectancy, and persistence. *Journal of Research in Personality, 16,* 409-418.
Sherif, M. (1966). *In common predicament: Social psychology of intergroup conflict and cooperation.* New York: Houghton Mifflin.
Siegman, A. W., & Reynolds, M. A. (1983). Self-monitoring and speech in feigned and unfeigned lying. *Journal of Personality and Social Psychology, 6,* 1325-1333.
Simard, L. (1981). Cross-cultural interaction. *Journal of Social Psychology, 113,* 171-192.
Simmel, G. (1950). The stranger. *The sociology of Georg Simmel* (K. Wolff, Ed. & Trans.). New York: Free Press.
Snyder, M. (1974). Self-monitoring of expressive behavior. *Journal of Personality and Social Psychology, 30,* 526-537.
Snyder, M. (1979). Self-monitoring processes. In L. Berkowitz (Ed.), *Advances in experimental social psychology* (Vol. 12, pp. 85-128). New York: Academic Press.
Snyder, M., Gangestad, S., & Simpson, J. (1983). Choosing friends as activity partners. *Journal of Personality and Social Psychology, 45,* 1061-1072.
Snyder, M., & Monson, T. (1975). Persons, situations, and the control of social behavior. *Journal of Personality and Social Behavior, 32,* 637-644.
Sodetani, L. L., & Gudykunst, W. B. (in press). The effects of surprising events on intercultural relationships. *Communication Research Reports.*
Stephan, W. G., & Stephan, C. W. (1985). Intergroup anxiety. *Journal of Social Issues, 41,* 157-166.
Stephenson, G. (1981). Intergroup bargaining and negotiation. In J. Turner & H. Giles (Eds.), *Intergroup behavior* (pp. 168-198). Chicago: University of Chicago Press.

Sudweeks, S., Gudykunst, W. B., Ting-Toomey, S., & Nishida, T. (1988, July). *Japanese-North American interpersonal relationship development.* Paper presented at the Fourth International Conference on Personal Relationships, Vancouver.

Sunnafrank, M. (1986). Predicted outcome value during initial interactions: A reformulation of uncertainty reduction theory. *Human Communication Research, 13,* 3-33.

Tajfel, H. (1978). Social categorization, social identity, and social comparison. In H. Tajfel (Ed.), *Differentiation between social groups* (pp. 61-76). London: Academic Press.

Tardy, C. H., & Hoseman, L. A. (1982). Self-monitoring and self-disclosure flexibility: A research note. *Western Journal of Speech Communication, 46,* 92-97.

Taylor, D. (1968). The development of interpersonal relationships: Social penetration processes. *Journal of Social Psychology, 75,* 79-90.

Taylor, D., & Altman, I. (1966). *Intimacy-scaled stimuli for use in studies of interpersonal relations* (Report No. 9). Washington, DC: Naval Medical Research Institute.

Ting-Toomey, S. (1981). Ethnic identify and close friendship in Chinese-American college students. *International Journal of Intercultural Relations, 5,* 383-406.

Ting-Toomey, S. (1985). Toward a theory of conflict and culture. In W. B. Gudykunst, L. P. Stewart, & S. Ting-Toomey (Eds.), *Communication, culture, and organizational processs* (pp. 71-86). Beverly Hills, CA: Sage.

Triandis, H. C. (1978). Some universals of social behavior. *Personality and Social Psychology Bulletin, 4,* 1-16.

Triandis, H. C. (1986). Collectivism vs. individualism: A reconceptualization of a basic concept in cross-cultural psychology. In C. Bagley & G. Verma (Eds.), *Personality, cognition, and values: Cross-cultural perspectives of childhood and adolescence* (pp. 57-89). London: Macmillan.

Tsujimura, A. (1987). Some characteristics of Japanese way of communication. In D. L. Kincaid (Ed.), *Communication theory from Eastern and Western perspectives.* New York: Academic Press.

Weick, K. (1979). *The social psychology of organizing* (2nd ed.). Reading, MA: Addison-Wesley.

Wetherall, M. (1982). Cross-cultural studies of minimal groups: Implications for the social identity theory of intergroup relations. In H. Tajfel (Ed.), *Social identity and intergroup relations* (pp. 207-240). Cambridge: Cambridge University Press.

Won-Doornink, M. (1979). On getting to know you: The association between stage of relationship and reciprocity of self-disclosure. *Journal of Experimental Social Psychology, 15,* 229-241.

Won-Doornink, M. (1985). Self-disclosure and reciprocity in conversation: A cross-national study. *Social Psychology Quarterly, 48,* 97-107.

Wright, P. H. (1978). Toward a theory of friendship based on a conception of self. *Human Communication Research, 4,* 196-207.

Yum, J. O. (1987a). Korean philosophy and communication. In D. Kincaid (Ed.), *Communication theory from Eastern and Western perspectives.* New York: Academic Press.

Yum, J. O. (1987b). The practice of uye-ri in interpersonal relationships in Korea. In D. Kincaid (Ed.), *Communication theory for Eastern and Western perspectives.* New York: Academic Press.

Uncertainty in Interpersonal Relationships: A Predicted Outcome Value Interpretation of Gudykunst's Research Program

MICHAEL SUNNAFRANK
Texas A & M University

UNARGUABLY the most prolific communication research program in the 1980s is being conducted by Gudykunst and his associates. This program examines cultural differences related to communication, and the effects these differences have on communication in the development of intracultural and intercultural relationships. These foci allow Gudykunst to advance our understanding of cultural and interpersonal communication processes, as well as the interrelationship of these processes.

Gudykunst's research tests various theoretical perspectives on interpersonal and intercultural communication. Social penetration theory (Altman & Taylor, 1973) plays a central role in several of his studies (Gudykunst, 1985a; Gudykunst & Nishida, 1983, 1986a, 1986b; Gudykunst, Nishida, & Chua, 1987). However, uncertainty reduction theory (Berger, 1979, 1987; Berger & Bradac, 1982; Berger & Calabrese, 1975) is used to inform and guide the majority of Gudykunst's work (Gudykunst, 1983a, 1983b, 1985b, 1985c, 1986; Gudykunst, Chua, & Gray, 1987; Gudykunst & Nishida, 1984, 1986a; Gudykunst, Nishida, & Chua, 1986; Gudykunst, Nishida, Koike, & Shiino, 1986; Gudykunst, Sodetani, & Sonoda, 1987; Gudykunst, Yang, & Nishida, 1985, 1987).

Gudykunst (this volume) interprets findings from his program as being supportive of uncertainty reduction theory. An alternative view suggests that the theoretical support provided may be equivocal. My own (Sunnafrank,

Correspondence and requests for reprints: Michael Sunnafrank, Department of Speech Communication, Texas A&M University, College Station, TX 77843.

Communication Yearbook 12, pp. 355-370

1986) review of uncertainty reduction research reveals limited, weak evidence for theoretical propositions. This review includes just two studies from Gudykunst's research program (Gudykunst & Nishida, 1984; Gudykunst, Yang, & Nishida, 1985), the results of which reflect the general pattern of weak theoretical support: While the overall uncertainty model received partial support, only three of 25 uncertainty reduction predictions tested in the two studies received consistent support. A more comprehensive review of Gudykunst's findings regarding support for specific uncertainty reduction propositions appears to be in order, and is provided in this commentary.

The focus for this review is supplied by my (Sunnafrank 1986) predicted outcome value theory. Basic assumptions and propositions of this perspective conflict with those of uncertainty reduction theory (Berger & Calabrese, 1975), suggesting that a reinterpretation of Gudykunst's findings from a predicted outcome value orientation might prove fruitful. This possibility is strengthened by Gudykunst, Nishida, and Schmidt's (1988) cross-cultural research, which provides consistent support for all predicted outcome value propositions tested.

As originally formulated, predicted outcome value theory is limited to initial interaction situations (Sunnafrank, 1986). Since much of the research conducted by Gudykunst and his associates involves more developed relationships, this commentary examines relational growth implications of the predicted outcome value position. The relative support for conflicting uncertainty reduction and predicted outcome value propositions provided by Gudykunst's research program are then examined. Although cultural influences are considered in this examination, the major concern of this commentary is on evaluating these contrasting theoretical positions regarding interpersonal communication.

PREDICTED OUTCOME VALUE THEORY

Predicted outcome value theory (Sunnafrank, 1986) presents 22 formal propositions and hypotheses regarding the interrelationships of variables addressed in Berger and Calabrese's (1975) original uncertainty reduction theory (URT). A total of 16 of the relationships posited in predicted outcome value (POV) theory conflict with corresponding uncertainty reduction axioms and theorems. Research evidence warrants a close examination of the POV alternative. My (Sunnafrank 1986) review of uncertainty reduction research demonstrates no support for URT propositions in approximately half of more than 100 tests conducted, and primarily weak support in the remaining tests. While no direct evidence regarding POV proposals is provided by this research, the great preponderance of findings are consistent with outcome value expectations.

Predicted outcome value theory posits that the primary relational goal of individuals is the maximization of their outcomes, an assumption consistent with various reward-costs orientations on interpersonal behavior (Altman & Taylor, 1973; Miller & Steinberg, 1975; Thibaut & Kelley, 1959). In order to meet this goal, the POV perspective assumes that individuals make predictions about the outcomes to be obtained in the relational future. Predicted outcome value theory further proposes that these predictions are employed to guide individuals' actions in a manner that would maximize their outcomes: Such predictions provide a basis for deciding whether to avoid, restrict, or seek future relational contact, and for determining how to proceed with the interaction to realize the most positive consequences.

I developed three general outcome value propositions that are directly relevant to uncertainty reduction theory (Sunnafrank, 1986):

> First, individuals should be more attracted to partners and relationships when greater predicted outcome values are expected in the relational future. Second, increasingly positive predicted outcomes will produces more communicative attempts to extend interaction and establish future contact. Conversely, increasingly negative predicted outcomes will result in communicative attempts to terminate or curtail the conversation and future contact. Finally, individuals will attempt to guide conversations toward topics expected to result in the most positive predicted outcomes. (pp. 10-11)

Predicted outcome value theory proposes that uncertainty reduction plays an important role in outcome-maximization processes. Obviously, uncertainty reduction regarding partners' likely actions and reactions should enhance one's perceived ability to predict outcome value alternatives, and to determine how to best serve outcome maximization goals. Reducing uncertainty about future relational behavior would, therefore, be an important vehicle for achieving the primary goal of increasing outcome values.

I employ this outcome value function of uncertainty reduction to reformulate the basic axioms proposed by Berger and Calabrese (1975). I argue that the original axioms are inaccurate, in part, because this formulation implicitly assumes uncertainty reduction produces positive interpersonal outcomes, and further relational development. Conversely, POV expects that reduced uncertainty could lead to either positive or negative outcome value predictions. While uncertainty reduction that results in partners mutually predicting positive outcome values should produce many of the relational consequences proposed by Berger and Calabrese (1975), decreased uncertainty that results in one or both partners predicting negative outcome values should generally produce opposite influences. As a result of the uncertainty reduction perspective's implicit positive bias, POV propositions generally agree with corresponding URT axioms when positive predicted outcome values are expected, but conflict when predicted outcome values are negative. In a recent chapter, Berger (1987) advances a similar position regarding the interrelationship of uncertainty reduction and outcome values, but generally limits his discussion to attraction (Axiom 7) while largely ignoring potential influences on the relationships specified in the remaining uncertainty reduction axioms.

Predicted outcome value and uncertainty reduction perspectives have developed as theories of initial interaction behavior. Most subsequent uncertainty reduction studies have attempted to generalize the basic URT axioms and theorems beyond initial acquaintance (e.g., Gudykunst, 1986; Gudykunst, Yang, & Nishida, 1985; Parks & Adelman, 1983), with mixed results. These results may be partially a result of inaccuracies in the relationships specified by URT axioms, regardless of acquaintance stage. It is also possible that the straightforward application of the specified initial interaction processes to more developed interpersonal relationships is unwarranted.

This possibility raises a similar concern regarding the potential applicability of POV propositions to later relational stages. Prior to examining the relative support for POV and URT provided by Gudykunst's research program (much of which focuses on these more developed relationships) it is necessary to briefly address two potentially important developmental influences on predicted outcome values: outcome values projected for available alternatives to a relationship, and differences between experienced and predicted outcome value levels in a relationship.

I have proposed that predicted outcome value levels are the primary determinant of change during initial interactions. Following Thibaut and Kelley (1959), I argue that subsequent change "may be more influenced by how these levels compare to those expected from alternative activities, when such activities are readily available" (Sunnafrank, 1986, p. 30). The POV assumption that individuals attempt to maximize their outcomes suggests that when individuals have two or more alternatives available to them, they will choose to engage in the alternative predicted to result in the most positive outcome values.

From this perspective, individuals should attempt to maintain or escalate relationship involvement levels only when that is the most positive activity available. In some cases, participating in a relationship with highly positive predicted outcome values might conflict with an activity projected to be even more attractive, while in other situations, relationships with negative outcome values might be the best alternative available. Attempts to generalize POV propositions beyond initial interactions will require assessing predicted outcome values for relationships relative to these available alternatives. It may be that this type of assessment would be relevant even prior to and during initial relational contact. For example, individuals may well make outcome comparisons among available alternatives in deciding whether or not to contact a particular stranger. Though this may occasionally be an important consideration, the influence of these comparisons and the need to assess this influence should increase substantially as relationships move beyond initial acquaintance.

It should be noted that the preceding position would lead to an expectation that most continuing relationships should exhibit generally positive predicted outcome values. Given this, and the fact that POV and URT propositions frequently agree when predicted outcome values are positive, research on existing interpersonal relationships may often support predictions from both theories. To assess the relative accuracy of such propositions, tests involving existing relationships known to possess both positive and negative predicted outcome value levels would be needed.

Another important source of influence in the development of interpersonal relationships is discrepancies between experienced and predicted outcome values. As relationships develop beyond initial interactions, participants have increasing opportunities to check the accuracy of their predictions. If experienced outcome values conform to expectations, earlier decisions about the partner, the relationship, and how to proceed would be confirmed. When experienced and predicted outcome values conflict, individuals may question and alter predicted outcome value levels. The influence of this discrepancy should depend on several factors; such as the magnitude of the discrepancy, how certain the individual had been of their previous predictions, whether the discrepancy is perceived as resulting from a basic misunderstanding of the partner, and the perceived likelihood of such discrepancies recurring.

Perhaps the most important influence of the predicted and experienced difference would stem from its direction. Experienced outcome values that vary in a positive direction from those predicted should result in more positive predicted outcome values for the relational future, while more negative experienced values should have the opposite effect. If the magnitude of this change is substantial, major relational changes are likely to follow.

Recent research on uncertainty-producing events in interpersonal relationships appears to support this POV interpretation. Planalp and Honeycutt's (1985) findings suggest that events reflecting an unexpected and negative shift in relational outcome values produce the expected negative relational consequences. Sodetani and Gudykunst's (in press) research confirms this, and further reveals that uncertainty-increasing events reflecting positive shifts may result in the positive relational consequences expected by predicted outcome value theory. Taken together, these findings support the position that a key to relational change is changing expectations concerning relational outcome values. Sodetani and Gudykunst's work strongly suggests that it is the direction of change in predicted outcome values—not change in uncertainty levels—that determines the direction of subsequent relational change.

This discussion of available alternatives and discrepancies between experienced and predicted outcome values indicates that only slight modifications of the POV perspective may be needed in applying it to relational stages beyond initial interaction. None of these modifications involves changing the three basic theoretical propositions. Given this, the relative support provided by Gudykunst's research program for URT axioms and their POV counterparts can now be examined.

GUDYKUNST'S RESEARCH PROGRAM

Gudykunst's findings have almost invariably been produced through variations on a single research method. Research participants from various cultures are asked to think of a real or imagined communicative relationship/encounter with an individual from their own or another culture. The researchers further specify some demographic characteristics of the person, and how well-acquainted the participants are to be with this individual (e.g., stranger, acquaintance, friend). Participants are asked to continue thinking of this individual while completing a questionnaire concerning their relationship. To assess cross-cultural variability on the measures of interest, responses of different cultural groups are examined and compared. In studies focusing on the influence of cultural similarity, responses to intracultural relations are compared to those obtained for intercultural relations. Major methodological differences between the studies in Gudykunst's program involve variations in the cultural groups and types of personal relationships examined, and in the measures taken.

Gudykunst and his associates systematically employ this method to examine several aspects of uncertainty reduction theory, including the associations specified in the original axioms (Berger & Calabrese, 1975). These axioms posit relationships between uncertainty level and amount of communication, nonverbal affiliative expressiveness, information seeking, intimacy level of communication content, reciprocity rate, similarity, and liking.

Berger and Calabrese (1975) propose a reciprocal causal relationship between uncertainty level and amount of verbal communication. (Axiom 1). This proposal posits that, in initial interactions, uncertainty is reduced by increasing the amount of verbal communication and that the resulting uncertainty reduction serves to further increase amounts of verbal communication. No research to date has examined the reciprocal causal nature of this relationship, but several studies from Gudykunst's program have tested for the predicted negative association between uncertainty level and amount of verbal communication—with mixed results.

Gudykunst's initial interaction research provides little support for Berger and Calabrese's Axiom 1. The only work reported is Gudykunst, Nishida, Koike, and Shiino's (1986) study of Japanese responses to language spoken in imagined intra- and intercultural interactions with strangers. Support for the posited relationship between amount of verbal communication and uncertainty level was observed in one of two intercultural conditions, but no support was forthcoming from either intracultural condition. These findings are consistent with previous research on U.S. samples which indicates that a negative association between amount of verbal communication and uncertainty level in initial interactions, if present, is weak (Clatterbuck, 1979).

Several tests of Axiom 1 in relationships beyond the initial interaction period are provided by Gudykunst's program. Gudykunst, Yang, and Nishida's (1985) cross-cultural research on acquaintance, friend, and dating relationships in Japan, Korea, and the United States provides support in only three of nine tests. Gudykunst, Sodetani, and Sonoda's (1987) examination of interethnic relations in Hawaii supports Axiom 1 with Caucasian, but not Japanese subjects. Gudykunst's (1985b) research on U.S. intercultural relationships provides evidence of the predicted association between amount of verbal communication and uncertainty level, as does Gudykunst's (1985c) U.S. data on intra- and intercultural relationships between both acquaintances and friends. However, support from this last study is equivocal since only one of four correlational tests reported is statistically significant. Overall, only 6 of 16 tests support Axiom 1 in existing relationships.

I have (Sunnafrank 1986) proposed an alternative view of the relationship between amount of communication and uncertainty reduction. Proposition 1 of POV predicts that when uncertainty reduction results in positive predicted outcome values, the amount of verbal communication will increase, but when it is associated with negative predicted outcome values, the amount of verbal communication will decrease. This proposition is based, in part, on the assumption that individuals will attempt to continue interaction and relationships with partners who are projected to provide positive outcomes, but they will attempt to curtail or end conversations and relationships with those expected to provide negative outcomes. Increasing the amount of verbal communication in positive situations, and decreasing it in negative situations would be one means of engaging in such attempts. Additionally, when attempts to continue or restrict the conversation are successful, the amount of verbal communication produced in the interaction and relationship would further conform to POV's Proposition 1 expectations.

This proposition was originally formulated to apply to early acquaintance situations in which initial uncertainty levels would be relatively high. Initial interaction findings reported above are consistent with the POV position that in such situations the relationship between amount of communication and uncertainty is determined by the value of predicted outcomes. Because neither strongly positive nor negative outcome value trends should be present in these situations, lack of support for an overall uncertainty-amount of verbal communication association would be expected. The relationship between amount of verbal communication and uncertainty should increase in complexity as acquaintance moves beyond initial interactions, as Berger (1987) points out. Even so, low levels of uncertainty associated with positive predicted outcome values should continue to produce greater amounts of verbal communication *than when associated with negative outcome values*. Comparisons of existing relationships with such differing predicted outcome values would be needed to support this speculation.

Axiom 2 of uncertainty reduction theory (Berger & Calabrese, 1975) proposes that increases in nonverbal affiliative expressiveness decrease uncertainty, which serves to further increase nonverbal affiliation. Research directly examining this association is limited to three studies from Gudykunst's program. Support is provided by Gudykunst, Sodetani, and Sonoda's (1987) examination of existing Japanese and Caucasian interethnic relations. Gudykunst and Nishida (1984) report a moderate association between intent to engage in nonverbal affiliative behaviors with an imagined stranger and attributional confidence for their Japanese sample, but not for their U.S. sample. Gudykunst, Nishida, Koike, and Shiino's (1986) work provides no support for Axiom 2 in either initial intra- or intercultural encounters for Japanese. Taken together, these results indicate that uncertainty level and nonverbal affiliative expressiveness may be negatively associated in ongoing interpersonal rélationships, but that such an association is unlikely in initial encounters.

Predicted outcome value theory (Sunnafrank, 1986) proposes that decreases in uncertainty increase nonverbal affiliative expressiveness when forecasted outcome values are positive, but that decreasing uncertainty produces decreases in these nonverbal behaviors when outcome values are negative (Proposition 2). When individuals project positive outcome values for a conversation or relationship, they should be expected to employ nonverbal affiliative behavior in an attempt to continue the relationship. Projections of negative outcomes should produce decreases in nonverbal affiliative behavior as individuals attempt to terminate or restrict the conversation or relationship. Therefore, decreasing uncertainty could lead to either increases or decreases in nonverbal affiliative expressiveness, depending on the associated predicted outcome value levels.

The general lack of support for URT, Axiom 2 in Gudykunst's initial interaction work (Gudykunst & Nishida, 1984; Gudykunst, Nishida, Koike, & Shiino, 1986), is unsurprising given this formulation. Subjects were given limited information about a stranger, and were then asked to report their intent to engage in nonverbal affiliative behaviors with that stranger. Some research participants may have responded to the information provided by projecting mildly positive predicted outcome values, with others projecting slightly negative values. In the former case, greater certainty would produce increases in nonverbal affiliation, and in the latter case, it would produce decreases. If such opposing effects had been present in these studies, they could well have canceled each other out. Moreover, many participants may have been unable to predict outcome values with the limited information available, suggesting that more uncertainty reduction would be required before influences on nonverbal affiliative expressiveness could be observed.

Gudykunst, Sodetani, and Sonoda's (1987) support for a negative association between uncertainty and nonverbal affiliative expressiveness in existing relationships is consistent with the POV position. As indicated earlier, ongoing relationships should generally manifest positive predicted outcome values. The more certain individuals are of their relational partners, the more certain they should be of these positive outcome value predictions. Decreased uncertainty of such outcomes should lead to more attempts to maintain relationships with such attempts including increases in nonverbal affiliative expressiveness. If existing relationships more often exhibit positive than negative predicted outcome values, uncertainty should generally be negatively associated with nonverbal affiliation. Of course, research that measures predicted outcome value levels would be needed to assess better the accuracy of this explanation.

A substantial amount of research, much of it provided by Gudykunst and his associates, focuses on the association between information seeking and uncertainty. Axiom 3 of uncertainty reduction theory (Berger & Calabrese, 1975) posits that high levels of uncertainty produce increases in information-seeking behavior, whereas decreases in uncertainty decrease information seeking. With few exceptions, tests produce either no support for this association or provide evidence of an unexpected negative relationship.

Research on initial interactions provides little support for Axiom 3. No support is provided by Gudykunst and Nishida's (1984) study of initial intra- and intercultural interactions in either the United States or Japan. Gudykunst, Nishida, Koike, and Shiino (1986) report supporting Axiom 3 in their study of Japanese intra- and intercultural first encounters. However, this support is weakened by the fact that information seeking, as measured by amount of interrogation, explained virtually no unique variance in attributional confidence in three of four tests conducted, and less than 1.5% in the remaining test. Two further initial interaction studies by Gudykunst (1983a, 1983b) provide evidence that the relationship between information seeking and uncertainty may be opposite to that proposed in Axiom 3. Four of nine tests reported in these studies indicate that subjects planned to ask an imagined stranger more questions when they were more certain about the stranger. The remaining tests conducted in these two studies provide no support for an information-seeking association to uncertainty.

Gudykunst's studies of ongoing relationships provide further evidence that the association between information seeking and uncertainty may be opposite to that proposed in Berger and Calabrese's (1975) formulation. Gudykunst, Yang, and Nishida (1985) report that acquaintance and friend (but not dating) relationships in Japan, Korea, and the United States manifest greater information seeking when partners are more certain of one another. Gudykunst's (1985b,c) studies of U.S. students' intra- and intercultural relations, and Gudykunst, Nishida, and Chua's (1986) findings regarding high context certainty among Japanese international students and their U.S.

acquaintances provides further support for such an association. Finally, Gudykunst, Sodetani, and Sonoda (1987) report no association between information-seeking and uncertainty in existing interethnic relationships.

It should be noted that these results are not as damaging to uncertainty reduction theory as they may appear. Most of the opposing findings come from existing relationships, not the initial interactions this axiom concerns. Moreover, these results are generally consistent with more recent uncertainty reduction explanations of information-seeking processes (Berger, 1979, 1987; Berger & Bradac, 1982). Even so, Gudykunst's findings appear to be more consistent with predicted outcome value expectations.

I have proposed that reduced uncertainty associated with positive predicted outcome values produces increases in information seeking, but when associated with negative values information seeking should decrease (Proposition 3). The use of many information-seeking strategies would prolong relational contact. Given this, Proposition 3 follows from the POV assumption that individuals attempt to maintain contact when outcome values are positive, and curtail or end contact when they are negative. This POV proposal differs from the previous ones in agreeing with the corresponding URT axiom when outcome values are negative, but disagreeing when these values are positive. Gudykunst's findings regarding ongoing relationships clearly support the POV alternative, granting the assumption that these relationships generally manifest positive predicted outcome values. His initial interaction research results are also consistent with Proposition 1, though adequate support would require an assessment of predicted outcome values.

Axiom 4 of uncertainty reduction theory (Berger and Calabrese, 1975) proposes that uncertainty level negatively influences intimacy of communication content. Results from Gudykunst's program consistently support this prediction for existing relationships, but not for relations at the initial acquaintance stage. In the only examination of this association in initial interactions, Gudykunst, Nishida, Koike, and Shiino's (1986) Japanese subject's exhibited no differences regarding their reported intent to self-disclose that were attributable to uncertainty level. However, findings from Gudykunst, Yang, and Nishida's (1985) Japanese sample support Axiom 4 expectations in acquaintance, friend, and dating relationships. Their U.S. and Korean samples exhibited the expected intimacy-uncertainty association in acquaintance and dating relationships, but not with friends. Interethnic research on existing Japanese-Caucasian relations (Gudykunst, Sodetani, and Sonoda, 1987), and Black-white relations (Gudykunst, 1986) further supports Axiom 4. Gudykunst's (1985b) intercultural findings, as well as his research (Gudykunst, 1985c) on U.S. intra- and intercultural relations again demonstrate the expected negative intimacy level-uncertainty association.

I have proposed that intimacy of communication content increases when uncertainty reduction is associated with positive predicted outcome values, and decreases when associated with negative predicted outcome values

(Proposition 4). This proposition is based, in part, on the assumption that increasing intimacy of self-disclosure reflects a desire to maintain or increase relational contact. Conversely, low intimacy levels should occur when individuals wish to end or curtail contact. Gudykunst, Nishida, Koike, and Shiino's (1986) findings for imagined initial encounters are consistent with this position. As previously argued, the research methods employed in this research would be expected to result in weakly formed predicted outcome values, at best. Moreover, both slightly positive and negative outcome values would be likely in these situations. Because these differing values would produce opposing intimacy effects, the initial interaction results from this study would be expected. Gudykunst's findings for ongoing relationships, assuming these relations exhibit primarily positive outcome values, are again consistent with Proposition 4.

Berger and Calabrese (1975) propose that uncertainty has a positive influence on reciprocity rate, with high uncertainty leading to high rates of reciprocity and low uncertainty producing low rates (Axiom 5). This is the least examined relationship from the original uncertainty formulation, with only one study from Gudykunst's program focusing on reciprocity rate. Gudykunst, Nishida, Koike, and Shiino (1986) claim support for this association in initial intra- and intercultural encounters. In imagined intracultural encounters with a stranger, Japanese subjects who were more certain about the stranger reported a greater likelihood of engaging in self-disclosure when the stranger did. The same association was observed in Japanese encounters with North American strangers when English was to be spoken, but not when Japanese was the language to be employed. Despite the preceding claim of support, these results appear to run counter to the prediction that uncertainty reduction decreases reciprocity rate. Berger and Calabrese's formulation, however, assumes that initial encounters need to proceed for some time before this effect would be observed. Given this, it is doubtful that the method employed in this study provided an adequate test of Axiom 5.

Proposition 5 of predicted outcome value theory predicts that uncertainty reduction associated with either positive or negative outcome values would produce decreases in reciprocity rate, though greater decreases are expected with negative values. While expectations regarding the association of uncertainty reduction and reciprocity rate are similar for positive and negative outcome values, POV proposes that different processes are involved in producing these results. In the case of negative predictions, individuals should reduce reciprocal exchanges in an attempt to end or curtail the conversation. Reciprocal communicative exchanges should continue in positive situations, but the *rate* of reciprocity should decline as length of speaking turns increases. As with Axiom 5, initial interactions would need to be observed to test this prediction.

Axiom 6 proposes that similarities between people decrease uncertainty and dissimilarities increase uncertainty. Gudykunst's initial acquaintance work provides little support for this prediction. No influence of manipulated attitudinal or cultural similarity on attributional confidence levels was observed in Gudykunst and Nishida's (1984) Japanese and U.S. samples. Gudykunst, Nishida, Koike, and Shiino (1986) report support for Axiom 6 in only one of four tests examining the influence of manipulated attitude similarity. Furthermore, these findings are consistent with Clatterbuck's (1979) summary that shows no support for Axiom 6 in several studies employing actual attitudinal similarities.

Much greater support for the similarity-uncertainty axiom is provided by research on existing relationships, particularly when those relationships beyond early acquaintance are considered. Gudykunst, Yang, and Nishida's (1985) Japanese, Korean, and U.S. samples provide no support for Axiom 6 with acquaintance relationships, but support from all three cultures for friendships. However, only their Japanese sample demonstrated a positive association between perceived attitude similarity and attributional confidence for dating relationships. Gudykunst (1985b) reports a positive association between attributional confidence and both cultural and perceived attitudinal similarity for U.S. intercultural relationships. Gudykunst's (1985c) study of U.S. intra- and intercultural relationships supports Axiom 6 regarding perceived attitudinal similarities between both friends and acquaintances. He also reports a positive cultural similarity association to attributional confidence for friends, though not for acquaintances. Gudykunst, Nishida, and Chua's (1986) study of Japanese international students and their U.S. acquaintances provides further support for a positive association between perceived similarity and certainty, as does Gudykunst, Sodetani, and Sonoda's (1987) interethnic study. Gudykunst (1986) reports support for a positive ethnic similarity-attributional confidence association in his study of ongoing intra- and interethnic relationships. Moreover, perceived similarities in this study were positively related to attributional confidence for whites' (but not Blacks') evaluations of existing intraethnic relationships, and for Blacks' (but not whites') evaluations of interethnic relationships.

Proposition 6 of predicted outcome value theory proposes that during initial acquaintance, both similarities and dissimilarities between persons reduce uncertainty, though similarities are expected to produce greater reduction in some situations. When initial interaction partners display similarities or dissimilarities of various kinds (e.g., ethnic, cultural, attitudinal), uncertainty should be reduced as long as individuals have knowledge of groups who display these same similarities or dissimilarities. Impressions individuals have of these others are likely to be tentatively applied to the partner. The more well-formed these impressions, the less uncertain individuals should be of these tentative judgments. In some cases, individuals may have more past experience with others from similar than from dissimilar backgrounds, and so be more certain of their attributions in such situations. Nevertheless, information indicating either similarity or dissimilarity should be uncertainty reducing, as long as it reflects a grouping for which the individual has an impression. This position is generally consistent with results from Gudykunst's initial interaction research.

Gudykunst's findings for ongoing relationships clearly indicate that Proposition 1 cannot be generalized beyond early acquaintance. Several of Gudykunst's (this volume) observations regarding similarity point to possible explanations for this lack of support. One reasonable possibility is that as relationships continue to develop, individuals discover that their predictions about dissimilar others are more likely to be inaccurate than predictions about similar others. That is, discrepancies (both positive and negative) between expected and predicted outcome values may occur more frequently in ongoing relationships between dissimilars. This would seem particularly likely in situations in which knowledge about the dissimilar groups the other belongs to is not extensive. Obviously, if individuals experience greater predictive failures in such relationships, uncertainty levels should remain relatively high.

Berger and Calabrese (1975) propose that uncertainty level negatively influences liking (Axiom 7). Gudykunst's research on existing relationships provides consistent support for this association, but findings on initial interactions are mixed. No significant association between attraction and attributional confidence was found in Gudykunst and Nishida's (1984) study of initial intra- and intercultural relations involving Japanese and North Americans. Gudykunst, Nishida, Koike, and Shiino's (1986) Japanese study provides support for Axiom 7 with initial intracultural, but not intercultural relations. Gudykunst, Yang, and Nishida's (1985) cross-cultural research provides support for Axiom 7 with acquaintance, friend, and dating relationships in all three cultures studied. Gudykunst's (1985b, 1985c) U.S. studies support this positive association for intra- and intercultural relations involving either acquaintances or friends. Finally, Gudykunst, Nishida, and Chua's (1986) research demonstrates support for the posited uncertainty-liking associations between Japanese and North American acquaintances.

Predicted outcome value theory (Sunnafrank, 1986) posits that liking increases when uncertainty reduction is associated with positive predicted outcome values, and decreases when uncertainty reduction is associated with negative outcome values (Proposition 7). This prediction is consistent with Gudykunst's initial interaction findings. Since the methods used in this research are unlikely to produce predominantly positive or negative predicted outcome values, his failure to find an uncertainty-liking association is not surprising. Gudykunst's findings for ongoing relationships clearly support Proposition 7, given the POV expectation that most continuing relationships manifest positive predicted outcome values.

CONCLUSION

Gudykunst's research program has made several significant advances in our understanding of how culture influences interpersonal communication processes. This work also provides the most thorough testing of uncertainty reduction theory (Berger & Calabrese, 1975), and its various expansions and modifications (Berger, 1979, 1987; Berger & Bradac, 1982; Gudykunst, 1985a; Gudykunst & Nishida, 1986a; Parks & Adelman, 1983). Gudykunst's findings have supported various aspects of these perspectives, and have supplied an important database for theoretical changes made in all of the most recent formulations. Some of these changes involve altering the relationships proposed in the basic axioms of Berger and Calabrese's perspective.

Predicted outcome value theory provides alternative propositions for all of these URT axioms, based on the assumption that individuals are interested primarily in increasing the value of their outcomes in relationships with others. This perspective posits that uncertainty reduction aids individuals in attaining this goal. Contrary to the implicit positive bias in the original axioms, I propose that uncertainty reduction may lead to predictions that either positive or negative outcomes will be experienced in relations with others. Results from Gudykunst's research program are generally supportive of this POV interpretation, and the propositions generated from it.

While the present review of Gudykunst's work supplies indirect support for POV proposals, research that directly assesses predicted outcome values is needed to test this perspective adequately. The recent development of a measure of predicted outcome values (Sunnafrank 1988) provides the opportunity to do this. Gudykunst, Nishida, and Schmidt's (1988) research employs this measure to test various POV proposals, with consistently supportive results. These findings supply additional evidence that future work on predicted outcome value theory may prove fruitful.

REFERENCES

Altman, I., & Taylor, D. (1973). *Social penetration: The development of interpersonal relationships.* New York: Holt, Rinehart & Winston.

Berger, C. R. (1979). Beyond initial interactions. In H. Giles & R. St. Clair (Eds.), *Language and social psychology* (pp. 122-144). Oxford: Basil Blackwell.

Berger, C. R. (1987). Communicating under uncertainty. In M. E. Roloff & G. R. Miller (Eds.), *Interpersonal processes* (pp. 39-62). Newbury Park, CA: Sage.

Berger, C. R., & Bradac, J. J. (1982). *Language and social knowledge: Uncertainty in interpersonal relations.* London: Edward Arnold.

Berger, C. R., & Calabrese, R. (1975). Some explorations in initial interactions and beyond: Toward a developmental theory of interpersonal communication. *Human Communication Research, 1,* 99-112.

Clatterbuck, G. W. (1979). Attributional confidence and uncertainty in initial interactions. *Human Communication Research, 5,* 147-157.

Gudykunst, W. B. (1983a). Similarities and differences in perceptions of initial intracultural and intercultural encounters. *Southern Speech Communication Journal*, XLIX, 49-65.

Gudykunst, W. B. (1983b). Uncertainty reduction and predictability of behavior in low- and high-context cultures. *Communication Quarterly, 31*, 49-55.

Gudykunst, W. B. (1985a). A model of uncertainty reduction in intercultural encounters. *Journal of Language and Social Psychology, 4*, 79-98.

Gudykunst, W. B. (1985b). An exploratory comparison of close intracultural and intercultural friendships. *Communication Quarterly, 33*, 270-273.

Gudykunst, W. B. (1985c). The influence of cultural similarity, type of relationship, and self-monitoring on uncertainty reduction processes. *Communication Monographs, 52*, 203-217.

Gudykunst, W. B. (1986). Ethnicity, type of relationship, and intraethnic and interethnic uncertainty reduction. In Y. Kim (Ed.), *Interethnic communication* (pp. 201-224). Beverly Hills, CA: Sage.

Gudykunst, W. B. (in press). Culture and communication in interpersonal relationships. In J. Anderson (Ed.), *Communication yearbook* (Vol. 12). Newbury Park, CA: Sage.

Gudykunst, W. B., Chua, E., & Gray A. (1987). Cultural dissimilarities and uncertainty reduction processes. In M. McLaughlin (Ed.), *Communication yearbook* (Vol. 10, pp. 456-469). Beverly Hills, CA: Sage.

Gudykunst, W. B., & Nishida, T. (1983). Social penetration in Japanese and North American friendships. In R. Bostrom (Ed.), *Communication yearbook* (Vol. 7, pp. 592-610). Beverly Hills, CA: Sage.

Gudykunst, W. B., & Nishida, T. (1984). Individual and cultural influences on uncertainty reduction. *Communication Monographs, 51*, 23-36.

Gudykunst, W. B., & Nishida, T. (1986a). Attributional confidence in low- and high-context cultures. *Human Communication Research, 12*, 525-549.

Gudykunst, W. B., & Nishida, T. (1986b). The influence of cultural variability on perceptions of communication behavior associated with relationship terms. *Human Communication Research, 13*, 147-166.

Gudykunst, W. B., Nishida, T., & Chua, E. (1986). Uncertainty reduction in Japanese-North American dyads. *Communication Research Reports, 3*, 39-46.

Gudykunst, W. B., Nishida, T., & Chua, E. (1987). Perceptions of social penetration in Japanese-North American dyads. *International Journal of Intercultural Relations, 51*, 256-278.

Gudykunst, W. B., Nishida, T., Koike, H., & Shiino, N. (1986). The influence of language on uncertainty reduction: An exploratory study of Japanese-Japanese and Japanese-North American interactions. In M. McLaughlin (Ed.), *Communication yearbook* (Vol. 9, pp. 555-575). Beverly Hills, CA: Sage.

Gudykunst, W. B., Nishida, T., & Schmidt, K. (1988). *Cultural, personality, and relational influences on uncertainty reduction in ingroup vs. outgroup and same vs. opposite sex relationships: Japan and the United States.* Paper presented at the International Communication Association Convention, New Orleans.

Gudykunst, W. B., Sodetani, L. L., & Sonoda, K. (1987). Uncertainty reduction in Japanese-American-Caucasian relationships in Hawaii. *Western Journal of Speech Communication, 51*, 256-278.

Gudykunst, W. B., Yang, S. M., & Nishida, T. (1985). A cross-cultural test of uncertainty reduction theory: Comparisons of acquaintance, friend, and dating relationships in Japan, Korea, and the United States. *Human Communication Research, 11*, 407-454.

Gudykunst, W. B., Yang, S. M., & Nishida, T. (1987). Cultural differences in self-consciousness and self-monitoring. *Communication Research, 14*, 7-36.

Miller, G. R., & Steinberg, M. (1975). *Between people.* Chicago: Science Research Associates.

Parks, M. R., & Adelman, M. B. (1983). Communication networks and the development of romantic relationships: An expansion of uncertainty reduction theory. *Human Communication Research, 10*, 55-80.

Planalp, S., & Honeycutt, J. (1985). Events that increase uncertainty in interpersonal relationships. *Human Communication Research, 11,* 593-604.

Sodetani, L. L., & Gudykunst, W. B. (in press). The effects of surprising events on intercultural relationships. *Communication Research Reports.*

Sunnafrank, M. (1986). Predicted outcome value during initial interactions: A reformulation of uncertainty reduction theory. *Human Communication Research, 13,* 3-33.

Sunnafrank, M. (1988). *Measuring predicted outcome values in initial interactions.* Unpublished manuscript.

Thibaut, J. W., & Kelly, H. H. (1959). *The social psychology of groups.* New York: John Wiley.

Culture and Interpersonal Relationship Development: Some Conceptual Issues

STELLA TING-TOOMEY
Arizona State University

INTERPERSONAL relationship development is a complex, multi-faceted process. it evolves and changes because of many intrinsic and extrinsic factors within and beyond the relationship. The relationship itself can transform the lives of the individuals in the relationship, and the individuals themselves can also actively monitor the progress of the relationship. The relationship transforms or develops, progresses or regresses within the larger social and cultural matrices.

In the span of the last 15 years, many theories have been developed to explain the interpersonal communication process (see for example, Knapp & Miller, 1985; Roloff & Miller, 1987). Among all the theories available, the uncertainty reduction theory and the social penetration theory are the two theories that have been used most often by intercultural communication researchers to explain cross-cultural and intercultural relationship developments (see Gudykunst's review in this volume). Consistent results have been found between the uncertainty reduction process and attraction across different types of relationships in different cultures (Gudykunst, Yang, & Nishida, 1985). Significant results have also been obtained between social penetration and various information-seeking strategies in different cultures (Gudykunst, 1983; Gudykunst & Nishida, 1984; Gudykunst, Yang, & Nishida, 1985). Edward T. Hall's (1976, 1983) low-context and high-context framework and Hofstede's (1980) cultural variability theory often have been used as the cultural grids that influence the various interpersonal encounter processes. Taken as a whole, the work of Gudykunst and his associates on uncertainty

Correspondence and requests for reprints: Stella Ting-Toomey, Department of Communication, Arizona State University, Tempe, AZ 85287.

Communication Yearbook 12, pp. 371-382

reduction and social penetration processes have advanced our understanding concerning cultural-specific information-seeking processes and the variables that affect interpersonal-intergroup attraction.

The objectives of this commentary are to examine some of the conceptual issues that undergird uncertainty reduction and social penetration theories, and to suggest some alternative ways to conceptualize intercultural-interpersonal relationship development.

CONCEPTUAL ISSUES

Uncertainty reduction theory and social penetration theory have been criticized on many grounds (Bochner, 1978, 1982, 1985a, 1985b; Cronen & Shuter, 1983; Delia, 1980; Kellermann, 1986; Planalp & Honeycutt, 1985; Sunnafrank, 1986; Ting-Toomey, 1983). Gudykunst himself (this volume) suggested that future work on the uncertainty reduction theory should "focus on uncertainty change in general rather than uncertainty reduction in particular." Altman, Vinsel, and Brown (1981), after years of research on the social penetration process, reconceptualize the social penetration theory from a dialectical perspective in which they hypothesize that "relationships can exhibit cyclical, reversible, and nonlinear processes, not necessarily only unidirectional and cumulative processes" (p.109). In his response to Sunnafrank's (1986) critique, Berger (1986) expresses surprise that it has taken over 10 years for someone to raise questions concerning uncertainty reduction theory, and he observes: "It is good that these questions are being raised. Scientific theories are constructed to be modified or discarded rather than accepted as dogma . . . . Not only has a formal theory been advanced to be challenged, the process of questioning has begun" (p. 35). It is in the spirit of raising questions that this section explores some of the fundamental issues that face uncertainty reduction and social penetration processes.

The five conceptual issues that will be discussed are: (1) the motivational base for the reduction of uncertainty; (2) that both uncertainty reduction and social penetration theories ignore relational changes and their subtle transformation processes; (3) that both theories ignore the dyadic effect of reciprocity; (4) that both theories ignore the larger social network contexts in which relationships are embedded; and (5) the assumptions of both theories, which reflect too well a Western-based ideology of intimacy.

Motivational Base for Uncertainty Reduction

Berger and Calabrese (1975) developed uncertainty reduction theory to explain communication phenomena in initial interactions. Two studies (Gudykunst, Yang, & Nishida, 1985; Parks & Adelman, 1983) have tested the theory in established romantic relationships and three types of cross-cultural relationships (acquaintanceship, friendship, and dating relationship) in

Japan, Korea, and the United States. However, the findings of both studies are still confined to the continuum of escalating relationships. Parks and Adelman (1983) found that uncertainty is associated with the overall level of relational stability. The more uncertain one is about his or her romantic partner, the greater the probability of relational termination. Gudykunst et al. (1985) discovered that the role of attributional confidence works differently for Japanese and Korean dating relationships in comparison to United States dating relationships. They conclude that the "lack of support for specific hypotheses in particular relationships in specific cultures undermines the generality of the model and suggests that revisions to the model are needed" (p. 448). Both studies deal with stable, established relationships and not with unstable, evolving relationships. Both studies deal with predefined relationship types rather than with the emergent relationship process. In addition, Berger (1979) also states that anticipated future interaction is one of the major conditions under which individuals try to reduce uncertainty. Kellermann's (1986) research, however, suggests that anticipated future interaction does not increase attempts to reduce uncertainty in initial interaction behavior. She concludes that while anticipation of future interaction may have a strong influence in passive settings prior to the actual first encounter of the individuals, it may not have a strong impact in active, information-rich environments.

Taken together, the bottom-line question is: What are the motivational bases for why individuals are propelled to reduce uncertainty in initial interaction? Beyond initial interactions, what comes next? Berger (1987) argues that reducing uncertainty is a function of "both the ability to predict and the ability to explain actions of other *and* of self" (p. 41). He (Berger, 1979) posits that a linear relationship exists between anticipation of future interaction and cognitive uncertainty. Kellermann (1986), however, questions the scope condition of the theory. She concludes:

> Because uncertainty reduction theory has an explicit boundary condition requiring the existence of high levels of uncertainty in an initial interaction, the applicability of the theory is severely curtailed if the antecedents to high uncertainty cannot be verified. Although high uncertainty may occur, the typical initial interaction may not be characterized by high uncertainty about the conversational partner. Inability to verify frequently occurring antecedents to high uncertainty limit the utility of the theory to explain behavior in initial encounters. (p. 66)

It has also been predicted that intercultural initial encounters include a high degree of uncertainty (Gudykunst, 1985). Although it is probably true that uncertainty exists in all types of encounters, not all individuals have the same baseline desire to reduce uncertainty in their relationships. Dispositional factors, situational factors, and cultural factors all come into play. Dispositional factors like tolerance for ambiguity may determine the individual's rates and pacing for the need for reducing relational uncertainty. Situational factors such as the context in which the individuals meet may act as a mediating variable between uncertainty reduction and relational anxiety. Cultural factors such as whether individuals come from a monochronic-time culture (time-bound culture) or a polychronic-time culture (time-fluid culture) may influence the attitudes of the intercultural dyads in reducing their uncertainty immediately or eventually.

In short, within and beyond initial interactions, we need to take a closer look at the motivational bases and a host of other variables that influence the uncertainty reduction process. We need to identify individuals who have a high urge to reduce uncertainty in their relationships with individuals who have a low urge to reduce uncertainty. Beyond initial interactions and well-established relationships, we need to test the theory in ambiguous, unstable relationships in which relationship definitions are not clear and communication patterns contain mixed signals. Finally, in the context of intercultural relationship development, we need to understand the cultural ideology, the cultural rhythm, and the cultural value that surrounds the concept of relational changes and evolution process. This then leads to our second point of discussion.

Relational Changes

Both uncertainty reduction theory and social penetration theory view interpersonal relationship development from a unidirectional perspective. Uncertainty reduction theory posits a "reciprocal relationship between uncertainty and attraction, with continued uncertainty reduction a function of the valence of affect toward one's partner" (Berger, 1987, p. 50). Implicit in the theory is the notion that reducing uncertainty leads to greater knowledge about the partner, and greater knowledge about the partner leads to increased interpersonal attraction. On the other hand, social penetration theory states that "people explore and reveal superficial, nonintimate aspects of themselves during the early stages of a relationship and that only gradually do they probe and disclose more personal, intimate aspects of their lives to another person" (Altman, Vinsel, & Brown, 1981, p. 109). Both theories are unidimensional because they study interpersonal relationship development from a one-way, cumulative pathway. An unrestricted uncertainty reduction process is essential to the interpersonal relationship development process, and an unrestricted mutual openness via self-disclosure is essential to the well-being of a relationship.

In reality, however, all relationships swing back and forth on a continuum between stability and change, openness and closedness, progression and regression. Relationship movements are made possible only by such oscillating and fluctuating actions and events in an interdependent relationship. As Bochner (1985a) succinctly concludes:

> The dialectical qualities of interpersonal communication make it obvious that things are not always what they seem: yet interactants sometimes are pressured to act as if things are. . . . Talk may inhibit what it exhibits—expressiveness mandating protectiveness, revealing necessitating concealing, openness petitioning discreation, weakness used to dominate, freedom as a constraint. Sometimes an interpersonal bond must be responsive to antagonistic pressures, making it very difficult for its members to function effectively. Interactants may feel required to be truthful but not insensitive, protective but not secretive, validating but not dishonest, spontaneous but not unpredictable. (p. 610)

Individuals involved in an interdependent interpersonal relationship have to face many relational paradoxes, dilemmas, and embedded emotions in their relationship development before their relationship reaches a certain level of stability or certainty. Stability in a relationship implies also the potential for changes in a relationship, and the existence of certainty also implies the polar opposite of uncertainty. Altman et al. (1981), in their reconceptualization of social penetration theory from a dialectical perspective, argue that:

> We assume that individuals are unique entities and sometimes desire to withdraw or not interact with others. Yet, they also sometimes wish to be in contact with others. The result is that they are motivated to be both open and closed. Similarly, we assume that people have differential desires at various times for stability and change in their social relationships. However, we also recognize that external factors affect the relative strength of openness-closedness and stability-change. Such influences take the form of social pressures exerted by others, societal norms and demands, and various environmental factors. (p. 13)

The dialectics of openness-closedness and stability-change operate simultaneously as a unified and dynamic system. Interpersonal relationship development involves the interplay of openness and closedness, and the oscillation between stability and change. Relationship development does not follow a unidirectional trajectory—from partial openness to complete openness, or from partial stability to complete stability. Interpersonal relationship development is a moving, dynamic process with cycles and spirals of open and closed patterns, and stable and change patterns. Couples who consistently synchronize their movements of openness and closedness, stability and change are more likely to move their relationship forward than are couples who are mismatched in their communication patterns.

Baxter and Wilmot (1985), in using a dialectical perspective in studying taboo topics in close relationship, found that concealment is at work over six primary types of "taboo topics": the state of the relationship, extra-relationship activity, relationship norms, prior relationships with opposite-sex parties, conflict-inducing topics, and negatively valenced self-disclosures. They concluded that taboo topics are just as evident "among relationships generally characterized by greater closeness (i.e., romantic relationships) as among less close relationships (i.e., platonic relationships)" (p. 265). In another study, Baxter (1984) analyzed 97 heterosexual romantic relationship breakups uncovering multiple trajectories of relational disengagement patterns rather than singular stages of relational dissolution process. Finally, Masheter and Harris (1986), in analyzing the communication patterns of a divorced couple who have become friends, concluded that relationship development oscillates between polar opposites (stability/changes, intimacy/detachment) and the integration of the polar opposites (stability/changes, intimacy/detachment). To study interpersonal relationship development *processes*, one has to attend to the sequences (and the embeddedness) of change and stability, and the sequences (and the embeddedness) of openness and closedness. Altman et al. (1981) recommend that researchers can examine the relationship between openness-closedness and stability-change through the dimensions of

> (1) the *frequency* with which participants shift from openness to closedness,
> (2) the *amplitude*, or absolute amount of openness-closedness,
> (3) the *regularity*, or redundancy with which given cyclical patterns recur, and
> (4) the *relative duration*, or proportion of time openness and closedness appear in a given cycle. Finally, stability-change patterns may differ in various content areas and modalities. (pp. 139-140)

To a certain degree, the same idea is expressed in Gudykunst's suggestion concerning the importance of studying the uncertainty change as a dialectical process rather than studying uncertainty reduction per se. In order to understand the concept of uncertainty in a relationship, one has to know something about the pattern of certainty in a relationship. What one partner views as an event of uncertainty in a relationship, another partner may view as an event of increasing certainty. We also need to view the study of certainty and uncertainty from both a cognitive and an affective angle. Cognitive certainty may not equate with affective certainty and vice versa. Gudykunst deals with this issue, in part, by including anxiety in his theoretical framework. Finally, we need to know the relational history of the dyads and the past relational histories of the individuals in order to account for the uncertainty reduction values, uncertainty reduction patterns, and the uncertainty reduction strategies used in the dyadic interaction.

A "process" approach to the study of either uncertainty reduction or social penetration should focus on the patterns of relational movements and the degree to which they are synchronized (or mismatched) throughout the initiation, maintenance, and termination of the relationship. Cultural norms and rules should also be taken into consideration when it involves the study of temporal qualities, pacing, and rhythms of the relationship progression process, and the gender issues that surround the relationship change process.

Dyadic Effect of Reciprocity

Most research on uncertainty reduction and social penetration processes involve self-report data or experimental data (e.g., Gudykunst, Nishida, & Chua, 1987; Gudykunst, Yoon, & Nishida, 1987; Kellermann, 1986; Parks & Adelman, 1983). Although the concept of "dyadic effect" of reciprocity has been investigated by a number of interpersonal communication researchers (e.g., Cappella, 1981; Dindia, 1982, 1985; Gottman, 1979) on nonverbal behavior and disclosure patterns, there have been only a limited number of cross-cultural communication studies (e.g., Won-Doornink, 1979, 1985) that explore the critical role of dyadic reciprocity in the uncertainty reduction process or the social penetration process. On the broader level, the norm of reciprocity states that "the receiver of a benefit is obligated to provide benefits to the giver" (Roloff, 1987, p. 13). On the specific level, the concept of *dyadic reciprocity* has been defined as mutual positive influence (Dindia, 1985), for example, self-disclosure begets self-disclosure. By defining reciprocity as mutual positive influence the definition also implies the possibility of mutual negative influence. Most intercultural uncertainty reduction and social penetration studies use self-report data, hence most studies have neglected totally the dyadic effect of reciprocity and its accompanying negotiation process. (Note, however, Gudykunst, Yang, and Nishida, 1985, do include reciprocity in the causal model.)

Although Berger and Calabrese (1975) posit that "high levels of uncertainty produce high rates of reciprocity [and] low levels of uncertainty produce low reciprocity rates" (p. 105) and that "the quality rather than the quantity of information exchanged between interactants should have a greater impact upon the reduction of mutual uncertainties" (Berger, 1987, p. 44), there is not any clear evidence concerning reciprocity rates, reciprocity patterns, and reciprocity information exchange in the intercultural uncertainty reduction process and in the longitudinal, intercultural social penetration process. We do not have data concerning the "mutual influencing" process of uncertainty reduction or uncertainty change, and we do not have clear evidence concerning the mutual progression and the mutual regression patterns of self-disclosure or information privacy-regulation patterns.

Relationship development, to a large degree, is a relational negotiation and a relational redefinition process. Unfortunately, the interactive dynamics of negotiation and the interpretive processes that are attached to the relational redefinition process have not been actively researched by intercultural communication scholars. Individuals, coming from different cultures, may hold different conceptualizations and expectations concerning how a relationship should be redefined and what constitutes appropriate or inappropriate behaviors in each relational stage. Their concerns for reciprocity of resource exchange may differ, and their concerns for different modalities and types of resource exchange may vary. Individuals coming from the high-context cultures such as China, Japan, or Korea (Hall, 1983), for example, may emphasize the nonverbal aspects of the uncertainty reciprocity process, whereas individuals coming from the low-context cultures such as Germany, Switzerland, or the United States may emphasize the verbal aspects of uncertainty reciprocity process. Individuals from high-context cultures may emphasize long-term reciprocity exchange, whereas individuals from low-context cultures may emphasize short-term reciprocity exchange. All these exchanges, however, depend on the types of relationships we are studying and the types of contexts in which the relationships evolve and change.

Context

Almost all studies on uncertainty reduction or social penetration processes call for the importance of incorporating context as a critical variable in the study of relational development and changes. Delia (1980) proposes that social contexts provide particular expectations and establish particular trajectories for relational development. He suggests that researchers should study relationship development as a natural accompaniment to ongoing activities in everyday living. Parks and Adelman (1983) point to the importance of studying the interaction between social network and dyadic relationship changes. They conclude:

> Relationships tend to develop in several directions at once as individual experiences, dyadic interactions, and patterns of network contact change together. . . . Participants must somehow synthesize all of these changes into an overall understanding of the relationship. Uncertainty might result when expected changes do not occur together. (p. 75)

The motivation to reduce uncertainty is not contingent on one or two factors. Rather, it involves a matrix of relational contexts and situational contexts. Relational contexts refer to the influence of family networks and friendship networks, and situational contexts refer to both the psychological and the physical characteristics of the setting. The formal-informal dimension of the setting and the warm-cold dimension of the setting may influence the affective process of uncertainty reduction, and the effectiveness of the uncertainty reduction process. Context also proscribes and prescribes what constitutes appropriate or inappropriate behaviors for relational disclosure, relational concealment, or the relational metacommunication process.

Culture

Social penetration theory derives its basic assumptions from the social exchange reward/cost model (Thibaut & Kelley, 1959). Cronen and Shuter (1983), however, argue that the "metaphor of the marketplace does not capture the subtlety and complexity of human relationships" (p. 92). Bochner (1985a) summarizes the three flaws in the reward/cost position:

> First, reward/cost principles are tautological; second, reward/cost principles attempt to reduce the irreducible; third, reward/cost principles oversimplify complex developmental process by implying that the same system of logic—the rational calculation of rewards and costs—operates at all levels (stages) of development. (pp. 578-579)

He concludes that the principle of reward/cost does not "provide an adequate or appropriate explanation for the developmental dynamics of interpersonal bonds" (p. 578).

The implicit goal in the uncertainty reduction process is to control one's environment via uncertainty reduction. The implicit objective in the social penetration self-disclosure process is to cultivate openness in a relationship. Both the themes of control and openness are themes that are highly valued by Western, individualistic cultures but not necessarily by Eastern, collectivistic cultures (Kincaid, 1987). Overall, individualistic cultures stress self-assertion over group-orientation, openness over implicitness, and relational control over relational fate. Conversely, collectivistic cultures emphasize group harmony over individual interests, concealment over revealment, and relational intuition over relational rationality. The fact that communication theory-development activities originate largely from Western, individualistic cultures, it is inevitable that terms and concepts that have been widely tested reflect a Western-based ideology of intimacy. Concepts like *relational intuition, relational fate,* and *relational letting go* are much more difficult to conceptualize and measure, and sound much too ambiguous and "soft" for rigorous scientific testing. This orientation, however, should not undercut the importance of studying such "fuzzy and ambiguous" concepts.

To develop a coherent theory of intercultural-interpersonal relationship development we need to incorporate the relevant taxonomies, salient terms, and sensitizing concepts of multiple cultures and multiple ethnic communities in order that comparison and contrast can be made between and among sets of cultures. Intercultural relationship development entails the active negotiation process of worldviews, values, and beliefs of individuals from different cultures. There are probably multiple relational pathways in reaching the same direction. The task at hand is to uncover these multiple pathways so that not one singular ideology of relationship development dominates our thinking at the expense of an alternative one.

CONCLUSION

Five conceptual issues that face the study of culture and interpersonal relationship development were discussed in this essay. These five issues are: (1) the motivational base for uncertainty reduction; (2) the issue of ignoring the study of the relational change and transformation process; (3) the issue of neglecting the study of relational negotiation patterns; (4) the issue of ignoring the study of context; and (5) the issue of a Western-based ideology of intimacy. Many of these issues, in one sense, are tied closely with intercultural methodological problems. Space does not allow a full-length discussion of these methological issues (see Gudykunst & Ting-Toomey, in press; Ting-Toomey, 1984; for overviews of these issues).

In sum, intercultural relationship development research is a wide-open field. Relational topics such as: (a) self, relationship development, and culture need to be critically examined; (b) the temporal dimensions of the intercultural relationship development process need to be addressed; (c) the multiple dialectics of the relational negotiation and the relational redefinition process need to be uncovered; (d) the cultural conditions that surround relational dilemmas and relational paradoxes need to be probed; and (e) the specific verbal and nonverbal patterns that accompany different spiraling phases of relationship development in different cultures need to be systematically explored and analyzed. Both qualitative and quantitative research is needed to study interpersonal relationship development, and greater collaborations among researchers from multiple cultures is needed in order for us to develop a fuller understanding of the richness and the complexity of the relational evolution process in different social and cultural systems.

REFERENCES

Altman, I., Vinsel, A., & Brown, B. (1981). Dialectical conceptions in social psychology: An application to social penetration and privacy regulation. In L. Berkowitz (Ed.), *Advances in experimental social psychology* (Vol. 14, pp. 107-160). New York: Academic Press.

Baxter, L. (1984). Trajectories of relationship disengagement. *Journal of Social and Personal Relationships, 1*, 29-48.

Baxter, L., & Wilmot, W. (1985). Taboo topics in close relationships. *Journal of Social and Personal Relationships, 2*, 253-269.

Berger, C. (1979). Beyond initial interactions. In H. Giles & R. St. Clair (Eds.), *Language and social psychology* (pp. 122-144). Oxford: Basil Blackwell.

Berger, C. (1986). Uncertain outcome values in predicted relationship: Uncertainty reduction theory then and now. *Human Communication Research, 13*, 34-38.

Berger, C. (1987). Communicating under uncertainty. In M. E. Roloff & G. R. Miller (Eds.), *Interpersonal processes: New directions in communication research* (pp. 39-62). Newbury Park, CA: Sage.

Berger, C., & Calabrese, R. (1975). Some explorations in initial interactions and beyond: Toward a developmental theory of interpersonal communication. *Human Communication Research, 1*, 99-112.

Bochner, A. (1978). On taking ourselves seriously: An analysis of some persistent problems and promising directions in interpersonal research. *Human Communication Research, 4*, 179-191.

Bochner, A. (1982). On the efficacy of openness in close relationships. In M. Burgoon (Ed.), *Communication yearbook 5*, (pp. 109-124). New Brunswick, NJ: Transaction.

Bochner, A. (1985a). The functions of human communication in interpersonal bonding. In C. Arnold & J. Bowers (Eds.), *Handbook of rhetorical and communication theory* (pp. 544-621). Boston, MA: Allyn & Bacon.

Bochner, A. (1985b). Perspectives on inquiry: Representation, conversation, and reflection. In M. Knapp & G. Miller (Eds.), *Handbook of interpersonal communication* (pp. 7-58). Beverly Hills, CA: Sage.

Cappella, J. (1981). Mutual influence in expressive behavior: Adult-adult and infant-adult dyadic interaction. *Psychological Bulletin, 89*, 101-132.

Cronen, V., & Shuter, R. (1983). Forming intercultural bonds. In W. Gudykunst (Ed.), *Intercultural communication theory: Current perspectives* (pp. 89-118). Beverly Hills, CA: Sage.

Delia, J. (1980). Some tentative thoughts concerning the study of interpersonal relationships and their development. *Western Journal of Speech Communication, 44*, 104-107.

Dindia, K. (1982). Reciprocity of self-disclosure: A sequential analysis. In M. Burgoon (Ed.), *Communication yearbook 6*, (pp. 506-530). Beverly Hills, CA: Sage.

Dindia, K. (1985). A functional approach to self-disclosure. In R. Street & J. Cappella (Eds.), *Sequence and pattern in communicative behaviour* (pp. 142-160). London: Edward Arnold.

Gottman, J. (1979). *Marital interaction: Experimental investigations*. New York: Academic Press.

Gudykunst, W. B. (1983).Uncertainty reduction and predictability of behavior in low- and high-context cultures. *Communication Quarterly, 31*, 49-55.

Gudykunst, W. B. (1985). The influence of cultural similarity, type of relationship, and self-monitoring on uncertainty reduction process. *Communication Monographs, 52*, 203-217.

Gudykunst, W. B., & Nishida, T. (1984). Individual and cultural influences on uncertainty reduction. *Communication Monographs, 51*, 23-36.

Gudykunst, W. B., Nishida, T., & Chua, E. (1987). Perceptions of social penetration in Japanese-North American dyads. *International Journal of Intercultural Relations, 51*, 256-278.

Gudykunst, W. B., & Ting-Toomey, S., with Chua, E. (in press). *Culture and interpersonal communication*. Newbury Park, CA: Sage.

Gudykunst, W. B., Yang, S. M., & Nishida, T. (1985). A cross-cultural test of uncertainty reduction theory: Comparisons of acquaintance, friend, and dating relationships in Japan, Korea, and the United States. *Human Communication Research, 11*, 407-454.

Gudykunst, W. B., Yoon, Y. C., & Nishida, T. (1987). The influence of individualism-collectivism on perceptions of communication in ingroup and outgroup relationships. *Communication Monographs, 54*, 295-306.

Hall, E. T. (1983). *The dance of life*. New York: Doubleday.

Hall, E. T. (1976). *Beyond culture*. New York: Doubleday.

Hofstede, G. (1980). *Culture's consequences*. Beverly Hills, CA: Sage.

Kellermann, K. (1986). Anticipation of future interaction and information exchange in initial interaction. *Human Communication Research, 13*, 41-75.

Kincaid, D. (Ed.). (1987). *Communication theory from Eastern and Western perspectives*. New York: Academic Press.

Knapp, M., & Miller, G. (Eds.). (1985). *Handbook of interpersonal communication*. Beverly Hills, CA: Sage.

Masheter, C., & Harris, L. (1986). From divorce to friendship: A study of dialectic relationship development. *Journal of Social and Personal Relationships, 3*, 177-189.

Parks, M. R., & Adelman, M. B. (1983). Communication networks and the development of romantic relationships: An expansion of uncertainty reduction theory. *Human Communication Research, 10*, 55-80.

Planalp, S., & Honeycutt, J. (1985). Events that increase uncertainty in interpersonal relationships. *Human Communication Research, 11*, 593-604.

Roloff, M. (1987). Communication and reciprocity within intimate relationships. In M. Roloff & G. Miller (Eds.), *Interpersonal processes: New directions in communication research* (pp. 11-38). Newbury Park, CA: Sage.

Roloff, M., & Miller, G. (Eds.). (1987). *Interpersonal process: New directions in communication research*. Newbury Park, CA: Sage.

Sunnafrank, M. (1986). Predicted outcome value during initial interactions: A reformulation of uncertainty reduction theory. *Human Communication Research, 13*, 3-33.

Thibaut, J., & Kelley, H. (1959). *The social psychology of groups*. New York: John Wiley.

Ting-Toomey, S. (1983, November). *Intracultural and intercultural encounters: A developmental perspective*. Paper presented at the Speech Communication Association convention, Washington, DC.

Ting-Toomey, S. (1984). Qualitative research: An overview. In W. Gudykunst & Y. Kim (Eds.), *Methods for intercultural communication research* (pp. 169-184). Beverly Hills, CA: Sage.

Won-Doornink, M. (1979). On getting to know you: The association between stage of relationship and reciprocity of self-disclosure. *Journal of Experimental Social Psychology, 15*, 229-241.

Won-Doornink, M. (1985). Self-disclosure and reciprocity in conversation: A cross-national study. *Social Psychology Quarterly, 48*, 97-107.

7 Cultural Identity and Modes of Communication

JAN SERVAES
Catholic University of Nijmegen

The concept of culture has long been virtually ignored in development and communication theories. In this chapter, a new perspective on culture has been developed. It defines cultures as social settings in which a certain reference framework has taken concrete form or has been institutionalized and orients and structures the interaction and communication of people within this historical context. Therefore, in the patterning of their social existence, people continually make principally unconscious choices that are directed by the applicable intracultural values and options. Cultural identity refers to the constitution and cultivation of a reality on the basis of particular values, a reality in which the value system and the social system are completely interwoven and imbued with the activity of each other. I focus on two aspects or levels of the relationship between forms of cultural identity and modes of production and communication that build upon this new perception of culture: (1) the micro level of culture and communication—the relationship between modes of communication and the social structure; and (2) the macro level of international communication—that is, the cultural imperialism problematic.

> Well, a hundred years ago, the white men wanted the Indians to go into prisons called "reservations," to give up their freedom to roam and hunt buffalo, to give up being Indians. Some tamely submitted and settled down behind the barbed wire of the agencies, but others did not. Those who went to the reservations to live like white men were called "friendlies." Those who would not go were called "hostiles." They were not hostile, really. They didn't want to fight; all they wanted was to be left alone to live the Indian way, which was a good way. But the soldiers would not leave them alone. Told by Rachel Strange Owl, Birney, Montana.
>
> —Erdoes and Ortiz (1984, pp. 264-265)

Since the Second World War, the idea of an emergent global village has slipped into scholarly discussions at regular intervals. In popular publications this idea has often been referred to as the universal Coca Cola or Mickey

Correspondence and requests for reprints: Jan Servaes, Catholic University of Nijmegen, Institute of Mass Communication, P. O. Box 9108, 6500 HK Nijmegan, The Netherlands.

Communication Yearbook 12, 383-416

AUTHOR'S NOTE: Special thanks are due to James Anderson, Alan Hancock, Bella Mody, and Dallas Smythe for their stimulating comments on earlier drafts of this text.

Mouse culture; in other words, as the Americanization of the world. Nevertheless, we still live in a culturally divided world.

Throughout history, societies and cultures have always, in one way or another, interacted with one another. With few exceptions, the general characteristic of such cultural interactions has been that they either maintained their integrity or developed a more diversified and richer pattern. Since the needs and values that various communities develop in divergent situations and environments are not the same, cultures manifest separate identities. As a consequence, our cultural awareness has become more global and historical.

Since the age of capitalism, however, this overall cultural diversity and autonomy has been threatened by mechanisms of Western cultural synchronization or "imperialism." Communication, in all its meanings and applications, played, and continues to play, a major role in this process. At the same time, in various parts of the world, one also observes, at distinct societal levels, an emerging countermovement that attempts to maintain and stimulate its cultural autonomy. In other words, generally because the living conditions of societies differ, culture is a phenomenon whose content differs from community to community.

Each culture operates out of its own logic. Therefore, each culture has to be analyzed on the basis of its own "logical" structure. Cross-cultural and intercultural communications are successful only when these logical foundations are understood and accepted as equal by the people concerned. The study of cultural identity should therefore concentrate on two levels simultaneously: providing accounts of other worlds from the inside, and reflecting about the epistemological basis of such accounts. As will be argued throughout this text, I advocate a convergence approach toward culture—the convergence of social dynamics and multidimensional interactions between internal and external factors. In this perspective the analysis of cultural identity presumes an insight into the basic cultural event, into the policy and practical options that are operational in the cultivation of the social system, and into the world view and ethos that inspire the people involved. Claude Lévi-Strauss (1966), often regarded as the father of structuralism, once called this approach "the science of the concrete."

The purpose of this text is not to make an exhaustive inventory of the problematic relationship between forms of cultural identity and modes of production of communication that build upon this new perspective. Rather, it attempts to clarify a few essential and often overlooked elements in the overall discussion on culture and communication. By adopting Armand Mattelart's (1979) definition of modes of communication, which includes (a) all of the production instruments, (b) working methods, and (c) all of the relations of productions established between individuals in the process of communication, I will focus mainly on the topic of cultural identity from two levels: (1) the micro level of culture and communication—the relationship between modes of communication and the social structure, and (2) the macro level of international communication—that is, the cultural imperialism problematic.

However, as the concept of culture has long been virtually ignored in the development and communication debate, I will start with a brief overview of three generations of thought on development problems. Only in the multiplicity paradigm (cf. infra), which searches for the necessary content and normative components for "another" development, does the concept of culture come into the picture again.

CHANGES IN DEVELOPMENT THINKING

> The unfolding dialectic of world history is entering its most comprehensive and perhaps most problematic phase—at once unnerving and creative. It heralds a process of mutation in the history of the human species, with far-reaching changes in the arrangement of human affairs: in the structuring of global power relations, in the encounter of civilizations, in several other areas such as class, region, ethnicity, and religion. And yet few, if any, seem to have a clue to the real nature of this transformation. (Kothari, 1984, p. 323)

During the late 1940s and 1950s most developmental thinkers stated that the problem of underdevelopment or "backwardness" could be solved by a more or less mechanical application of the economic and political system in the West to countries in the Third World, under the assumption that the difference was one of degree rather than of kind. This mainly economically-oriented perspective ultimately developed into the modernization and growth theory. As a result of the general intellectual "revolution" that took place in the mid-1960s, this Eurocentric look on development was challenged by Latin American social scientists, and a theory dealing with dependency and underdevelopment was born. This dependency approach formed part of a general structuralist reorientation in social sciences. The *dependistas* were primarily concerned with the effects of dependency in peripheral countries, but implicit in their analysis was the idea that development and underdevelopment must be understood in the context of the world system, a view that has been strengthened as the recent worldwide stock market crisis shows the degree to which the world economy has become a reality.

The need for a more global analysis has become apparent. Contrary to the more economically and politically oriented views of the modernization and dependency theories, the central idea in what I perceive as an emergent third paradigm is that there is no universal path to development, that development must be conceived of as an integral, multidimensional, and dialectic process that can differ from one community to another. In other words, every nation must find its own strategy.[1] At the same time, this claim implies that the problem of development is a relative one, and no part of the world can claim to be developed in all aspects. Therefore, the discussion on the degree and scope of inter- (in)dependence is connected with the content of development. According to this view, "another" development could be defined as need-oriented, endogenous, self-reliant, ecologically sound, based on participatory democracy and structural transformations. This new perspective on development might be defined as "multiplicity in one world" (see Servaes, 1986a, 1986b, 1987c).

One World, Many Cultures

This new approach on development emerged from the criticism of the modernization and dependency paradigms. The common starting point here is the examination of the changes from a "bottom-up" perspective, from the self-development of the local community. The basic assumption is that there are no nations that function completely autonomously and that are completely self-sufficient, nor are there nations whose development is exclusively determined by external factors. Every community is dependent upon others in one way or another, both in form and in degree. Thus a framework was sought within which both the center and periphery could be studied separately and in their mutual relationship. According to Arno Addo (1985), "as we move from Eurocentric consciousness to world-system consciousness, our categories and concepts must be reconsidered in the light of rendering them usable at the world-system level" (p.25). The impetus for this new approach stems from at least two interdisciplinary theories: the economic world system analysis and the anthropological "coupling" of the forms of production approach.

The best known representative of the former trend is Immanuel Wallerstein (1974, 1979, 1980, 1983), who argues that the fundamental traits of the capitalist world system have remained virtually unchanged since the sixteenth century, that a small number of Center countries enter into functional relationships with peripheral and semiperipheral nations, that the developmental dynamic is determined internally and not externally, and that the hope for fundamental changes in certain states can be called almost nonexistent so long as the world capitalism system does not collapse.

According to other authors (e.g., Hyden, 1983; Laclau & Mouffe, 1985; Petras, 1978; Salama & Tissier, 1982; Taylor, 1979; Thomas, 1984; or Vogler, 1985) the interpretations of this group seem to stress the dynamic of the capitalist system one-sidedly, as a universally explanatory principle. From the viewpoint of these authors, it is more a matter of a multiple dynamic: In the margin of the capitalist system, all kinds of pre- or noncapitalistic organizational patterns maintain their own coherency and significance. Therefore, these authors are more interested in what is happening within the boundaries of a country or nation in which they examine class and ethnic struggles, the varying contiguous forms of production, populist and nationalist trends, and the functioning of ideologies as social processes:

> The contemporary reality . . . must be analyzed from within historical materialism as a social formation which is dominated by an articulation of (at least) two modes of production—a capitalist and a non-capitalist mode—in

> which the former is, or is becoming, increasingly dominant over the other. (Taylor, 1979, p. 101-102)

Therefore, one returns to the old discussion on Asiatic or precapitalist modes of production (Godelier, 1973; Hindess & Hirst, 1975; Lubasz, 1985).

It is not surprising that this view prevails among anthropologists, especially those who are doing research in Africa (Fonkoue, 1985; Meillassoux, 1975, 1986; Rey, 1976). It is precisely in Africa, where old forms of organization, however much transformed, still seem to form a real obstacle to the effects of capitalist relationships. These forms of economic organization and production are often defined by the term *conviviality.* In this respect, two research areas from the work of the anthropologists are important: their studies on the organization and development of local groups, communities, and social structures in general; and their analyses of the "informal sectors" in society. They stress the special autonomy of superstructural institutions in the precapitalist forms of production and the coupling of forms of production and its particular role after decolonization. From this position, it appears that all kinds of noneconomic factors, such as cultural principles (like kinship and religion) which gave the old forms of production shape, still have a direct influence in this coupling.

A fascinating integration of the two viewpoints is given by Osvaldo Sunkel and Edmundo Feunzalida (1980) with their transnationalization thesis, which can be summarized in four points; (a) the capitalist system has changed from an international to a transnational structure with the transnational corporations as the most significant actors; (b) the most striking feature of the actual system is the polarized development of transnationalization on the one hand, and national disintegration on the other; (c) of particular interest is the emphasis on culture that is the main stimulator of a new transnational community of people from different nations, but with similar values and ideas, as well as patterns of behavior; (d) at the same time, the national societies are generating a variety of counterprocesses that assert national and/or subnational values—sometimes reactionary, sometimes progressive. In other words, the concentration on this dialectical relation between (mainly transnational) integration and (mainly national) disintegration leads to liberating as well as oppressive processes on several levels of a particular nation.[2]

Culture and Development

The changes within development thinking in general and its related consequences for the theory and practice of development can also be traced in issues dealing with cultural development. Roy Preiswerk (1980), for instance, attempted to evaluate the degree and level of cultural identity, self-reliance, and basic needs in a multiple development perspective. His thesis is that these aspects can be applied in a suppressing or negative as well as liberative or

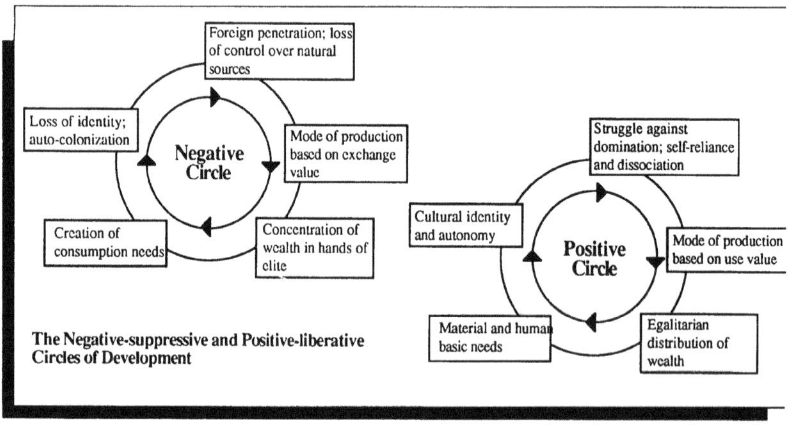

Figure 7.1

positive way (see Figure 7.1). A positive-liberating interpretation of the concept of cultural identity may, among other aspects, imply a positive orientation toward historical values, norms, and institutions; the resistance to excessive external influence; the rejection of values, institutions, and forms that destroy social cohesion; and the adaptation of forms of production so that they favor the specificity of human and local social development. On the other hand, a negative-dominating interpretation of cultural identity may include the use of traditional values and norms, or arguments emphasizing cultural "uniqueness" to legitimize marginalization or the existing status quo. Like Sunkel and Feunzalida, Preiswerk sees both processes at work simultaneously (see also Escobar, 1985; Jamal, 1984; Tehranian, 1985, in press; Wignaraja, 1977, 1986; Worsley, 1984; Yearwood, 1987).

The Many Faces of Power

As noted, another important aspect of the development debate is the concept of power. Although most social scientists reckon that the power concept is essential for the understanding of social reality, it is often not defined and, therefore, interpreted differently. This confusion is mainly due to the multidimensionality of the concept of power.

The traditional interpretation of the power concept refers to material or perceived possessions in a narrow as well as a broad meaning, that is, a property or possession that is handled by actors in a mainly intentional, direct, or indirect manner. Max Weber's definition, which describes power as the capability of one individual or social group to impose its will, despite the objections of others, is often quoted in this context (see, e.g., Perroux, 1983). One can find such a static perception in different functionalist as well as classic

Marxist theories. In such definitions power is one-sidedly situated with the "power holders." Their position of power rests on a conflict relationship that can be "resolved" only by consensus on one side or by struggle on the other. Critical social philosophers and poststructuralists have pointed out the limitations of such a power concept. Michel Foucault (1966, 1975, 1977, 1980), Anthony Giddens (1978, 1981, 1984), and Jürgen Habermas (1981, 1985), for example, state that the relationship between power and conflict is of an accidental nature. They nevertheless do not deny that the exercise of power is an asymmetrical phenomenon, but instead believe that power is "all embracing" and "all mighty" and has to be coupled with the concept of "interest." Power and conflict often go together, so they argue, but this union is not because one logically implies the other, but because power has to be seen in concert with the pursuit of interest. While power is a characteristic of every form of human interaction, contrapositions of interests are not, meaning that power is a dual concept that can be interpreted in two ways. Looking at power in a static way, there are those who have power and those who endure power. But if interpreted in a dynamic way, one could say that even the powerless exercise power over the powerful. In other words, the exercise of power is not the same as suppression.

> Thus power concerns the possible effectuated and asymmetrically divided ability of one actor (power holder) to put into order, inside a specific interaction system, the alternatives of actions of one or more actors (power subjects). Power centers around the capability to regulate and structure the actions inside asymmetrical relations. (Laermans, 1985, p. 131, my translation)

A NEW PERSPECTIVE ON CULTURE

> Clearly, the possibility of cultural sociology is connected (1) with the fact of culture itself becoming problematic, (2) with the emergence of a science that makes the social process, as such, the object of investigation, and (3) with the genesis of a specific method and new orientation to cultural formations, which found its scientific expression in the study of ideology. None of the three originates within science; instead they codify something produced by life itself. It is appropriate to our dynamic conception to endeavour to locate the origins and development of these factors in the total process. (Mannheim, 1982, p. 278)

The meaning of concepts and symbols, as well as the use of language, as such, is culture-bound. Culture is a complex phenomenon that can be interpreted in a narrow or broad sense. I want to reject the viewpoint that conceives of culture as only a partial phenomenon of the social reality and thus considers cultural sociology a subdiscipline of the social sciences. I am of the opinion that cultural sociology derives its special character not so much from a specific object field, but from a specific perspective on society.

In this sense, cultures can be defined as social settings in which a certain reference framework has taken concrete form or has been institutionalized and orients and structures the interaction and communication of people within this historical context. The classic distinction between structure and culture as an empirical duality becomes meaningless. All structures are cultural products and all culture gives structure. This intrinsic bond with a society in which actions are full of value makes all social facts cultural goods. Social facts, like institutions, behavioral patterns, normative systems, structures, and societal models, are construed and cultivated in the light of certain values, preferences, or options that have developed in society in response to certain common needs or problems. With the concept of culture, one therefore also means material and immaterial aspects of a certain way of life, passed on and corroborated via socialization processes (e.g., school, media, church) to the members of that society. The reproduction of any social organization entails a basic correspondence between processes of "subjection" and "qualification." This basic social functioning of subjection/qualification involves three fundamental modes of ideological interpolation. Ideologies subject and qualify subjects by telling them, relating them to, and making them recognize: (a) what exists and what does not exist (i.e., a sense of identity); (b) what is good and bad (i.e., normalization); and (c) what is possible and impossible (i.e., a logic of conservation versus a logic of change). Ideological interpolations are made all the time, everywhere, and by everybody. However, even though ideological interpolations occur everywhere, they tend to cluster at nodal points in the ongoing social process that one could call ideological institutions, or apparatuses, which are both discursive and nondiscursive (Servaes, 1981). This process through which knowledge is transmitted is never linear. It is linked to power in conscious and unconscious ways; it is sporadic and ubiquitous and transcends national and cultural boundaries: "Culture is the deposit of knowledge, experiences, beliefs, values, attitudes, meanings, hierarchies, religion, timing, roles, spatial relations, concepts of the universe, and material objects and possessions through individual and group striving" (Samovar, Porter, & Jain, 1981, p. 24). It not only concerns decisions about good and evil and so on, but also the way we eat, live, or dress. In this sense, culture can be described as a social setting in which a certain reference framework has found its basis or is institutionalized and that orients and structures the interaction and communication of the people within that context. Therefore, various cultures also manifest different identities. Three empirical dimensions can be distinguished in such reference frameworks: a worldview (Weltanschauung), a value system, and a system of symbolic representation.

As argued, ideological institutions or apparatuses fulfill a key role here. They are forms of behavior that are crystallized on the basis of social acceptance into more or less standardized, self-evident routines and that can work as both negative-repressing and as positive-liberating. They exist in strategies or relations of forces supporting, and supported by, types of knowledge that are both discursive and nondiscursive. They form clusters of institutions that have an impact on and influence each other and that are distinct from others by their own identity. The term *cultural identity* refers to two complementary phenomena: on the one hand, an inward sense of association or identification with a specific culture or subculture; on the other hand, an outward tendency within a specific culture to share a sense of what it has in common with other cultures and of what distinguishes it from other cultures. Birgitta Leander (1986), editorializing in the special and last issue of *Culture: Dialogue Between the Peoples of the World*, writes:

> The major characteristic with regard to awareness of identity in Latin America is the integration of multiple influences, both external and internal, forming a cultural whole in which, despite countless local and regional variations, common features are identifiable throughout the continent. (p. 16)

The construction of cultural or regional identifications, as illustrated by Peter Putnis (1987) in the case of the Queensland identity in Australia, is not only made in the propositional attitudes of outsiders, but also in the performative attitudes of the insiders. Like all social processes, these processes are not purely rational or preplanned events. Thus culture must be seen as the unintended result of an interweaving of the behavior of a group of people who interrelate and interact with each other.[3]

Emic or Etic

Instead of starting a discussion about the positive or negative, objective or subjective interpretation of a culture, anthropologists usually distinguish between an *emic* and an *etic* approach:

> Emic operations have as their hallmark the elevation of the native informant to the status of the ultimate judge of the adequacy of the observer's descriptions and analyses. The test of the adequacy of emic analyses is their ability to generate statements the native accepts as real, meaningful, or appropriate. . . . Etic operations have as their hallmark the elevation of observers to the status of ultimate judges and concepts used in descriptions and analyses. The test of adequacy of etic accounts is simply their ability to generate scientifically productive theories about the causes of sociocultural differences and similarities. (Harris, 1980, p. 32)

In this context I would like to plead for an emic position. However, as Clifford Geertz (1973) warns, this is an extremely difficult approach to accomplish: "We begin with our interpretations of what our informants are up to, or think they are up to, and then systematize" (p. 15). Therefore, I fully agree with Sari Thomas (1982) when she argues that "it is at the very least naive to assume that such frames of reference, theories, models or paradigms can ever be entirely emic. The notion of data collection for its own sake and without paradigmatic bias is no less than scientific romanticism" (p. 79). For this reason, Geertz prefers the notions of "experience-near" and "experience-far" to the emic and etic concepts. The former are internal to a language or culture and are derived from the latter that are posed as universal or scientific (cf. the distinction between phonemic and phonetic sounds in language use).

Furthermore, Geert Hofstede (1980) and Peter Kloos (1984) for example, eloquently point out that there are different kinds of knowledge: Some regularities in human behavior are explainable on the basis of culture-specific laws, other on the basis of generally valid laws. Because their epistemological status differs, these two kinds of knowledge also imply two kinds of rules. In the case of culture-specific rules, one speaks of moral rules that have a normative character; the generally applicable laws have a more natural-scientific character. The laws of the forms of production, for example, cannot be changed; the laws that underlie the production relationships, however, may well be changed. Moreover, as explained by Marsella, Devos, and Hsu (1985), human behavior can be analyzed on a number of levels. To better locate the modes of analysis from an etic versus emic point of view, they consequently distinguish the various levels of approach on which contemporary social science takes place and the focus of attention on the self in a given culture (p. 4). (For more details, see also Abdel-Malek, 1984; Barley, 1986; Eilers, 1986; Fuglesang, 1982; Society for International Development 1987).

The Dynamic of Culture

Another essential feature of culture is its dynamic character:

> La culture est la synthèse dynamique, au niveau de la conscience de l'individu ou de la collectivité, de la réalité historique, matérielle et spirituelle, d'une société ou d'un groupe humain, des relations prévalant aussi bien entre l'homme et la nature qu'entre les hommes et entre les catégories sociales. Les manifestations culturelles sont les différentes formes par lesquelles cette synthèse s'exprime, individuellement ou collectivement, à chaque étape de l'évolution de la société ou du groupe humain en question. (Cabral, 1980, p. 186)
>
> Culture is the dynamic synthesis, both at the consciousness level of the individual or the collectivity, of the historically conceived material or spiritual reality of a society or social group. This dynamic synthesis conditions the relationships between mankind and nature as well as between people and between social categories (institutions). Cultural manifestations are the distinct forms through which this synthesis is expressed, individually and collectively, at each stage of development of the given society or social group (my translation).

Edward Hall (1973) distinguishes between three states that together constitute processes of cultural change—a formal, an informal, and a technical state. "These states are constantly fluid, shifting one into the other—

formal activity tends to become informal, informal tends toward the technical, and very often the technical will take on the trappings of a new formal system" (p. 90). As a classical example of these constantly shifting formal, informal, and technical states, one often refers to the concept of time in different cultures (see Hall, 1983).

This dynamic character of a culture finds good expression in an historical analysis such as Said's (1985). His captivating overview of the way in which Asian societies and philosophies were perceived by the West starts from the thesis

> that the essential aspects of modern Orientalist theory and praxis (from which present-day Orientalism derives) can be understood, not as a sudden access of objective knowledge about the Orient, but as a set of structures inherited from the past, secularized, redisposed, and re-formed by such disciplines as philology, which in turn were naturalized, modernized, and laicized substitutes for (or versions of) Christian supernaturalism. In the form of new texts and ideas, the East was accommodated to these structures. (Said, 1985, p. 122)[4]

Interlude

To summarize this new perspective on culture I would like to emphasize once again that culture is not only the visible, nonnatural environment of the person, but primarily his or her normative context. As culture mediates all human perceptions of nature, an understanding of these mediations is a much more important key to explaining human events than is mere knowledge of such limits. In other words, the natural world is also part of our culture, as are ideas and values. In the patterning of their social existence, people continually make principally unconscious choices that are directed by the applicable intracultural values and options. The social reality can then be seen as a reality constituted and cultivated on the basis of particular values, a reality in which the value system and the social system are completely interwoven and imbued with the activity of each other. Cultures derive an "identity" from the fact that a common world view and ethos are active in the network of institutions or apparatuses of which they consist. This "identity" differs from culture to culture. Consequently, honor, power, love, and fear are defined and enacted through cultural forms that may differ widely from one culture to another. The task for a researcher is to reveal these distinctive structures of meaning. In other words, in the study of concrete examples of cultural identity, one must be attentive to the following aspects: (a) the characteristics and dimensions of the cultural reference framework (i.e., the world view, the ethos, and their symbolic representation); (b) the interaction and interrelation with the environment of power and interests; and (c) the "ideological apparatuses" by which the cultural reference framework is produced, and through which it is at the same time disseminated.

WESTERN AND ASIATIC MODES OF COMMUNICATION

East is East, West is West, and never the twain shall meet

—Rudyard Kipling

This section will first summarize a few characteristics of what can be called a Western versus an Asiatic mode of communication (see Servaes, 1987a). Such an attempt, however, cannot be undertaken without an explicit warning: As has been argued by many scholars, bringing Western and Asian culture face-to-face is not only ambitious, but also given to simplistic impressions. With regard to the Western and Asian concept of self, for instance, Frank Johnson (1985) summarizes the problems inherent in attempting systematic comparisons between "East" and "West." False antitheses and monolithic comparisons can easily slip into the cliché generalization and overstatement of the obvious. He, therefore, cautions:

> First, generalizations stressing differences between East and West gloss over the diversity within both Eastern and Western traditions themselves—over different eras, among different cultures, and as these traditions are differentially experienced by individuals. Second, such comparisons between East and West necessarily set aside civilizations and nations whose traditions have not been recorded in a manner permitting equivalent representation. (pp. 91-92)

These risks are particularly high in condensed versions of cross-cultural comparison, such as this text. Therefore, the following should be perceived as ideal-typical cases of which the extremes are underlined in order to accentuate the typicalness of each mode of communication.

While outlining the Western mode of communication, I had the Anglo-Saxon culture, to which I belong, in mind as the framework of reference. My appreciation of the defined Asiatic mode of communication is based upon experiences in these cultures in which Confucian and Buddhist influences play a major part. In each culture I have been trying to search for the archetypes rather than for the formal and often officially propagated manifestations of a culture. More than in the West, and in a way because of the Western influences, one can observe in Asia a pronounced difference between the "written" and "unwritten" cultures (Hsiung, 1985; Taylor, 1986; Terwiel, 1984). For example, all Asian governments subscribe to the universal United Nations' Declarations that were issued after the Second World War by Western governments and that were based mainly on Western ideas and philosophies. However, the reality in many of these countries is often completely different. Confucian concepts such as harmony and hierarchy are in blazing contrast to the Western principles of conflict and democracy. Further, the three basic principles of Buddhism (Rajavaramuni, 1983), such as *Anijjang* (everything is perpetually changing), *Dukhkang* (life is full of suffering), and *Anatta* (everything is relative; certainty does not exist), differ greatly from the static, optimistic, and "ideal-utopian" principles on which the Western way of thinking is built. John Walsh (1973) summarizes these differences as follows:

> One of the basic differences between Eastern and Western cultures is that the Eastern are dominated by the concept of harmony; the Western by power. In the East, it is said, knowledge is for the sake of living in better and closer harmony with nature and man; in the West, knowledge is for the sake of controlling peace and order is a prime value; in the West, achieving the things that power makes possible is considered by many as a primary goal. (p. 82)

Language as Culture and Power

Language is an instrument of communication and power. People communicate by means of language. But at the same time, language arises out of the social matrix of power relationships in a given nation (Fuglesang, 1984; Pattanayak, 1986; Rahim, 1986). Linguistic misunderstandings are mainly a result not of linguistic incompetence, but to the difference in social and cultural patterns between communicating groups or individuals. One does "understand" the other, but one does not always comprehend.

In many Asian languages there is a distinction made between so-called levels of speech according to age, social status, and patterns of social interaction. One has to use other titles and forms of addressing when one approaches a younger or elder, a higher- or lower-ranked person. This kind of hierarchical language use has gradually disappeared in the West. Misunderstandings can be of a verbal and of a nonverbal nature. The impact of nonverbal communication forms cannot be underestimated. According to Klopf and Park (1982), only 35% of the social meaning in a face-to-face conversation is imparted verbally, more than 55% in a nonverbal way (i.e., by making use of space and time, body language, and so on).

There is something more involved than just the grammatical competence in the Chomskyian meaning. Of importance are the social use and the social and cultural context in which the language appears. Myung-Seok Park (1979, p. 29) calls this broader notion of linguistic competence the "communicative competence" of a language. A language cannot be separated from its social-cultural context. In different cultures the same words or concepts can have different connotative, contextual, or figurative meanings and evoke idiomatic or metaphoric expressions. The word *fat,* for instance, has a positive connotation in most Asian societies, it shows the person's well-being and wealth. In the West, however, the word is interpreted mainly in a negative way. In the West, the owl is a symbol for wisdom, in the East it is regarded as a stupid bird (for more of these examples, see Klopf, 1981). Rahim (1984) explores the full consequences that these differences have on international communications, while McCreary and Blanchfield (1986) analyze the patterns of discourse in negotiations between Japanese and U.S. companies.

O-Young Lee (1967) concludes that Asian languages have developed on the basis of auditive interpretation (listening) and emotion (pathos) and take into account the "aura" of things. Because of this, Asian languages are more colorful and poetic than are Indo-European languages that are based on visual ascertainment (seeing) and rationation (logos): "A culture of the eye is intellectual, rational, theoretical and active, while a culture of the ear is emotional, sensitive, intuitive and passive" (Lee, 1967, p. 43).

I or We

An essential difference between Western and Asian society is the position of the individual and, consequently, the conception of self. While Western culture is characterized by a strong self-image, in the Asian context, group consciousness plays a much bigger part. Geertz (1973), for instance, in his influential essay on Bali, describes how Balinese act as if persons are impersonal sets of roles, in which all individuality and emotional volatility are systematically repressed. Their notion of self is quite different from the one described by Freud (1951). Freud demonstrated that one can trace out systematic interrelationships between conscious understandings of social relations, unconscious dynamics, and the ways ambigious, flexible symbols are turned into almost deterministic patterns of cultural logic. Therefore, Westerners are I-orientated:

> Their behavior is largely determined by their perception of self, a concept we define as the identity, personality, or individualism of a given person as distinct from all other people. For them, the self is a unifying concept. It provides a perspective in thinking, a direction for activity, a source of motivation, a locus in decision-making and a limit to group involvement. (Stewart, 1972, p. 75)

Asians, on the other hand, are we-orientated. They get their identity from the position they hold in the group. In Geertz's study, the Balinese tried to establish smooth and formal interpersonal relationships in which the presentation of the self is affectless and determined by the social group. A typical example is the Asian way of addressing people. A Westerner writes first his Christian name, then his surname, followed by street, town, and country. Asians do it the other way around. Agehananda Bharati (1985), for instance, points out that when one asks for a Hindu's identity, he will give you his caste and his village as well as his name. There is a Sanskrit formula that starts with lineage, family, house, and ends with one's personal name. In this presentational formula the empirical self comes last.

In other words, Asians are submerged, so to speak, in the group, and find themselves lost and powerless as individuals when the link with the group is taken away or does not exist:

> The predominant value is congeniality in social interactions based on relations among individuals rather than on the individual himself. A network of

> obligations among members of a group is the point of reference, not the self. In Oriental cultures, people's behavior is directed first to maintaining affiliation in groups and congenial social relations. Goals that could be personally rewarding to the individual are only of secondary importance. (Klopf & Park, 1982, p. 30)

Only after the Asian knows someone's status, age, sex, and so on (these are often the first questions that are asked of a foreigner and are regarded as "indiscreet" by a Westerner), he or she will be capable of communicating, of addressing the conversational partner in the "appropriate" cultural way.

Social Relations

Social relations patterns, as well, are perceived and shown differently. Social stratification exists, of course, in the East as well as in the West. But whereas it is not accentuated in the West—moreover, in interpersonal communication one often attempts to construct a (often feigned) horizontal and equal relationship—hierarchic relations still exist and are explicitly emphasized in the East. Appearances, such as clothes and etiquette, play a major role. The Confucian ethic, for instance, attaches a lot of importance to tradition and manners. One individual is not equal to another, one is always of a higher or lower rank or status. This ranking applies to every social form or organization—family, enterprise, or school. In China, this performance of rank is called *li,* and involves the ability to value the position one has to take up in each specific relationship pattern and consequentially to be able to follow the right ritual. An investigation into the way in which the Chinese Communist Party is organized and operates on the basis of Confucian principles, would, in my opinion, yield many revealing views about modern-day China.

Even in more formal relations and modernistic institutions these patterns of communication are carried on. Yong-Bok Ko (1979) refers to Weber's three forms of administration—traditional, charismatic, and legal government—and states that Korean society, although formally a legal government, is dominated by hierarchic and feudal conventions, and that the authorities justify in emotional and superstitious arguments, rather than rational ones.

> The fact that the organizational structure of political parties is based not on the from-below pattern but on the from-above pattern or, at best, on a compromise between the two, exposes an inversion of value the like of which can be found in the phenomenon that the master comes first to be obeyed by the masses. As we often find in National Assembly elections, the fame of candidates, the degree of their personal acquaintance with voters, and their personal ties are more decisive than their ability. This discloses that an emotional rather than rational atmosphere prevails in politics. The fact that politicians have their own world and they are poorly equipped with elasticity so as to embrace heretics indicates that Korean politics is still not far from nepotism and factionalism. (Ko, 1979, p. 173)

In my opinion, this political pattern is also true in other Asiatic countries and in sectors such as commerce or industry as well. Asians feel themselves, less than do Westerners, drawn by political programs; they follow charismatic leaders with whom they can identify emotionally. In business matters as well, Asians follow a hierarchic, time consuming, and indirect pattern of communication, in which immediate friends or "group members" act as intermediaries. Don McCreary and Robert Blanchfield (1986) analyzed the patterns of discourse in negotiations between Japanese and U.S. companies. They arrived at the conclusion that the negotiation is complicated and dependent upon several constructs unique to the homogeneous Japanese people and culture, and that three constructs are particularly crucial: (1) *amae* (a social hierarchy of dependency relationships), (2) *haragei* (a culturally based set of paralinguistic cues coupled with superficially misleading verbal arguments with multiple semantic readings), and (3) the pragmatics of formal negotiation that concern special patterns of discourse in regard to speaking versus writing, colloquial versus formal language, responsibility spread in decision making, and translation/interpretation difficulties. They conclude that

> phatic communication, the communication and build-up of personal trust, must be included from negotiating day one. Conversation, seemingly about nothing of consequence, that is, family backgrounds, likes and dislikes, and employment history, tests the foreign negotiator's trustworthiness, how much respect and credibility is due him, and how much he is committed to a long-term outlook. (McCreary & Blanchfield, 1986, p. 156)

Because of this difference, less import is attached to a number of values that in the Western world are considered very important, such as the equality of men and women, or democracy. On the other hand, other values and norms, such as respect for one's elder, or loyalty to the group are given a more important place in the East. Therefore, Deleury (1978) argues, the Western concept of parliamentary democracy is incompatible with a Hindu society, while Kolm (1984) claims that Marxism is more closely related to Buddhism than to Western liberal principles.

Fançois Perroux (1983), however, doubts the relevance of this sort of comparison and puts forward a Weberian and anti-Weberian model.

> At most and at best, Weber's model is a sociological construct of little real benefit even in the investigation of cultures that differ from our own. What do we gain by labelling an Oriental or African culture as "charismatic" or "traditional" when it stems from a living faith? (p. 121)

And he adds that the new and "another" development movement in the North and the South:

> If it is not to lead to the world's going up in flames, [it] must at least adopt a line of research, a guiding principle and, basing itself on the anti-Weber model, a course of slow, patient and cumulative advance. (Perroux, 1983, p. 124)

Aristotle Versus Plato

The Asiatic mode of communication is indirect and implicit, the Western, direct and explicit. In Asian communication processes, a lot is supposed and "implicitly said." Westerners insist on making very explicit arrangements and have almost no ear for nonverbal forms of expression. Therefore, Westerners use language in an instrumental way and emphasize therewith the exchange of ideas and thoughts. The more emotionally involved and poetic Asian is less direct. In an instrumental pattern of communication, one defends one's opinion in an assertive way. Westerners attempt to convince their listeners by way of rational, Aristotelian argumentation. The end product, the message, is the most important part of the communication process. The communication is considered a success if the public has understood the "message." Whether or not the public agrees to the underlying viewpoint in the message is for a Western communicator of second importance. While Westerners start a conversation with a definite goal, (i.e., they want to state or obtain something material or immaterial), for Asians the emotional exchange, the being together, the pleasure of communicating are equally important. In interpersonal communication, Asians will try to assess the feelings and state of mind of those present. They do not want to bring the harmony of the group into danger, and thus will give their opinion in an indirect way. Not the product, or the message, but the process is of importance; hence, for instance, the totally different perceptions with regard to work and leisure time. In the West, they are regarded as two separate aspects of life; but not so in the East.

So the Asiatic mode of communication can be labeled as defensive and situational. The conversation is often abruptly stopped, or the subject changed without any obvious reason, as soon as the speaker feels that his listener does not totally agree with his point of view or that his feelings might have been hurt. Asians attempt to reach a "total communication." If this is not possible they prefer "no communication" to the Western compromise of "partial communication."

Whereas the Western mode of communication concentrates on the "encoding" of issues, and is, as such, sender or communicator orientated, the Asian mode of communication attaches more attention to the "decoding" problems of messages and is, as such, receiver- or public-oriented. Whereas the Westerner does actively look "for the truth" and is convinced that this can be achieved on the basis of a logical argumentation, the Asian accepts that the "truth" will be "revealed" when he or she is ready for it or, in other words, when enough knowledge and insight has been accumulated. The attitude is passive; data collection and argumentation—two essential elements in a Western mode of communication—are often missing. On the other hand, the action orientation of Westerners dictates their attitude with regards to nature and technology, they want to command and control these, while Asians try to achieve a harmonious relationship with both. Therefore, in more general terms, the vision of intuition, rationalism, and empiricism is in both modes of communication totally different (for more details see Chu, 1986; Contractor,

East	West
sociocultural system (emphasis on)	
cosmocentrical	anthropocentrical
self is part of group	self is central
hierarchy/assymetrical	
horizontal/symmetrical	
harmony	power/conflict
being	doing
mode of communication (emphasis on)	
Platonic	Aristotelian
pathos prevails	logos prevails
indirect	direct
intermediate	face-to-face
situational	instrumental
receiver-oriented	communicator-oriented
dialectic/cyclic/dialogic	linear/monologic
total	partial
poetical/nonverbal	explicit/verbal
deductive/accepting	inductive/analyzing
affective	assertive
relative statements	absolute statements
form	content

Figure 7.2 The main differences between the Asiatic and Western sociocultural and communicative patterns.

Fulk, Monge, & Singhai, 1986; Dissanayake, 1982, 1985; Dissanayake & Said, 1983; Itty, 1984; Tehranian, in press; White & Nair, 1986).

By way of summary, I have attempted to bring together the fundamental differences between the Asiatic and Western social-cultural organization and communication modes in Figure 7.2.

CULTURAL IMPERIALISM AND THE MASS MEDIA

> The level of analysis employed for understanding the implications of the mass media at the international, as opposed to the national and individual level, has remained frozen at the stage of intellectual development achieved by communications [*sic*] research in the first three or four decades of this century. (Tracey, 1985, p. 44)

The debate on cultural or media imperialism has focused mainly on the international domination of the so-called periphery or Third World by the Center of First World. This domination occurs through a combination of power components, that is, military, economics, politics, culture, and so forth. The specific components of the domination of any nation at a given point in time vary from those of another as a result of the variations, including the resources of the Center powers, the nature or structure of the Periphery nation, and the degree of resistance to domination. Nowadays the cultural and communication components have become of great importance in continuing the dependent relationships. Because, as many scholars argue, we stand within the rather paradoxical situation that, as the Third World begins to emancipate itself economically and politically, cultural dominance increases. Whereas the former colonialist was largely out to plunder economically profitable areas and showed only moderate interest in political administration, the technological evolution of the communication media have contributed to a cultural and ideological dependence. A relatively old but still very appropriate definition of media imperialism is the one used by Boyd-Barrett (1977):

> The process whereby the ownership, structure, distribution or content of the media in any one country are singly or together subject to substantial external pressures from the media interests of any other country [nation] or countries [nations] without proportionate reciprocation of influence by the country so affected. (p. 117)

Building on this definition and Galtung's (1980) discussion of imperialism, we can distinguish between four mechanisms of imperialism: exploitation, penetration though a bridgehead (i.e., the peripheral elite), fragmentation, and marginalization. While exploitation is seen as the major source of inequality in this world, the three other mechanisms can be conceived as supporting factors, though not all are necessary. In other words, their influence can be both direct and indirect, either of an objectively measurable or subjectively perceptible nature (see Servaes, 1983; 1986c).

Some minor work on the motion of imperialism may be necessary. Cees Hamelink (1978, 1983) gives preference to the concept of cultural synchronization over the more common cultural imperialism idea. In his opinion, cultural imperialism is the most frequent, but not exclusive, form in which cultural synchronization occurs. For cultural synchronization can take place without any overt imperialistic relations. (I tend to agree with this view and have tested it in the case of Thailand, a country that has never been colonized [Servaes, 1985; 1987b].)

Modes of Influence

One can distinguish between different modes of influence by the degree of intentionality that precedes them or with which they are accepted. According to Boyd-Barrett (1977, 1982), the international communication process consists of four major interrelated components: (a) the shape of the communication vehicle, involving a specific technology at the consumer end, and a typical range and balance of communication contexts; (b) a set of industrial arrangements for the continuation of media production, involving given structural relationships and financial facilities; (c) a body of values about ideal practice; and (d) specific media contents. Lee (1980), among others, adds a fifth component when emphasizing the importance of historical analysis.

Among those scholars who are particularly interested in studying the so-called shape of the communication vehicle are Sidney Head (1985), and Elihu Katz (1973, 1977). These scholars argue that radio and television were developed mainly in the United States, specifically as one-way communication media for domestic distribution. Yet neither of these features were absolutely necessary as technological or market terms. This one-way character of broadcasting media, that is, the goal of nonstop broadcasting, the orientation toward a large, mass audience, and the striving for up-to-the-minute news, has become the dominant "shape" for the rest of the world. This standardization is sustained by a technological infrastructure developed largely in the United States. Although some developing countries have begun to manufacture their own receiver sets, all are dependent on imports for the expensive production and distribution technology supplied by transnational companies.

In this respect, language also must be seen as more than a vehicle of communication. Developing a national language is, therefore, very closely tied to the whole question of national identity (see e.g., De Sousa, 1974; Khubchandani, 1983). The organizational and financial structure that lies behind the shape of a communication vehicle is equally subject to export and dissemination. The form of the export or dissemination is not always direct, but may be of an indirect nature through advertising, technology transfer, the control of banking facilities, the dissemination of values or contents, and so on. (For a general appraisal, see Becker, 1984; Cvjeticanin, 1985; Hancock, 1984; Moriarty, 1984; or Servaes, 1987e.)

It is in the software (programming), management, and evaluation domains that the threats to cultural autonomy and local adaptations are most acute because, once a nation accepts another's concepts of what constitutes "professional," "responsible," or "appropriate" use of any communication medium, its room for cultural adaptation and experimentation may be seriously compromised.

Values of practice can be either explicit and visible rules of behavior in media organizations or implicit assumptions. Examples of values of practice include the idealized principles of "objectivity" and "impartiality" in news reporting; assumptions about the most appropriate forms of technology for specific media tasks (e.g., in encouraging the adoption of educational TV by developing countries); and/or assumptions about what constitutes a "good" TV series. Peter Golding (1977) and Karol Jakubowicz (1986), among others, explain how Western values of practice can be exported and disseminated through three mechanisms: the just mentioned institutional transfer, training and education, and the diffusion of occupational ideologies. The export and dissemination of media products, including form and content, is probably the most visible form of Western domination and penetration in the Periphery. It has resulted in a substantial body of research on general as well as more specific cases that attempt to explore how particular media structures and products function as importers of cultural and consumption values and promoters of (foreign, mainly Western) economic and political interests. The most outstanding work in this tradition, which has had the greatest influence on the international scene, is the study by the International Commission for the Study of Communication Problems, edited by Sean MacBride (1980).[5]

Media Imperialism Reconsidered

Many authors, among them advocates of the cultural imperialism approach, have recognized its shortcomings and urged that the approach be redefined and reexamined. Owing mainly to the fact that research in the international communication area, on the one hand, is still in its infancy (Hur, 1982), and, on the other hand, that it deals with rather complex realities, one may say that the media imperialism thesis needs further empirical examination. There is an urgent need for more quantitative but especially qualitative research. Most of the studies on the imbalance and one-way flow do not go far beyond quantitative aspects: They show how information, ideas, entertainment, capital, and hardware flow between nations and media institutions, and, therefore, cause imbalances between Center and Periphery nations, as well as disparities within regions and countries (between rural and urban areas, between linguistic or ethnic majorities and minorities, and between rich and poor groups or classes).

But, besides these necessary quantitative research findings, one also needs more detailed information on the qualitative aspects, such as, cultural and ideological components, or the impact of external (mainly Western) influences on local communities. This kind of research is not widespread in this research tradition.

> The level of generality of most of the "cultural dependency" literature does not clarify the specific dynamics of the ideological process and its effects on Latin American peoples. The specification of how ideological action takes place, and whom it affects and how, is often overlooked. (Sarti, 1981, p. 323)

In other words, most dependistas take for granted that together with the huge volume of Western communication messages, a conservative and capitalist ideology and consumptive culture will be introduced simultaneously. Such a view ignores some of the basic truths about communication as they are developed in the multiplicity paradigm. Far from being a top-down phenomenon only, foreign mass media interact with local networks in what can be named a coercive/seductive way, and, therefore, have radically different effects and meanings in different cultural settings. Far from being passive recipients, audiences are actively involved in the construction of meaning around the media they consume.

As documented by Boyd (1984, 1985), Chu (1985), Goonasekera (1987), Laing (1986), Mattelart (1983), Tracey (1985), or Ugboajah (1985), one can observe at least two interrelated developments. First, there is a tendency to import cultural content and develop local imitations, and, second, many Third World communicators and organizations are using the imported media technologies to attempt to forge a more autonomous culture, independent of but, at the same time, borrowing from the Western culture. The idea of an international media software convergence is, therefore, rendered weak. Furthermore, as is the case in the West, one observes that in spite of the better production quality, the majority of local audiences prefer programs produced in their own culture. This preference is based on, at least, language and cultural affinity. Therefore, imported media can have a "boomerang effect," conveying precisely the opposite consequence to that presumed by purveyors or observers on the surface.

Another related problem concerns the absence of a so-called intranational analysis. Dependistas put too much emphasis on the contradictions at the international level, and accordingly overlook the existing contradictions at the national level between the interests of the state and the media owners and between the government and the population. For example, in Latin America, Motta (1984) points out, state intervention in national affairs has increased overall. This process of capitalist state intervention has produced authoritarian, mostly military, governments that have centralized decision making:

> First, the government controls the creation, distribution, and operation of mass media, as well as the flow of messages. The control takes many forms— station licensing, broadcasting regulations, and censorship . . . . This type of control seeks to depoliticize and demobilize society. Second, the government widely circulates official messages in order to mobilize the population toward state ends and to legitimize itself. (pp. 384-385)

The political result of the dependency view, the critics state, is to turn attention away from these internal class relations and focus it on the Center, which is held responsible for existing social inequality and injustice.

One has to accept that "internal" and "external" factors inhibiting development do not exist independently of each other. Thus, in order to understand and develop a proper strategy, one must have an understanding of the class relationships of any particular peripheral social formation and the ways in which these structures articulate with the Center, on the one hand, and the producing classes in the Third World, on the other. To dismiss Third World ruling classes, for example, as mere puppets whose interests are always mechanically synonymous with those of the Center is to ignore the realities of a much more complex relationship. The very unevenness and contradictory nature of the capitalist development process necessarily produces a constantly changing relationship. So, for instance, Sinclair (1986), in his analysis of the Mexican case, arrives at the conclusion that broadcasting owners not only

resist attempts by the state to assert its authority, but actually draw legitimacy from the state's own activities in the media sphere. An important transition taking place in many countries is the strengthening of the traditional culture at grass-roots levels. As has been argued previously, "tradional" should not only be viewed in a conservative way but also as having progressive connotations. Therefore, one can observe the growth of dualistic communication structures (Malik, 1980; Wang & Dissanayake, 1984). Adaptation of traditional media for education and social action are encouraged because of their cultural values and their inexpensiveness:

> Folk media are grounded on indigenous culture produced and consumed by members of a group. They reinforce the values of the group. They are visible cultural features, often strictly conventional, by which social relationships and a world view are maintained and defined. They take on many forms and are rich in symbolism. (Ugboajah, 1985, p. 172)

A logical approach for societies and culture that are concerned about the hegemony of culturally imperialistic Western media, therefore, could be to develop sets of "alternative," "countercultural," or "demythologizing" integrated media that could use external media technologies and products for radically different purposes (such as those described by Constantino, 1978; Nettleford, 1979; and Tehranian, 1984).

Robert Graff (1983) summarizes this new perspective on the role of media and culture in development as follows:

> First, total control over modern communication channels—press, broadcasting, education, and bureaucracy—does not ensure control of all the communication networks in a given society. Nor does control of the mass media ensure support for the controlling forces, nor for any mobilization around their objectives, nor for the effective repression of opposition. Second, no government or ruler is able to operate effectively, to control, censor, or to play the role of gatekeeper with regard to all communications networks at all times in a given society.... Third, both alternate and parallel networks exist in every society by definition. Obviously, they are not always active.... Fourth, the fact that alternate and parallel networks often function through structures and channels does not mean that such networks must necessarily be religious, as in Iran. They can function through political, national or class structures ... [and] can also be based upon secular, cultural, artistic, or folkloric channels.... Fifth, alternate and parallel networks feature a highly participatory character, high rates of credibility, and, in Emile Durkheim's terms, a strong organic integration with other institutions deeply rooted in that society. In contrast, the modern mass media, having been mechanically transplanted from abroad into Third World societies, enjoy varying and limited rates of penetration. They are seldom truly integrated into institutional structures, as occurs in Western societies. Finally, modern mass media and alternate or parallel networks are not mutually exclusive by definition. They can be effectively combined, provided a functional division of

> labor is established between them, and provided the limits of the mass media are recognized. (p. 74-76)

Not Only a Third World Concern

It should be clear that the discussion of dependency and cultural imperialism cannot be seen as only a Third World concern. Many authors (see LeDuc, 1983; Littunen, 1980; or Webster, 1984) argue that the newer technological developments, such as Direct Broadcasting Satellite (DBS) systems, will initially have their greatest impact within the so-called developed world.

> The problem of dependency and cultural identity, especially in broadcasting, has been prominent in the relationship between Canada and the U.S. At a time that official U.S. policies are moving toward the dismantling of regulatory restrictions in favour of free market competition and deregulation, Canada is still heavily relying upon government regulations. These different approaches profoundly reflect differences in traditions in the two countries. Canadians may have greater trust and confidence in government than Americans do . . . . In the U.S. the role of the state in the regulation of broadcasting must always be tested in the light of the First Amendment guarantee of "freedom of speech," whereas until 1982 there was in Canada no similar bench mark embedded in a written constitutional instrument. (Zolf, 1987, pp. 1-2)

However, this difference does not mean that Canada's response to the foreign technical influx is protectionism, but the strengthening of the domestic cultural industries. Canada has sought a workable balance between freedom of access to a multiplicity of international programming and the imperatives necessary for maintaining a national cultural identity. Their aim is not only to control the hardware but also the software. Therefore, only Canadian nationals are entitled to own broadcasting systems and 60% of the television and 30% of the radio programming has to be Canadian-produced. In order to stimulate Canadian content in the media, the government directly and indirectly encourages local productions through subsidies and tax deductions.

The Canadian federal government in 1984 appointed a special task force to investigate the ways in which a new federal broadcasting policy could be implemented. According to their latest report (1986) the three fundamental points that have to guide the Canadian national broadcasting strategy are (a) all peoples and all nationals have an interest in promoting diversity; (b) people will have access to international programming (this is a factor beyond control in many Third World nations); and (c) "choice" for Canadians is meaningless unless it also includes programming that reinforces the cultural heritage of all Canadians (see also Audley, 1983; Canadian-U.S. Conference on Communications Policy, 1983; Desaulniers, 1987; Therrien, 1980). The task force calls for increasing Canadian content on the air, and for creating several new networks via pay-TV and cable. These would be commercial-free.

The overall policy objective, therefore, is that Canadian programs must, in general, reflect Canadian experience and the social, visual, and linguistic idioms of the country. At the same time, it is assumed that Canadian broadcasting should provide quality programs that speak to universal themes—programs of widespread appeal that can compete both domestically and internationally. In order to meet these goals the Canadian Broadcasting Corporation (CBC, 1985), in its latest proposal to the Federal Task Force on Broadcasting Policy, advocates a number of restrictive and stimulative policy measures to increase Canadian content and change viewers' orientation. It calls for the removal of American commercial programs from the CBC network and argues that 90% of the programs on the CBC services should be Canadian. The CBC also urges that the government set an overall national target of more than 50% domestic programming by 1990 on public as well as privately owned stations. However, despite an ability to pronounce these kinds of policy statements at frequent intervals, Canada has had enormous difficulty implementing such policies. Robin Mansell (1984), for instance, convincingly shows how institutional and structural factors that generally have received little attention condition the effectiveness of government intervention.

A similar discussion is taking place in Western Europe. In 1984 the Commission of the European Communities published a "Green Paper" on the establishment of a common market for broadcasting, especially by satellite and by cable. The purpose of the report was threefold: to demonstrate the importance of broadcasting for European integration and, in particular, for the free democratic structure of the European Communities; to illustrate the significance of the EC Treaty for those responsible for producing, broadcasting, and retransmitting radio and TV programs, and for those receiving such programs; and to submit for public discussion the Commission's thinking on the approximation of certain aspects of Member States' broadcasting and copyright laws (Schwartz, 1985). Although the report claims to present a detailed analysis of the technical, sociocultural, economic and legal aspects of broadcasting and related topics in the respective EC countries, it focuses mainly on the economic and legal aspects of broadcasting policies. As the title of the report—Television without Frontiers—may indicate, it advocates total freedom to provide services across borders and emphasizes the need to harmonize national legislations. This move would imply the opening up of intracommunity frontiers for national programs and the establishment of a common market for broadcasters and audiences. Most researchers, in a reaction to these EC deregulation proposals, fear the cultural synchronization in European television of the future with more services and more competition. A total liberalization will favor mainly economic interests toward commercialization and privatization. Therefore, they propose strategies to preserve

European culture and values, and to stimulate domestic production movements in Europe instead of relying on imports, particularly from the United States. Wolfgang Hoffmann-Riem (1986, 1987) elaborates the concept of pluriformity, which is often used in debates on national cultural identity and indigenous programming. He concludes that the internationalization and commercialization of programming takes place in both private and public broadcasting systems. Small and centrally located countries, like Belgium, the Netherlands, or Switzerland, are very vulnerable to these developments. Referring to the Canadian case, I argue (see Servaes, 1988) that these countries, in order to defend their cultural identity, should give priority to supporting their public service broadcasting systems both financially and legally: financially, to improve their programming so that everybody could have an appropriate chance under equal conditions; legally, by imposing regulations that stimulate and promote national and regional initiatives, for instance by propagating coproductions among similar language broadcasting stations. (For an overview of these issues, see Forrest, 1987; McQuail & Siune, 1986; Pragnell, 1985.)

BY WAY OF CONCLUSION

In this text I have argued that the classic materialist-idealist distinction between political economy and interpretative approaches has become outdated. Analysis should involve the relative power-linked articulations and conflicts over ideologies, world views, moral codes, and the locally bounded conditions of knowledge and competence. Although all social research presumes a hermeneutic moment, often it remains latent because researcher and research inhabit a common cultural milieu. Moreover, it is in the study of the unintended consequences of action and the creation of meaning that some of the most distinctive tasks of the social sciences in general and communication studies in particular are to be found. At least two types of unintended influences can be distinguished: first the unconscious ones, and second, influences conditioned by the context in which the different forms of social action take place. Without disqualifying and underestimating the significance of other research contributions I would like to advocate the following research design. What I have in mind is a text that takes as its subject not a concentrated group of people in a community, affected in one way or another by politico-economic forces, but the "system" itself—the political and economic processes, encompassing different locales, or even different continents. This research project must be centered around two problem areas. First, it must be determined what actors or interest groups on the one hand, and what factors or structural constraints on the other hand, exercise influence from above. These influences can transform, reinforce, or weaken each other. What is required is a much more precise analysis of influence patterns that function from the top down by means of power in the broad sense. With this focus, the role of the state also becomes more central.

The second problem area is the grass-roots reaction to this influence. Research must be focused on the rational objectives of target groups and social movements. The difference from traditional anthropological research should be that the choice of the symbolic order for the research is determined by key concepts, such as reproduction and labor. It is not the more or less chance differences in rational objectives that are interesting, but the systematic tendencies and the thereby generalizable differences. This interest implies that the choice of the place and the context of research cannot be at random but must be based on macrostructural insights. There is the danger that the research area will be selected on the basis of practical reasons rather than theoretical considerations. This research can be performed on small-scale, large-scale, as well as integrated levels. In all cases one needs to break through artificial boundaries of distinct media and communication systems in search of those elements that constitute the ideological order of power/empowerment and domination/emancipation, which is the historical outcome of (class) struggle. The main target of this new approach is social groups or movements with a concern for public issues like ecology, social justice, peace, education, human rights, civic action, and so on. This type of social grouping transcends the notion of political parties or interest groups as traditionally understood and conceived. The guiding principle of these groups is to proceed from a bottom-up perspective, rather than from the top down as is the case in the classic power structure that disregards the views of the masses and is therefore elite-oriented. The most effective forms of mobilization of these social groups and movements are rooted in popular cultural and ideological expressions in both interpersonal and mass communication. Their greatest ontological challenge is the political rationality of traditional knowledge, or, as Orlando Fals Borda (1985b, p. 2) calls it, "the rediscovery of forms of wisdom that have become obscured or discarded by Cartesian methods and Kantian empirical presuppositions." In other words, the goal of these social movements is political in the old sense of the word. Therefore, I (Servaes, 1987c) have advocated a more dialectic and multicentered perception of power and cultural factors in the context of communication and development in which I distinguished between three problem areas: the mutual dependency between the macro level of the society or a given structure, and the micro level of the social actions involved; the position and the autonomy of organized subjects; and the relationship of domination, dependency, and subordination versus liberation, selective participation, and emancipation of power and interest contrapositions. However, a combination of all these factors must consist of not only the formulation of knowledge, but also of the influencing of those who can do more with knowledge than can the researchers themselves because they have more power at their disposal. Therefore, the political relevance of the advocated perspective on culture and development has a chance to succeed only if an organic bond can be forged, internationally, between the grass-roots movement in the West and in the Third World, and nationally, between those groups that are aiming for a more just and more efficient communication and societal order.

NOTES

1. In this text I am using the concept of *nation* as defined by Tran Van Dinh (1987, p. 109): "A nation is a community characterized by cultural cohesion and communality of identity." Van Dinh rejects the more commonly used term *nation-state* "because it has neither a clear analytical purpose nor a generally understood popular meaning." Instead of nation-states he prefers the term *countries*, and *state* to designate *government*.

2. In Servaes (1987d), I combined an adjusted version of Sunkel and Fuenzalida's transnationalization thesis with Johan Galtung's (1980) six types, or aspects, of (possible) dependent relationships in order to achieve a conceptual framework for the analysis of relationships between processes of integration, disintegration, and reintegration at the various levels of a specific societal system, and for the study of the internal versus external variables and/or positive versus negative factors that determine the processes of power and empowerment in society.

3. Those who are familiar with newer cultural approaches may have observed that I heavily defend the views of people like Peter Berger (1967), Pierce Bourdieu (1979), Michel Foucault (1980), Clifford Geertz (1973), Goran Therborn (1980), Claude Lévi-Strauss (1966), Marshall Sahlins (1976), and Raymond Williams (1981), to whom I refer the reader for more details.

4. Daniel Boorstin's (1986) historical account of man's search to know his world and himself is a similar study. For more general assessments, see Glenn and Glenn (1981), Gudykunst (1983, 1985), Gudykunst and Nishida (1986), Kim (1984), and Van Nieuwenhuyze (1984).

5. For more comprehensive assessments of the dependency literature, see, Alrabaa (1986), Fejes (1981, 1986), Moschner (1982), or Servaes (1987d).

REFERENCES

Abel-Malek, A., & Pandeya A. M. (Eds.). (1984). *Intellectual creativity in endogenous culture*. Tokyo: United Nations University Press.

Addo, A. (1985). Beyond Eurocentricity: Transformation and transformational responsibility. In A. Addo, S. Amin, G. Aseniero et al. (Eds.), *Development as social transformation: Reflections on the global problematique*. London: Hodder & Stoughton.

Alrabaa, S. (1986). Western mass media hegemony over the Third World. *Communications, 12*, (1).

Audley, P. (1983). *Canada's cultural industries: Broadcasting, publishing, records and film*. Toronto: Lorimer.

Barley, N. (1986). *The innocent anthropologist*. Harmondsworth: Penguin.

Becker, J. (Ed.). (1984). *Information technology and a new international order*. Lund, Sweden: Studentlitteratur.

Berger, P., & Luckmann, T. (1967). *The social construction of reality*. New York: Doubleday.

Bharati, A. (1985). The Self in Hindu thought and action. In A. Marsella, G. Devos, & F. Hsu (Eds.), *Culture and self: Asian and Western perspectives* (pp. 185-230). London: Tavistock.

Boorstin, D. (1986). *The discoverers*. Harmondsworth: Penguin.

Borda, O. F. (Ed.). (1985a). *The challenge of social change*. London: Sage.

Borda, O. F. (1985b). *A rediscovery of wisdom as power.* Paper presented at the World Conference of the Society for International Development, Rome.

Bourdieu, P. (1979). *La distinction: Critique sociale du jugement.* Paris: Minuit.

Boyd-Barrett, J. (1977). Media imperialism: Towards an international framework for the analysis of media systems. In J. Curran, M. Gurevitch, & J. Woollacott (Eds.), *Mass communication and society.* London: EdwardArnold.

Boyd-Barrett, J. (1982). Cultural dependency and the mass media. In M. Gurevitch, T. Bennett, J. Curran, & J. Woollacott (Eds.), *Culture, society and the media* (pp. 174-198). London: Methuen.

Boyd, D. (1984). The Janus effect: Imported television entertainment programming in developing countries. *Critical Studies in Mass Communications, 1,* 379-391.

Boyd, D., & Straubhaar, J. (1985, Winter). Development impact of the home video cassette recorder on Third World countries. *Journal of Broadcasting & Electronic Media, 29,* (1), 5-21.

Cabral, A. (1980). *Unité de lutte.* Paris: Maspero.

Canadian Broadcasting Corporation (1985). *Let's do it! A vision of Canadian broadcasting.* Ottawa: Author.

Chu, C. (1985). *Satellite age and cultural identity.* Paper presented at the Symposium on International Satellite and Cable TV Law, Los Angeles.

Chu, C. (1986). Mass communication theory: The Chinese perspective. *Media Asia, 13,* (1).

Commission of the European Communities (1984). *Television without frontiers: Green paper on the establishment of the common market for broadcasting, especially by satellite and cable.* Brussels: EC.

Constantino, R. (1978). *Neocolonial identity and counter consciousness.* London: Merlin.

Contractor, N., Fulk, J., Monge, P., & Singhal, A. (1986, October-December). Cultural assumptions that influence the implementation of communication technologies. *Vikalpa, 11,* 4.

Cvjeticanin, B. (1985). *L'identité culturelle et le développement technologique dans les pays en développement.* Paper presented at the Conference of the Society for International Development, Rome.

Deleury, G. (1978). *Le modèle hindou.* Paris: Hachette.

Desaulniers, J. P. (1987). What does Canada want? or L'Histoire sans leçon. *Media, Culture and Society, 9,* 149-157.

De Sousa, E. (1974). *Portuguese colonialism in Africa.* Paris: UNESCO.

Dissanayake, W. (1981). Development and communication: Four approaches. *Media Asia, 8,* (4).

Dissanayake, W. (1982). The phenomenology of verbal communication: A classical Indian view. *Semiotica, 41,* 1-4.

Dissanayake, W., & Said, A. R. (Eds.). (1983). *Communications research and cultural values.* Singapore: Asian Mass Communication and Information Center.

Dissanayake, W. (1985). *The need for the study of Asian approaches to communication.* Paper presented at the AMIC Conference on Asian Communication Theories, Bangkok.

Eilers, F. J. (1986). *Towards ethno-communication.* Sankt Augustin: Intercultural Communication Research Unit.

Erdoes, R., & Ortiz, A. (Eds.). (1984). *American Indian myths and legends.* New York: Pantheon.

Escobar, A. (1985). Discourse and power in development: Michel Foucault and the relevance of his work to the Third World. *Alternatives, 10,* (3).

Fejes, F. (1981). Media imperialism: An assessment. *Media, Culture and Society, 3,* 281-289.

Fejes, F. (1986). *Imperialism, media and the good neighbor.* Norwood, NJ: Ablex.

Fonkoue, J. (1985). *Difference et identité.* Paris: Silex.

Forrest, A. (1987). La dimension culturelle de la Communaute Européenne. *Revue du Marche Commun, 307,* 326-332.

Foucault, M. (1966). *Les mots et les choses: Une archéologie des sciences humaines.* Paris: Gallimard.
Foucault, M. (1975). *Surveiller et punir: Naissance de la prison.* Paris: Gallimard.
Foucault, M. (1977). *Language, counter-memory, practice.* New York: Cornell University Press.
Foucault, M. (1980). *Power/knowledge: Selected interviews and other writings 1972-1977.* Brighton: Harvester.
Freud, S. (1951). *Civilization and its discontents.* New York: Norton.
Fry, V., & Fry, D. (1987). *Toward a communicative view of the production of meaning.* Paper presented at the annual meeting of the International Communication Association, Montreal.
Fuglesang, A. (1982). *About understanding: Ideas and observations on cross-cultural communication.* Upsala: Dag Hammerskjold Foundation.
Fuglesang, A. (1984). The myth of people's ignorance. *Development Dialogue, 1-2.*
Galtung, J. (1980). *The true worlds: A transnational perspective.* New York: Free Press.
Geertz, C. (1973). *The interpretation of cultures.* New York: Basic Books.
Giddens, A. (1978). *Studies in social and political theory.* London: Hutchinson.
Giddens, A. (1979). *Central problems in social theory.* London: Macmillan.
Giddens, A. (1981). *A contemporary critique of historical materialism.* London: Macmillan.
Giddens, A. (1984). *The constitution of society: Outline of the theory of structuration.* Berkeley: University of California Press.
Glenn, E., & Gleen, C. (1981). *Man and mankind: Conflict and communication between cultures.* Norwood, NJ: Ablex.
Godelier, M. (1973). *Horizon, trajets marxistes en anthropologie.* Paris: Maspero.
Golding, P. (1977). Media professionalism in the Third World: The transfer of an ideology. In J. Curran, M. Gurevitch, & J. Woollacott (Eds.), *Mass communication and society.* London: Edward Arnold.
Goonasekera, A. (1987). The influence of television on cultural values: With special reference to Third World countries. *Media Asia, 14,* 1.
Graff, R. (Ed.). (1983). *Communications for national development: Lessons from experience.* Cambridge: Oelgeschlager, Gunn & Hain.
Gudykunst, W. (Ed.). (1983). *Intercultural communication theory: Current perspectives.* Beverly Hills, CA: Sage.
Gudykunst, W. (1985). Intercultural communications: Current status and proposed directions. In B. Dervin & M. Voigt (Eds.), *Progress in communication science* (Vol. 6). Norwood, NJ: Ablex.
Gudykunst, W., & Nishida, T. (1986). The influence of cultural variability on perceptions of communication behaviour associated with relationship terms. *Human Communication Research, 13,* 525-549.
Habermas, J. (1981). *Theorie des kommunikativen Handelns* (Vols. I, II). Frankfurt: Suhrkamp.
Habermas, J. (1985). *Der philosophische Diskurs der Moderne.* Frankfurt: Suhrkamp.
Hall, E. (1973). *The silent language.* New York: Doubleday.
Hall, E. (1983). *The dance of life: The other dimension of time.* New York: Doubleday.
Hamelink, C. (1978). *Derde Wereld en culturele emancipatie.* Baarn: Het Wereldvenster.
Hamelink, C. (1983). *Cultural autonomy in global communications: Planning national information policy.* New York: Longman.
Hancock, A. (Ed.). (1984). *Technology transfer and communication.* Paris: UNESCO.
Harris, M. (1980). *Cultural materialism: The struggle for a science of culture.* New York: Vintage.
Head, S. (1985). *World broadcasting systems: A comparative analysis.* Belmont: Wadsworth.
Hindess, B., & Hirst, P. (1975). *Pre-capitalist modes of production.* London: Routledge & Kegan Paul.
Hoffmann-Riem, W. (1986). Internationale Medienmarkte—Nationale Rundfunkordnungen: Anmerkungen zu Entwicklungstendenzen in Medienbereich. *Rundfunk und Fernsehen, 34,* 57-72.

Hoffmann-Riem, W. (1987). National identity and cultural values: Broadcasting safeguards. *Journal of Broadcasting and Electronic Media, 31,* 57-72.
Hofstede, G. (1980). *Culture's consequences: International differences in work-related values.* London: Sage.
Hsiung, J. (Ed.). (1985). *Human rights in East Asia: A cultural perspective.* New York: Paragon House Publishers.
Hur, K. (1982). International mass communication research: A critical review of theory and methods. In M. Burgoon (Ed.), *Communication yearbook 6* (pp. 531-554). London: Sage.
Hyden, G. (1983). *No shortcuts to progress.* London: Heinemann.
Itty, C. (Ed.). (1984). *Searching for Asian paradigms.* Bangkok: Asian Cultural Forum on Development.
Jakubowicz, K. (1986). Broadcasting and cultural identity in Black Africa: Can they go together? *The Third Channel, 2,* 1.
Jamal, A. (1984). The cultural dimensions of development: National cultural values versus transnational cultural domination. *Development Dialogue, 1,* 76-82.
Johnson, F. (1985). The Western concept of self. In A. Marsella, G. Devos, & F. Hsu (Eds.), *Culture and Self: Asian and Western perspectives.* (pp. 91-138). London: Tavistock.
Katz, E. (1973). Television as a horseless carriage. In G. Gerbner, L. Gross, & W. Melody (Eds.), *Communication technology and social policy: Understanding the new "cultural revolution".* (pp. 381-391). New York: John Wiley.
Katz, E., & Wedell, G. (1977). *Broadcasting in the Third World: Promise and performance.* Cambridge: Harvard University Press.
Khubchandani, L. M. (1983). *Plural languages, plural cultures: Communication, identity, and sociopolitical change in contemporary India.* Honolulu: East-West Center.
Kim, Y. (1984). Searching for creative integration. In W. Gudykunst & Y. Kim (Eds.), *Methods for intercultural communication research.* Beverly Hills, CA: Sage.
Klopf, D. (1981). *Interacting in groups: Theory and practice.* Englewood, CO: Morton.
Klopf, D., & Park, M. S. (1982). *Cross-cultural communication: An introduction to the fundamentals.* Seoul: Han Shin.
Kloos, P. (1984). *Antropologie als wetenschap.* Muiderberg: Coutinho.
Ko, Y. B. (1979). Principal-subordinate relationship. In M. S. Park (Ed.), *Communication styles in two different cultures: Korean and American.* Seoul: Han Shin.
Kolm, S. (1984). Marxisme et bouddhisme. *Cahiers Internationaux de Sociologie, 77,* 339-360.
Kothari, R. (1984). Peace in an age of transformation. In R. Walker (Ed.), *Culture, ideology, and world order.* Boulder, CO: Westview.
Laclau, E., & Mouffe, C. (1985). *Hegemony and socialist strategy.* London: Verso.
Laermans, R. (1985). De vele gezichten van de machtselementen voor een sociologisch machtsbegrip. In W. Dumon (Ed.), *Sociale (on)gelijkheid.* Louvain: Sociological Research Institute.
Laing, D. (1986). The music industry and the "cultural imperialism" thesis. *Media, Culture and Society, 8,* 331-341.
Leander, B. (1986). Cultural identity in Latin America. In *Cultures: Dialogue Between the Peoples of the World.* Paris: UNESCO.
LeDuc, D. (1983). Direct broadcasting satellites: Parallel policy patterns in Europe and the United States. *Journal of Broadcasting, 27,* 99-118.
Lee, C. C. (1980). *Media imperialism reconsidered: The homogenizing of television culture.* London: Sage.
Lee, O. Y. (1967). *In this earth and in that wind.* Seoul: Hollym.
Lévi-Strauss , C. (1966). *The savage mind.* London: Weidenfeld & Nicolson.
Littunen, Y. (1980). Cultural problems of direct satellite broadcasting. *International Social Science Journal, 32,* 2.
Lubasz, H. (1985). Marx's concept of the Asiatic mode of production. In D. Banerjee (Ed.), *Marxian theory and the Third World.* New Delhi: Sage.

MacBride, S. (Ed.). (1980). *Many voices, one world: Communication and society.* Paris: UNESCO.
Malik, M. (1980). *Traditional forms of communication and the mass media in India.* Paris: UNESCO.
Mannheim, K. (1982). *Structures of thinking.* London: Routledge & Kegan Paul.
Mansell, R. (1984). *Industrial strategies in the communication/information sector: An analysis of contradictions in Canadian policy and performance.* Vancouver: Simon Fraser University.
Marcus, G., & Fischer, M. (1986). *Anthropology as cultural critique: An experimental moment in the human sciences.* Chicago: University of Chicago Press.
Marsella, A., Devos, G., & Hsu, F. (Eds.). (1985). *Culture and Self: Asian and Western perspectives.* London: Tavistock.
Mattelart, A. (1979). For a class analysis of communication. In A. Mattelart, & S. Siegelaub (Eds.), *Communication and class struggle: Vol 1. Capitalism, imperialism* (pp. 23-70). New York: International General.
Mattelart, A. (1983). *Transnationals and the Third World: The struggle for culture.* South Hadley, MA: Bergin & Garvey.
Mattelart, A., Delcourt, X., & Mattelart, M. (1983). *La culture contre la democratie? L'audiovisuel à l'heure transnationale.* Paris: La Decouverte.
McCreary, D., & Blanchfield, R. (1986). The art of Japanese negotiation. In N. Schweda-Nicholson (Ed.), *Languages in the international perspective.* Norwood: Ablex.
McQuail, D., & Siune, K. (Eds.). (1986). *New media politics: Comparative perspectives in Western Europe.* London: Sage.
Meillassoux, C. (1975). *Femmes, greniers et capitaux.* Paris: Maspero.
Meillassoux, C. (1986). *Anthropologie de l'esclavage.* Paris: Presses Universitaires de France.
Moriarty, G. E. (1984). *New technologies and their impact on broadcasting.* Paper presented at the AIBD Seminar on Broadcasting in the '80s, Kuala Lumpur.
Moschner, M. (1982). *Fernsehen in Latineamerika.* Frankfurt: Lang.
Motta G. L. (1984). National communication policies: Grass roots alternatives. In G. Gerbner & M. Siefert (Eds.), *World communications.* New York: Longman.
Nettleford, R. (1979). *Cultural action and social change: The case of Jamaica. An essay in Caribbean cultural identity.* Ottawa: International Development Research Centre.
Park, M. S. (Ed.). (1979). *Communication styles in two different countries: Korean and American.* Seoul: Han Shin.
Pattanayak, D. P. (1986). Communication: Perspectives from the developing world. In N. Schweda-Nicholson (Ed.), *Languages in the international perspectives.* Norwood: Ablex.
Perroux, F. (1983). *A new concept of development.* Paris: UNESCO.
Petras, J. (1978). *Critical perspectives on imperialism and social class in the Third World.* New York: Monthly Review Press.
Pragnell, A. (1985). *Television in Europe: Quality and values in a time of change.* Manchester: European Institute for the Media.
Preiswerk, R. (1980). Identité culturelle, self-reliance et besoins fondamentaux. In P. Spitz & J. Galtung, *Il fault manger pour vivre . . .* Paris: Presses Universitaires de France.
Putnis, P. (1987). *The construction of regional identity: An Australian case study.* Paper presented at the annual meeting of the International Communication Association, Montreal.
Rahim, S. (1984). *Understanding cultural problems in transnational information flow.* Paper Forum of the Japan Society for Communication and Information Research, Tokyo.
Rahim, S. (1986). Language as power apparatus: Observations on English and cultural policy in nineteenth-century India. *World Englishes, 5*(2/3), 231-239.
Rajavaramuni, P. (1983). *Social dimension of Buddhism in contemporary Thailand.* Bangkok: Thai Khadi Suksa.
Rey, P. (1976). *Capitalisme négrier: La marche des paysans vers le proletariat.* Paris: Maspero.
Sahlins, M. (1976). *Culture and practical reason.* Chicago: The University of Chicago Press.
Said, E. (1985). *Orientalism.* Harmondsworth: Penguin.

Salama, P., & Tissier, P. (1982). *L'Industrialisation dans le sous-développement.* Paris: Maspero.
Samovar, L., Porter, R., & Jain, J. (1981). *Understanding intercultural communication.* Belmont: Wadsworth.
Sarti, I. (1981). Communication and cultural dependency: A misconception. In E. McAnany, J. Schnitman, & N. Janus (Eds.), *Communication and social structure.* New York: Praeger.
Schwartz, I. (1985). The policy of the Commission of the European Communities with respect to broadcasting. *EBU Review, 36,* 6.
Servaes, J. (1981). *Idéologie et pouvoir: Notes pour une théorie matérialiste de l'idéologie.* Louvain: CeCoWe.
Servaes, J. (1983). *Communication and development: Some theoretical remarks.* Louvain: Acco.
Servaes, J. (1985). Film in Thailand. In W. Hesling & L. Van Poecke (Eds.), *Communicatie: Van teken tot medium.* Louvain: Leuven University Press.
Servaes, J. (1986a). Development theory and communication policy. *European Journal of Communication, 1,* 2.
Servaes, J. (1986b). Communication and development paradigms: An overview. *Media Asia, 13,* 3.
Servaes, J. (1986c). Cultural identity and the mass media in the Third World. *The Third Channel, 2,* 1.
Servaes, J. (1987a). De westerse en Aziatische communicatiewijze. *Kultuurleven, 54,* 1.
Servaes, J. (1987b). Cultuur in Thailand. Achter het masker van de Thaise glimlach. *Streven, 54,* 5.
Servaes, J. (1987c). *The past forty years—and the next: Towards another development communication policy.* Paper presented at the Conference on Communication and Change, Honolulu.
Servaes, J. (1987d). *Media aid: Naar een ander communicatie—en ontwikkelingsbeleid.* Louvain: Acco.
Servaes, J. (1987e). *Technology transfer and development communication.* Paper presented at the Unesco International Seminar on the Application of Communication Technology in Education among Developing Countries, Kuala Lumpur.
Servaes, J., & Drijvers, J. (1988). *Cultural identity and media policies in Belgium: A regional, national and European perspective.* Paper presented at the IAMCR Conference, Barcelona.
Sinclair, J. (1986). Dependent development and broadcasting: "The Mexican formula." *Media, Culture and Society, 8,* 81-101.
Singer, K. (1973). *Mirror, sword and jewel.* London: Croom Helm.
Stewart, E. C. (1972). *American cultural patterns: A cross-cultural perspective.* Belmont: Intercultural Network.
Sunkel, O., & Fuenzalida, E. (1980). La transnacionalizacion del capitalismo y el desarrollo nacional. In O. Sunkel, E. Fuenzalida, F. Cardoso et al. (Eds.), *Transnacionalizacion y dependencia.* Madrid: Ediciones Cultura Hispania.
Taylor, C. (1986). Human rights: The legal culture. In P. Ricoeur (Ed.), *Philosophical foundations of human rights.* Paris: UNESCO.
Taylor, J. (1979). *From modernization to modes of production.* London: Macmillan.
Tehranian, M. (1984). Communication and revolution in Asia: Western domination and cultural resistance in Japan and Iran. *Keio Communication Review, 5.*
Tehranian, M. (1985). *Electronic democracy: Information technologies and democratic projects.* Paris: UNESCO.
Tehranian, M. (in press). *Communitarian democracy.* Norwood: Ablex.
Terwiel, B. (1984). Formal structure and informal rules: An historical perspective on hierarchy, bondage and patron-client relationship. In H. Ten Brummelhuis & J. Kemp (Eds.), *Strategies and structures in Thai society.* Amsterdam: Anthropologisch-Sociologisch Centrum.
Therborn, G. (1980). *The ideology of power and the power of ideology.* London: Verso.
Therrien, R. (Ed.). (1980). *The 1980's. A decade of diversity: Broadcasting, satellites and pay-TV.* Ottawa: CRTC.

Thomas, C. (1984). *The rise of the authoritarian state in peripheral societies.* London: Heinemann.

Thomas, S. (1982). Some problems of the paradigm in communication theory. In D. C. Whitney & E. Wartella (Eds.), *Mass communication review yearbook* (Vol. 3, pp. 79-96). London: Sage.

Thompson, J. B. (1984). *Studies in the theory of ideology.* Cambridge: Polity Press.

Tracey, M. (1985). The poisoned chalice? International television and the idea of dominance. *Daedalus, 114,* 4.

Ugboajah, F. (Ed.). (1985). *Mass communication, culture and society in West Africa.* Munich: Saur.

Van Dinh, T. (1987). *Independence, liberation, revolution: An approach to the understanding of the Third World.* Norwood: Ablex.

Van Nieuwenhuijze, C. A. O. (Ed.). (1984). *Development regardless of culture?* The Hague: Institute of Social Studies.

Vogler, C. (1985). *The nation state: The neglected dimension of class.* Hants: Gower.

Wallerstein, I. (1974). *The modern world system: Capitalist agriculture and the origins of the European world economy in the 16th century.* New York: Academic Press.

Wallerstein, I. (1979). *The capitalist world economy.* Cambridge: University Press.

Wallerstein, I. (1980). *The modern world system II: Mercantilism and the consolidation of the European world economy 1600-1750.* New York: Academic Press.

Wallerstein, I. (1983). *Historical capitalism.* London: Verso.

Walsh, J. (1973). *Intercultural education in the community of man.* Honolulu: University of Hawaii Press.

Wang, G., & Dissanayake, W. (Eds.). (1984). *Continuity and change in communication systems.* Norwood: Ablex.

Webster, D. (1984). Direct broadcast satellites: Proximity, sovereignty and national identity. *Foreign Affairs, 62,* 5.

White, S., & Nair, K. S. (1986). *Hierarchical thinking and acting: A deterrent in development of human resources and communication systems in Third World organizations.* Paper presented at the annual meeting of the International Communication Association, Chicago.

Wignaraja, P. (1977). From the the village to the global order. *Development Dialogue, 1.*

Wignaraja, P. (1986, May). *Lessons for sustainable development in Asia.* Paper presented to the United Nations University Asian Regional Perspectives Project, Beijing.

Williams, R. (1981). *Culture.* Glasgow: Fontana.

Worsley, P. (1984). *The three worlds: Culture and development.* London: Weidenfeld & Nicolson.

Wuthnow, R., Davidson-Hunter J., Bergesen A., & Kurzweil E. (1984). *Cultural analysis: The work of Peter Berger, Mary Douglas, Michel Foucault and Jürgen Habermas.* London: Routledge & Kegan Paul.

Canadian-U.S. Conference on Communications Policy (1983). *Cultures in collision: The interaction of Canadian and U.S. television broadcast policies.* New York: Praeger.

Supply and Services Canada (1986). *Report of the Task Force on Broadcasting Policy.* Ottawa: Canada: Author.

Society for International Development (1987). Culture and ethnicity. *Development: Journal of the Society for International Development, 1.*

Yearwood, G. (1987). Cultural development and Third World cinema, *Gazette, 39,* 47-70.

Zolf, D. (1987). *The regulation of broadcasting in Canada and the United States: Straws in the wind.* Paper presented at the annual meeting of the International Communication Association, Montreal.

The Relationship Between Cultural Identity and Modes of Communication

CEES J. HAMELINK
University of Amsterdam

THE chapter by Jan Servaes addresses a complex problem and contributes to an eventful debate that has caused considerable academic and political commotion in the past decade. At stake is the exploration of the relationship between cultural identity and modes of communication.

Essential for understanding the contribution by Servaes are: (a) an understanding of culture that combines insight into the basic cultural event with both the policy options that are operational in cultivating a social system and the "Weltanschauung" that motivates the people involved; (b) the distinction between micro-level and macro-level analysis of cultural identity; and (c) a broad understanding of modes of communication (following Mattelart). The argument proceeds from the critical analysis of the paradigms that dominate the discourse on communication and development to the proposal to focus on culture as normative context. The latter implies that the aspects to be attended in the study of cultural identity are: the cultural frame of reference, the interaction of culture and power, and the ideological apparatuses that produce and disseminate the cultural frame of reference. Dealing with the micro- and macro-level analysis, Servaes illustrates the juxtaposition of Asian versus Western modes of communication and the phenomenon of cultural imperialism. The chapter is completed by advocating a research design for further study.

In response to this contribution I am inclined to propose a somewhat different approach to the same question of culture and communication. This

Correspondence and requests for reprints: Cees J. Hamelink, University of Amsterdam, Department of Communication, Oost-Indisch Huis, Oude Hoogstraat 24, 1012 CE Amsterdam, The Netherlands.

Communication Yearbook 12, 417-426

approach does not necessarily undermine Servaes's work but it offers a different perspective in interpreting the complexities under analysis. My argument questions the adequacy of the key thematic concept *cultural identity* in proposing to structure the modes of communication differently, and concludes with the research questions that follow from the argument.

CRITIQUE OF CULTURAL IDENTITY

Cultural identity has become a crucial concept in the debates on international communication, development communication and culture, and communication. In July 1988, for example, the scientific conference of the IAMCR (International Association for Mass Communication Research) had as its main theme "Mass Communication and Cultural Identity." Both academic and political publications use the concept generously and, in general, with the implicit assumption that the community addressed knows unequivocally what is meant. Illustrative is the report by the International Commission for the Study of Communication Problems (Paris: UNESCO, 1980). The cultural identity concept shows up on many pages without any proper definition.

The usefulness of cultural identity as a concept is taken for granted and the analytical concerns are directed toward such questions as "How is cultural identity threatened?" or "How can cultural identity be preserved?" Servaes offers little in defense of the concept and seems to be unconcerned about the adequacy of a notion that dominates his chapter.

I would like to propose that cultural identity is an inadequate and misleading concept and that the academic debate would do well to delete it. My defense for this position proceeds along the following lines.

First, on a basic level, one could define cultural identity as an analogue to the identity of human beings, that is, identity would be understood as the individual personality, the set of distinct features that tells us what and who the individual is. Cultural identity would consequently refer to "what a culture is." This reference to the personality of a culture does imply the assumption that we could isolate an identifiable subject of a culture and that this subject would have distinct features.

This assumption raises two problems. In the first place, there is the question of the collective subject of the phenomenon that (in many different ways) is defined as "culture." It seems doubtful to me that any such subject we might select (be it a nation or an ethnic community) can be identified in terms of "the" culture of this collectivity. It would seem more likely that apart from a few closed or secret societies most subjects would be from many different cultures. This presumption is important because one often finds references in the literature to the culture of a "country," when it would seem more realistic to propound that any country has many different cultures.

The second problem is whether we can identify the individuality of a culture and establish a cultural personality vis-à-vis other distinctly recognizable cultural personalities. Is it possible to think of the uncontestable features that distinguish culture A from culture B? Does "A" culture exist? Or can we refer only to myriad forms through which human beings express the ways in which they cope with their environments? And are these forms so varied—even within small communities—that the notion of "A" culture suggests a coherence that reflects the mental constructs of the observer and not the empirical reality of the participants? What we call the culture of a collective subject is an effort in which many lines converge and diverge, dominate and suffer, emerge and disappear. Any phenomenon that we describe as culture has, in reality, a set of many different identities. Any culture is many different expressions to many different people. To talk about "the" identity of "a" culture is unnecessarily restrictive and deceptive because it suggests a clarity and unanimity that in fact do not exist. The literature tends to refer to the original identity of every culture. However, it seems more realistic to think of every culture as having many identities.

Second, identity presupposes the usage of a series of characteristics that converge into the individual personality. At which point do such features constitute a personality? This constitution may largely depend upon the type of identity one searches for. At least three types can be distinguished for our discussion.

First, there is the *passport* identity that needs only a minimal description of such features as name, sex, age, place of birth, and place of residence. This identity facilitates a superficial recognition. Passport identities of collectivities are well known from the arbitrary and distorted features through which international travelers will describe their confrontations with foreign cultures.

A second type of identity is the *fingerprint* identity. This identity characterizes the subject through one feature only, but one that provides an absolutely unique identification. The fingerprint may unequivocally identify the criminal offender, it reveals little to nothing about human personality. Even if it were possible to single out such identification for a collective subject (and I have argued we cannot), we would still know little about that culture's personality.

The third type of identity is the *sociological* identity. This identity describes the subject through a series of social expressions, such as conventions, customs, rites, and ceremonies, that a collectivity employs in its social existence. The social scientist (notably the anthropologist) could describe these features and claim that the totality of these expressions would make up the personality of a collectivity. However, what constitutes the totality? All the manifest and latent expressions? All the current and past expressions? All the dominant and suppressed expressions? Which expressions are characteristics? Who defines this? The observer? But the observation is too distant and always arbitrary, distorted, and contestable. The participant? But the participation is too close and always arbitrary, distorted, and contestable. Moreover, could cultural personality sufficiently be described through the cultural expressions that represent the masks through which a collectivity enables its members to hide their real selves from one another?

The sociological significance of cultural expressions is largely that they help us to hide who we really are, and enable us to not expose ourselves unduly to others. Culture, to a large degree, protects those who are behind the masks. There is a school of thought in the psychology of personality that stresses the origin of the notion of *persona* (in Latin) as meaning a mask or a role an actor performs. Is this sufficient? Are we the masks we wear? Are cultures to be equated with the smoke screens they erect? Is there life behind the masks? Is the personality not precisely what the mask attempts to hide? This is a relevant question because masks as "cultural identities" may have been chosen by collective subjects as a function of a specific protest even though the mask was recognized as a very inadequate characterization. Black cultural identity, for example, was not defined naturally but was enforced upon a part of the human species in order to defend themselves against those who gave them this identity in the first place. Thus Sartre (1960) writes, "It is the anti-Semite who makes the Jew" (p. 69). And Fanon (1986) tells us, "It is the racist who creates his inferior" (p. 92).

The next problem refers to the possibility that what is referred to as cultural identity is imposed upon a collective subject for control purposes. The usage of the concept can be an instrument convenient to the distribution and execution of power. It forces all members into the straitjacket of an undisputed loyalty to unquestioned social objectives and measures. It supports the sentiment of communalism that is dangerously oppressive toward the dissident insider and expansionist toward the nonaccommodating outsider. In the latter sense, the acceptance of a cultural identity serves the expansionist ethnocentrism of collectivities that may feel quite justified in launching a holy war in the name of their culture.

When we accept the notion that a collective subject has an identity, we have to accept a generalization in which judgments are applied to all individual members of the collectivity. If the same labels are used for members of a group, however, they are perceived as more alike than they really are. This distortion seriously inhibits differentiated perception and thinking, the lack of which could easily reinforce prejudicial stereotypes and legitimize discriminatory conduct.

A critical problem with the use of the concept of collectivity is, finally, that cultural identity focuses almost exclusively on the contents of culture ("what a culture is") when this is not the crux of the matter. Fundamentally, it is not decided what precisely a culture is. More important is "how" people develop their modes of coping with the environment. This does not deny that cultural choices per se do matter, but I would like to claim that it is of overriding interest "how cultural choices are made." In this vein, one could argue that the adoption of foreign elements in a culture may not be a problem, it may even support the survival of a community or, at least, of some dissident faction in that community. What matters is that more often than not the subjects never had a choice in the first place. The existing relations of power (colonial and neocolonial) determined the space for cultur al development. Focusing upon the problem of *cultural identity* (as most contributors to the debate do) neglects the more pressing problems of *cultural development*.

CULTURAL DEVELOPMENT

In addition to the proposal to remove the concept of cultural identity from the current debate, I would submit that we need a critical analytical inquiry into the problem of conditions for cultural development. How do we want cultural development to take place and can conditions be established that would guide policymaking on cultural development as useful criteria? I would argue that for any subject of cultural development, the following three conditions are essential: *dynamism*, *diversity*, and *dispute*.

Dynamism

For any collectivity the environment changes, for example, the number of its members or its access to resources. What is adequate at one time turns out to be fully inappropriate in case such changes occur. The increasing complexity of the environment, for example, demands an adaptation in cultural expressions in order to survive. Static cultures disappear. Culture is not the holdings of a museum: A collection of precious treasures that need to be preserved. It is rather the continuous dialectical process in which the human environment and modes of coping with this environment interact with each other, mutually influence each other, and change in the process.

Diversity

Once systems become monolithic they become vulnerable to decay. The erosion of diversity seriously threatens ecological systems, for example. The more diverse an ecosystem is, the more stable it is. As certain species develop in extreme ways at the cost of others, diversity decreases, the complexity of the system diminishes, and it becomes less defensible against erosion. The more diversity a group allows, the more successful the process of independent cultural development is.

Dispute

The elements of dynamism and diversity already imply the need for collectivities to tolerate the development of various personalities. Since this seems basic, I argue this criterion somewhat further using the model of Rawls's (1973) original position. The original position is a hypothetical situation

> of which essential features are that no one knows his or her place in society, his or her class position or social status, nor does anyone know his or her fortune in the distribution of natural assets and abilities, his or her intelligence, his or her strength and the like. Since all are similarly situated and no one is able to design principles to favor his particular condition, the principles of justice are the result of a fair agreement. (p. 12)

It can be suggested that if people in the original position (behind the veil of ignorance) would have to express a preference for conditions for cultural development, they would choose the option of continuous dispute. Given the fact that they do not know what position they would be in, dominant or dissident, they would ask that all cultural choices be disputed in order to exclude the possibility that certain interests could decide on behalf of all the others what choices to make. In the original position, people would probably not risk repression. They might, however, leave open the possibility of competing choices, noting that they might want their potential dissident choice to be not only not repressed, but to have the chance of it reaching the agenda of public discourse and even gaining a wider acceptance. Therefore, the minimal demand would be the possibility of open dispute.[1]

CONTRARY FORCES

If we accept these conditions as policy guidelines, then it is pertinent to take a close look at those forces that may resist dynamism, diversity, and dispute. Moreover, it would be necessary to analyze which specific interests are served by such forces. Combining the conditions for cultural development in a collective subject with those forces that (from inside as well as from outside the collectivity) resist these conditions, the following matrix emerges:

Conditions/forces	Internal	External
dynamism	conformism	exotism
diversity	fundamentalism	globalism
dispute	paternalism	ethnocentrism

These forces are not merely mental constructs, they are guided by interests and they are functional to a specific distribution of wealth and power in a collectivity. These concepts need further analysis; only a beginning can be made here.

Conformism

This concept represents the demand for conformity to the dominant norms that may range from ways of dressing to loyalty to the flag. Changing the norms usually leads to the rejection of the individual who tries to change and to the maintenance of the norm. Conformism hampers dynamism as it insists on leaving the status quo untouched. This resistance clearly serves the interests of those in command and keeps the underprivileged in their place. It obstructs social change since it insists that the existing arrangements are the most appropriate ones. Conformism is particularly effective when it is accepted by those at the bottom of the social hierarchy. This acceptance conveniently justifies the way in which power is distributed.

Fundamentalism

This force serves the interests of those who claim spiritual leadership and pretend to hold the uncontestable truth. It obviously cannot tolerate a diversity of viewpoints that would implicitly challenge the exclusivity of its claims.

Paternalism

This force makes dispute superfluous. Paternal care is taken and there is no need to contest it. This care obviously serves the interests of patriarchal power (whoever the patriarch may be).

Exotism

This force serves the perception of the outsider who needs the cult of the "noble savage": unchangeable and exploitable for a variety of commercial purposes. Exotic exploitation hampers cultural development. The identity it has decided upon for the other has to remain static. The black man should forever smile. The Asian woman serves sex tourism best when she remains subservient, dexterous, and mysterious.

Globalism

This force suggests the homogeneity of the world. It attempts to negate the rich diversity of cultural expressions and serves the global marketing needs of the largest transnational merchants.

Ethnocentrism

This force negates the need of a continuous dispute since it unequivocally establishes the superiority of its own position. It serves the power of those who define others as inferior, since this conveniently legitimizes the exploitation of the inferior. Ethnocentric prejudices (such as racist stereotypes) serve a social function: They assist the powerful to maintain their advantageous position.

BY WAY OF CONCLUSION

In summary, I have argued that the focal point of analytic inquiry should not be cultural identity but the conditions for cultural development and the interest-guided forces that resist these conditions.

The next step in the analysis then would be to study how communication relates to the conditions of cultural development and the forces of resistance. The relationship of communication and cultural development is particularly relevant since communication itself is both cultural expression and carrier of cultural expressions. When we link communication with the conditions of cultural development the implication is that modes of communication would have to reflect dynamism, diversity, and dispute. These conditions would be the yardsticks by which current modes of communication could be judged as to their contribution to cultural development. When we link communication with the forces of resistance, the implication is that modes of communication, if they are to serve cultural development, should not be instrumental to these forces. This seems a relevant and timely judgment, precisely because, in the reality of many collectivities, communication modes operate in the service of conformism, fundamentalism, paternalism, exotism, globalism, and ethnocentrism. In further analysis we would have to face questions such as "which specific modes of communication are prone to serve forces that resist cultural development," or "which specific modes of communication can support cultural development?" To investigate these questions we need to find a systematic distinction between communication modes. Here I would propose we use as an analytic tool a matrix that looks at communication both as process and as institution. Communication processes could be distinguished in terms of the institutional versus individual character of the source they emanate from and in terms of the institutional versus individual definition of the messages they carry.

MATRIX I.
Communication-as-Process

Source definition	Institutional	Individual
institutional	distribution	registration
individual	consultation	conversation

In Matrix I four distinct patterns of communication as process emerge in the format of distributional, registrative, consultative, and conversational modes. In the distributional mode, institutions produce and distribute messages and determine when and how this happens. In the registrative mode, the message may have the individual as source, but an institution defines when and how the message is collected and processed. In the consultative mode, individuals may communicate with collections of messages that are captured and processed by institutions. In the conversational mode, individuals communicate directly with each other.

Communication processes are incorporated in various institutional modes and they can be distinguished as in Matrix II in accordance with their method of exploitation and nature of control.

MATRIX II.
Communication-as-Institution

Ways of Exploitation:		Commercial	Noncommercial
nature of control:	public	1	2
	private	4	3

There are four dominant modes by which either public or private interests control commercial or noncommercial forms of communication as a process. In quadrant one, we find public institutions that operate communication media for commercial purposes; in two, there is the more common type of publicly owned, noncommercial media; in three, there are private institutions (such as churches) that exploit nonprofit media; and in four, we encounter the well-known format of private entrepreneurs operating commercial media. I would suggest that the combination of these two matrices offers an adequate basis for the further analysis of the relationships between communication and cultural development.

Concluding from this argument as presented in response to Jan Servaes's chapter, the following research priorities would emerge: (a) the analysis of the conditions of the cultural development; (b) the analysis of the relationship between cultural development and the distribution of power; (c) the analysis of the relationship between the distribution of power and modes of communication both as process and as institution; and (d) the analysis of the relationship between modes of communication and the conditions for cultural development.

NOTE

1. This is a more dynamic situation than the possible option of mere tolerance. In Rawls's argument, people in the original position would opt for equal liberties and equal opportunities. I am inclined to think this is too naive. It is not realistic to assume that even in ignorance human beings (an aggressive species) would not keep a back door open to competitive conduct.

REFERENCES

Fanon, F. (1986). *Black skin, white masks*. London: Pluto.
International Commission for the Study of Communication Problems (UNESCO, MacBride Commission) (1980). *Many voices, one world*. Paris: UNESCO.
Rawls, J. (1973). *A theory of justice*. Oxford: Oxford University Press.
Sartre, J. P. (1960). *Anti-Semite and Jew*. New York: Grove.

Poststructuralist Concepts in Culture and Communication

SYED A. RAHIM
Institute of Culture and Communication
East-West Center Honolulu

THE problem of interrelationships among culture, communication, modernity, and development is a common concern in contemporary social sciences and humanities. Scholarly works on this problem in the field of communication and culture have drawn conceptual and methodological resources from political economy, sociology, psychology, anthropology, and semiotics. The chapter under discussion here has maintained that tradition. I want to follow it, and hope to extend it by tapping less explored resources including certain ideas, concepts, methods, and, most importantly, criticism, produced by literary theories and language philosophy. Servaes's chapter raises some problems and issues that offer real possibilities for sharpening and enriching the discourse on communication and cultural identity by introducing certain concepts and ideas, and critical tones from contemporary studies in literature and culture. The main thrust of my commentary on his chapter will be toward extending that discourse.

In his concluding remarks on research, Servaes emphasizes the need for analyzing "the relative power-linked articulations and conflicts over ideologies, world-views, moral codes, and the locally bounded conditions of knowledge and competence." He refers to the problems of meanings production, contexts of social action, autonomy of organized subjects, symbolic orders reproducing labor, forms of knowledge, and ideological expressions in the folk and popular cultures, and domination, dependency, and liberation. How can we better organize these problems into a common

Correspondence and requests for reprints: Syed A. Rahim, East-West Center, 1777 East-West Road, Honolulu, HI 96848.

Communication Yearbook 12, 427-434

conceptual framework? In his chapter, Servaes seems to be aiming at a structuralist framework. How well will that work and what kinds of problems will that framework face? I want to keep these questions in mind while probing the ideas discussed in his chapter, and offer a few suggestions.

Contemporary approaches to literary theory and criticism—Russian formalism, Anglo-American new criticism, phenomenology, hermeneutics, structuralism, poststructuralism—confront two central problems. The first problem is how to *interpret* a particular literary text (a poem or a novel) in its own terms, so that interpretation does not depend on interpreter's intuition alone or on factors external to the text. The second problem is how to *explain* the production of literary texts (not publications) in general, and the production of meanings by such texts. How and to what extent can the process of literary production be related to previous texts, and to philosophical, historical, economic, social, and psychological determinants of cultural practices?

In the passing of literary theory from formalism to poststructuralism, the focus has been shifting from the first problem to the second problem, with the first problem more or less subsumed under the second. Another significant development is that the preoccupation with poetics and linguistics is giving way to a focus on the languages of discourse, and the philosophical and epistemological basis of speech, writing, and modes of communication. Within the broad categories of approaches mentioned, there are, of course, different theoretical positions—neo-Marxist, psychoanalytical, reader-response, deconstructive, feminist, and others. But all of them are more or less concerned with problems of interpretation and cultural productivity.

What is the relevance of literary theory and criticism for our discussion on culture and communication? To answer this let me adapt the well known Chomskyan question on linguistic competence by substituting the word *language* for "culture" in his statement: How is it possible that an individual having only a fragmentary knowledge and experience of his culture can identify himself with and confidently operate within that culture? A Chomskyan answer to this question would be that the individual born and raised in that culture has genetically acquired the innate competence to be in his culture. An outsider, or a culturally marginalized individual, lacking cultural competence, will have great difficulty in speaking the language of that culture. A Lévi-Straussian answer would refer to a set of universal, fundamental, unconsciously shared codes of communication that are inscribed in the human brain, of which the specific culture under consideration is one particular manifestation. An Althusserian explanation would point out the process of ideological subjection of individuals through ideological state apparatuses, particularly educational and mass media institutions. A Derridean approach would probably begin by deconstructing the question itself in order to expose traces of Western logocentric values, the belief in some ultimate presence, essence, or deep reality, hidden in the question, that inevitably leads to the kind of answers given by those other scholars. If we imagine how Michel Foucault would deal with the same problem, we would see a totally different approach. For Foucault, the concept of innate competence is unnecessary. He would ignore the quest for universal or first principle; he would examine the history of forms of knowledge and modes of communication by which culture is constituted and individuals are made its subject. In contemporary literary theory and criticism, these various explanations are hotly debated. Given the fact that the field of culture and communication is close to, and even overlaps the field of literature, we should be aware of what is happening there.

Structuralism has made a major impact on literary theory and cultural study. From a structuralist point of view, literature and culture are seen as products of underlying (mostly unconscious) conceptual structures, the elements of which, their differential rules, codes, and conventions produce the phenomenon under observation. Saussurian structural linguistics (Saussure, 1959) provided a powerful instrument for conceptualizing such structures; and Lévi-Strauss (1963, 1966) made an exemplary use of that in his structural anthropology. Structuralism invented a technology of analysis and interpretation of symbolic orders and signifying systems. That analysis was anticipated in the Russian formalist theory of literature (Lemon & Harvey, 1965), and developed later in various works of Barthes, Genette, Greimas, Jacobson, Todorov, and others (Culler, 1975; Jefferson & Robey, 1982).

Structuralism was instrumental in reinforcing the autonomous status of literary and cultural studies by developing concepts and methods from within, and reducing dependence on other disciplines and authorities. Structuralism insists that human meaning in communication and culture is the outcome of a production process within various shared systems of signification, primarily language and discourse. But the quest of hardcore structuralism for fundamental, universal, invariant codes or themes led it toward a kind of reductionism of its own making. By ignoring the historical and material process of social transformation, and by bracketing the human subject and his or her lived experience in society, structuralism moved away from the task of explaining the play of meanings in communication and cultural practices (Eagleton, 1983, p. 109).

In his chapter, Servaes compares and contrasts Eastern and Western culture and communication, and presents two "ideal-typical" sets of concepts or categories designating the two cultures. I see in that a real danger of stepping into the structuralist reductionism trap. I am not suggesting that such differentiation between cultures is unproductive. In structuralist terms, the meanings of cultures can be revealed only in their differences or differentials. My concern is about prefixing absolute categories based on traditional authority, such as the classical texts of Confucianism, or Buddhism, or Plato, or Aristotle. It is necessary to examine cultural archetypes in order to understand the historical process of cultural production, and to determine what and how much of the traces of archetypal values are actually present in the contemporary manifestation of culture and modes of communication. But to claim, for instance, that "harmony" has primacy in the Eastern culture as against "power/conflict" in the Western culture is to lock the door on the critical study of culture and communication. One can contest this claim by pointing out that in Western classical music, harmony is central, as against melody in Eastern classical music, and that in both Eastern and Western modern music those codes are constantly violated. In rural Asia, litigations over property rights, power struggles in village politics, and communal and ethnic conflicts are endemic. Yet to the extent that a Confucian worldview is active, for instance in China, one cannot ignore the concept of harmony. But it is essential to recognize that in Confucian methodology a conceptual opposition (harmony/conflict) is thought of as a whole in which the opposing elements complement each other; one does not think of choosing one and rejecting the other element; both are necessary for the whole because in the whole, the opposition is harmonized.

"One world, many cultures." According to Servaes this is the essence of the emerging approach to development, the call for a new paradigm. There is certainly a change in development thinking in general, which is evident in new theories that attempt to integrate cultural factors. The negative-suppressive and positive-liberative theory of Preiswerk cited in the chapter is an example of that move. Servaes also mentions the transnationalization thesis of Sunkel and Fueazalida, that integrates world economic system theory and anthropological production forms theory.

In a recent study of development theory in transition, Blomstrom and Hettne (1984) discussed current theories under the category "modern structural approach." Their review shows how the transition from modernization theory to dependency and postdependency theories of development has been marked by a shift of focus from development to underdevelopment. The reason for this shift is that the new theories discard the notion of development as a wholesale transfer of Western industrial models to developing countries. The problem has been redefined as explaining the lack of development, or economic growth of a particular kind, in terms of structural relations of economic, social, and cultural factors between the center and the periphery of world economic system, and within national economies. This broadening of the base and reformulation of the problem have produced encouraging results and a better understanding of the dynamics of development and underdevelopment.

However, it should be pointed out that these structural theories of development are essentially economic theories. Their central concern is with structural analysis of the modes of production at the national as well as the transnational level and their relationships. The problem addressed in Servaes's chapter—cultural identity and modes of communication—is at most a secondary concern of the structural theories of development. But by drawing an analogy, one can gain insights and formulate the questions of cultural study in a different way. For instance, the problem can be defined as cultural identity crisis, or loss of identity, in the midst of the world system economic development and its unpredictable short-term rising and falling trend. One can raise questions about the role of the telecommunications revolution in that cultural crisis.

In this context the concept of power becomes of crucial importance, specifically, the power of information, telecommunications, and computer networks to forge new asymmetrical relations between the center and the periphery. In recent years, this movement has been a topic of considerable debate and discussion in various national and international forums. But the result has been inconclusive. Development theory, particularly the new version of modernization theory of the information society, has done more in arguing the case of telecommunication as a means of production than as a mode of cultural development. The new modernization theory defines information and telecommunication as strategic factors of production in the world economic system, but fails to explain its cultural implications.

I want to make explicit a point hinted at in Servaes's perceptive discussion on "a new perspective on culture." This point refers to "culture itself becoming problematic." What this statement essentially means to me is that cultural and communicative practices need to be considered as contested sites. The production and reproduction of cultural identity are continuing processes of struggle, and modes of communication play a distinctive role in those processes. Even in the Enlightenment view of culture, elaborated by Rousseau and Kant, the notion of contestation is implied. As Bloom (1987) points out, the word *culture* sums up the human response to the nature-society tension. Today there is a continuing struggle between two views of culture—one emphasizing universality and the cosmopolitan nature of culture, and the other emphasizing nationalistic and particularistic aspects (Bloom, 1987, p. 185-193). But the contestation is much more pervasive than Bloom would have us believe. It is active within a nation—between communities, ethnic and racial groups, economic classes, genders and generations, and, of course, between nations. One of the most important cultural consequences of economic and political modernization is that cultural contestations are sharpened, intensified, and even raised to a crisis level, as development accelerates material and symbolic transactions among the contestants.

Viewed from this perspective, culture is a terrain expropriated from nature, in which contending individuals and groups differentiated by race, religion, caste, class, profession, gender, generation, and language necessarily coexist with each other in various forms of domination/dependency relations. It is an active site of cooperation, competition, and contest in the production and exchange of goods and services, establishment and change of social relations, legislation and enforcement of law and order, formulation and sharing of moral and ethical values, creation and dissemination of knowledge and information, and manipulation of power and authority relations by men and women. Therefore, when one conceptualizes culture as a symbolic and signifying structure, it is essential to think of that as a structure of a system in which the concepts of the subject, self, and identity are not only central, but privileged, sites of contestation. Furthermore, the competition and contest is both internal and external, manifested in relations within a national culture as well as between national cultures. From this point of view the main question for research is: how cultural hegemony of a dominant class, or race, or ethnic group is established and maintained, and what role communication plays in that process. But this question necessarily gives rise to its opposite: How do the dominated respond, and how do they initiate their own strategy to undermine hegemony from inside? How do they make use of or why do they fail to make use of the same means of communication and education instituted by the hegemonic class to establish their own identity and autonomous voice?

The notion of cultural or media "imperialism," based primarily on macro-level studies of the imbalances of information and media program flow, certainly needs reconsideration. I am in agreement with Servaes's analysis of this issue, particularly his point that the foreign mass media "have radically different effects and meanings in different cultural settings," and that target audiences play an active role in that process. It will be most interesting to study why and how certain national mass media (American Public Television, Indian Television) appropriate techniques and ideas from a foreign medium (the BBC), and with what cultural effects. I think that the notion of "imperialism" will be of little use in that kind of study. The West is not accused of literary imperialism, although English or French literature has greatly influenced many other national literatures. But the mass media seems to be more susceptible to the charge of imperialism. Is it because the media are more closely connected with economics than with literature? This problem is complicated because the media perform multiple functions, and the media institutions are owned and controlled by larger corporations or governmental agencies. The autonomy of media institutions is fragile, and under constant threat. The media cannot withdraw from economic and political struggles, it is a part of them.

After reviewing current concerns about media development in Canada and western Europe, Servaes argues for stronger financial and legal support for the public service media. I am not sure how strengthening public service media, if it means more centralization, will enhance media autonomy. Alternatively, a media strategy aimed at decentralizing power, permitting many voices to speak independently of each other and establishing true dialogues, should help cultural development by articulating diversity. Developments in modern communication technology, particularly the rapid growth of "little media," seems to offer the possibility of an infrastructure for such a strategy.

In advocating a research approach in the concluding section of his chapter Servaes says, "What I have in mind is a text . . . the 'system' itself—the political and economic processes encompassing different locales, or even different continents." Then, after identifying two research problem areas—structural influence on and grass-roots reactions of target groups—he adds, "The difference from traditional anthropological research should be that the choice of the symbolic order for the research is determined by key concepts, such as reproduction and labor." He points out that the targets of that research approach are "social groups and movements with a concern for public issues like ecology, social justice, peace, education, human rights, civic action and so on." Unfortunately, his exposition in this part of the chapter is so sketchy that the reader is likely to feel disappointed.

However, I take liberty in reading those brief statements as an attempt to define the problem in the following terms. The formation of certain social groups and movements around contemporary public issues is an active response to the cultural identity crisis going on in all parts of the world. The voices of those groups and movements constitute a discursive system in which the meanings of cultural crisis and its proposed solutions are represented, debated, and contested. The local, national, or international discourses produced by those movements are then appropriate units of analysis for research. The latter can be justified in terms of Habermas's theory of communicative action that takes speech acts (verbal and written, but behavioral modes of communication can also be included) as the unit of cultural analysis (Habermas, 1979; Wuthnow, Hunter, Bergesen, & Kurzweil, 1984, p. 199). The purpose of analysis is, of course, not statistical description, paraphrasing, or interpretation of contents, but to reveal the underlying process of structuration signifying social action and performative behavior. How the words and pictures, the speech acts and visual signs are woven in discourse to represent what aspects of the social movement in what plane of meanings with what effects the discourse, in fact, has in driving the movement in which directions are rich areas of research.

There are some theoretical difficulties in this kind of an approach, because questions are raised about discourse as practice and power, its internal and external relationships, the transformational principle defining discourse's representation of reality, the place of the subject, and the relationship among and between signifiers and signifieds. In the contemporary intellectual movement called poststructuralism and in the literary theory and criticism following that tradition, such questions are of central concern. I think that Servaes' research project will benefit from exploring ideas and concepts developed in poststructuralist theory and criticism. Specifically, I consider that deconstructive criticism, the theory of the text, psychoanalytical theory of poetry, and the dialogical theory of the novel are among the unexplored sources of new ideas and concepts. There is no space in this brief commentary for a detailed discussion on the uses of poststructuralist concepts in culture and communication research. But, in concluding my commentary, I should like to mention a few important concepts and their sources for the benefit of readers interested in pursuing the subject: *blindness and insights,* in the rhetoric of discourse (de Man, 1983); *deconstruction of logocentric first principles* upon which 'discourses and meanings are constructed (Derrida, 1976); *texts* as structural units of discourse, and *texts* as *signifying practice* and *productivity* (Barthes, 1975, 1981); *the anxiety of influence* as the driving psychic force factor in the production of contending discourse (poetry) that is counterpoised to the dominant discourse (poetry) it wants to overcome and surpass (H. Bloom, 1973, 1976); and discourse in the novel as *dialogized representation,* on a higher plane, of *social heteroglossia* (Bakhtin, 1981, 1984).

REFERENCES

Bakhtin, M. (1981). *The dialogical imagination* (M. Holquist, Ed.; C. Emerson & M. Holquist, Trans.). Austin: University of Texas Press.

Bakhtin, M. (1984). *Problems of Dostoevsky's poetics* (C. Emerson, Trans.). Minneapolis: University of Minnesota Press.

Bakhtin, M. (1984). *Rabelais and his world* (H. Iswolsky, Trans.). Bloomington: Indiana University Press.

Barthes, R. (1975). *The pleasure of the text* (R. Miller, Trans.). New York: Hill & Wang.

Barthes, R. (1981). The theory of the text. In R. Young (Ed.), *Untying the text: A poststructuralist reader.* Boston: Routledge & Kegan Paul.

Blomstrom, M., & Hettne, B. (1984). *Development theory in transition: The dependency debate and beyond.* London: Zed.

Bloom, A. D. (1987). *The closing of the American mind.* New York: Simon & Schuster.

Bloom, H. (1973). *The anxiety of influence: A theory of poetry.* New York: Oxford University Press.

Bloom, H. (1976). *Poetry and repression.* New Haven, CT: Yale University Press.

Culler, J. (1975). *Structural poetics.* Ithaca, NY: Cornell University Press.

de Man, P. (1983). *Blindness and insights: Essays in the rhetoric of contemporary criticism.* Minneapolis: University of Minnesota Press.

Derrida, J. (1976). *Of grammatology* (G. C. Spivak, Trans.). Baltimore: Johns Hopkins University Press.

Eagleton, T. (1983). *Literary theory: An introduction.* Minneapolis: University of Minnesota Press.

Habermas, J. (1979). *Communication and evolution of society* (T. McCarthy, Trans.). Boston: Beacon Press.

Jefferson, A., Robey D., & Forgacs D. (1982). *Modern literary theory.* New York: Barnes & Noble Books.

Lemon, L. T., & Reis M. J. (Eds.). (1965). *Russian formalist criticism.* Lincoln: University of Nebraska Press.

Lévi-Strauss, C. (1963). *Structural anthropology* (C. Jacobson & B. G. Schoepf, Trans.). New York: Basic Books.

Lévi-Strauss, C. (1966). *The savage mind* (G. Widenfeld, Trans.). Chicago: University of Chicago Press.

Saussure, F. De (1959). *Course in general linguistics* (W. Baskin, Trans.). New York: Philosophical Library.

Wuthnow, R., Hunter J. D., Bergesen A., & Kurzweil E. (1984). *Cultural analysis.* New York: Routledge & Kegan Paul.

SECTION 3

TECHNOLOGY AND COMMUNICATION SYSTEMS

8 Issues and Concepts in Research on Computer-Mediated Communication Systems

RONALD E. RICE
University of Southern California

Computers and telecommunications networks have converged to provide a new category of communication media: computer-mediated communication systems (CMCS). The increasing development and application of these systems is matched by increasing research concerning their uses and implications. However, it is often difficult to integrate this body of research across disciplines, technologies, and research processes. Further, such research is often too narrowly focused. This chapter suggests four dimensions of research—stakeholders, goals, analytical domain, and tools—that scholars may use to guide and expand future studies of CMCS.

THE study of the uses and effects of computer-mediated communication systems (CMCS) has been drawing increased attention from researchers in a variety of disciplines—communication, information science, psychology, computer science, education, and management science, among others.[1] Besides the varied methodologies of these disciplines, studies of different kinds of CMCS—videotext, audiotext, personal computers, computer conferencing, word processing, computer bulletin boards, office information systems, and electronic and voice mail—tend to emphasize technological idiosyncrasies rather than communication commonalities. Finally, much of the insights to date about use and implications of CMCS is integrally bound up in, and confounded with, the research processes applied

AUTHOR'S NOTE: I would like to acknowledge the helpful comments of anonymous reviewers and Stephen Acker, James Anderson, Jim Danowski, and Susan Eastman on earlier drafts of this chapter. Some initial ideas for this chapter were presented in a paper coauthored with Jim Danowski at the International Communication Association, Minneapolis, May 1981.

Correspondence and requests for reprints: Ronald E. Rice, Annenberg School of Communications, University of Southern California, Los Angeles, CA 90089.

Communication Yearbook 12, 436-476

in specific studies. Thus the developing body of research on the uses and implications of CMCS reflects variations in three areas: disciplinary paradigms, technological distinctions, and evaluation approaches.

This chapter suggests a framework for integrating the contributions of these three streams of knowledge about CMCS, by focusing on and elaborating four general dimensions: stakeholders, goals, analytical domains, and tools. The presentation here is an initial attempt to identify broad categories of dimensions and their components, and to discuss some of their assumptions and possibly conflicting interpretations. Awareness of the existence and interaction of these dimensions may lead to more systematic research that considers influences, constraints, and implications of CMCS, and relationships among them. Such an approach is in line with conclusions of Danzinger, Dutton, Kling, and Kraemer (1982) and others that "computing (in general) is more accurately viewed as a 'package' that includes many complex social and technical elements."

Section 1 defines the communication perspective of this chapter by identifying CMCS as one of four basic applications of computers. Then it describes the characteristics and contributions of CMCS in the context of media in general. Section 2 provides an overview of the four dimensions, with some examples of their use and interaction. Section 3 outlines the range of stakeholders who might fund, conduct, oppose, or await CMCS applications and research. Section 4 notes some possible goals or criteria of CMCS research. Section 5 identifies domains of analysis. Section 6 considers tools of the research process, including designs, data, and methods of analysis of particular relevance to the study of CMCS. Section 7 discusses two examples of how applying the framework can identify alternative perspectives on CMCS and the concept of information. Section 8 summarizes the idea that components of the suggested dimensions interact within a given dimension, and across dimensions. Section 9 concludes by discussing implications of this framework for the study of CMCS.

DEFINING CMCS AND THE SCOPE OF THE CHAPTER

To begin, it is necessary to identify and define the specific focus of this chapter. Based upon a typology of general communication activities developed by Bordewijk and van Kamm (1982) and McQuail (1986), we can see that the wide and rapidly growing uses of computers for the processing and exchange of information include (1) allocution (processing of transactional information for forms and records, management information systems, computer-generated music and art), (2) registration (online polling, computer-based patient diagnostic systems), (3) consultation (computer-assisted instruction, information retrieval from online databases, video games), and (4) conversation (communication between individuals via computer systems). The first and

		Source of Information	
		System	Individual
Source of control of timing and choice of information	System	"allocation"— offer of information for immediate use and later processing Example: batch transaction processing	"registration"— collection of information available to or about individuals Example: online voting
	Individual	"consultation"— selective use of stored information Example: computer-aided instruction, management information systems, online databases	"conversation"— exchange of information between individuals Example: electronic messaging, computer conferencing, computer bulletin boards, some videotex

Figure 8.1 Typology of uses of computers for communication activities. Adapted from Bordewijk and van Kamm (1982) and McQuail (1986).

third categories represent the bulk of research so far on the organizational and social implications of computers (see, for example, Danzinger & Kraemer, 1986, or Kling, 1980). (See Figure 8.1.)

Reasonable people may well categorize all these activities as communication of one degree or another. For instance, all of these examples involve the exchange of information by means of computers, perhaps interactively. However, only the "conversation" category usually involves an interactive *relationship* directly among individuals or groups of individuals. (This distinction may be debated of course: does the user of an online database communicate with the person who abstracted and indexed the articles, or is the user simply reading sets of information retrieved by combinations of search terms?) This chapter primarily considers studies and concepts appropriate to the research of computer applications in the "conversation" category as focusing on conversational aspects emphasizes the attributes of computers that are common to other communication media. This category comprises computer-mediated communication systems (CMCS), media that facilitate the exchange of semantic content, transmitted through telecommunication networks, processed through one or more computers, between individuals and among groups who in one way or another can be identified as such.

CMCS involve *telecommunication networks*, part of larger systems that allow interactive exchanges among sets of users at different places. CMCS also facilitate the *processing* of the content of human communication. In this context, processing means the ability to use the algorithmic, computational, and data-handling capabilities of a computer to alter the input, conversion, or output of content either directly by the user by submitting commands to the system's computer or indirectly, by storing, indexing, editing, retrieving, and distributing the content. The networking and processing aspects of CMCS heavily influence the four sets of media characteristics. It is the *convergence* of telecommunications networks and computers that makes CMCS distinct, say, from personal computers and word processors: In isolation, they cannot be used for direct communication among multiple individuals.

Two forms of CMCS are electronic messaging (EM) and computer conferencing (CC). The simplest use of CC is similar to using an EM system: sending a private message from one user to another. Recent developments in EM include voice mail, in which voice communications are digitized and stored until the other communication participants retrieve and listen to those messages, and perhaps further process them by forwarding, copying, or storing. CC systems provide structured access to shared files by one or more users. CC systems are more group-oriented than are EM systems. One example is a computer bulletin board system (CBBS) that allows users to post a message for all or some subset of users on the system to read. In full CC systems, content may include short notes, personal messages, headlines, data, reports, drafts of articles, and open discussions of technical and social topics, and support online polling and tabulation, partitioning of memory for joint authoring of documents, electronic publishing, retrieval of information by the use of indices, alteration of information in content or display format, selection of transmission and reception time and location, prioritizing access by individuals to real-time conferences, and more. Thus the most complex CMCS are difficult to distinguish from systems intended to augment the activities of knowledge workers or integrated office automation systems.

One way to assess the potential significance of CMCS is to compare them to prior communication media. Media can be said to differ with respect to a variety of generic characteristics (Rice, 1987b):

(1) Freedom from constraints as determined by: the need to know target receiver, the ability of the sender to select the target, the ability of the receiver to select the medium and content, the need for participants to be using the medium at the same time or to be in the same location, and the ability of participants to store the contents in the medium, retrieve the contents from the medium, or use the medium to reprocess the content.

(2) Mode or technical band width indicated by the ability to communicate physical proximity, gestures, paralinguistic cues, semantic connotations, semantic denotations.

(3) Feedback and interactivity shown by the number of prior communication loops reflected in the most recent exchange, the quickness of response, the ability to terminate the interaction, and the sequential nature of communication among several individuals.

(4) *Network flows* indicated in the pattern of distribution of the communication, control of and access to the communication system and content, and the effect of particular positions or roles in the pattern of distribution.

For example, a letter requires the sender to know at least the address of the target, allows the receiver to choose whether and when to open the medium and select what to read but not to choose other content, does not require the communicants to be in the same place or to share the letter at the same time, does store the content for later use but does not provide ways to reprocess or retrieve selected aspects of the content or combine the content with other information without reentry of the material.

CMCS differ significantly from a letter with respect to freedom from constraints. CMCS do not always require that the sender know the address or even the existence of potential receivers (or may identify them by means other than name and address), can allow the receiver to choose when and whether to read or respond to the communication, can allow the receiver to decide not only what to read but how to retrieve it in association with other information, do not require the participants to be using the system in the same place or the same time, can store the content for later use, provide ways to reprocess or redistribute selected aspects of the content to one or numerous other individuals, but are generally still too inaccessible or expensive for most individuals.

Even from the simplistic comparison of letters and CMCS on the characteristics of freedom from constraints, we can see that CMCS are an additional kind of communication medium with advantages and disadvantages, appropriate and inappropriate uses, and common and unique characteristics, perhaps a blend of interpersonal and mass media. Because of these characteristics and communication aspects, research on CMCS must not only consider traditional issues and concepts, but also consider newer and additional ones. The following sections consider four such sources of these considerations: stakeholders, goals, domains, and tools.

OVERVIEW OF DIMENSIONS

Research on CMCS can be seen as the product of four interacting dimensions (Figure 8.2), as follows:

(1) *stakeholders*: actors or agencies who have an interest in or claim to the outcome of specific research, and particularly actors who initiate and/or fund given research activities;

(2) *goals* or criteria: what is to be studied, the purposes of the system, audiences of the research, what constitutes "positive" or "negative" results (criteria here are used not as significance levels or decision rules, but as standards).

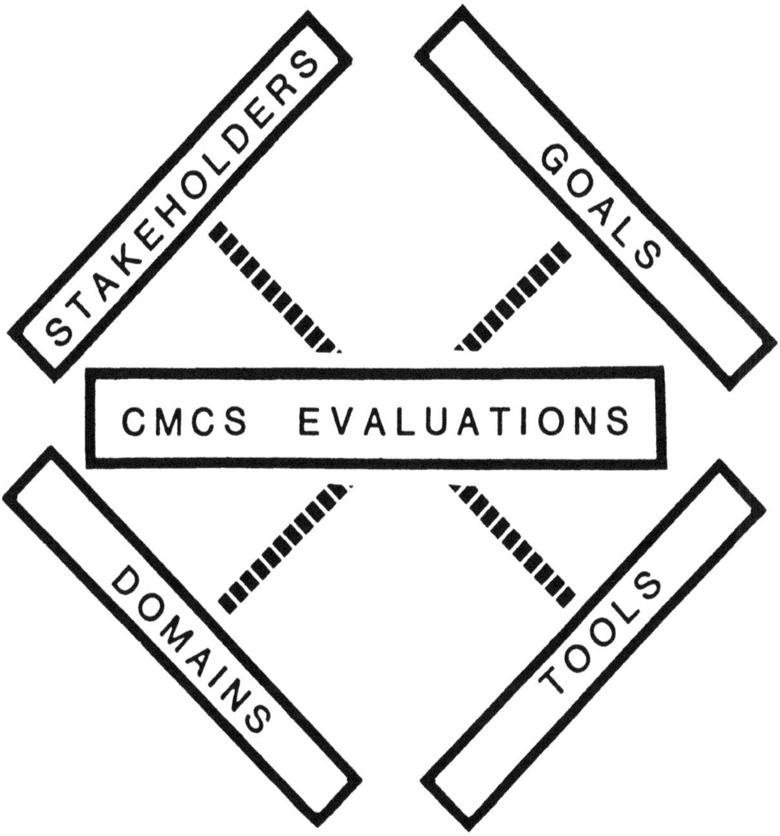

Figure 8.2 Interaction of dimensions of social evaluations of CMCS.

(3) *domains*: the levels of complexity, relationship, or organization at which the communication process takes place;

(4) *tools*: the research designs, kinds of data, and methods of inquiry and analysis that researchers apply.

For example, research on the use of a CMCS designed to understand the convergence of meaning among participants might focus on users as the primary stakeholders, explicitness of metacommunication as the primary goal, dyadic interaction as the primary domain, and content analysis as the primary tool.

The four dimensions discussed in this chapter—stakeholders, domains, goals, and tools—capture some of the process and content of social research of CMCS to date. Technical evaluations and their relevant dimensions, though also important, will not be considered in this chapter. But researchers of the development, diffusion, implementation, use, applications, implications, meaning, and nature of CMCS may improve the utility and relevance of their efforts by identifying which actors and forces within each of these dimensions are playing a role and which dimensions are interacting to bias or constrain the research.

STAKEHOLDERS

Stakeholders were defined earlier as actors or agencies who have an interest in or claim to the outcome of a specific research. They differ in their finances, political security, constraints, expertise, goals, research, and criteria. Consider, for example, a system vendor with an extensive development investment in a new CMCS, a manager of information systems on a tight budget, and a group of innovative employees who have no prior experience in computing: They all differ significantly on these factors and will have greatly different criteria of success and stakes in the outcome. Further, the identity or the attributes of stakeholders may change over time, leading in one case to the eventual rejection of a computer system that had been initially adopted (Dutton, 1981).

The stakeholder approach rejects the notion of isolated, independent researchers assessing a nonpoliticized, somehow "objective" project. Instead, stakeholders should be either a significant focus or significant participants in evaluation activities (see, for example, the March 1983 issue of *New Directions for Program Evaluation*; Majchrzak, 1984; Mitroff, 1983). Identifying and involving significant stakeholders is important in assuring that the final research results will be contextualized and useful, but also that possible recommendations will be more likely to be accepted. Some recommended stages in stakeholder analysis include:

(1) identify initial and additional stakeholders, including cultural and psychological forms;
(2) determine definitions, values, assumptions, and power held by these stakeholders;
(3) assess the willingness of various stakeholders to change with respect to the topics of interest;
(4) explore ways that stakeholders expect to use the research; and
(5) rate the acceptability and implementability of classes of potential recommendations.

Murray (1983) summarizes the benefits and disadvantages of the stakeholder approach to research:

> The stakeholder approach is a useful device for getting the leading players to cooperate, for understanding a program intimately, for attracting attention to interim evaluation findings, and perhaps even for getting decision makers to take evaluation findings into account when they make decisions. [It also] carries

> a high price tag. The intense, continual personal interactions that it requires with all the parties... are both its strength and its danger. (pp. 59-60)

One of these dangers is that stakeholders involved early on will influence who should formulate the research questions and who should have the opportunity to ask which questions. What is asked naturally limits what can be answered. For example, administrators rarely involved word processing operators in decisions about initial system acquisition or implementation strategies because of demands on their time and assumptions about clerical workers (Johnson & Rice, 1987). This approach ignores the need for divergent views and user involvement in systems design (Bostrom & Heinen, 1977 a, b). Possible researcher bias is influenced by both political and pragmatic processes in choosing the researcher and the extent to which the researcher participates in the design, implementation, and use of the system. The danger of bias seems particularly likely when the researcher "is dependent on the project being evaluated or the funders . . . not only for access to data (permission to observe, etc.) but also for the continuation of employment" (Cook & McAnany, 1979).

Many stakeholders reject or downgrade "theoretical" components of research. The proper balance between theory and practice is, of course, a very subtle and complex issue. Perhaps the main difficulty is assuming that they *are* separate. Theory can help determine what to look for, what constitutes change, what forms "new" awareness might take. Planning is, after all, one form of applied theory. The researcher brought in to "evaluate," *post hoc,* a new system may experience considerable frustration in seeing the results used to bolster the prior predispositions of those in control rather than to test theoretical expectations. On the other hand, systems managers and users need useful and implementable implications of research and either are not sufficiently aware of the implications of research design for achieving these goals or do not have the time and resources to implement before/after or treatment/control designs. While many of the perceived gaps between practicality and rigor may well be insurmountable given the different cultures, goals, and training of evaluators and users (widely defined), there seems to be at least two ways to improve the situation.

The first is to identify ongoing issues of importance to stakeholders rather than just situation-specific issues for evaluation. Recent analyses of enduring strategic and managerial issues in computers and communication are discussed by Culnan and Bair (1983) and Dickson, Leitheser, Wetherbe, and Nechis (1984). The second is to show how research efforts provide more insights into these top agenda issues than do hurried, ad hoc estimations. This effort requires an awareness of past research as well as an understanding of what represents convincing evidence for those stakeholders.

Involving stakeholders and their concerns in research efforts may help to identify perspectives and assumptions that may be unknowingly guiding system introduction, management, and evaluation. Kling (1980) suggests that there are two broad perspectives permeating analyses of computing: systems rationalism and segmented institutionalism. Each perspective reflects assumptions of different sets of stakeholders, influences what is analyzed and how the results are interpreted, and effects the design and implementation of a CMCS as well as the research process itself.

Systems rationalism includes three variants, emphasizing technical experts, managers, or users respectively. Systems rationalism focuses on rational design and use of the system, managed for efficiency and possibly user satisfaction, with the assumption that consensus (perhaps in the form of hierarchical authority accepted by organizational members) is possible. An extreme example occurs when highly trained system designers establish criteria for success based solely on system performance measures such as throughput, cost, and downtime. Another example is when traditional measures of cost are used to evaluate the worth of a new communication system. This particular example is explored in greater detail in the section on information.

Segmented institutionalism, on the other hand, assumes instead that the meaning of a particular system is socially constructed, that organizational politics serve to protect resources, conflict is pervasive because social structure is stratified. This perspective focuses on pluralism of interpretation and interests of the various stakeholders who are part of the social milieu of system use. Potentially severe organizational conflicts resulting from the introduction of CMCS might be more readily understood and avoided by identifying different organizational positions or individual members and how they interpret the potential system.

General categories of potential stakeholders in CMCS evaluation include the following actors, as listed in Table 8.1:

(1) Macrosupporters. Macrosupporters are those agencies, institutions, and organizations that fund evaluations of CMCS. There seem to be three general models for macrosupport of CMCS: research and development (R & D) grants, industry-university collaboration, and proprietary studies.

The first model is the traditional grant for research and development of a model or a specific system for governmental or policy-related purposes. The National Science Foundation (NSF) and the Department of Defense are two major sources of such funds (Bamford & Savin, 1978). The early development of CMCS (Hiltz & Turoff, 1981), ARPANET and packet switching (Roberts, 1978) and online databases (Schiller, 1982) were stimulated by requirements for defense and national emergencies.

Perhaps the best example of the R & D grant model is the continued evolution of the Electronic Information Exchange System (EIES) developed by Murray Turoff (New Jersey Institute of Technology) and evaluated by Roxanne Hiltz (Upsala College and NJIT). EIES has been funded largely by the National Science Foundation (NSF) and the Annenberg/CPB Program.

TABLE 8.1

Stakeholders
Macrosupporters
Regulators
Social analysts
Industries and vendors
Administrators and system designers
Users
Researchers

While the initial development of the prototype system was motivated by national economic policy and funded through the Office of Emergency Preparedness, the major stimulus came from NSF's interest in using information systems to increase research productivity and diffusion of scientific and technical information, especially within invisible colleges (Crane, 1972; Tombaugh, 1984). This thrust led to a large number of studies of the use of EIES by nonprofit university or government researchers (see Kerr & Hiltz, 1982; Hiltz, 1983). In a sense, this funding source and the nature of many of the studies seem perfectly matched. However, what might appear to be a reasonable match of resources and respondents has in fact weakened the influence of this program of research. Management and communication researchers alike have questioned the generalizability of results from "unrealistically priced" CMCS used by "atypical" R & D scientists. Further, the longevity of the system and the research program leads some critics to dismiss the relevance of the results on the ground that EIES is no longer a "leading edge" system. However, one may well argue that until a system represents easily available technology and has been used by a large number of people over time, results cannot be generalizable.

A related example of this R & D grant model is the support of cross-national studies by nonprofit international agencies such as UNESCO (1980). Precisely because of its multiple stakeholders, such research has difficulty arriving at conclusions that are not obscured by the diplomatic need to compromise. The goal of such support is often the articulation of ideological principles and the description of trends and current conditions (such as the extent of transborder information flows or difference in regulatory polices toward technical communication standards). Such evaluations clearly provide baselines for further debate.

The second model, industry-university collaboration, may be represented by the research of the Institute for the Future (Johansen, 1984; Johansen, Vallee, & Spangler, 1979; Tydeman, Lipinski, Adler, Nyhan, & Zwimpfer, 1982) and the School of Social Science at Carnegie-Mellon University (Kiesler, 1986; Kiesler, Siegel, & McGuire, 1984; Sproull, 1986). Both of these institutions work extensively with corporate organizations that provide equipment and financial resources as well as research sites, but also receive government grants and publish many of their results in academic journals. This shifting blend of the agendas of corporations and nonprofit research institutes avoids the more monolithic focus of the EIES effort and provides conclusions that are more generalizable for organizational communication research and practice. However, certain aspects of results from such studies are considered proprietary and thus are inaccessible to the wider scholarly community. Further, the primary audience for such research, as well as the populations to which the results are generalizable, are often limited to managers and management researchers. One may criticize such research for not being generalizable to any person not part of a formal, Fortune-500 organization. Of course, most of this research and its associated methods are administrative in nature and not especially critical.

The third model is the proprietary study done for a specific company or industry, either as in-house projects or multiclient reports. Because the value of these studies is a global overview of markets and industries, and summaries of information are not generally available, their reports tend to focus on either technological and financial reviews or provide generalizations about trends based upon strategic analyses and market penetration. Proprietary research cannot advance theory much because it does not encourage replication or external critique of its methods and data.

(2) Regulators of resources, rights, and laws. As stakeholders, regulators, such as the Federal Communications Commission, Federal Trade Commission, World Administrative Radio Conference, International Telecommunications Union, and State Public Utilities Commissions (and other agencies which regulate businesses in general), constrain or change the jurisdiction or goals of telecommunications system evaluations. The convergence of computing and communication technologies is creating new battlegrounds and uncertainties for regulators as well as vendors (see Compaine, 1984; De Sola Pool, 1983; Robinson, 1978). Lack of uniform standards for EM systems, for example, prevents not only interconnections across systems and countries, but generates different sets of system functions, which make evaluation replications and generalizations difficult (Panko, 1981a). Policymakers are interested in who should have access, who should be funded, data flow regulations (Schiller, 1982), copyright issues (Keplinger, 1980); and privacy and secrecy (Rule, 1974; Westin & Baker, 1972) may set the agenda for system evaluations. For example, Palmer (1981) relates how Swedish statutes concerning freedom of information required detailed descriptions of the kind of content and records structure information that systems would contain before they could operate; because the content of CMCS is unknown before use, the Swedish COM system was stymied until the policy could be revised.

(3) Social analysts. These are generally interested in the social use and effects of computers in general and occasionally CMCS in particular, as opponents, proponents, or technological forecasters. Such authors include

Bush (1945), Beniger (1986), Ganley and Ganley (1982), Hiltz and Turoff (1978), Kling (1980), Martin (1981), Mosco (1982), Moshowitz (1976), Parker (1976), Rice and Associates (1984), Schiller (1982), Weizenbaum (1976), Wessel (1976), among others.

(4) Industries, vendors, and system designers. These overlap in their interests. Systems designers working for vendors are sensitive to research on programming languages, human-computer interfaces, software, operating systems, databases, communications, human factors, and the like (Ellis & Nutt, 1980; Ramsey & Grimes, 1983; Rouse, 1975). Technical evaluations of system performance (Carlson, 1974; Svoboda, 1976; and the journal *Performance Evaluation*) are better understood and more pervasive than are social evaluations (Hamilton & Chervany, 1981). Indeed, it is this imbalance between technical and social aspects of design and implementation that advocates of the sociotechnical systems perspective attempt to address. Bostrom and Heinen (1977a, 1977b) call upon system designers to inspect their assumptions about the level of involvement, ownership, and knowledge that users can provide; Pava (1983) argues that information work presents new challenges for both designers and managers to match technological and social systems.

(5) Administrators. Administrators have many interests at stake concerning CMCS: (a) Institutional directors, such as library planners, must redefine their services and needs to respond to technological opportunities and threats (ASIS, 1980); (b) system directors and managers tend to be cost-oriented, have a procomputer bias and be concerned with budgets, short-term time frames, organizational goals, management policies and mandates, and prioritization of use and support; (c) programmers and support staff will emphasize error statistics, new services, customer support, flexible and forgiving languages, documentation, as well as informed users; (d) moderators of computer conferences might desire information on how CC may facilitate or impede group decision making, level of participation by the conference members, access to past transcripts of the conference, relative appropriateness of other media, and technical obstacles (Kerr, 1986).

(6) "Users." This includes a wide array of stakeholders: (a) Potential users include service communities, those unfamiliar with computers such as students and the disadvantaged. Many potential users first have to overcome obstacles such as physical distance to the system, inequitable pricing strategies, insufficient education, general attitudes toward computers, misunderstanding of information needs, difficult human-machine interface, lack of control over the content, and so on; (b) organizations and institutions can include the individual representing an organization (raising issues of effects on workers, and alteration of the individual's role and status); the organization using CMCS as part of society (institutions such as schools, universities, and libraries); and social concerns (such as occupational dislocation and industry-wide needs for skills training); (c) groups, involving questions of group

dynamics, effects of the group's task, or the emergence of leadership; (d) users' social networks (raising issues of altered living patterns, decreased sociability, increased communication networks, increased knowledge gaps between those communicating by using CMCS and those not); (e) current individual users (who might be concerned about satisfaction with the system and its ergonomics, their anxiety about learning new systems, access to information in the system, changes in their attitudes and roles, and so on).

(7) Researchers. Researchers, of course, have their own skills, needs, norms, constraints, and goals in research activities. Needs may range from making contributions to knowledge to increasing their status in a discipline. Norms include what are considered "acceptable" research topics and the kinds of methodological tools brought to bear. And these norms shift as researchers bring new theories and tools to bear upon important topics and as different paradigms gain adherents. For example, there is a growing dissatisfaction with studies that do not include insights gained from qualitative or contextual analyses and with studies that focus solely on individual levels of analysis. Constraints may be inadequate funding or limited access to an appropriate field setting. Goals may be the testing of theory, improved system implementation, or increased chances of tenure.

GOALS

The goals or criteria of a research effort specify what is to be analyzed, what the purpose of the system and the research is, what constitutes "positive" or "negative" results. Goals constitute the motivations for conducting the research and using its results. Tools, discussed in Section 6, constitute the ways of gathering evidence for, and the criteria for assessing the conclusions of, such research. The major distinction among categories of research goals is whether they are formative or summative (Table 8.2).

Formative Research

Formative research about CMCS acquires information useful in designing and improving project components, and provides feedback during the design, implementation, and use of the system. The EIES developers (Hiltz & Turoff, 1978) consider formative research a fundamental part of system development. EIES includes a computer language for developing customized communication structures, online consultants who apply users' suggestions and problems to the continued redesign of the system and continuing evaluation projects that provide the foundations for training and satisfaction of CMCS users.

Formative research raises such issues as, Why are you doing this? Or, why do these users find this system so difficult? Or, what is the goal of this evaluation? These questions are clearly political and may be quite different in

TABLE 8.2

Goals
Formative evaluation
needs assessments
ongoing systems design
implementation
evaluation of research process
Summative evaluation
distribution of resources
functionality
political process
knowledge
actualization
information-processing skills
problems and tasks
structure
sensation
cost
symbolism

character than the questions of summative research. An ongoing series of research projects may profit from formative analysis, which asks such questions as these: What are the effects of evaluation itself? Will a CMCS be reinterpreted by various stakeholders after the recommendations suggested by the formative results are implemented? (For a further discussion, see Acher, this volume.)

Summative Research

Summative research aims to summarize how the system affected those involved with the system as well as the wider social context, including intended and unintended effects, and to detect to what extent the system's goals were achieved. Summative research typically attempts to determine causal processes leading to those effects and goals. Intensity and duration of effects are measured as well as the extent to which the intended project treatment was in fact delivered (Suchman, 1967). For example, Kerr and Hiltz (1982) argue persuasively that having *access* to a CMCS, *using* it, and *accepting* it are very different components of system delivery, so they must be measured explicitly and separately. Culnan (1984) also discusses the concept of access with respect to office information systems. She concludes that accessibility encompasses physical access to a terminal, the actual information system, the command language, and the ability to retrieve the desired information successfully.

The following list suggests social dimensions of summative evaluation goals for CMCS; other dimensions for the evaluation of computer and information systems have been suggested by Carlson (1974) and Kling (1984).

(1) Resource distribution, equity, and participation: Studies of CC systems usage show increased equality of participation by users compared to similar users in face-to-face situations (Hiltz & Turoff, 1978; Kerr & Hiltz, 1982; Rice & Associates, 1984, chap. 6). The presence of computer-based networks do not always guarantee that users gain the full positive benefits of such systems, or even guarantee that the general effects *are* positive. For example, as previously noted, users must first gain access to such systems, and then must also gain access to information and other users on these systems. "Access" usually requires financial resources, cultural support, and prior knowledge about the availability and operational logistics of a particular system. Thus it is necessary to analyze "the structure of social inequality and the consequent differential access to key communication resources across the population" (Golding & Murdock, 1986, pp. 71), and constraints owing to infrastructure, technology, economics, sociocultural norms, and politics (Vitalari & Venkatesh, 1986) before we can adequately talk about "increased choice" from the new media on a societal level. Further, Lowi (1983) argues that computer communications can simultaneously increase individuals' power and the flow of information as well as increase the public's susceptibility to manipulation by those who control large systems and the origination of information. For example, the increased ability to narrowcast information and target audiences by distribution lists or system directories could lead to a fragmentation of attitudes and the development of separate interest groups which may become empowered by their unity or isolated by their lack of awareness of other publics (Lowi, 1983; Rice, 1987a). Schiller (1982) and Mosco (1982) claim that international information networks support the increased economic domination of lesser developed countries by multinationals.

Issues of resource allocation may even determine which projects are worth evaluating. Goals of both efficiency and ethics demand an analysis of the trade-off between using scarce resources to evaluate a project or using them to provide more services. If a project involves fairly familiar ground or if the likelihood is small that the treatment (or system, for example) being evaluated will be widely implemented, then the resources may well be better spent elsewhere.

(2) Functionality: What is the user doing, or what does the user want or have to do? What can the medium do for the user? Within an organization, functionality is constrained by organizational climate, policies on efficiency and productivity, history of innovation, responsiveness to workers, and so on. A recent analysis of the diffusion of the intelligent telephone (PBX) in two divisions of a large organization showed that only nine out of more than 100 phone functions were used in a year, and three of those represented most

usage; organizational politics and insufficient training contributed to this low functionality (Rice & Manross, 1986).

(3) Political process: What role does or could CMCS play in creating an informed public, providing access to congressional representatives, distributing community information, and stimulating grassroots activity, or developing information resources? One example is the EIES Legitech group (see Hiltz & Turoff, 1978), which responds to queries from one state's agency staff with another state's staff experience in the matter. Another example is the use of computer bulletin board systems (CBBS) by constituents to participate in political discussions with their elected representatives. Garramone, Harris, and Anderson (1986) applied a uses and gratifications model to understanding the use of a political CBBS based in a university near a state capitol. Personal identity and surveillance (communicating with others about political issues) were the most commonly mentioned motivations for general use of the system, while those who actively placed messages on the system reported the greatest personal identity satisfaction. Haight and Rubinyi (1983) found that community groups used computers to augment and improve their local operations, but rarely used the systems to communicate with other community groups. (With the decreased cost and increased diffusion of computers and bulletin board software, this situation may have changed significantly since 1982.)

(4) Knowledge: How do CMCS play a part in the progression of a bit to data to information to knowledge to wisdom in creating, accessing, sharing, expanding, valuing knowledge, and experience bases? This move is of particular interest to research communities: Hiltz (1983) argues that CMCS can increase the amount and distribution of scientific and technical information, but scientific norms and individual's expectations often limit this potential.

(5) Actualization: What are the possible roles of CMCS in well-being, religion, spirit, human potential, life-styles? The Japanese are the trend-setters in evaluating effects of information and its technologies on these measures of quality of life in the information society (see Edelstein, Bowes, & Harsel, 1978, and especially Bowes, 1981).

(6) Information processing skills: How do individuals, groups, and organizations represent, encode, transmit, and decode information? Some aspects include management of information load and related stress, ability to adapt to processing asynchronous rather than simultaneous exchanges, performing multiple tasks through multiple media, constraints on reflective thinking due to rapid turnaround, and development of computer literacy. Zuboff (1982) argues that office workers must be trained to think in more abstract ways because office automation systems do not allow visual or tactile organization of information. Rice (1982) argues that human information-processing limits lead individuals to more instrumental and reciprocal use of CMCS.

(7) Problems: How can CMCS help—or hinder—individuals in handling and solving individual, group, and social problems and tasks (Paisley, 1980)? Research shows that CMCS have considerable and consistent effects on group decision making (Rice & Associates, 1984, chap. 6).

(8) Structure: How might the use of CMCS change the magnitude and distribution of relations among users, and effects of these changes on users' roles and behavior? Freeman (1980), for example, analyzed the effect of CMCS on users' social networks. He found that although theory predicted that no new strong links between participants ("close friend" compared to "acquaintance") could develop from using the system if the relationships did not already have the potential to do so (based upon common educational institutions, colleagues, research interests, and so on), several participants who had no prior potential linkages did become very close. Further, these larger clusters of "close friends" became more differentiated from the remaining social structure represented by the participants in the computer conference.

(9) Sensation: How might CMCS interact with physical and emotional arousal, pleasure and pain, including direct effects as well as indirect effects on other activities, such as the use of communication systems to relieve tension arising from other activities or to compensate for or respond to information from other experimental domains? Theories of uses and gratifications derived from these media include the possibility that many people use media out of habit or for the pleasure of "consumption" (Rice & Associates, 1984, chap. 5; Urban, 1984).

(10) Cost: What are the fixed and variable costs of hardware, software, training, operation, maintenance. Panko, for example, has provided several detailed economic analyses of electronic mail systems (1980, 1981b, 1985; Bair, 1978, 1980; Rice & Associates, 1984, chap. 8). In general, dollar costs of computing, particularly in decentralized systems, are underestimated (King & Kraemer, 1981) and social costs are rarely even estimated. For example, Strassman (1985) argues that only a moderate percentage of the total first-year cost for an end-user workstation is attributable to the obvious costs of acquisition. Other costs include training, supplies, overhead, telecommunications, software, support staff, furniture, organizational learning, implementation, uncertainty, and conflicts. (See the information section for an elaboration of this point.)

(11) Symbolism: What are the symbolic and political reasons for justifying the implementation of a CMCS, or for CMCS research? For example, organizational evaluation of a pilot electronic mail system, when long-range policy has already mandated extensive implementation and specific results will not alter this decision, may defuse possible resistance. Having access to a CMCS may be important to creating an image of an "informed" and "innovative" professional (see Feldman & March, 1981, for a discussion of the symbolic uses of information).

DOMAINS

A domain is the level of complexity or organization at which the computer-mediated communication relationship is evaluated. Domain is used rather than "level of analysis" to emphasize the sphere of communication behavior, rather than just the analytical unit chosen by the researcher. As Rogers and Kincaid (1981, chap. 2) argue, much communication research has assumed a linear model of communication, audiences comprised of noninteracting individuals, and the absence of constraining social structures. Particularly because CMCS support interactions among changing sets of individuals who can structure their communications, distinctions among domains are appropriate and necessary. Research efforts should be explicit about which domains are being studied. Stakeholders may be concerned about resources in different domains and users may experience varied benefits and disadvantages in different domains. A single domain, the boundary between domains, an individual's behavior throughout several domains, the interaction of domains across two or more individuals, and so on, constitute the kinds of research areas possible. The metastudy of the existence and forms of these domains is one of the possible goals of analysis. All the following domains may interact, of course: An *individual's* use of CMCS is likely to be hampered by *national* standards and access regulations owing to concerns about data flows and control of telecommunications markets (Panko, 1985; Shipley, Shipley, & Wigand, 1985). Possible domains and particular examples, as summarized in Table 8.3, include the following:

(1) The individual. In this domain, psychological, emotional, physiological, and behavioral aspects of CMCS use and effects are studied typically by aggregating responses from a sample of system users (potential, actual, or a control group), or by conducting a case study of specific users. Changes in the amount or channels of communication attributed to, or the role of user's attitudes in the level of, use of a CMCS (Miller & Nichols, 1981; Rice & Associates, 1984, chap. 9; Tapscott, 1982) are typical topics.

(2) Dyads. These are two individuals who participate in, or are identified through, a particular communication process. Here, asymmetry, reciprocity, source, direction, and amount of communications between two individuals or sets of individuals are typical topics. Gutek (1982), for example, spent a year studying the work relationship of one secretary-manager dyad before, during, and after the implementation and removal of an office CMCS. Gutek based her study design on the assumption that the relationship between the two was a rich source for understanding the use and interpretations of CMCS.

(3) Roles. This includes sender, transmitter, isolate, group member, gatekeeper, leader, occupation, organizational position, social status, and so on. The particular role may influence an individual's access to a CMCS (for example, top university administrators had first access to an EM system in order to encourage later adoption by subordinates—Rice & Case, 1983), while

TABLE 8.3

Domains
Individual
Dyads
Roles
Groups
Organizations and institutions
Societal relations

the nature of one's CMCS usage may determine which role that individual occupies in an information environment (Rice, 1987a).

(4) Groups. These range from triads to portions of "invisible colleges." The dynamics of group decision making are altered when members communicate through CMCS (see Rice & Associates, 1984, chap. 6); one group of geographically dispersed researchers intensified their personal networks by using CMCS (Freeman, 1980).

(5) Organizations and institutions. These are collections of individuals and relationships that have constraints and goals different from those of their constituent individuals. Organizations can change those constraints by using CMCS, for example, to support telecommuting programs (Nilles, Carlson, Gray, & Hanneman, 1976), or to redefine the nature of information work (Johnson & Rice, 1987). Frameworks for identifying types of, and relationships among, effects of CMCS in the organizational domain have been suggested by Giuliano (1982), Simon (1973), and Olson and Lucas (1982).

(6) Societal relations. These range from community computer bulletin boards and public CMCS services (Glossbrenner, 1983) to wired cities (Dutton & Kraemer, 1985), networked nations (Dordick, Bradley, & Nanus, 1981; Hiltz & Turoff, 1978; Martin, 1981), information economies, and a global world information order.

As an example of some of the implications of emphasizing one or more particular domains in the study of CMCS, consider one of the more widely accepted concepts of societal relations concerning information and communication technologies: the "information economy."

Many authors and researchers have argued that the economies of the United States, Japan, and several European countries have, in the last decade, become predominantly information-based. That is, the information sector, rather than the service, industrial, or agricultural sector, represents the largest component (over 50% in the United States) of the national economy. This predominance may be measured by labor employed, capital invested, or outputs produced, but also may be indicated by the continued exponential growth in scientific and technical information, by the continued diffusion of a wide variety of information technologies, by diverse access to and consumption of media products, and by the convergence of computing and communication technologies (Bell, 1976, 1981; Beniger, 1986; Huber, 1984; Ito, 1981; Machlup, 1962; Porat, 1977; Price, 1963).

While these and similar measures do indicate a clear growth in information-related activities, there is considerable debate not only about the benefits of such a transition, but also about the extent of the transition. For example, Weizenbaum (1981) rejects not so much the concept itself, but more the underlying assumptions about the information society that lead many authors to herald its development. Weizenbaum criticizes Simon's (1981) faith in humans' use of computer technology to generate new knowledge that is accountable, understandable or humane. He argues that the rise of the information society is paramount to an abdication of human control of human reason, that computers can be used to communicate facts but not understanding, and that those theoretically in control may use such systems for their own ends or may not even understand how the information was created or used. Marien (1985) makes a different kind of critique: he argues that whatever changes are associated with the information economy, they cannot be acclaimed "revolutionary." There are arguably many other current developments that are far more revolutionary, such as genetic engineering. Schement and Lievrouw's (1987) volume contains basic questions as to the extent and nature of the change in work that the information revolution is supposed to support.

Schiller (1982), UNESCO (1980), and others argue that there *is* a major transformation of economies and perhaps societies associated with the development of information technologies, but that it is primarily symptomatic of the continuing trends of industrial nations, multinational corporations, and advanced capitalism. That is, shifts toward information economies expand the realms for economic and cultural domination, increase social and economic differentiation, and increase the privatization and control of information itself (Mehra, 1987; Schiller, 1985; Traber, 1986). Thus the terms *information economy* or *information revolution* are problematic and can represent very contradictory moral, economic, and social visions. Evaluations of CMCS in this domain must be careful to analyze the assumptions behind both traditional and new measures of job categories, information flows, economic development, and societal influences on and outcomes of communication technologies.

Relationships are fundamental in the use and understanding of CMCS. Research studies should identify relevant domains and their interaction.

TOOLS: DESIGN, DATA, AND METHODS

There is a wide variety of issues related to the choice and use of tools in CMCS research (Williams, Rice, & Rogers, 1988). This section does not intend to provide a survey of tools and data sources generally available, but

TABLE 8.4

Tools: Design, Data and Methods
Designs:
issues of sampling randomization
controlled experiments
panel and time-series studies
quasi-experimental field trials
surveys
focus groups
case studies
benchmark comparisons
impact assessments
Data:
literature reviews
observations (participant or remote)
interviews
questionnaire responses
open-ended comments from questionnaires or focus groups
archival data
unobtrusive measures
computer-monitored data
system transcripts
Methods of Analysis:
description
content analysis
interpretive
critical
univariate and multivariate techniques
network analysis
activity analysis
change over time

notes a few issues particularly relevant to designs, data, and methods in CMCS research, as listed in Table 8.4. We here consider one or two examples in each of three major categories: design, data, and analysis.

Design

(A) Appropriate designs. There has already been considerable work, not only in research on CMCS, but in identifying appropriate designs and methods for the study of CMCS. A fairly comprehensive typology of approaches and variables has been developed by Johansen, Miller, and Vallee (1974). Their typology included (a) controlled lab experiments, (b) quasi-experiments, (c) directed field trials, (d) open-ended trials, (e) survey research, and (f) impact assessment of, for example, scenarios, simulations, and models. These are standard alternatives open to any research project, but the authors cross-reference the numerous studies of CMCS of which they were aware by these alternatives (Johansen, Vallee, & Spangler, 1979, pp. 166-191). Johan-

sen, Vallee, and Spangler (1979) expanded the 1974 typology of variables by developing the pioneering work of Bailey, Nordlie, and Sistrunk (1963). The revised typology consisted of five sets of group communication attributes—medium, task, rules, person, and group (Johansen, Miller, & Vallee, 1974, p. 16)—and was part of a very detailed and useful schema that incorporated the analysis of changes over time in a group's use of a CMCS and associated outcomes (Vallee, Johansen, Randolph, & Hastings, 1974, p. 25).

Case studies, participant observation, and descriptive analyses are useful research tools to provide ethnographic and interpretive insights into the use and meaning of CMCS (Hiltz & Turoff, 1978; see also Erlandson, 1980 and Rice, 1984). In these approaches, the evaluator may be a group participant, and the analysis chronicles the group's passage through time and difficulties, revealing external and internal obstacles or factors, the social aspects of jointly working on a task via computer, and other situational processes that perhaps could never be adequately measured or predicted. The question of potential bias looms large, as the controversy over stakeholder analysis emphasizes, but system designers, managers, and users of CMCS may be keenly interested in the kinds of insights possible from the approach. Further, transcripts from interviews and actual system sessions provide examples of problems or possibilities that use the language, symbols, and criteria that are immediately interpretable and usable to stakeholders in the particular setting. For example, Hiemstra (1983) used focus groups, content analysis, and personal interviews to extract underlying themes in discussions about office automation, and then analyzed relations among these themes.

(B) Generalizability. The goals of a particular project will influence the value of particular research designs. For example, if generalizability has been established as one of the research goals, then the value of summative research is affected by the extent to which findings are convincing and ecologically valid. Satisfying these and other criteria is traditionally a function of subject and treatment randomization and study design. Suchman (1967) emphasizes that (a) effect, (b) adequacy, and (c) process of the impact must be discussed in order to gauge the generalizability of the effect.

As defined by Suchman, *effect* is the amount of significant impact, typically specified by subgroup. Very large groups will typically show significant effects; the lack of significant effects in small groups may not indicate no impact, only low statistical power. Many studies of organizational use of CMCS are limited to small or convenience samples, owing to the pilot nature of the system, a desire to have an identifiable and task-related set of users, or poor questionnaire response rate.

Adequacy is the meaningfulness and duration of the impact. A valid and statistically significant effect may not be very meaningful to the stakeholders, or may not last very long. For example, a study of the uses and effects of an agricultural videotext system showed statistically significant relationships, but the variance explained (10%) was not large enough for the policy recommendations to be meaningful for the program administrators (Rice & Paisley, 1982). Poor design may make generalizability risky or misleading. Short-term effects may appear overnight, or other important effects, such as the change in users' attitudes toward computers and the appropriateness of CMCS for certain tasks, may develop only in the long run (Hiltz & Turoff, 1981). Or the kinds of users who have early access to a CMCS system are not likely to be typical of users who gain later access to a system.

Process is Suchman's term for specification or contingency analysis: the specification of the social and psychological factors that mediate or impede effects. For example, Rice (1982) found that task-orientation was a major determinant of a group's wider participation in a nationwide CMCS.

These criteria are discussed in the context of positivist social science approaches, but interpretive and critical approaches are also concerned with effect, adequacy, and process, but without a necessary concern with statistical inference and quantification. For example, effect may involve the determination of the extent of access to a CMCS by a particular social or organizational group (Haight & Rubinyi, 1983). Adequacy may involve the analysis of ongoing and indirect social changes brought about by pervasive telecommunication networks (Rice, 1987a; Schiller, 1982). Process is a main focus of interpretive analysis, intended to uncover the ways in which a system comes to be used, controlled, or changed (Kling & Scacchi, 1980). From this paradigm, generalizability to a particular *population* is not necessarily the goal, but to enduring *issues* or deeper social structures.

(C) Control and randomization. Because of the several stakeholders and domains involved in a particular CMCS, it often is not obvious which experimental or quasi-experimental designs could be used or are appropriate (Cook & Campbell, 1979). In the case of CMCS, whether in homes, communities, or organizations, it seems highly unrealistic, if not impractical, to select users randomly. Not only do most studies analyze self-selected users, but the value of CMCS is fundamentally based upon the interactions among a network of users. That is, by definition, random sampling seems an inappropriate way to study such communication systems. There are also ethical issues, as with many research designs, such as who (randomly) would get access to the system? Do those who do not have access continue to suffer from problems that the system is supposed to solve?

Then too, there is the question of whether there can ever be a true randomized control group when individuals and organizations are actively using CMCS for their ongoing work. However, controlled and quasi-experiments involving specific groups of new as well as experienced users have been conducted to compare how groups use different media in decision-making processes or in conducting normal organizational conmmunications (Bair, 1978; Kerr & Hiltz, 1982; Rice & Associates, 1984, chap. 6; Tapscott, 1982, p. 207). The controlled experiments are often conducted online, using a CMCS which presents the treatments and collects and analyzes the data, and involve variables, such as the complexity of task, communication channel, prior familiarity of subjects, time to decision, consensus reached, satisfaction, and so on.

The CMCS is conceptually a treatment or an intervening variable, and must be considered as only one of many possible channels of communication (such as telephone, memo, face-to-face, letters and reports, video, interpersonal, psychic). Analyses taking this treatment into account have led to the considerable knowledge we now have in cross-media comparisons in various domains (Johansen, 1977; Short, Williams, & Christie, 1976). Indeed, research might place more emphasis on understanding the role of media diversity and media choice in influencing the use and effects of CMCS.

Data

The presence of a computer in many new media systems creates new opportunities for the kinds of data that can be collected and analyzed. That is, both content and flows can be collected by the system itself, enabling analyses of a full census of users, of transcripts of content, of interactions among large sets of users, and of content and flows over time (Penniman & Dominick, 1980; Rice & Borgman, 1983). Such data avoid problems of measurement error, developing enumeration lists, missing responses, and discrepancies between respondents' actual usage of a system and their reported usage. Indeed, the availability of measures of actual CMCS communication behavior has provided more fuel to the attitude-behavior consistency controversy (Berger & Roloff, 1980). While some have argued that communication behavior (as measured by computer-monitored usage data) is not necessarily the criterion against which self-report data should be evaluated, and that they probably measure different aspects of usage, the debate has raised the question as to the underlying assumption social science has held about interview and questionnaire data. That is, if these two sources of data *do* diverge, this divergence is a different question from whether attitudes are good predictors of behavior. Rather, the question is whether we have too easily accepted the assumption that respondents' self-reports are valid reports of anything other than rather enduring but otherwise unfounded opinions (Bernard, Killworth, Kronenfeld, & Sailer, 1984).

CMCS, as new sources of data, may help us better understand the biases and differential predictability of reported versus actual communication behavior (Ettema, 1985). On the other hand, simple measures of number of log-ons or hours on-line may summarize CMCS usage, but say nothing about function, user satisfaction, or political conflict about the meaning and implications of the system. For example, Ettema (1984) argued that videotext users who operate the system more effectively may also use the system less, precisely because they achieve their information needs quickly: usage can be negatively correlated with reported satisfaction or benefits, but that does not mean that the system should be removed!

Methods of Analysis

(A) Content analysis. The content of communications via CMCS has not received sufficient study, in spite of the fact that precisely because the medium can keep a record of the content there are opportunities to measure the kinds of content and interaction exchanged by CMCS users. Further, most analyses of organizational systems assume that the content of the systems is objective, routine, and unproblematic information used to perform rational tasks, or that CMCS are inherently impersonal and inappropriate for social topics. Exceptions have been studies of the subjective evaluations of the uses and value of the content by system users (Ives, Olson, & Baroudi, 1983). Steinfield's (1986a) analysis of a large organization's use of electronic messaging showed that the social uses of the medium were in fact frequent, and quite important, especially to newer employees who used the system to learn about the organization's social and business norms.

Another strand of research has focused on the consequences of the limited range of nonverbal communication content possible in CMCS (Rice & Associates, 1984; Rice & Love, 1987). Sproull and Kiesler (1986) found that the content of an organizational electronic messaging system indicated that people were more self-absorbed in system messages than in face-to-face communication, that hierarchical boundaries are crossed more in electronic communication, users tend to violate organizational norms more in electronic messaging behavior, and much of the content was new information that was not otherwise available. Hiemstra (1982) applied Goffman's theory of "presentation of self" in human communications to the transcripts of a series of CMCS sessions, and found, with only a few exceptions, very similar patterns of "face-saving" behavior. Other content analyses of CMCS transcripts are more descriptive and anecdotal (Philips, 1982).

Some studies of CMCS have specifically focused on the interaction between flows and content in CMCS. Danowski (1982) evaluated the content of community computer bulletin board messages to suggest applications of discussion leadership that could lead to optimal convergence of participants around a topic or around a participant. Automated content analysis revealed linkages of topics across messages. The linkages were then scaled via metric multidimensional analysis, and possible related topic clusters were extracted. The goal was to be able to train group leaders to recognize these clusters, or sequential patterns, and perhaps steer discussion back to the task via topics closer to the stated goals of the conference. Clearly, different stakeholders would hold very different opinions as to the utility or even ethics of such research. A related approach has been the analysis of "threads of discourse" or the multiple themes that often coexist in CMCS (Black, Levin, Mehan, & Quinn, 1983).

(B) Network analysis. Another CMCS research approach emphasizes the importance of the domains and involves the analysis of communication patterns in organizations. One methodology appropriate to communication

flow analysis is network analysis (Aldrich, 1979; Farace, Monge, & Russell, 1977; Goldhaber, Yates, Porter, & Lesniak, 1978; Rogers & Kincaid, 1981). Network analysis can be used to describe (or "audit") the communication flows and roles at dyadic, group, organizational, and societal domains, and to test theories of organizational communication. Lowenstein (1979), Rice and Richards (1985) and Tapscott (1982) give detailed procedures for collecting and measuring network variables for evaluating CMCS design, use, and consequences.

A network-oriented evaluation might measure communication flows before, during, and after the implementation of a CMCS, for example, to determine whether the technology assists the development of desired communication flows, whether other organizational media (memos, face-to-face conversations, meetings, visitations, telephone calls, conference travel, and so on) are affected, whether certain tasks are performed better in these altered communication patterns, whether the same information can be handled in fewer transformations among media, whether the same information can be shared and accessed with less cost, or whether decision making is centralized or decentralized (and the desirability of either of these). Rice (1982) and Rice and Barnett (1985) used computer-monitored data to show how, over time, task-focused research groups using a nationwide CMCS were more likely to become and remain "isolates," while nontask groups were more likely to remain as information-rich "carriers." Network indices, such as the ratio of within-group to system-wide communication, were useful indicators of potential group cohesion or dissolution. Metric multidimensional scaling procedures were used to determine the effect of groups' entry and exit upon the larger CMCS network. Thus network analysis as one research tool seems to provide helpful insight into important goals, at a variety of domains, to inform a number of stakeholders.

(C) The nature of change. Traditional designs assume that pre- and posttest measures simply detect the difference, along a fixed scale, in variables between two time periods. More rigorous designs would collect data over time to understand how patterns of use and consequences develop, how the sociotechnical system responds to the shock of new communication structures, and how users develop new patterns of communication networks. However, if hypotheses that using a CMCS actually changes the nature of work and alters one's communication environment are correct, then evaluations must also measure changes in the *scales* and *dimensions* upon which respondents base their responses. Golembiewski (1986), among others, has suggested a framework for measuring such changes, called alpha, beta, and gamma change. Alpha change is the traditional measure of change: variation along specific intervals in a given scale. Beta change indicates that the intervals and boundaries of the scale have changed, so identical scale ratings do not indicate identical attitudes or behaviors. Gamma change involves reevaluation of the scale: It may be measuring something else entirely after the treatment. In one

study of an organizational CMCS, workers' notions of what effectiveness meant, as well as the extent to which workers were effective at different tasks and how effective one could actually be in performing those tasks, changed after the system was implemented and respondents had used it for a period of time (Mohrman & Novelli, 1983). Another study of a large-scale CMCS showed that users' attitudes toward the system became more positive, and their use of different functions expanded, as the individuals passed through different thresholds of usage (Hiltz & Turoff, 1981).

There are at least three major implications from such evidence that change is a fundamental part of CMCS. One is that social evaluations of CMCS should use tools—quantitative or qualitative—that allow the collection and analysis of data over time. The second is that different stages in the life cycle both of the system and of individuals' usage patterns should be analyzed separately. The third is that analyses should test whether the dimensions on which users evaluate their usage and the consequences of CMCS have changed over time. Although the first implication is well recognized by communication researchers, it is still infrequently practiced. The second two implications are as yet extremely rare in CMCS research.

INFORMATION AND CMCS

Dervin (1981) and Rogers and Kincaid (1981, chap. 2) have well summarized the growing rejection of a linear model of communication (Shannon & Weaver, 1949) and conceptions of information as objective content sent by one party to be received and consumed as fact by a passive, mass audience. While the denotative meaning of communicated content clearly *is* highly significant and relevant, and while many audiences value and *are* satisfied by the mass media, this concept of information has dominated much of CMCS research. Further, this conceptualization tends to limit research to the domain of individual communication behavior (the user as an isolated processor of information, or the recipients of messages as homogeneous "accounts"). Hirschheim (1985) argues that this "analytical" perspective tends to focus on communication tasks as rational and overt instead of political and nondeterministic, on organizations as structures instead of agents and cultures, on communication actions as manifest behavior instead of socially constructed meaning, on quantitative rather than qualitative tools, and on analysis instead of understanding meanings. Focusing on the information exchanged via CMCS as an interpreted social good can lead to very different goals, system designs, and communication applications (Rice & Parker, 1979).

This section, then, takes the opportunity briefly to investigate this changing concept of information with respect to several aspects of the four evaluative dimensions as applied to CMCS. The first section considers how stakeholders who conceptualize information as an objective commodity may be misled by narrow goals. The second section considers how a wider conceptualization of information exchange as an interpretive activity, along with wider domains and appropriate evaluative tools, can lead to new system designs and applications of CMCS.

Information as an Economic Object

A narrow conceptualization of information—information as a commodity with an objective price set by market mechanisms—constrains the kinds of information that will be evaluated as appropriate or valuable (Johnson & Rice, 1987). This bias is particularly likely when stakeholders, their goals, and their evaluation tools emphasize cost and efficiency while ignoring the meaning, context, and purpose of the content communicated by system users. Stakeholders who use the criteria of traditional economic goals to justify or evaluate CMCS are often unaware of the underlying assumptions about the nature of information and consequent problems or contradictions (Hall, 1981). These assumptions and their reanalyses are presented as follows:

(1) Assumption: In a particular market, the production of all firms, and the consumption of all individuals, are independent.

Reanalysis: (a) Creators and owners of specific information are hard to identify, so benefits and costs from the final product cannot be fully or correctly allocated. Therefore, information (such as new knowledge exchanged through a CMCS) will be underproduced, unless outcome criteria are based upon production of material units (a tangible product, such as a bound report), in which case it will be overproduced. (b) Because information, unlike physical commodities, can often be separated from its physical medium, additional consumers generally create few additional costs but are also difficult to exclude. This characteristic means that information that is valuable will not be communicated in sufficient quantities unless it is subsidized or tightly controlled. For example, evaluations of the Institute for the Future's PLANET computer conferencing system, in which most field trial participants paid for usage (Johansen, Vallee, & Spangler, 1979), and the New Jersey Institute of Technology's EIES system, in which most participants did not pay (Hiltz & Turoff, 1978), showed that subsidized users evaluated the systems positively, but decreased or stopped usage when they had to bear the full costs. (c) A different version of this problem is that consumption of information does not necessarily deplete it; information, therefore, may grow or decline in value in ways unrelated to consumption and may appreciate or depreciate at a nonlinear rate. (d) Communicating certain information may change the value of other information, or lead to redistribution of resources. Thus the value of content at one point in time may have little to do with the value of the content at a later point in time. Thus, for situations in which the value of the communication must be confirmed, face-to-face interaction, even if subject to greater constraints and involving greater costs in time and energy, will be preferred over CMCS, because receipt of and reply to an electronic message cannot be guaranteed within a prespecified time interval.

(2) Assumption: All actors have sufficient information to make optimal choices.

Reanalysis: (a) Because of (1a), the value and consequences of information are uncertain. (b) Because this value is uncertain, full evaluation of the worth of some communicated content is possible only through direct consumption (listening, purchase, reading, and so on). Since this evaluation requires some cost in status, money, or time, indirect consumption mechanisms have arisen to help reduce this problem (Aldrich, 1979; Baligh & Richartz, 1964; Williamson, 1979). Indirect evaluations in academic communication include publishing in or reading only refereed articles in high quality journals within one's discipline, publishing or reading review articles, reading publications by well-known authors, and inspecting the reference list before deciding to read an article. Applying this process to CMCS research, we can begin to understand why nearly 40% of those with free access to a nationwide CMCS declined to use it on personal cost/benefit grounds (Kerr & Hiltz, 1982). Some individuals responded that they derived greater benefits from their limited time and energy using other media and channels. Others, assessing the value of CMCS for supporting and extending an invisible college of researchers, feared that other users might appropriate their ideas into research before they could establish ownership and reward through publications. Therefore, they underinvested in scholarly innovation in the uncontrolled information marketplace of the CMCS.

(3) *Assumption*: No one buyer or seller can affect the price of a product.

Reanalysis: (a) The costs of communicating some content are so high that mechanisms such as patents and academic tenure have been established to guarantee returns on long-term investments and to influence the price for subsequent users and potential market entrants. (b) Because information is easily replicated once created, in some situations distribution and marketing costs become predominant considerations, leading to natural monopolies. This consideration is one of the reasons that multinational CMCS are unlikely to support a truly free flow of information: They are more likely to consolidate control and stratify users' access to information (Golding & Murdock, 1986; Mosco, 1982).

(4) *Assumption:* In an efficient market, the price of a product reflects its marginal value after costs are recovered. The classic evaluation approach typically measures economic efficiency as an increase in an output/input ratio, through increased outputs and/or decreased inputs. One form of efficiency is *cost avoidance*; for example, after the implementation of a CMCS, fewer telephone circuits, clerical workers, or business trips are necessary, so communication costs will be avoided in the future.

Reanalysis: (a) Because the costs of producing the information, the costs of the medium used to transmit the information, and the value of the information to a particular stakeholder are generally unrelated, the actual price paid or costs saved are misleading criteria for evaluating whether a CMCS achieved specific goals. In general, the huge investment in social systems (relationships, status, norms, expectations, patterns of communication) vastly overwhelms the actual costs and possibly the returns from new communication technology. Therefore, evaluations should consider a variety of stakeholders and goals in order to understand the contexts for use and outcomes of CMCS. For example, Markus (1987) shows that organizations that "charge back" for a CMCS, based upon cost-recovery methods imposed by stakeholders in accounting and data processing departments, in fact are stifling the adoption process by encouraging potential users to continue using currently "free" or easily accountable media, such as copying machines, telephones, and paper memos. The influential stakeholders (the data processing department) in the organization that Markus studied never included the users' or the wider organization's goals in their set of evaluation goals.

Information as an Interpretative Activity

Paradoxically, precisely because CMCS have media characteristics derived from both telecommunication networks and computer processing, there is the potential not only to analyze them using tools based upon a different conceptualization of information but also to design them to support more interpretivist communication processes in multiple domains.

Considering first the question of domains and tools, one characteristic of CMCS that makes them particularly different from interpersonal and mass media is the ability to support *group* communication processes. While discussions of EM tend to emphasize the ability to *send* a message easily to one or more other users, conferencing and bulletin board systems enable prescribed or emergent groups to communicate jointly—collaboratively creating meaning out of diverse sources of information, commenting on and editing messages and documents, indicating ways in which individual opinions may diverge from the common material, and possibly continually evolving the group's shared experiences and meaning. Thus the interactive and processual nature of both the act and content of communication can be emphasized in CMCS research by tools such as network analysis and longitudinal data.

The interpretivist approach to communication can also be used to understand interaction among individuals and groups in organizations (Hirschheim, 1985). General approaches include:

(a) considering work roles as sets of rights and duties, or social contracts, that govern social behavior in ways that fit the sources and content of current beliefs;

(b) analyzing decision-making as the content, process, and location of examining a problem and creating meaning, based on a mixture of evidence, intuition, analysis, and value judgments;

(c) understanding the transactions involved in acquiring, exchanging, and distributing information and the collective or hierarchical sources (such as policies, rituals, and ceremonies) of those transaction mechanisms (Williamson, 1979); and

(d) identifying how communication mediates people's intentions and behaviors, either through defensible, valid reasons or by vested interests and conventions (Habermas, 1984). This language action approach argues that subjective bias, physical constraints, distortions of information by social conditions, and lack of awareness of intention and implications for performance all create obstacles to intersubjective intelligibility of communications.

For example, Hiemstra (1983) identified meanings of the set of terms associated with "information technology" in four organizations. The evaluative dimensions of conversations about CMCS included *fast/slow, dynamic/static, patent/impatient, young/old, future/past, creative/routine, mysterious/obvious, exciting/dull.* Extremes of users (clericals versus computer operators) and technology (typewriters versus computer terminals) are arranged along these dimensions. Information technology is referred to in metaphors such as *magic, toys,* and *moving objects.*

The interpretivist approach seems to raise serious challenges not only to the CMCS research, but also to the validity of communication through such systems. The prevalent argument is that CMCS, because of their bandwidth limitations, cannot convey much of the nonverbal and social communication among individuals and will thus reinforce the conceptualization of information as rational, objective content to be transferred from one person to another. While this position is subject to considerable debate just on the basis of the kinds of communication that *do* occur in CMCS (see Sproull & Kiesler, 1986; Rice & Associates, 1984; Rice & Love, 1987), it is perhaps more important to realize that the computer-processing capabilities can be used to *emphasize* these language actions rather than to suppress or limit them. Further, tools such as network analysis, content analysis, and participant observation are appropriate tools for understanding communication as an interactive process of convergence (Rogers & Kincaid, 1981).

Indeed, CMCS provide opportunities for individual, social, and technical mechanisms to explicitly or subtly structure and filter the flow, content, and exchange of communication (Hiltz & Turoff, 1985). In the more narrow context of group decision making, there is considerable research activity in designing capabilities in such systems for agenda-setting, decision-modeling, and structured group methods (Delphi analysis, group polling, nominal group techniques, brainstorming, interaction rules, and feedback to group members; DeSanctis & Gallupe, 1987).

The need to remove the obstacles to understanding intention has been the expressed rationale of some system designers behind the development of the *Coordinator* CMC system (Flores & Winograd, 1986; Winograd, 1984). The system allows individuals and groups to identify their communication intent—facts, requests, offers, commitments, and expressions—in the structure of their exchanges by associating categories of intention with the content, choosing from directories of individuals sharing common discussion topics, or establishing follow-up messages appropriate to the intentions. These and other capabilities allow shifting groups of users to make explicit their communication acts and reduce the negative mediation of communication between intention and behavior.

INTERACTION OF COMPONENTS OF DIMENSIONS

Specific components of each dimension can interact with other components in the same dimension and in other dimensions to create a matrix of cells representing potential social realities and areas of research.

Interaction Within a Dimension

For example, different users have different stakeholder roles which may interact. Consider the use of CMCS in educational settings (Black, Levin, Mehan, & Quinn, 1983; Hiltz, 1986; Quinn, Mehan, Levin, & Black, 1983; Welsch, 1982). The institution has needs, such as providing services across campuses and clientele (for example, evening students and distance learners), and in situations of insufficient classroom space. Faculty who need to match their scheduling constraints with their desires to provide assistance to large classes, often would like to share their comments with the full class or even colleagues, and enjoy reading neatly printed papers. Students need access to courses and faculty without having to move or leave work, need increased interaction not only with faculty but also with other students, may have difficulty with understanding classroom discussion if their language skills are not sufficient, and enjoy their ability to revise and to have a valid version of the assignment. Studies have shown that the nature of instructional communication changes: Rather than the typical interaction between teacher and student that consists of linear and hierarchical questions and responses, there is more sharing of information and more group discussion among students, a greater perception of participative learning, more simultaneous threads of discourse, increased evaluations of students' comments by other students, and longer and more complex sentences in students' responses. The needs of each category of user, however, may conflict with the constraints of technological resources, system reliability and accessibility, evaluation standards, norms of privacy, computer literary, attitudes toward technology, and perhaps the needs of other categories of users.

Interactions Across Dimensions

Components of one dimension can be used to facilitate—or constrain—the use of components in another dimension. For example, in their description of the sociotechnical approach to total system design, Bostrom & Heinen

(1977a) argue first for a formative evaluation of managers' or system designers' assumptions (such as seeing people only as inefficient information processors with insufficient information, underestimating the amount of legitimate responsibility users have for changing a system, optimizing the system at the cost of the organization, overlooking users as part of the design process, seeing the development process as rational and static, and using limited implementation techniques). Once these are identified, other research efforts can be applied to create both an improved organizational environment and a useful information system (Bostrom & Heinen, 1977b).

Constraints Across Dimensions

If few studies represent a particular interaction of components in several dimensions, we might well ask whether that interaction is uninteresting or difficult, or whether support for research on an aspect in one dimensions is not forthcoming for some reason relating to an aspect of another dimension. For example, Kerr and Hiltz (1982) conclude that there are few *empirical* studies of CMCS in the *societal* domain, in contrast to research in individual and group domains.

One reason for this dearth of studies is that such research requires longitudinal, multiple-source data in the industrial or societal domain. Such data are difficult to come by and analysis cannot easily disentangle the influences of other pervasive social changes. Another reason is that administrators, respondents, or funding agencies may resist the collection of necessary data such as network rosters or computer-monitored data because of concerns over confidentiality or scarce programming resources. It may be difficult to justify research at all to managers who must account for the use of employees' time, users who do not really make fine distinctions among the media they use in daily life, or unions that criticize the collection of job activity measures.

Traditional social science designs and tools also may be preventing stakeholders from setting goals that are more useful to them but can be achieved only by other sources of insights, such as computer-monitored data, archival data, in-depth interviews, focus groups, participant observation, interpretive narratives, or participative redesign of the system. For some stakeholders, causality may be of interest on a local level only, because funding decisions are largely political, or may be irrelevant precisely because the *concept* of causality is seen as an epistemological and ideological bias. For example, King, Kling, Kraemer, Scacchi, and their colleagues at the University of Irvine have rejected causality in favor of concepts such as *social action, evolutionary systems,* and the *web of computing* to understand the ongoing processes of design, usage and application of computing systems (Kling & Scacchi, 1980).

For others, insights from a case study may be sufficient and generalizability of little concern—circumstances particularly true for most proprietary office automation studies, because the associated competitive environments create conflicting goals for different stakeholders. Two sets of stakeholders may remain uninterested in CMCS research for opposite reasons: users, because the proposed research does not address their practical needs, and theoreticians, because the analysis of actual systems is seen as too applied. Clearly, the different goals of these and other stakeholders influence the cost-benefit ratio of any proposed research effort.

Further, it is difficult to disambiguate the influences on, contexts of, and societal aspects associated with large-scale CMCS. For these and other reasons, some stakeholders feel that case studies, economic and demographic approaches, and political analyses seem generally more suited to this interaction across dimensions than the more traditional social science research methods (see, for example, Forester, 1980; Kling, 1984; Lowi, 1983; Mosco, 1982; Schiller, 1982). Some of these studies are part of analyses or critiques of the "information society" as a whole.

CONCLUSION

This chapter began by postulating that the developing body of research on the uses and implications of CMCS reflects a variety of disciplinary paradigms, technological distinctions, and evaluation approaches. Awareness of the four dimensions of social evaluations of CMCS suggested in this chapter—stakeholders, domains, goals, and tools—can aid in understanding how ideological, social, economic, political, technical, organizational, and individual factors constrain or expand the uses and implications of this new medium of human communication. The suggested framework for social evaluations of CMCS may be used to identify how different academic disciplines make different assumptions about the acceptability or familiarity of certain topics and methods in CMCS research. It may be used to provide common dimensions with which to evaluate different forms of communication technologies. And it may be used to identify in what ways the evaluative process may be confounded with the results used by managers or community groups to guide their use of CMCS, or with the evidence used by researchers in extending their own research into the use and implications of a new communication medium.

This preliminary framework has been applied to a specific and perhaps narrow aspect of communication and computer technology. Other aspects of human communication that are experiencing the convergence of these two technologies, such as providing instruction, the delivery of health services, the retrieval of database information, or the computerization of political campaigns may well be considered by a similar framework, or may require expansions and alterations of the framework. Further, the dimensions of social research of CMCS should be joined with the technical and economic dimensions to provide a more complete framework. However, because

CMCS directly facilitate communication among individuals, and because the extant social science literature on CMCS is so widely dispersed, the present four-dimensional framework for identifying issues and concepts in social evaluation of CMCS may provide a focused and helpful beginning.

NOTE

1. Reviews of the nature of CMCS and research on their uses and effects may be found in Hiltz and Turoff (1978), Kerr and Hiltz (1982), Hiltz (1983, 1985), Johansen, Vallee, and Spangler (1979), Kiesler, Siegel, and McGuire (1984), Rice (1980b), Rice and Associates (1984), Steinfield (1986b), Tapscott (1982), Vallee (1984), and Uhlig, Farber, and Bair (1979).

REFERENCES

Aldrich, H. (1979). *Organizations and environments.* Englewood Cliffs, NJ: Prentice-Hall.

ASIS (1980). Perspectives on library networks and resource sharing (Special Issue). *Journal of American Society for Information Science, 31*(6), 404-445.

Bailey, G., Nordlie, P., & Sistrunk, F. (1963). *Teleconferencing: Literature review, field studies and working papers* (RP P-133). Washington, DC: Institute for Defense Analysis.

Bair, J. (1978), Productivity assessment of office systems technology. *Proceedings of trends and applications: 1978 distributed processing* (pp. 12-17). New York: IEEE.

Bair, J. (1980). An analysis of organizational productivity in the use of electronic office systems. *American society for information science proceedings* (Vol. 43, pp. 4-9). Anaheim, CA: ASIS.

Baligh, H., & Richartz, L. (1964). An analysis of vertical market structures. *Management Science, 10,* 667-689.

Bamford, H., & Savin, W. (1978). Electronic information exchange: The National Science Foundation's developing role. *Bulletin of ASIS, 4,* 12-13.

Bell, D. (1981). The social framework of the information society. In T. Forester (Ed.), *The microelectronics revolution* (pp. 500-549). Cambridge: MIT Press.

Bell, D. (1976). *The coming of post-industrial society.* New York: Basic Books.

Beniger, J. (1986). *The control revolution.* Cambridge, MA: Harvard University Press.

Berger, C., & Roloff, M. (1980). Social cognition, self-awareness and interpersonal communication. In B. Dervin & M. Voigt (Eds.), *Progress in communication sciences* (Vol. 2, pp. 2-49). Norwood, NJ: Ablex.

Bernard, H., Killworth, P., Kronenfeld, D., & Sailer, L. (1984). The problem of informant accuracy: The validity of retrospective data. *Annual Review of Anthropology, 13,* 495-517.

Black, S., Levin, J., Mehan, H., & Quinn, C. (1983). Real and non-real time interaction: Unraveling multiple threads of discourse. *Discourse Processes, 6,* 59-75.

Bordewijk, J., & van Kaam, B. (1982). *Allocutie.* Baarn, the Netherlands: Bosch & Keuning.

Bostrom, R., & Heinen, J. (1977a, September). MIS problems and failures: A sociotechnical perspective. Part I: The causes. *MIS Quarterly,* 17-32.

Bostrom, R., & Heinen, J. (1977b, December). MIS problems and failures: A socio-technical perspective. Part II: The application of socio-technical theory. *MIS Quarterly,* 11-28.

Bowes, J. (1981). Japan's approach to an information society: A critical perspective. In G. Wilhoit & H. de Bock (Eds.), *Mass communication review yearbook,* (Vol. 2, pp. 699-710). Beverly Hills, CA: Sage.

Bush, V. (1945). As we may think. *Atlantic Monthly, 176,* 101-108.

Carlson, E. (1974, March). Evaluating the impact of information systems. *Management Informatics, 3,* 56-67.

Compaine, B. (Ed.). (1984). *Understanding new media.* Cambridge, MA: Ballanger.
Cook, T., & McAnany, E. (1979). Recent U. S. experiences in evaluation research with implications for Latin America. In R. Klein et al. (Eds.), *Evaluating the impact of nutrition health programs* (pp. 39-97). New York: Plenum.
Cook, T., & Campbell, D. (1979). *Quasi-experimentation: Design and analysis issues for field settings.* Chicago: Rand-McNally.
Crane, D. (1972). *Invisible colleges: Diffusion of knowledge in scientific communities.* Chicago: University of Chicago Press.
Culnan, M. (1984). The dimensions of accessibility to online information: Implications for implementing office information systems. *ACM Transactions on Office Information Systems, 2*(2), 141-150.
Culnan, M., & Bair, J. (1983). Human communication needs and organizational productivity: The potential impacts of office automation. *Journal of the American Society for Information Science, 34*(3), 218-224.
Danowski, J. (1982). Computer-mediated communication: A network analysis using a CBBS conference. In M. Burgoon (Ed.), *Communication yearbook 6* (pp. 905-924). Beverly Hills, CA: Sage.
Danzinger, J., Dutton, W., Kling, R., & Kraemer, K. (1982). *Computers and politics: High technology in American local government.* New York: Columbia University Press.
Danzinger, J., & Kraemer, K. (1986). *People and computers: The impacts of computing on end users in organizations.* New York: Columbia University Press.
Dervin, B. (1981). Mass communicating: Changing conceptions of the audience. In R. E. Rice & W. Paisley (Eds.), *Public communication campaigns* (pp. 71-88). Beverly Hills, CA: Sage.
DeSanctis, G., & Gallupe, R. (1987). A foundation for the study of group decision support systems. *Management Science, 33,* 589-609.
De Sola Pool, I. (1983). *Technologies of freedom.* Cambridge, MA: Belknap.
Dickson, G., Leitheser, R., Wetherbe, J., & Nechis, M. (1984). Key information systems issues for the 1980s. *MIS Quarterly, 8*(3), 135-159.
Dordick, H., Bradley, H., & Nanus, B. (1982). *The emerging network marketplace.* Norwood, NJ: Ablex.
Dutton, W. (1981). The rejection of an innovation: The political environment of a computer-based model. *Systems, Objectives and Solutions, 1,* 179-201.
Dutton, W., & Kraemer, K. (Eds.), (1985). *Advanced wired cities.* Englewood Cliffs, NJ: Prentice-Hall.
Edelstein, A., Bowes, J., & Harsel, S. (1978). *Information societies: Comparing the Japanese and American experiences.* Seattle: University of Washington Press.
Ellis, C., & Nutt, G. (1980). Office information systems and computer science. *Computing Surveys, 1*(12), 27-60.
Erlandson, R. (1980). The participant observer role in systems methodologies. *IEEE Transactions on Systems, Man and Cybernetics, SMC 10-1,* 16-19.
Ettema, J. (1984). Videotex for market information: A survey of prototype users. *New Directions in Program Evaluation, 23,* 5-22.
Ettema, J. (1985). Explaining information system use with system-monitored vs. self-reported use measures. *Public Opinion Quarterly, 49,* 381-387.
Farace, R., Monge, P., & Russell, H. (1977). *Communicating and organizing.* Menlo Park, CA: Addison-Wesley.
Feldman, M., & March, J. (1981). Information in organizations as signal and symbol. *Administrative Science Quarterly,* 26, 171-186.
Flores, F., & Winograd, T. (1986). *Computers and cognition.* Norwood, NJ: Ablex.
Forester, T. (Ed.). (1980). *The microelectronics revolution.* Cambridge: MIT Press.
Freeman, L. (1980). Q-analysis and the structure of friendship networks. *International Journal of Man-Machine Studies, 3*(12), 367-378.
Ganley, O., & Ganley, G. (1982). *To inform or to control? The new communications networks.* New York: McGraw-Hill.

Garramone, G., Harris, A., & Anderson, R. (1986). Uses of political computer bulletin boards. *Journal of Broadcasting and Electronic Media, 30*(3), 325-339.

Giuliano, V. (1982). The mechanization of office work. *Scientific American, 247*(3), 148-165.

Glossbrenner, A. (1983). *The complete handbook of personal computer communications.* New York: St. Martin's Press.

Goldhaber, J., Yates, M., Porter, D., & Lesniak, R. (1978). Organizational communication: 1978. *Human Communication Research, 5*(1), 76-96.

Golding, P., & Murdock, G. (1986). Unequal information: Access and exclusion in the new communications market place. In M. Ferguson (Ed.), *New communication technologies and the public interest* (pp. 71-83). Beverly Hills, CA: Sage.

Golembiewski, R. (1986). Contours in social change: Elemental graphics and a surrogate variable for gamma change. *Academy of Management Review, 11*(3), 550-566.

Gutek, B. (1982). Effects of office of the future technology on users: Results of a longitudinal field study. In G. Mensch & R. Niehaus (Eds.), *Work, organizations and technological change.* New York: Plenum.

Habermas, J. (1984). *The theory of communicative action: Vol. 1. Reason and the rationalization of society* (T. McCarthy, Trans.). Boston: Beacon Press.

Haight, T., & Rubinyi, R. (1983). How community groups use computers. *Journal of Communication, 33*(1), 109-117.

Hall, K. (1981). The economic nature of information. *The Information Society, 2*(1), 143-166.

Hamilton, S., & Chervany, N. (1981). Evaluating information system effectiveness. Part I: Comparing evaluation approaches. *MIS Quarterly, 5*(3), 55-69.

Hiemstra, G. (1982). Teleconferencing, concern for face, and organizational culture. In M. Burgoon (Ed.), *Communication yearbook 6* (pp. 874-904). Beverly Hills, CA: Sage.

Hiemstra, G. (1983). You say you want a revolution? "Information technology" in organizations. In R. Bostrom (Ed.), *Communication yearbook 7* (pp. 802-827). Beverly Hills, CA: Sage.

Hiltz, S. R. (1982). Experiments and experiences with computerized conferencing. In R. Landua, J. Bair, & J. Siegman (Eds.), *Emerging office systems* (pp. 182-204). Norwood, NJ: Ablex.

Hiltz, S. R. (1983). *Online communities: A case study of the office of the future.* Norwood, NJ: Ablex.

Hiltz, S. R. (1985). Teleconferencing: Recent developments in computer-mediated communication and other technologies. In A. Cawkell (Ed.), *International handbook of information technology and office systems.* Amsterdam: Elsevier-North Holland.

Hiltz, S. R. (1986). The "virtual classroom": Using computer-mediated communication for university teaching. *Journal of Communication, 36*(2), 95-104.

Hiltz, S. R. & Turoff, M. (1978). *Network nation: The network nation.* New York: Addison-Wesley.

Hiltz, S. R., & Turoff, M. (1981). Evolution of user behavior in a computerized conferencing system. *Communications of the ACM, 11*(24), 739-751.

Hiltz, S. R., & Turoff, M. (1985). Structuring computer-mediated communication systems to avoid information overload. *Communications of the ACM, 7*(28), 680-689.

Hirschheim, R. (1985). *Office automation: A social and organizational perspective.* New York: John Wiley.

Huber, G. (1984). The nature and design of post-industrial organizations. *Management Science, 8*(30), 928-951.

Ives, B., Olson, M., & Baroudi, M. (1983). The measurement of user information satisfaction. *Communications of the ACM, 10*(26), 785-793.

Ito, Y. (1981). The "Johoka Shakai" approach to the study of communication in Japan. In G. Wilhoit & H. de Bock (Eds.), *Mass communication review yearbook* (Vol. 2, pp. 671-698). Beverly Hills, CA: Sage.

Johansen, R. (1977). Social evaluations of teleconferencing. *Telecommunications Policy, 5*(1), 395-419.

Johansen, R. (1984). *Teleconferencing and beyond.* New York: McGraw-Hill.

Johansen, R., Miller, R., & Vallee, J. (1974, August). Human communication through electronic media: Fundamental choices and social effects. *Educational Technology*, pp. 7-20.

Johansen, R., Vallee, J., & Spangler, K. (1979). *Electronic meetings: Technical alternatives and social choices.* New York: Addison-Wesley.

Johnson, B., & Rice, R. E. (1987). *Managing organizational innovation: The evolution from word processing to office information systems.* New York: Columbia University Press.

Keplinger, M. (1980). Copyright and information technology. In M. Williams (Ed.), *Annual review of information science and technology* (Vol. 15, pp. 3-34). White Plains, NY: Knowledge Industry Publications.

Kerr, E. (1986). Electronic leadership: A guide to moderating online conferences. *IEEE transactions on professional communications,* PC 29, 1, 12-18.

Kerr, E., & Hiltz, S. R. (1982), *Computer-mediated communication systems.* New York: Academic Press.

Kiesler, S. (1986, January-February). Thinking ahead: The hidden messages in computer networks. *Harvard Business Review,* pp. 46-59.

Kiesler, S., Siegel, J., & McGuire, T. (1984). Social psychological aspects of computer-mediated communication. *American Psychologist, 39*(10), 1123-1134.

King, J., & Kraemer, K. (1981). Cost as a social impact of information technology. In M. Moss (Ed.), *Telecommunications and productivity* (pp. 93-130). Reading, MA: Addison-Wesley.

Kling, R. (1980), Social analyses of computing: Theoretical perspectives in recent empirical research. *Computing Surveys, 12*(1), 61-110.

Kling, R. (1984, June). Assimilating social values in computer-based technologies. *Telecommunications Policy,* pp. 127-147.

Kling, R., & Scacchi, W. (1980). Computing as social action: The social dynamics of computing in complex organizations. *Advances in Computers, 19,* 249-327.

Lowenstein, R. (1979). *Office system studies.* White Plains, NY: International Business Machines Corp.

Lowi, T. (1983). The political impact of information technology. In T. Forester (Ed.), *The microelectronics revolution* (pp. 453-472). Cambridge: MIT Press.

Machlup, F. (1962). *The production and distribution of knowledge in the United States.* Princeton, NJ: Princeton University Press.

Majchrzak, A. (1984). *Methods for policy research. Applied social research methods series* (Vol. 3) Beverly Hills, CA: Sage.

Marien, M. (1985). Some questions for the information society. In T. Forester (Ed.), *The information technology revolution* (pp. 648-660). Cambridge: MIT Press.

Markus, M. L. (1987). Chargeback as an implementation tactic for office communication systems. *Interfaces, 17,* 54-63.

Martin, J. (1981). *Telematic society: A challenge or tomorrow.* Englewood Cliffs, NJ: Prentice-Hall.

McQuail, D. (1986). Is media theory adequate to the challenge of new communications technologies? In M. Ferguson (Ed.), *New communication technologies and the public interest* (pp. 1-17). Beverly Hills, CA: Sage.

Mehra, A. (1987). *Free flow of information.* Westport, CT: Greenwood Press.

Miller, J., & Nichols, M. (1981). An update in a longitudinal study of the adoption of an electronic mail system. In G. Reeves & J. Sweigart (Eds.), *Thirteenth annual proceedings of the American Institute for Decision Sciences,* Boston, (Vol. 1, pp. 218-200).

Mitroff, I. (1983). *Stakeholders of the organizational mind.* San Francisco: Jossey-Bass.

Mohrman, A., Jr., & Novelli, L. (1983). *Adaptively researching the impacts of information processing technologies in the office.* Paper presented at the Academy of Management conference, New York, 1982.

Mosco, V. (1982). *Pushbutton fantasies: Critical perspectives on videotex and information technology.* Norwood, NJ: Ablex.

Moshowitz, A. (1976). *The conquest of will: Information processing in human affairs.* Reading, MA: Addison-Wesley.

Murray, C. (1983). Stakeholders as deck chairs. *New Directions in Program Evaluation, 17,* 59-62.

Nicholson, R. (1985). Usage patterns in an integrated voice and data communications system. *ACM Transactions on Office Information Systems, 3*(3), 307-314.

Nilles, J., Carlson, F., Gray, P., & Hanneman, G. (1976). *The telecommunication-transportation tradeoff.* New York: John Wiley.

Olson, M., & Lucas, H., Jr. (1982). The impact of office automation on the organization: Some implications for research and practice. *Communications of the ACM, 25,* 838-847.

Paisley, W. (1980). Information and work. In B. Dervin & M. Voigt (Eds.), *Progress in communication sciences* (Vol. 2, pp. 113-166). Norwood, NJ: Ablex.

Palmer, E. (1981). Shaping persuasive messages with formative research. In R. E. Rice & W. Paisley (Eds.), *Public communication campaigns* (pp. 227-238). Beverly Hills, CA: Sage.

Panko, R. (1980, August 25). The EMS revolution. *Computerworld,* pp. 19, 34, 45-56.

Panko, R. (1981a). Standards for electronic message systems. *Telecommunications Policy, 5*(3), 181-197.

Panko, R. (1981b). The cost of EMS. *Computer Networks, 5,* 35-46.

Panko, R. (1985). Electronic mail. In K. Takle-Quinn (Ed.), *Advances in office automation.* New York: John Wiley.

Parker, E. (1976). Social implications of computer/telecoms systems. *Telecommunications Policy, 1*(1), 3-20.

Pava, C. (1983). *Managing new office technology.* New York: Free Press.

Penniman, W., & Dominick, W. (1980). Monitoring and evaluation of on-line information system usage. *Information Processing and Management, 116,* 17-35.

Philips, A. (1982). Computer conferencing: Success or failure? *Systems, Objectives, Solutions, 4*(2), 203-218.

Porat, M. (1977). *The information economy: Definition and measurement.* Washington, DC: Government Printing Office.

Price, D. de S. (1963), *Little science, big science.* New York: Columbia University Press.

Quinn, C., Mehan, H., Levin, J., & Black, S. (1983). Real education in non-real time: The use of electronic message systems for instruction. *Instructional Science, 11,* 313-327.

Ramsey, H., & Grimes, J. (1983). Human factors in interactive computer dialog. In M. William (Ed.), *Annual review of information science and technology* (Vol. 18, pp. 29-60). White Plains, NY: Knowledge Industry.

Rice, R. E. (1980a). Impacts of organizational and interpersonal computer-mediated communication. In M. Williams (Ed.), *Annual review of information science and technology* (Vol. 16, pp. 221-249). White Plains, NY: Knowledge Industry.

Rice, R. E. (1980b). Computer conferencing. In B. Dervin & M. Voigt (Eds.), *Progress in communication sciences* (Vol. 2, pp. 215-240). Norwood, NJ: Ablex.

Rice, R. E. (1982). Communication networking in computer conferencing systems: A longitudinal study of group roles and system structure. In M. Burgoon (Ed.), *Communication yearbook 6* (pp. 925-944). Beverly Hills, CA: Sage.

Rice, R. E. (1984). Evaluating new media systems. *New Directions in Program Evaluation, 23,* 53-72.

Rice, R. E. (1987a). Communication technologies, human communication networks and social structure in the information society. In J. Schement & L. Lievrouw (Eds.), *Competing visions, complex realities: Social aspects of the information society.* Norwood, NJ: Ablex.

Rice, R. E. (1987b). Computer-mediated communications systems and organizational innovation. *Journal of Communication, 37*(4), 65-94.

Rice, R. E., & Associates (1984). *The new media: Communication, research, technology.* Beverly Hills, CA: Sage.

Rice, R. E., & Barnett, G. (1985). Group communication networking in an information environment In M. McLaughlin (Ed.), *Communication yearbook 9* (pp. 315-326). Beverly Hills, CA: Sage.
Rice, R. E., & Borgman, C. (1983). The use of computer-monitored data for information science and communication research. *Journal of the American Society for Information Science, 4*(34), 247-256.
Rice, R. E., & Case, D. (1983). Computer-based messaging in the university organization: A description of use and utility. *Journal of Communication, 33*(1), 131-152.
Rice, R. E., & Love, G. (1987). Electronic emotion: Socio-emotional content in a computer-mediated communication network. *Communication Research, 14*(1), 85-105.
Rice, R. E., & Manross, G. (1986). The relationships of job category to the adoption of organizational communication technology. In M. McLaughlin (Ed.), *Communication yearbook 10.* Beverly Hills, CA: Sage.
Rice, R. E., & Paisley, W. (1982). The green thumb videotext experiment: Evaluation and policy implications. *Telecommunications Policy, 6*(3), 223-236.
Rice, R. E., & Parker, E. (1979). Telecommunications alternatives for developing countries. *Journal of Communication, 4*(29), 125-136.
Rice, R. E., & Richards, R. (1985). Overview of communication network analysis methods. In B. Dervin & M. Voigt (Eds.), *Progress in communication sciences* (Vol. 6, pp. 105-165). Norwood, NJ: Ablex.
Roberts, L. (1978). The evolution of packet switching. *IEEE Proceedings, 66*(11), 1307-1314.
Robinson, G. (Ed.). (1978). *Communications for tomorrow: Policy perspectives for the 1980s.* New York: Praeger.
Rogers, E., & Kincaid, L. (1981). *Communication network analysis.* New York: Free Press.
Rouse, W. (1975). Design of man-computer interfaces for on-line interactive systems. *Proceedings of the IEEE, 6*(63), 847-857.
Rule, J. (1974). *Private lives and public surveillance: Social control in the computer age.* New York: Schocken.
Salvaggio, J. (1985). Information technology and social problems: Four international models. In B. Ruben (Ed.), *Information and behavior* (Vol. 1, pp. 428-454). New Brunswick, NJ: Transaction Books.
Schement, J., & Lievrouw, L. (Eds.). (1987). *Competing visions, complex realities: Social aspects of the information society.* Norwood, NJ: Ablex.
Schiller, H. (1982). *Who knows? Information in the age of the Fortune 500.* Norwood, NJ: Ablex.
Schiller, H. (1985). Privatizing the public sector: The information connection. In B. Ruben (Ed.), *Information and behavior* (Vol. 1, pp. 387-405). New Brunswick, NJ: Transaction Books.
Shannon, C., & Weaver, W. (1949). *The mathematical theory of communication.* Urbana, IL: University of Illinois Press.
Shipley, C., Shipley, D., & Wigand, R. (1985). Corporate transborder data flow and national policy in developing countries. In B. Ruben (Ed.), *Information and behavior* (Vol. 1, pp. 455-480). New Brunswick, NJ: Transaction Books.
Short, J., Williams, E., & Christie, B. (1976). *The social psychology of telecommunications.* New York: John Wiley.
Simon, H. (1981). What computers mean for man and society. In T. Forester (Ed.), *The microelectronics revolution.* Cambridge: MIT Press.
Simon, H. (1973). Applying information technology to organizational design. *Public Administration Review, 3*(33), 268-278.
Sproull, L. (1986). Using electronic mail for data collection in organizational research. *Academy of Management Journal, 29*(1), 159-169.
Sproull, L., & Kiesler, S. (1986). Reducing social context cues: Electronic mail in organizational communication. *Management Science, 32*(11), 1492-1512.

Steinfield, C. (1986a). Explaining task and socio-emotional use of computer-mediated communication in an organizational setting. In M. McLaughlin (Ed.), *Communication yearbook 9* (pp. 777-804). Beverly Hills, CA: Sage.

Steinfield, C. (1986b). Computer-mediated communication systems. In M. Williams (Ed.), *Annual review of information science and technology* (Vol. 21, pp. 167-202). White Plains, NY: Knowledge Industry.

Strassman, P. (1985). *The information payoff: The transformation of work in the electronic age.* New York: Macmillan.

Suchman, E. (1967). *Evaluative research.* New York: Russell Sage Foundation.

Svoboda, L. (1976). *Computer performance measurement and evaluation methods: Analysis and applications.* New York: American Elsevier.

Tapscott, D. (1982). *Office automation: A user-driven method.* New York: Plenum.

Tombaugh, J. (1984). Evaluation of an international scientific computer-based conference. *Journal of Social Issues, 40*(3), 129-144.

Traber, M. (Ed.). (1986). *The myth of the information revolution.* Beverly Hills, CA: Sage.

Tydeman, J., Lipinski, H., Adler, R., Nyhan, M., & Zwimpfer, L. (1982). *Teletext and videotex in the United States.* New York: McGraw-Hill.

Uhlig, R., Farber, D., & Bair, J. (1979). *The office of the future: Communications and computers.* New York: North-Holland.

UNESCO International Commission for the Study of Communication Problems (MacBride Commission) (1980). *Many voices, one world.* Paris: UNESCO.

Urban, C. (1984). Factors influencing media consumption: A survey of the literature. In B. Compaine (Ed.), *Understanding new media* (pp. 213-282). Cambridge, MA: Ballenger.

Vallee, J. (1984). *Computer messaging systems.* New York: McGraw-Hill.

Vallee, J., Johansen, R., Randolph, R., & Hastings, A. (1974). *Group communication through computers: Vol. 2. A study of social effects.* Menlo Park, CA: Institute for the Future.

Vitalari, N., & Venkatesh, A. (1986). Computing in the home: Implications for the provision of government services. *Computers, environments and urban systems.* Manuscript submitted for publication.

Weizenbaum, J. (1981). Where are we going? Questions for Simon. In T. Forester (Ed.), *The microelectronics revolution* (pp. 434-438). Cambridge: MIT Press.

Weizenbaum, J. (1976). *Computer power and human reason: From judgment to calculation.* San Francisco: Freeman.

Welsch, L. (1982). Using electronic mail as a teaching tool. *Communications of the ACM, 23*(2), 105-108.

Wessel, M. (1976). *Freedom's edge: The computer threat to society.* Reading, MA: Addison-Wesley.

Westin, A., & Baker, M. (1972). *Databanks in a free society: Computers, record-keeping, and privacy.* New York: Quadrangle.

Williams, F., Rice, R. E., & Rogers, E. M. (1988). *New methods and new media.* New York: Free Press.

Williamson, O. (1979). Transaction cost economics: The governance of contractual relations. *The Journal of Law and Economics, 22,* 233-261.

Winograd, T. (1984, September). Computer software for working with language. *Scientific American* (pp. 131-145).

Zuboff, S. (1982). New worlds of computer-mediated work. *Harvard Business Review, 5*(60), 142-152.

Classifying Mediated Communication Systems

CARRIE HEETER
Michigan State University

COMMUNICATION researchers must establish perspectives for studying new communication technologies that extend theory and results beyond the boundaries of any particular technology or implementation. In his chapter, Rice proposes a framework for organizing multidisciplinary research on uses and implications of computer mediated communication systems (CMCS). He focuses on classifying the research rather than the systems. I concur that there is a need to integrate research across disciplines and media systems. I see Rice's chapter as a very useful reminder of the illusion of objectivity and as an important step toward classification dimensions for mediated communication systems research. It would be useful if every methods section addressed the kinds of issues he raises. I contend, however, that detailed specification of the particular mediated communication system under study is even more crucial to generalizing across studies than is classification of the research project.

Section 1 of this commentary will extend the scope of Rice's framework's from computer mediated communication systems to all mediated communication systems. Section 2 will propose a distinction between classifying media systems and classifying media system research. Section 3 will discuss the importance of detailed descriptions of media systems for generalizing across studies. Section 4 will review other media system classification schemata. Section 5 will propose and apply a schema based on two traditional communication variables: function and channel. Section 6 will discuss extensions of that schema.

Correspondence and requests for reprints: Carrie Heeter, Communication Technology Laboratory, 287 Communication Arts, Michigan State University, East Lansing, MI 48824.

Communication Yearbook 12, 477-489

DEFINING MEDIATED COMMUNICATION SYSTEMS

Rice's recommendations are relevant beyond any narrow definition of computer mediated communication systems. He proposes a framework that he describes as being primarily appropriate to research on computer applications that allow "conversation" between individuals and among groups. These types of CMCS are part of the broader taxonomy of all mediated communication systems. Rice's dimensions of stakeholders, goals, domains, and tools are as meaningful to television, videotext or CB radio as they are to interpersonal communication over CMCS. Broadening the perspective strengthens Rice's case, enhancing the scope and value of comparability across studies that the framework was intended to enable.

One problem in comparing research across media systems is vocabulary. Distinctions between medium, channel, and technology are often confused. The result is lack of differentiation between these elements. Channel was initially defined in communication models as the sense or combination of five senses along which communication occurred. Berlo's (1969) Source-Message-Channel-Receiver model of communication elaborated on channel as sight, sound, smell, hearing, touch. In some studies, channel is used synonymously with medium, for example, television is described as one channel, and radio and movies as other channels of communication. Applying Berlo's definition of channel, television and movies both use audio-visual channels, whereas radio uses only audio. To permit vocabulary to clarify rather than confuse, I suggest that channel be used exclusively under its original definition: *the combination of senses over which messages in a media system can be sent and received.*

The phrase *medium of communication* is used often as a synonym for communication technology, discouraging recognition of the diversity of mediated communication systems that might make use of a technology. For example, television is referred to as a medium of communication. Television is also a class of technology that involves two-dimensional electronic representation of moving visual images and synchronous sound. There are many variations of basic television technology currently available. A television signal may reach a screen via traditional broadcast of VHF or UHF signals, or be delivered via coaxial cable, fiber optics, satellite, or microwave to an entire community or to selected business locations. In addition to forms of broadcasting, television signals can come from a home VCR or be linked directly from camera to monitor. Further, television can be used as a two-way technology for interpersonal communication (i.e., video phones and teleconferencing) in which participants at different locations each originate and receive a television signal. All of these media systems are applications of television technology. *Communication technology should be used to refer to a class of hardware, software, and distribution networks from which media systems can be created.*

A medium is something interposed between other things. One dictionary definition of medium is a person who links beings in the spiritual world with those inhabiting the physical world. Rice's chapter helps to emphasize that most of what we call communication media are complex media systems, replete with political, social, economic, and technological complexities. The term *mediated communication system* (or *media system*) is a more evocative descriptor than *medium* to encompass the technological, social, and economic structures surrounding a broad class or particular instance of communication media. All mediated communication systems are composed of diverse distribution networks, hardware, and software that enable and constrain communication. There are players (or stakeholders) who implement, operate, study, use, and are affected by the media systems. Media systems are designed to enable certain functions (or goals) and may also serve other (perhaps unintended) goals. Over time, norms of content and use patterns are likely to evolve for a media system.

CLASSIFYING MEDIA SYSTEMS OR MEDIA SYSTEM RESEARCH

Rice suggests that use and implication findings of media systems research are bound up in, and confounded with, the research process. The first dimension identified is *stakeholders*. For both stakeholders and goals, I think it is important to separate analysis of the media system from analysis of the research process. Rice's dimensions are intended to be applied to the research process. Clearly the most direct stakeholders in the research process are those who are aware of the research project and recognize that they have a stake in the process and outcomes—including those conducting, funding, and approving the research. In some way, anyone involved in any way with the media system could be considered a stakeholder in the research process. These may include system developers, system operators, information providers, users, regulators, and competitors. However, in most cases these less direct "stakeholders" will not even be aware that research is being conducted. It is important that research reports acknowledge their funding sources and relationship to system operators and users. It is also important to identify in a research report the stakeholders involved in the particular media system.

The second dimension is identification of *goals*. Again, I would distinguish analysis of the goals of the media system from the goals of the research. Media systems are designed to achieve particular goals. System operators, information providers, and users all have different goals. Researchers also have particular goals. In research, the hypotheses and literature review articulate the bias and expectations of the researcher (intentional of unintentional). Rice's list of 11 dimensions of summative evaluation goals for CMCS pulls together multidisciplinary perspectives ranging from the role of CMCS in actualizing the human spirit to analysis of fixed and variable costs of operating a CMCS to the symbolic and political reasons for justifying implementation of a CMCS. This potpourri of research goals is not usually discussed in one chapter. A major weakness of the presentation of goals is the lack of any attempt to organize and make sense out of the many perspectives that are listed.

Domains and tools (Rice's third and fourth dimensions) are classifications more commonly applied to research than stakeholders and goals. His articulation of types and his review of research along a rich collection of domains and tools is informative and enlightening. It would be interesting and worthwhile to apply those ideas using metaanalysis to consider the impact of tools and domain on research findings.

WHY CATEGORIZE MEDIA SYSTEMS?

The nature of media systems is changing in ways that have important implications for research. When researchers first began to study mediated communication, the media systems they studied were few in number and relatively ubiquitous and homogeneous. Wartella and Reeves (1985) reviewed historical research trends for children and media and were "impressed by the overwhelming similarity in the research studies from epoch to epoch, with a new technology substituted as the object of concern." The same types of research questions were applied to movies, then radio, then television. The list of new technologies that could now follow the same repetitive pattern of research is prohibitively vast. Thus the proliferation of technologies demands research theories and findings that can generalize across diverse media systems. This need is voiced by Chen (1984), as follows:

> Future research on television, microcomputers, and other media can benefit by moving away from a view of these media as distinct packages of technology to a focus on the specific features of these media that are linked to specific child outcomes. . . . Research that looks beyond the technology of each new medium to its underlying content and symbols will enable theoretical progress that does not stop at the borders of each machine. (p. 284)

But media systems are also smaller in scope and less homogeneous than traditional media systems as movies, radio, and television once were. An electronic mail system operated within a company is one implementation of an electronic mail media system. That system will be different from another electronic mail system operated by another company, which will be different from a national electronic mail system. The differences may or may not be an obstacle to generalizing across electronic mail media systems, but unless the differences are articulated and examined, generalizations across those systems may not be justified. With the new media systems there is a need to identify the essential elements that are common, as well as distinct, across different implementations of media systems. Chaffee (Rogers & Chaffee, 1983) suggests that one of the challenges of behavioral researchers is that we "now find ourselves studying structural factors and historical contexts" (p. 22). Rogers (Rogers & Chaffee, 1983) now finds himself "disappointed with a research paper that doesn't tell us about the communication system being investigated, even though the effects data may be handled very well" (p. 22).

REVIEW OF OTHER MEDIA SYSTEM CLASSIFICATION SCHEMAS

Rice's chapter calls for identification of the stakeholders and goals of media systems. Others (including Rice) have proposed classification systems for differentiating media systems.

Paisley and Chen (1982) characterized computer media systems by presentation features, inputting and command features, and content features. They adapted Bretz's (1971) attributes. *Presentation features* include display rate, character resolution, use of upper/lower case, line length, number of lines per screen, graphic resolution, motion, color, music, and sound effects. *Inputting and command features* include keyboards, keypads, other input devices, menus, other structured choices, and command languages. *Content features* consist of instructional software, text files, message files, and other databases.

The features Paisley and Chen developed are specific to media systems that are based on computers. Beyond classifying attributes as relating to display, interaction, or content realms, there appears to be no attempt to group attributes by underlying factors of conceptual concern. They identify individual components of computers rather than underlying factors. For example, the importance of line length, lines per screen, character resolution and upper/lower case display may relate to the amount of information available per screen of text, and its readability. These underlying concerns are not articulated, therefore the attributes are less suggestive of meaningful research than they could be. Amount of information available is a richer concept than upper/lower case display. Further, the list of features is not a taxonomy in the hard science tradition: It cannot be used to classify computer media systems into a small number of discrete, meaningful categories.

Daft and Lengel (1984) developed a system for assessing the "information richness" of media system (See Figure 1). They conceptualized richness as the "potential information-carrying capacity of data." Four constructs were used to determine richness: the speed of feedback, channels employed, personalness of the source and the form of language employed. Daft and Lengel's focus was on media systems' use in business for interpersonal communication. Rapidity of feedback refers to the speed with which a response to a message can be received. Face-to-face communication is considered instantaneous, whereas mail is considered very slow. There are three levels of channel. Full visual and

Information Richness	Medium	Feedback	Channel	Source	Language
HIGH	face-to-face	immediate	visual, audio	personal	body, natural
	telephone	fast	audio	personal	natural
	written, personal	slow	limited visual	personal	natural
	written, formal	very slow	limited visual	impersonal	natural
LOW	numeric, formal	very slow	limited visual	impersonal	numeric

Figure 1 Daft and Lengel's information richness schema.

audio is available in face-to-face communication. The next level is audio only, with telephones. The final level is labeled limited visual (which they do not define). Sources may be personal or impersonal and language forms employed may include body language, natural language, or numeric language. Face-to-face communication is most information rich, with immediate feedback, visual and audio channels, personal sources, and natural and body languages. Numeric, formal communication (e.g., a computer output) is the least information rich, with very slow feedback, limited visual channel, impersonal source, and numeric language.

Daft and Lengel define a continuum for comparing interpersonal communication media systems. An advantage of their schema is that it organizes a diverse set of information concepts and suggests interrelationships. A problem with the continuum they propose is that the dimensions are arguably not linear. To say that audio is more rich than limited video and less rich than full visual is one perspective. Also the components for constructing the continuum are not independent. The availability of body language seems to be directly related to whether a visual channel is available. Some of the components are external attributes of the media system. Others, such as whether the source of a communication is personal or impersonal, could actually vary within any medium, depending on who the source and receiver are for each communication. There can be a formal, impersonal, face-to-face meeting or an impersonal telephone call (e.g., randomly selected phone interview).

Rice and Williams (1984) offered a more general list of constructs which may vary across media systems:

(1) *Stimulus-conveying restrictions* refer to the channel limitations imposed by a media system (e.g., audio only).

(2) *Channel redundancy* is a combination of channel limitations and content. In order to have the potential to carry the same content over two or more sensory channels, a media system must carry information over two or more channels (e.g., sight and sound). Further, to have channel redundancy, the same content must be offered over both channels. While Rice and

Williams do not discuss the intricacies of channel redundancy, note that true redundancy is rarely achieved, except, perhaps, when the same words that are spoken appear visually in text form.

(3) *Potential for interactivity* is defined as the potential for immediate, two-way interpersonal exchange over a media system. This exchange requires a technical configuration of a media system that allows for interpersonal communication *and* allows it to occur immediately.

(4) *Social presence* refers to how users of a media system would fill in such semantic differentials as *sociable-unsociable, sensitive-insensitive, warm-cold* and *personal-impersonal.* The mean score of the summed scales equals the social presence.

(5) *Privacy* is a user's "consciousness of whether "outside" individuals may monitor and exchange." Greater perceived privacy is presumed to enhance the potential of a media system to become "personalized."

(6) *Familiarity* is measured by subjective ratings of different media that, according to Rice, "may be as much a consequence of our restricted use of the medium as of the physical restrictions a given technology may impose." Familiarity with media systems probably has a major impact on how study respondents rate other attributes of that media system. In fact, familiarity or experience with different media systems may have as much influence on subjective ratings of the utility of new technologies for performing various functions as the technological attributes of that media system. Rice also cites Phillips's (1984) study of the subjective ratings of different media as to their familiarity (combining inexpensive, old, and common), importance (important, time saving, necessary), and personalness (personal and private).

Applying Rice and William's categories, privacy, familiarity, and social presence are based on user perceptions and thus can be reported only if they have been empirically assessed as part of the study. These categories are, therefore, not useful in comparing studies that do not include surveys of users or have not asked those particular questions of users. Channel redundancy relates to a combination of whether the system can transmit multiple channels to allow channel redundancy and to whether a particular piece of content is communicated simultaneously over two or more channels. The potential for interactivity and stimulus-conveying restrictions are characteristics that are either technically possible or not possible over a media system.

CLASSIFYING MEDIA SYSTEMS BY FUNCTION AND CHANNEL

The number of different dimensions along which media systems could be classified is overwhelming. This fact is a major impediment to uniform reporting of media system features in research that would permit comparison across studies. A general guideline would be to urge researchers (and editors) to err on the side of providing too much rather than too little information about the media system being studied. Of particular interest would be descriptions of the technology (networks, hardware, and software) that enable and constrain communication; players (or stakeholders) who implement, operate, study, use, and are affected by the media system; functions (or goals) that the media system is intended to serve; and norms of content and use.

At the same time, standardized reporting of basic media system information would be extremely useful. In choosing dimensions of importance from infinite possibilities for classification, I refer to the original theories of models of communication that launched our discipline. I will propose and apply a standardized classification system based on two traditional communication concepts: function and channel.

Function

Communication research has traditionally distinguished among intrapersonal, interpersonal, and mass communication. Older media systems tend to perform a single communication function, while some newer media systems integrate two or all three functions.

Information retrieval media systems allow mass communication, delivering information from a person or group to a mass of users. Broadcast television carries programming to millions of households simultaneously. Teletext carries pages of information to many users at different times.

Messaging media systems allow interpersonal communication by permitting users to send messages to one or a small number of particular other users. For example, telephones are typically used to connect one person to another and allow both to provide and receive information.

Media systems under the category of *information processing* extend the concept of intrapersonal communication, allowing a user to extend thought and perform transactions by providing information that the media system acts upon in some way to alter or produce new information that is a result of action taken on the information provided. Word processors and video games are examples of information processing media systems. Their purpose is not to enable electronic messaging or mass information retrieval. Instead, they are tools for thought, for work, or for play.

Integrated media systems can perform multiple functions. Videotext services often permit users to send electronic mail as well as to retrieve information on a variety of topics.

To examine the utility of communication function for understanding media systems, hypothetical mediated communication systems will be classified as performing any or all of the three traditional communication fuctions. Figure 2 shows the classification of 53 media systems by communication function. Classifications derive directly from assumptions about the nature of each hypothetical media system. For example, by definition, the hypothetical media system labeled broadcast television normally allows for mass information retrieval and not interpersonal or intrapersonal service. The

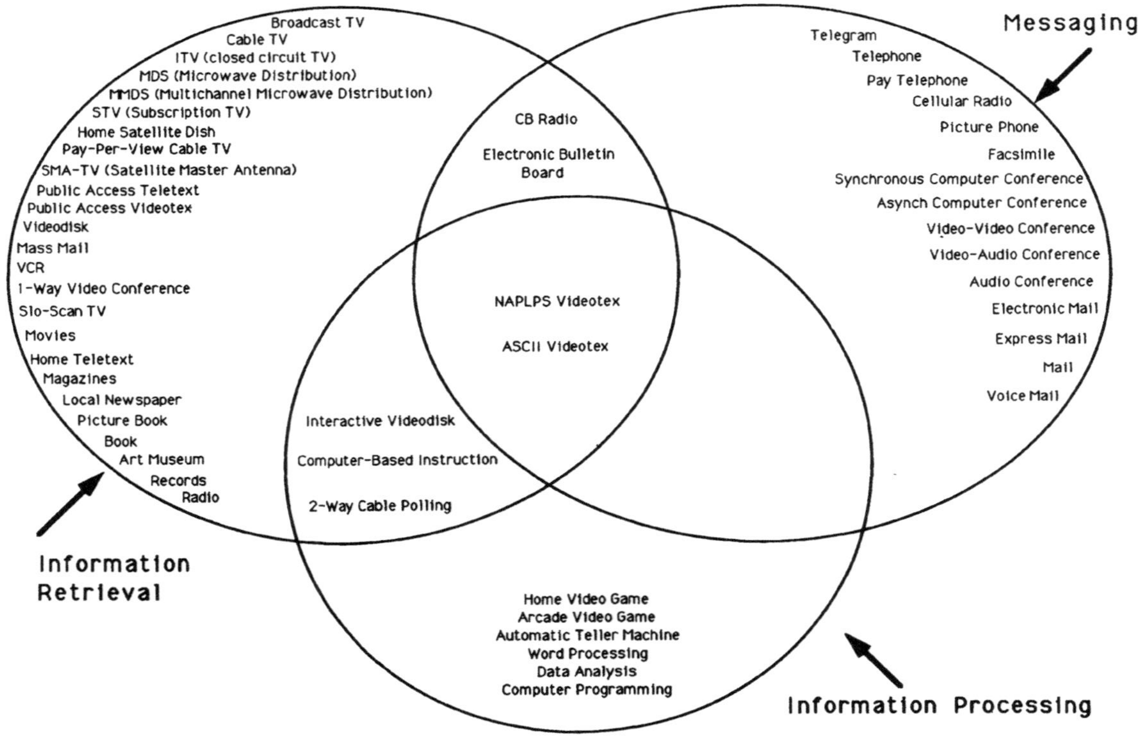

Figure 2 Classification of 53 hypothetical media systems by function.

process of classifying media systems by function is synonymous with explicity defining the media system. If there is an argument about the validity of a classification, it is likely to be an argument about the classifier's definition of the media system.

Information retrieval media systems include various permutations of broadcast, cable, satellite, and microwave television and traditional mass media (books, radio, records, newspapers, and so on). Teletext and public access videotext are also pure information retrieval services. One way to classify media systems that can perform multiple functions is to consider each function as a distinct media system. For example, mail is classified as an interpersonal media system, mass mail is classified as a mass media system because the players and functions are quite different.

Classification is based on normal uses of a media system. One-way teleconferences are typically used to disseminate information to a large mass of users at one or more remote sites. One-way teleconferencing technology can be, but rarely is, used to reach a single individual or small group. Therefore, one-way teleconferencing is classified as an information retrieval media system. Similarly, teletext services could be elaborately programmed to simulate information processing in addition to information retrieval. If this usage were common, then that type of teletext systems could be considered distinct from the straight information retrieval teletext systems. Finally, an art museum is included as an unusual example of mediated information retrieval, to test the robustness of the taxonomy.

Messaging media systems include various person-to-person and group conferencing systems, from telephone to express mail to computer conferencing.

Information processing is currently the smallest category, consisting of video games, word processing and data processing, automated teller machines, and computer programming.

In general, the categories are discrete. Of the 53 media systems classified, 46 fit under a single category. Most media systems specialize in one of the three information exchange functions. However, at least seven relatively new technologies confound the coding system because they integrate two or more functions. For example, interactive videodisk training and computer-based instruction combine the function of reaching a mass of individuals with the same content and the information processing function of anticipating individual responses to programmed questions and providing feedback. In the case of mail, mass mail was treated as a separate system from interpersonal mail. And programmed teletext systems would be distinct from information retrieval teletext. But with computer-based instruction (CBI) the same user engages in information retrieval and information processing from moment to moment. It is harder to argue that there are two separate media systems. Likewise, audience polling over two-way cable television offers mass mediated content to users, but also processes the information they provide and responds to it. Electronic bulletin board systems permit mediated interpersonal information exchange but also can be used to provide mass information to all users of the service. Integrated media systems such as some videotext systems actually permit all three modes of information exchange. As wideband transmission becomes more available and information processing more sophisticated, integrated systems will become more widespread and even more integrated.

Channel

Limitations on the sensory channels over which information can be communicated vary widely across media systems and constrain the type of information available on a media system. A broad distinction is whether auditory or visual or both types of information can be exchanged over a media system. More detailed classification can also be conducted, differentiating visual information exchange into full motion video, still images, graphics, and text. Audio can be broken down into full audio and limited sounds. These categories were chosen to represent important distinctions in the types of symbol systems with which communication could take place and to correspond to meaningful technical differences in media systems. The four types of visual information (text, graphics, pictures, and full motion video) are one way of describing the visual symbols used in media systems. Text refers to written language. Full motion video is usually the least abstract visual representation, followed by pictures, and finally graphics, the most abstract of the three. Auditory information may include speech and music, or it may be limited by the technology to occasional noises. Finer distinctions of bandwidth are also possible but perhaps not necessary at this point.

One approach to channel classification would be to determine whether or not each channel category is technically possible over a particular media system. However, it would be more informative to also take into account norms of communication for that system. For example, even though it is technically possible to transmit text and graphics over broadcast television, the majority of such content is full motion video. Theoretically, it would be possible to assign proportions to each channel subcategory to describe relative, normative emphasis on each channel mode of communication over a particular media system. If a channel mode is technically impossible over a media system, the proportion for that category would, of course, be zero. One could conduct content analysis of each media system to determine accurate proportions.

IMPLICATIONS FOR RESEARCH

This commentary has attempted to establish the need for a perspective on media systems that accounts for the diversity of types of systems currently in

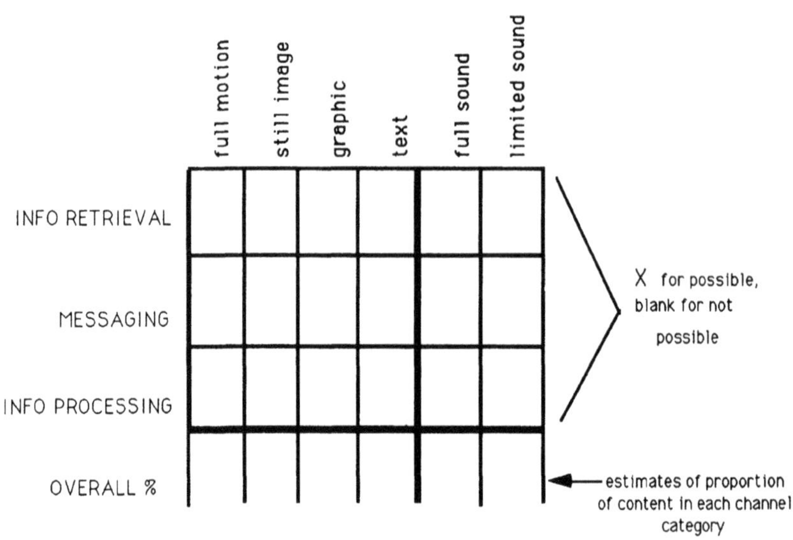

Figure 3 Media system classification table.

use. In agreement with Rice, the specification of the media system research framework, and particularly, the media system under study is called for. A specific, basic schema for classifying media systems by function and channel was introduced and demonstrated for 53 hypothetical media systems. The analysis began with classification and went on to examine relationships between function and channel. Those relationships may be based on technological convenience, or it may be that certain channels and modes of interactivity are more conducive to certain functions. For example, are audio and text more important in interpersonal information exchange than are graphics, pictures, and full motion video, or has technology simply denied access to these video forms until now? Will the graphic and pictorial language forms develop further when technologies are widely available for home use?

It is important that a simple classification schema be used across all articles on mediated communication systems. Suggesting that each author conduct a content analysis of the media system along with the research project is unrealistic and will certainly never meet the goal of uniform, comparable, regular reporting of information about the communication system.

Figure 3 presents a media systems classification table that, if present in all research methods sections, could facilitate cross-system and cross-study comparison. Future work should carefully expand the classification schema to include interactivity, ease of use, human interface protocols, user choice, and other communication variables.

REFERENCES

Berlo, D. (1969). *The process of communication.* New York: Holt, Rinehart & Winston.

Bretz, R. (1971). *A taxonomy of communication media* (Report R-697-NLM/PR Rand Corporation). Englewood Cliffs: Educational Technology.

Chen, M. (1984). Computers in the lives of our children: Looking back on a generation of television research. In R. Rice & Associates (Eds.), *The new media: Communication, research and technology* (pp.169-286). Beverly Hills, CA: Sage.

Daft, R., & Lengel, R. (1984). Information richness: A new approach to managerial behavior and organizational design. *Research in Organizational Behavior, 6,* 191-233.

Paisley, W., & Chen, M. (1982). *Children and electronic text: Challenges and opportunities of the new literacy.* Stanford, CA: Stanford University Institute for Communication Research.

Phillips, A. (1984). Attitude correlates of selected media technologies: A pilot study. In R. Rice & Associates (Eds.), *The new media: Communication, research, and technology.* Beverly Hills, CA: Sage.

Rice, R., & Williams, F. (1984). Theories old and new: The study of new media. In R. Rice & Associates (Eds.), *The new media: Communication, research, and technology.* Beverly Hills, CA: Sage.

Rogers, E., & Chaffee, S. (1983). Communication as an academic discipline: A dialogue. *Journal of Communication,* 33, 18-30.

Short, J., Williams, E., & Christie, B. (1984). The social psychology of telecommunications. In R. Rice & Associates (Eds.), *The new media: Communication, research and technology.* Beverly Hills, CA: Sage.

Wartella, E., & Reeves, B. (1985). Historical trends in research on children and the media: 1900-1960. *Journal of Communication, 35,* 118-133.

Commentary on Issues and Concepts in Research on Computer-Mediated Communication Systems

JEROME JOHNSTON
University of Michigan

IN his chapter on Computer-Mediated Communication Systems (CMCS), Rice notes that the body of research on the uses and implications of CMCS is unusually diverse, reflecting wide-ranging goals and disciplinary orientations of those who have conducted studies on this topic. Over the years, Rice's own publications on CMCS have played an important role for academics in the field of communication by synthesizing literature from sources outside the mainstream of the communication field. In this chapter, he attempts to provide a framework that can be used to both understand the existing diversity and guide future research. This is a laudable goal. But I would like to argue that there is a basic diversity of goals between communication researchers with their theoretical orientation and those researchers who identify with the field of program evaluation. Second, the stakeholder notion, which arose in the field of program evaluation, is impractical because it diffuses focus and interest. Third, on the topic of tools, I want to argue for increased use of qualitative strategies to study a phenomenon as fast-changing and novel as CMCS.

PROGRAM EVALUATION

As a research tradition, program evaluation dates back to the mid-1960s, the time of Lyndon Johnson and the social programs of the Great Society. The

Correspondence and requests for reprints: Jerome Johnston, School of Education, University of Michigan, Ann Arbor, MI 48109.

Communication Yearbook 12, 490-497

field burgeoned in 1965 when Robert Kennedy included a requirement for program evaluation in the legislation that created the Head Start program. He felt that an annual public evaluation of every local Head Start program would serve to empower the local poor and inform them of whether the federal money had been spent in ways that served their interests. Following this call, several other pieces of legislation in the 1960s contained evaluation components as well. But there were no evaluation specialists in the federal bureaucracy. Program officers in the various federal departments needing evaluations sought expertise from academia. Those responding were most frequently academics in the fields of education, psychology, and political science. As a field, evaluation grew rapidly throughout the late 1960s and the 1970s paralleling the demand for greater accountability in the delivery of services—especially educational services (McLaughlin, 1974). The major topics of study were social programs in education, mental health, public health, welfare, and crime and justice. The major goal was accountability—providing evidence for the success or failure of a social program. The major variables were receipt of service by the target audience, satisfaction, and alteration of the target group's well-being in areas such as educational achievement, income, housing, and social adjustment. (See Glass, 1976, and other volumes in the series, *Evaluation Studies Review Annual.*) While not atheoretical, most evaluation studies are not theory driven, unless the theories are about strategies for social intervention or social-science knowledge usage.

A distinction is made in the evaluation literature between formative and summative research. As originally formulated by Scriven (1967), formative research is part of a product development process. It seeks to collect data in a timely fashion in order to improve the potential of the product to be accepted and to achieve its intended impact. For example, formative research in educational television seeks, at various stages (story board, script development, pilot production), to assess the appeal and comprehensibility of the product (Baker, 1974; Johnston, 1984).

Summative evaluation is designed to assess whether a mature program—one that is well tested and relatively stable in its design—delivers what it promises. It is built around pre/post designs in which a naive group experiences an experimental program of specified characteristics. Based on comparison with a control group on differences in test performance before and after the program, a judgment is made about the effectiveness of the intervention.

STAKEHOLDERS

Typically, evaluations are funded by one group that has a "stake" in the program itself. The most common interest of the founder is to know whether the program achieves its goals. While there are impartial funders (e.g., NSF), quite frequently, groups that fund an intervention have an interest in obtaining evidence to show that the funds were wisely spent—that the program does work, because such evidence can then be used to defend past or proposed expenditures. The bias is not always intended; sometimes it is a function of having too narrow a focus on the problem to be solved and the nature of the solution under test.

To counter this potential for bias, the notion of stakeholder research arose in the late 1970s. Those who advocate this approach argue that evaluative information is power, and that evaluations of significant interventions should be designed to collect information that serves the needs of the full range of groups that have some stake in the program's success or failure. They argue that an evaluation needs to be attentive to the information needs of the program's proponents and enemies. In a pluralistic society, most social programs have a variety of stakeholders, although many of them do not recognize evaluative information as an important commodity in working through their social benefits. On the other hand, CMCS has a clearer set of stakeholders. Manufacturers of CMC systems have a stake in their acceptance and proliferation, and consumers have a stake in accurate assessment of the cost/benefit ratios of using CMCS.

The stakeholder notion has never included scholars among the list of potential stakeholders. It has always referred to other political entities—groups having a stake (enhanced well-being of one kind or another) in the outcome of the evaluation. Academics, however, clearly have a stake in the theoretical contributions of the evaluation study. Design has become contested. Frequently, when academics have been involved in program evaluations of CMCS their interest in theoretical variables have been tolerated by sponsors, but only after assuring them that basic cost-benefit questions will be answered within the design and measurement plan.

But there is a fundamental problem with the stakeholder approach. As a former advocate and practitioner of the stakeholder approach (Johnston, 1978), I have concluded that it is impractical. Those with experience in program evaluation know the difficulty of dealing with the basic four stakeholders: the funder, the program's designers, the delivery agents, and the targets of the program. Funders of an evaluation are rarely interested in defining the evaluation so that it serves multiple constituencies in addition to that of the funding agency. In addition to political interests the agency might hold, stakeholder evaluations inevitably cost more, because they require more time by the research staff throughout the research process. Few agencies are interested in the extra cost. There are exceptions. Congress (Office of Technology Assessment; Institute for Program Evaluation) and the National Science Foundation have taken a broad perspective, but only when it was perceived that society had a stake in knowing the relative value of a social program or a new technology.

Another limitation of the stakeholder approach relates to the researcher and his or her values and interests. Rarely are the rewards for the evaluator—especially if he or she is an academic—enhanced by serving the information needs of various constituencies. Stakeholder research by its very nature is an extended process. It inevitably focuses on the collection of data on many issues that are of limited theoretical interest to the research community with which the researcher identifies. This eclecticism limits the opportunities to publish in a timely fashion those results that are valued by one's primary academic department.

While the stakeholder approach has intuitive appeal, it has a number of impracticalities for communication researchers. Similarly, the practical orientation of most program evaluations of CMCS may constrain scholars in undesirable ways.

METHODOLOGY

The majority of research done on CMCS has been in the quantitative survey research tradition, as opposed to the qualitative case study tradition. In Rice's chapter there are references to only three qualitative research studies. Yet characteristics of CMCS and the patterns of their use provide ample reason to expand the use of case study techniques. As Rice points out, CMCS is a new and evolving technology. As such, its use is characterized by small groups of early adopters who experiment with new (and rapidly changing) systems. They adapt their work behavior experimentally to discover how and whether the technology can enhance their productivity in ways that justify the new technology. Should a particular implementation of CMCS prove its worth, then use will likely increase and communication patterns will change in ways that are new and frequently unknown to the researcher at the time the initial measurement is designed. As Golembiewski (1986) points out, this type of change threatens the design, measurement, and analysis strategies most frequently used by quantitative researchers. This section considers the typical strategies of quantitative survey research, and evaluates them in light of the characteristics of CMCS and the goals of studies on the topic. It then provides some examples of the kinds of information that case study research can provide uniquely, arguing not that this research tradition ought to replace the survey approach, but complement it.

Survey research with scientific sampling of respondents is used to collect information from a representative sample of some population. Done properly, it can yield point estimates of great accuracy with a relatively small proportion of the population of interest. The accuracy depends on having a population of known characteristics. In conducting a survey, it is assumed that each member of the population could provide useful information. With rare events (e.g., computer use or CMCS use), a filtering technique can be used in a multistage operation to ensure that only appropriate respondents are asked to complete a questionnaire or participate in an interview.

The design of measures for survey operations depend on the researcher having a clear notion of the constructs of interest (e.g., usage, communication flow, and gratifications) and operationalizing these with a series of questions for which validity and reliability can be established. Typically, the construct has a limited number of dimensions within it, each of which is scalar in the sense that respondents can indicate their position on the scale (minutes of use, high-low satisfaction, and so on). Cross-time studies look for change on these scales, but assume that the dimensions themselves have a constant meaning for respondents. Or, if not constant, that the researcher will know enough about the changed meaning of the construct at various points in time to adjust the measurement accordingly.

The CMCS is an evolving technology. New technological capabilities constantly change the very character of the CMCS and, therefore, its meaning for users. Even with stable systems, CMCS provide new ways of communicating for users, and increasing use has the potential to alter users' entire conception of what communication is all about in the full range of media he or she uses. To the extent that this possibility is true, cross-time measures based on an initial operationalization of concepts have the potential to miss the change.

My recent research has been investigating a phenomenon with similar characteristics: the evolving use of microcomputers in higher education.[1] The guiding questions include an important quantitative question: the amount that faculty from different disciplines incorporate computer-based learning activities into the design of instruction. Other questions are concerned with the meaning this new technology has for faculty and students alike: What were early adopters trying to accomplish when they incorporated the computer into their courses? How did their students respond to the computer-based activities? And how did the faculty and student's conception of the computer's role change as they acquired increasing experience with it? These goals were consonant with an overarching goal of trying to shape the future by showing administrators and late adopters the potentials and liabilities of computer technology for education.

The research strategy selected was a video case study of several higher education institutions. The first stage involved conducting a census of all faculty on a campus and ascertaining with a short questionnaire whether they were users of computers in their teaching. Users supplied some details about the nature of the use. From this census, early and recent adopters were selected to meet several sampling rules. The selected respondents were interviewed on videotape following—but not totally constrained by—a structured interview schedule. The interview itself was followed by visitations to sites where the computers were used, rule-guided videotaping of the context, and selected interviews with students and faculty colleagues who were not users of the technology.

The interviews accomplished two things that a more traditional survey approach would not. Many informants with extensive experience in the institution could summarize the institutional experience in ways that would be very time-consuming for an outsider with a survey instrument directed to the entire faculty. Because informants may not have conducted a scientific survey themselves, there may be inaccuracy in some of their estimates or reports. But validity is always acquired at some cost. Reports from one informant can always be written up and circulated to other informants for verification. A second advantage was the gaining of perceptual insights from individuals at various stages of adoption. The insights that came from some of the extended interviews captured dimensions of meaning that were unanticipated by the researchers at the beginning of the study.

In this excerpt, an assistant dean captures the essence of the computer revolution on his campus (Johnston & Gardner, 1987).

> The faculty are taking a growing interest in the use of computers for instructional purposes. And for the most part, what one sees now are some visible pioneers (a dozen or, perhaps, a half dozen people in the literature college) who are one to two years into the application of microcomputers to instruction in the large courses. Instruction in small advanced courses has been going on for a very long time at the university, but for the freshmen and sophomore kinds of courses, the big developments have been in the last couple of years.[2]

In this next statement, a faculty member summarizes new experience with 500 students, a group that would have taken inordinate resources to study separately:

> Probably the ultimate verification of this positive attitude of the students comes from the fact that there's a very, very extensive use of the Study Center by the students. Now this is an entirely supplemental facility. We do not require that they use these programs. There is no attendance taken. We don't keep track of how often they've used it. This is entirely voluntary and supplemental, and yet we find that there's a very intensive use of the Study Center, especially as the exam draws closer. At times we'll have waiting lists of 100-150 people trying to get in to use these computer programs. So we know they want to use the material, that they're using it very intensively.[2]

Based on several years of experience this same instructor provided clues about the nature of the impact that were quite subtle, and had not been among the hypotheses of the researchers.

> I've also noted that there seems to be less anxiety around exam time in this course. Prior to having the Study Center, students were always asking questions about what's going to be on the exam, and didn't know how to study because they really didn't know what to expect.
>
> By providing all this material based on problem solving skills, they can find out what it is we expect and get experience in trying to attempt to solve these kinds of problems. They feel much more secure that they know what to expect when they come in to take the exam.[2]

In this next interview, a student in this class provides a new understanding of how computer-based tutorials can alter the basic learning model of mastery of lectures and text. It's in her search for words to explain the shifting conception of learning/instruction that we gain this understanding.

> These [computer-based tutorials] are different in the way that I can go [to the Study Center], and I can put my books away, and I can do the questions, and it'll be kind of like creating a test situation. Whereas in other places at lecture, they're giving you information, and you're just receiving it. Here you're kind of interacting with it, and that way it helps me a lot for the test. The computer lessons are like more applied, and the lecture and the textbook can give you the information, and when you take it to the Study Center, it's more like you're applying the information.[2]

The quote does not establish the extent to which other students shared this perception; that information would require a traditional sample survey of the entire class.

In another example, a professor of political science uses a CMCS to carry on a semester-long simulation of roles played in international conflicts. Here a student explains how the computer conferencing system represents a different kind of communication act than do live simulations.

> The computer gives you a chance to really structure your arguments logically and make sure those arguments are consistent. Also, you're not as likely to let emotions fly during confrontations.[2]

Any of the previous examples could themselves become separate studies of the role and impact of computers in education. (Indeed, the Study Center became just that—a year-long study of the impact on students [Johnston & Kleinsmith, 1987].) But, with an evolving technology and limited resources, such studies might not be completed in time to provide an integrated picture of the diverse ways in which computers can affect the character of educational experiences.

Research methodologies must match the overall goals of the research. Many of the goals of CMCS research can be well served by case studies, especially when point estimates and variance analysis are not required. Case studies can provide efficiency in the case of complex organizational innovation. Coupled with traditional sampling techniques, it is useful to study early adopters of innovations. The use of structured interview and observation can provide a quality of insight frequently not possible with structured questionnaires. The limitation of the methodology rests largely in generalizability, although verification procedures can help in this regard. But much of CMCS research does not require the reliability sought in sample surveys. There is greater need for deep understanding of complex, diverse, and shifting perceptions of the CMCS user communities.

NOTES

1. The research is contained in a series of videotaped case studies. There are three videotapes covering three separate contexts: The Electronic Classroom at The University of Michigan, The Electronic Classroom in the Regional Teaching University, The Electronic Classroom in the Community College. A fourth videotape—The Electronic Classroom in Higher Education—looks across five institutions. A printed report—Educational Computing in Higher Education: The Issues—contains transcripts of the four videos and methodological notes about the video case study. These are available for a fee from The National Center for Research to Improve Postsecondary Teaching and Learning, The University of Michigan, 2400 School of Education, Ann Arbor, MI 48109-1259.
2. Transcribed by author from videotape.

REFERENCES

Baker, E. (1974). Formative evaluation of instruction. In J. W. Popham (Ed.), *Evaluation in education: Current applications* (pp. 531-585). Berkeley, CA: McCutcheon.

Glass, G. V. (Ed.). (1976). *Evaluation studies review annual.* Newbury Park, CA: Sage.

Golembiewski, R. (1986). Contours in social change: Elemental graphics and a surrogate variable for gamma change. *Academy of Management Review, 11,* 550-566.

Johnston, J. (1978, March). *What we know about the researcher and research methods in evaluation.* Paper presented at a symposium, Using evaluation results in planning: Alternative views of the decision-maker and the evaluator, at the meeting of the American Educational Research Association, Toronto, Canada.

Johnston, J. (Ed.). (1984). *New directions in program evaluation: Sourcebook No. 23. Evaluating the new information technologies.* San Francisco: Jossey-Bass.

Johnston, J. (1984). Evaluation approaches for the new information technologies. In J. Johnston (Ed.), *New directions in program evaluation: Sourcebook No. 23. Evaluation the new information technologies* (pp. 73-87). San Francisco: Jossey-Bass.

Johnston, J., & Gardner, S. (Producers & Directors). (1987). *The electronic classroom at the University of Michigan* (video). Ann Arbor: University of Michigan (National Center for Research to Improve Postsecondary Teaching and Learning).

Johnston, J., & Kleinsmith, L. (1987). *Computers in higher education: The biology tutorials.* Ann Arbor: University of Michigan (Institute for Social Research).

McLaughlin, M. W. (1974). *Evaluation and reform: The Elementary and Secondary Education Act of 1965, Title I.* Santa Monica, CA: Rand Corporation.

Scriven, M. (1967). *The methodology of evaluation* (AERA Monograph Series on Curriculum Evaluation No. 1). Chicago: Rand McNally.

9 Designing Communication Systems for Human Systems: Values and Assumptions of "Socially Open Architecture"

STEPHEN R. ACKER
Ohio State University

This chapter describes *socially open architecture* as an approach to designing technology-based communication systems. It argues that designers must pursue a "principle of incompleteness," which recognizes that design is never finished; rather it is "brought to form" in a variety of ways within different social contexts. Concrete examples of socially open architecture and the implications of the designer's assumptions in the implementation and social effects of technology are presented.

TO a great extent, communication technologies are the outcomes of how designers assess the process of human communication. When a school board member, or the resident technology guru of an organization, selects a configuration of computers and modems, videoconference system components, or other communication technology, he or she has chosen more than metal cases wrapped around microprocessors. Rather, the system implementer has established an interactive relationship between his or her community and the designer, and the assumptions about communication that each brings to the relationship.

The designer's assumptions about human communication have a powerful effect on how the relationship between person and machine is first established and later developed. These assumptions are designed into the machine and lie dormant until activated in the user's environment. Much like a competent human communicator able to modify these a priori assumptions through interaction, technologies designed to adapt to the user's environment should find more acceptance in the social setting of system use than should a less

AUTHOR'S NOTE: I would like to acknowledge my debt to James Anderson, Joseph Foley, Eric Fredin, and Diana Gagnon for many helpful comments on earlier drafts of this chapter.

Correspondence and requests for reprints: Stephen R. Acker, Department of Communication, Ohio State University, 205 Derby Hall, 154 North Oval Mall, Columbus, OH 43210-1360.

Communication Yearbook 12, 498-532

flexibly designed system. This chapter attempts to identify some of the critical features of this process of design and the integral connection of these design features to the process of implementing—finding social acceptance for—new communication technologies. Of particular importance are the assumptions that the designers make about (1) the purposes for the technological innovation, and (2) about the users, both as individual information processors and as persons embedded in larger social contexts.

One consequence of highlighting the importance of the designer's assumptions is that it redefines the arguments surrounding technological determinism, that machinery per se drives social change. If the machines that come to market are seen as reifications of the assumptions and goals of designers, the process of social change becomes the dialectic between one set of social assumptions (the designers') and another set of social assumptions (the policymakers' and users' of the technologies). From this perspective, social change is driven by the interactions of the designers' goals (derived from assumptions) and those of the user communities. Also, this perspective extends the role of the system designer beyond packaging a product to be released as "finished" into society. Instead, the designer is seen as a "match maker," one who creates potential relationships that will evolve over time.

Since this chapter takes as its starting premise that the goals and assumptions of designers are important, it is consistent for the author to offer one set of goals and assumptions that he feels are constructive for guiding the design process. These motivating principles are value-laden, and their usefulness will be related to the degree of agreement between the author's and individual reader's assessments of how social and technological systems *should* interact. This value system is described by the phrase *socially open architecture* and includes a particular set of assumptions about the purposes of technology and the individual and social characteristics of users. The principles of socially open architecture will be elaborated in the middle sections, and several examples of technological systems designed according to these principles conclude the chapter.

This chapter covers a number of issues that, on first reading, may seem to be loosely coupled. Restating the goal and then associating the upcoming sections with this goal, may help organize the content and prestructure the argument. The goal is to consider design as an open-ended process that is heavily influenced by the individual designer's assumptions about who will use the technology and what the technology is supposed to do for the user. The design horizon must be viewed as extending beyond the product release phase.

The first assumption that structures this chapter is that the importance of design must be justified to the audience of communication researchers. This premise is based on the lack of design literature in the field of communication, substantiated by Roger's (1986) observation that: "Seldom is communication research explicitly involved in designing communication technology. The main role of communication researchers in studying the new media has been to carry out post hoc evaluations. This passive role is very limited" (p. 219). This assumption motivates the Design and Evaluation Research for Implementers section (Section 2) that extends the issues of design into the realm of implementation, an area of demonstrated interest to communication scholars. The conclusion reached is that if one important purpose of research is to assist decision makers, field studies and laboratory studies provide incomplete data for the purpose of charting action. Without pursuing research as a "complementary triad" of (1) laboratory, (2) field and (3) design research, the contribution of each to answering the very difficult and real question of "What should we do?" is weakened.

The next section, Action Science and the Discipline of Design, (Section 3) presents one framework for the study of design. It lays out broad assumptions about human beings as social actors and how research settings can capture the realism of their interactions.

Section 4, Cybernetic Versus Homeostatic Foundations, discusses the distinctions between systems yoked to a standard through cybernetic feedback systems (i.e., self-correcting toward a norm), and systems driven by homeostatic feedback responding toward the emergent (i.e., stable under conditions of change). This section includes many of the author's assumptions about the purposes of machine.

Section 5, The Influence of Social Context on Design, is about the need for technology to adapt to the social environment of the user. This section confines itself to work and educational environments, but the role of social context in technological design can be demonstrated in personal habitats as well.

Section 6, The Individual User, examines assumptions about the designer's conceptual representation of the user and the design guidelines derived from these "user models."

Section 7, Designs of Incompleteness, presents several design projects premised on the arguments presented in earlier sections. This section emphasizes the role of social context in the ultimate culmination of the design process.

Section 8, Summary and Conclusions, integrates material from the opening sections and offers suggestions for future design research.

DESIGN AND EVALUATION RESEARCH FOR IMPLEMENTERS

The decisions of designers are often mass produced and then distributed into a multitude of different user contexts. Different contexts require different implementation strategies for successful integration of the technology into the social system.

Both system implementers and system designers must make decisions about how the technology and its users will interact as a sociotechnical system. This section proposes that the dominant forms of research in new media technologies, field studies, and laboratory experiments, must be complemented by design research concepts to contribute meaningfully to the real world struggles of implementers charged with introducing technological systems into social systems.

The essence of the argument is that the system implementer fulfills a role much closer to that of a designer than to that of a field researcher or laboratory researcher. The similarity between the implementer and designer is in their common subjective experience of creating a new environment rather than retrospectively or clinically evaluating an existing environment. Without a designer's perspective, the implementer can easily misuse the existing evaluation research in his or her decision-making process.

One useful definition of design is that it is a process through which a conceptual solution to a problem is concretely realized (Carnall & Medland, 1984). As in the case of implementers, the designer observes how previous designs have been accepted by users (field research) as well as how particular design features influence the use of a design under carefully controlled circumstances (laboratory research). The other source of information used by designers is their poorly articulated but heavily relied on "intuition," a global form of knowledge developed through training and previous personal involvement in design. This intuition is the gestalt of the designer's assumptions about users, their social contexts, and the applications of their design as concrete technologies (see Schon, 1983).

Because of the socialization of designers and the structures of the institutions within which they work, intuition is sanctioned as a viable source of data for decision making (Schon, 1985; but see Newall & Card, 1985, for a dissenting opinion). In contrast to the designer's environment, implementers of new technologies often work within organizations that demand bureaucratized reasoning, a process that insists on formalized and routine decision making (Peccei & Guest, 1984). To the extent that the definition of *design,* "a process through which a conceptual solution to a problem is concretely realized," also describes *implementation,* the implementer who is not permitted to argue from intuition and whose cognitive responses emerge *only* in the process of action (Nadin, 1988), is severely handicapped.

As a consequence of the preferred form of argument sanctioned by bureaucratized organizations, implementers of new technology often must justify their decisions by citing previous field or experimental studies. Often this locus of justification becomes internalized as a sense of accountability on the part of the implementer, and a desire to reach back to previous events for evidence. In short, decision makers largely have been trained to find similarities with other situations rather than to look for the novelty in the situations in which they are currently operating (Argyris & Schon, 1978).

The problem with justification based on the past hinges on whether the past truly is similar to the present. The recommendations and generalizations that come out of a post hoc evaluation are applicable within the particular context that defined the evaluation setting. In a sense, evaluation research aggregates particular contexts as "historical findings," of which the usefulness for guiding future actions depends on the stability of both the technology and the social system. Because nearly all communication technologies are experiencing rapid design evolution and because the social systems into which the innovations are being introduced have not made routine the use of most technologies, the social and technological systems are both very unstable. Consequently, using evaluation results as the basis for decision making, as in the case of a manager's need to select which technological system to purchase, is problematic, and becomes increasingly so as system implementation is projected further into the future.

The following discussion about computer conferencing illustrates some of the difficulties of applying past evaluations as if the environment that characterizes the present were adequately represented in previous research settings. The conclusion drawn is that past evaluations are poor predictors of future relationships between technical and social systems. Instead, the principal contribution of summative evaluations is to identify important variables to be addressed in subsequent design evolutions. From the implementer's perspective, evaluation research may be more helpful in identifying likely problems than in suggesting likely solutions.

Computer Conferencing and the Notion of Lexical Vestiges

The literature on computer-mediated communication provides a specific example of the dilemma of using evaluation research to guide action in a fluid technological environment. A sampling of the pre-1987 literature would suggest this set of conclusions:

(1) Computer communication might weaken social influence because of the absence of nonverbal communication (Dobos & Grieve, 1985).
(2) Messages are depersonalized because communicators must imagine their audience (Kiesler, Siegel, & McGuire, 1984).
(3) Group communication is inhibited by computer conferencing's linearity (Hiltz & Turoff, 1978).
(4) Reactions of participants are difficult to gauge because one cannot monitor the nonverbals of others during discourse (Phillips, 1983).
(5) "Even a memo, with its letterhead and chosen form, carries more nonverbal information than does a message on the screen." (Eckholm, 1984, p. C1).

The generalization derived from this literature on computer conferencing is that the medium's weakness in conveying nonverbal cues reduces the social presence of the communicators. An implementer informed of this literature would be hard pressed to justify computer conferencing for collaborative interactions requiring high levels of social presence, such as group negotiations.

However, as established as this generalization has become, published studies seldom describe the age or the operating characteristics of the system used in the research supporting this conclusion. Without an adequate description of the technological systems on which these conclusions are based, individuals considering current system configurations cannot use these evaluation findings to inform their decision making. Only by guessing that the foregoing systems were text-only, simplex systems, would an implementer be in position to infer that the computer conferencing system used by Apple Computer to conduct its 1985 annual report to stockholders (January 22, 1986) might differ from those described, might challenge the metafinding that computers cannot convey nonverbal information, and thus that computer conferencing systems might serve for the purpose of negotiation.

The 1986 Apple stockholders' conference was "simulcast" as a live meeting and as a computer conference using VMCO, a Macintosh software package designed by Robert Perez. Two of the distinguishing features of VMCO are that the computer conference supports voice synthesis and presents a visualization of the conference (Perez, 1985).

In a VMCO conference, the Macintosh screen displays a large conference table surrounded by 20 chairs. Conference participants "occupy" a chair by placing an icon of themselves in a chair. These icons can be customized to reflect recognizable features of a participant such as the appearance of glasses, beards, and so on. Each icon has eight faces that register nonverbal reactions, such as boredom, anger, or suprise. By toggling their face icons, several participants can register simultaneously their reaction to a statement "on the floor" (see Figure 9.1).

It is reasonable to expect that the rules that "define" text-only computer conference systems operate differently in a VMCO conference and that negotiation and other forms of collaborative inquiry are viable considerations for the use of computer conferencing (Mooney, 1988). However, potential system implementers unfamiliar with VMCO might decide not to implement computer conferencing for its lack of social presence. Studying "flies in amber" does still the "blooming, buzzing confusion" (James, 1890/1950), but at some cost to our appreciation of evolution.

One can conclude that evaluation findings in fast changing areas of technology contain only "lexical vestiges"—these descriptive traces of immature technologies, since supplanted by a new state of the art. For these evaluations to benefit both implementers and designers, more attention must be paid to fully presenting the technical characteristics of the system being evaluated. From this carefully constructed base, the outcomes of these field evaluations could stimulate redesign of systems rather than be considered final assessments of a technology's capability.

ACTION SCIENCE AND THE DISCIPLINE OF DESIGN

To the extent one goal of research is to guide decision making in complex, changing environments, a methodology oriented toward addressing unique

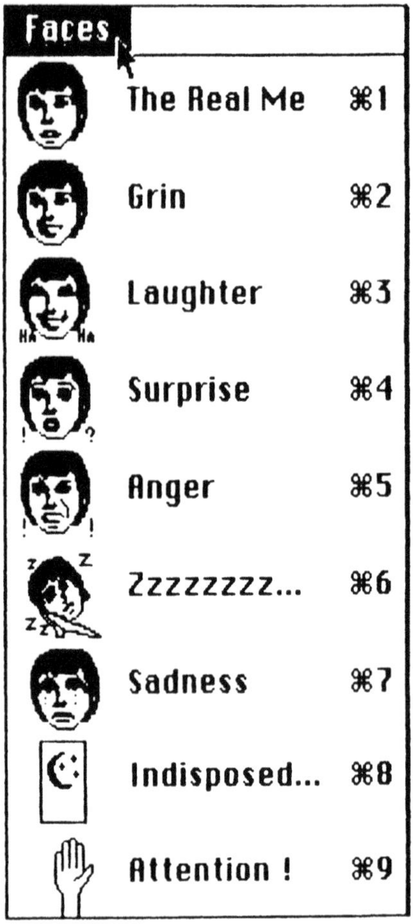

Figure 9.1 Each member of a VMCO computer conference can register his or her response to a "statement on the floor" by presenting one of these faces at the participant's place at the conference table. This default file can be customized to reflect a participant's recognizable features.

aspects of the interrelated social and technical systems may complement methodologies seeking to generalize across systems. Adhering to this goal legitimizes intuition, defined as reasons, whether or not articulated, invested in action appropriate to the moment (Nadin, 1988). This orientation characterizes the design process, and forms the basis for a method of inquiry known as *action science.*

One approach to understanding action science is to contrast it to hypothetico-deductive "normal" science. Argyris, Putnam, and Smith (1985) characterize the goal of normal science as describing reality as accurately as possible. In normal science, the emphasis is on this description rather than on changing reality. Once an adequate description has been obtained, the concerned scientist may propose an intervention to bring about a desired change, but this intervention is not the scientist's purpose for doing the research.

In contrast, action science is explicitly goal driven; its purpose is to solve problems and to generate action toward desired ends. The action scientist enters the research process to create change. Lewin (1948) pointed out that trying to change the world is an excellent approach to trying to understand it, and to that extent action research shares a common motivation with normal science. However, the distinction remains that action scientists "ready themselves in anticipation" of a process rather than come to an event with script in hand. Action science "invents" a description of the process as it unfolds. Action precedes description, rather than the reverse (Argyris, Putnam, & Smith, 1985).

Action science assumes that individuals model the world in cause-effect relationships, and that action is motivated by a desire to cause certain effects (achieve certain goals). Goal-driven action emerges through stages. First, a short list of possible actions is generated. This stage is called the discovery process, also known as the *design of action* phase. From among the alternatives conceived during discovery, the one most likely to achieve a desired end is selected. This selection represents the *decision* stage of action.

The importance of the design of action phase is that humans seldom make "optimum" decisions; rather they make *reasonable* decisions (Simon, 1982). Design is central to decision making because action is governed by this primacy principle: People search for an action to the point that an acceptable one, not necessarily the best one, has been found. Simon (1982) refers to this process as *satisficing*, or finding an action that is satisfactory though not necessarily ideal.

A productive discovery phase implies rapid and successful generation of adequate decision alternatives, because once a workable solution to the problem has been found further search will be abandoned. If this model of human decision making is accurate, the importance of the discovery process is elevated. Every action, as well as the success of every action, is constrained by an initial set of alternatives contemplated in the discovery phase.

The systematic study of design is the study of this discovery phase of action. Design organizes a poorly structured problem (Argyris, Putnam, & Smith, 1985). The way a system is designed establishes probabilities among possible actions by weighting the likelihood of selection of each alternative within the set of those actions initially contemplated. Different designs favor different actions. The goal of design is to foreground an adequate set of alternatives to make a problem actionable. Design emphasizes this problem definition and assumes that the goal of identifying a single problem solution in any final sense is unattainable. New contingencies will redirect the problem definition, and design must be adaptable to permit the expression of the redirected, goal-driven behavior.

Considering the environment as an "emergent" phenomenon undergoing constant change, rather than a stable environment amenable to a fixed description, underlies the action science community's demand for situational relevance, and simultaneously is at odds with the community of normal science's demand for generalizability. Design involves probabilistically structuring emergent environments at the expense of replicability. This feature of the design process has led to design being criticized for lack of rigor. Alternately, one could argue that an inappropriate epistemology is being invoked for assessing design findings.

As argued earlier, an implementer may be advantaged by being informed through multiple epistemologies. For example, another premise of action science favoring "just in time" research methods is that contingencies in the environment form the basis for the decisions of actors (Argyris, Putnam, & Smith, 1985). While decision making certainly can be informed by experimental research, the *ceteris paribus* caveat of laboratory work—all things, or contingencies, equal—raises concerns. And although action science and the experimental paradigm are both premised on cause-effect relationships, action science assumes that the social actors' assessments of the contingencies are what exacts the relationships between cause and effect. In contrast, experimental research uncovers cause-effect relationships by holding contingencies fixed. For the action scientist, the laboratory experiment offers one restricted set of contingencies from which the ability to generalize is problematic. Instead, action research concentrates on the environmental contingencies on the belief that how the context is evaluated will dictate the action strategy.

Implementing an "Intelligent" Phone System

An example of how "variable isolating" and "contingency isolating" research approaches can inform action differently can be seen in the efforts of a large midwestern university to replace a Centrex (five button) phone system with an intelligent (software configured) telephone system.

Early in the implementation process, the training department added new personnel and established an ambitious schedule for offering training on the features of the new phone system to a campus community of perhaps 10,000 faculty and staff. The underlying assumption of the implementation team, based on numerous on-site visitations to other universities installing new phone systems and a review of the literature, was that training on the system was a prerequisite for users to establish proficiency on the new phones. It further was argued that the complexity of the new phones, capable of 104 separate operations, supported the need for training. Through this literature review and reasoning process, pretraining was isolated as a relevant variable related to successful system implementation.

An early needs assessment allowed the implementers to package the telephone's many functions into useful (and smaller) subsets and define users as single-line or multiline (e.g., switchboard) users. Confident of their assessment of the situation, the trainers first developed hour-long training sessions targeted at these different user groups, then heavily promoted attendance through campus mail and the university newspaper. Every effort was made to offer the sessions at convenient times and to groups small enough to promote hands-on experience.

After several months of offering training, the implementation team observed that although staff attendance was satisfactory, the level of faculty participation was disappointing. Still convinced that training was essential, the implementation team continued to pursue the strategy of introducing faculty to the system through training sessions. They devised the innovative tactic of modularizing the training classroom and bringing it onto the premises of various departments. They further encouraged faculty attendance by soliciting support letters from deans and senior administrators. Despite these genuine attempts, faculty attendance at training sessions remained minuscule.

Throughout this implementation phase, an alternate, design-based approach had been presented. From a design perspective, three contingencies argued against offering training sessions for faculty. The first contingency was the unlikelihood that faculty could fathom a need for training on a device they had used successfully for many years. Second, faculty members would probably not publicly disclose their possible ignorance of how to use a telephone by attending a group training session. And third, based only on informal observations of where telephones tended to be placed on the desk of faculty members, the telephone was a "background" technology that emerged into relevance only when it rang or when it was used to call someone else.

The design-based conclusion was that telephone training should exist precisely like the telephone, as a latent potential in the environment, and not be foregrounded through training sessions. When needed, this latent potential could be activated in two ways. First, an instruction card would be carefully designed to assist faculty with using the phone's features and be placed beneath every phone. Much like an elaborate version of the phone instructions found in every hotel room, this card would direct the user, at the specific time the information was needed, on the operations for using the conference call, call-waiting, line-camping, and so on—features offered by the new system. Additionally, rather than hire several trainers, it was proposed that an operator be funded full time to serve as a "hotline" consultant.

While this design "solution" (structuring alternatives probabilistically) in no way contradicted the benefits of universal training, it highlighted the environmental contingencies in which the system usage problem was embedded. The operative contingency in this case was that faculty were unmoveable in their opposition to attending training. The design approach, "readiness in anticipation," invested the implementation resources in a latently responsive environment that connected the sociotechnical system on a "when needed" basis rather than a "will need" assumption.

Sociotechnical Analysis and Socially Open Architecture

This telephone example illustrates several principles of design research and reintroduces the phrase *sociotechnical system*. Based on the assumptions of action science, a methodology known as *sociotechnical analysis* has developed to match technical systems with social systems. The method traces its origin to the Tavistok group in England and cofounder Eric Trist's work with introducing new technology to the coal mining industry (Trist, Higgens, Murray, & Pollock, 1963). The problem Trist faced was that coal output fell when new production equipment was introduced, even though the new methods were clearly technologically superior to the old mining techniques. Trist found that by involving the miners in redesigning their approach to their work, the promise of the new design was realized and led to a substantial rise in output.

Traditional sociotechnical analysis (STS) advocates a process of scanning the technological environment, scanning the social environment, and consulting with workers to address the problems introduced by the shift to new technology (Pava, 1983). Through this process of problem definition, the researcher allows the community to construct its own appropriate responses rather than proposing exogenous solutions. In this process, STS works backwards from organizational or societal problems toward theory. The action research tradition is "learning by doing" (Pava, 1986) and involves nesting action within the systems that influence its implementation. This approach supports a design architecture open to the influence of the social system as well as subsequent technical advances.

Creating open architecture in the design of communication systems begins with scanning both the social and technological environments. A first step in the social scan is to examine the dynamics of human interaction within the organization. The designer first determines the organization members' expectations about how their organization functions (called their theories *of action*). The designer must then anticipate the set of possible responses (or actions) toward the technology from the organization's members based on their theories of action. Often, these action theories will differ from what the agent *espouses* in an interview situation. For example, in the case of the intelligent phone system, no faculty member would argue that training wasn't valuable (espoused theory), members simply wouldn't attend training sessions (theories in action). When individuals' theories in action differ from their espoused theories, the initial goal of design is to help individuals see the apparent contradictions in their actions and the explanation they present for their actions. Once this level of self-reflection has been achieved, it is possible for the individuals to try to change how they act to achieve their stated goals more successfully (Argyris & Schon, 1978).

The challenge of designing communication systems for organizations is integrating an understanding of this adaptation process into the technology. Since no design should be considered static and finished at the time of its release, how the system can evolve after implementation must be considered from the earliest stage of system design. The phrase *socially open architecture* is intended to convey that successful design of technology follows a *principle of incompleteness* in which the technology does not determine how it will be used but instead its function is completed by the system users. Technologies that require the social system to complete them are adaptive in a manner similar to systems described by the conventional meaning of "open architecture," that a technology can assimilate future hardware innovations. Socially open architecture uses the "social system" to direct the use of the technology, thereby assimilating future social innovations.

In combination, the designer's assumptions about the technological and social systems guide the design process. Communication occurs in an interdependent system of socially contextualized individuals and media with technologically defined characteristics. Unfortunately, the process by which technological and social systems adapt to each other is sequential rather than simultaneous; difficult rather than easy, and expensive rather than cost-free. A new communication technology is first designed based on inferences about the user group. Only after the technology has been introduced does the social system either accommodate to it or reject it. If the social system rejects the innovation it is often after a frustrating and expensive attempt at implementation.

The next section contrasts technologies that are decoupled from the social system (called *cybernetic systems*) with those that are bound with the social system (called *homeostatic systems*). It will be argued that the foundational assumptions of cybernetics measurably contribute to the problems of successfully implementing technological systems within social systems.

CYBERNETIC VERSUS HOMEOSTATIC FOUNDATIONS

A *cybernetic* system uses feedback to regulate its response relative to an established norm often instantiated in the technology. The classic example of a cybernetic system is a thermostatically controlled heater. The output of the heater is referenced to a fixed temperature. When the temperature falls to a specified degree, the heater turns on to bring the temperature up to the reference. If the temperature in the environment is above the norm, the thermostat directs the heater to turn off to allow the temperature to drop back toward the norm.

Homeostatic systems use feedback for the purpose of establishing internal equilibrium. In a homeostatic system, the reference point is not fixed, but implies a calculus of stability. Biological systems tend to be homeostatic. For example, muscle groups convert more energy when the environment demands exertion. Then, during rest, a new equilibrium is established in which the reduced activity is balanced with less energy conversion. The key point is that homeostatic systems can establish equilibrium at different points, whereas cybernetic systems drive events toward a fixed point.

The distinction between cybernetic and homeostatic systems is placed in a social context in Beniger's (1986) discussion of the information society. He describes the information society as an extension of the industrial revolution, rather than a new social form that has grown out of the revolution in computer design. Communication systems designed on the premises of the industrial revolution would share concepts with Taylorism, a management philosophy associated with a particular social structure for managing work.

Taylorism organizes activity by breaking a process into small, discrete parts. Efficiency is obtained by identifying a single best way to achieve a goal and then establishing control mechanisms to assure that this single best way is invariably replicated. This premise has been actualized by splitting the planning function for some effort from the activities carried out in the service of that task. In many instances, management has reserved the planning function and delegated to workers the responsibility of executing the plan (Schoonhoven, 1986).

The classic example of Taylorism is the assembly line, in which time-motion experts set the speed of the moving conveyer belt and required normative procedures for rapidly accomplishing tasks. However, offices of the 1920s often reflected the same ideas; with work stations linked by pneumatic tubes (similar to today's local area networks?), secretarial output set with the help of mechanical word counters that advanced when the space bar was hit, and water fountains located minimum distances from desk clusters (Leuder, 1986). Braverman (1974) argued that the sedentary nature of office work reflects Taylorist principles of keeping all materials within reach to avoid unnecessary movement and the need of the employee to leave the work station. In short, a Taylorist definition of efficiency reached beyond the manufacturing environment.

As industrialization speeded up the production cycle, the need to coordinate and control the passage of intermediate products *between* stages of production grew in importance. As each discrete operation in the conversion process became faster, the way in which transitions between stages in production were handled came to determine the system's overall output. To increase efficiency, the "handoffs" among the interrelated, but autonomous, actors at the boundaries in the production-consumption cycle had to be brought under control (managed).

The rise in the importance of boundary conditions motivated and paralleled the invention of more technologically sophisticated control systems to manage them. Communication systems, often technologically based, create these transfer mechanisms between human subsystems. These technologies enact their control through feedback, with one system adjusting its activities based on information exchanged with the other. When the feedback systems are cybernetic in nature, they tend to standardize actions of the autonomous actors at the boundaries. In contrast, homeostatic systems incorporate the autonomous actors under the assumption of *equifinality*, that there are multiple paths to a specified end (Schoonhoven, 1986).

It is reasonable to argue with Beniger (1986) that *systems* are driven toward efficiency, a goal of maximizing output for a specified set of inputs. He uses the term *teleonomic* (p. 41) to locate the manifestation of this desired end state of efficiency in structured information, or the system's *program*. This locus of control requires systems in which actions to reach desired end states are generated within program constraints. From this perspective, the overall output of the sociotechnical system reflects the end goals of the information technology cybernetically activated within the goal states of the social enterprise.

The principles of homeostatic design invest the locus of control in teleologically driven individuals rather than the teleonomically structured programs. The important distinction between teleonomic and teleologic is that the teleonomic program precreates, or *harbors*, the exchange mechanisms that drive behavior toward goals. In contrast, teleological change is less deterministic in that it is *invented* during the goal-seeking process. Homeostatic systems seek *responsiveness*, at the possible cost of *efficiency*.

Work can be premised on the classical definition of efficiency or on the expectation that responsiveness provides a more productive management philosophy. Organizations that subscribe to homeostatic rather than cybernetic mechanisms for controlling work differ fundamentally in how the relationship between technology and workers is maintained. Communication technologies, through which the control of the work process is maintained, will contribute differently to the work process as a function of the organization's approach to controlling work.

Cybernetic Organizations

In his arguments against socially decoupled design, Hirschhorn (1984) cites the utility industry as relying excessively on cybernetic thinking. His account of the Three-Mile Island nuclear accident provides a compelling example of how overreliance on self-correcting machine mechanisms can create a near disaster. The following overview is extracted from Hirschhorn (1984; pp. 75-80). The extended editorial "play" the example is given reflects the potentially serious consequences of misplacing the locus of control in the technological side of the sociotechnical system.

At Three-Mile Island, the nuclear reactor was designed so that the core was bathed in water, which, because it came in contact with the nuclear reaction, became hot and radioactive. Another water bath, the secondary cooling system, jackets this primary water bath and removes the heat from the primary bath while leaving the radioactivity isolated. The heat located in this second bath generates steam that is the source of power produced by the nuclear reactor.

While cleaning the reactor, maintenance workers accidentally jammed the valve that exchanged the hot water for cold water in the secondary cooling system. Without a fresh supply of cold water, there was no way to remove the heat from the secondary bath and, by extension, the primary cooling system. A meltdown became imminent.

The reactor's feedback system sensed the heat build-up and automatically shut down the reactor core and turned on an emergency pump to force cool water into the secondary cooling system. Both this system and another backup failed, but the control panel light falsely informed the human operator that the back-ups were operating. Shortly, other indicators contradicted the faulty panel light, but the operators, far removed from true control of the technological system, had no obvious way to choose among the contradictory data. *The occurrence of a nuclear meltdown was prevented only because the system sustained itself long enough for a design team to come on site and accurately diagnose the problem.*

Homeostatic Organizations

Cybernetic controls emerged in the early days of the industrial society. Today, information industries, and increasingly all other industries, are typified not by the well-defined linear processes of the assembly line, but by adaptive processes in which feedback guides and coordinates inventions of the work group (Pava, 1986). This redefinition of work implies new responsibilities for the individual worker and has implications for the redesign of the technologies integrated into the workplace.

An illustrative example can be found in the organizational philosophy driving the latest "industrial revolution:" *flexible manufacturing systems* (FMS). Factories that have adopted FMS techniques are designed to use highly automated processes to accomplish small, customized, production runs, rather than large-scale mass production. Their efficiency is a direct function of their capacity to adapt rapidly to changing demands, a capacity directly linked to the control systems afforded the work force.

The FMS process relies heavily on robotics and is designed to run 24 hours a day, largely untended by humans. Dramatic shifts have occurred with respect to the makeup of the labor force in FMS environments. Jaikumar

(1986) identifies representative FMS factory work forces as having 40% of the membership college educated and having three engineers for every production worker.

The FMS is designed by a team of workers that spends its energy anticipating contingencies and planning responses appropriate for changes in the factory's work orders. The engineers make continual programming changes to keep the robots supplied with the proper materials and the needed instructions to properly assemble the materials into finished products. Outside of such activities as loading parts bins with different components, production workers allocate their time mainly to testing and refining the machine-driven operations. Although many components of the technology-only side of FMS are cybernetic in design, the overall sociotechnical system is truly homeostatic.

The conclusions about how the FMS production process is constituted are instructive. First, the intellectual competence of the work force and its ability to constantly accommodate to novel circumstances is essential for success. The worker serves as the control system over the machine and succeeds when the machine reliably performs its function. In the FMS environment, the communication systems serve to reunite the planning and performance of work and invest decision making in the on-floor worker. The system is designed to emphasize the importance of the human operator.

To summarize the theme of this section, cybernetic design reflects excessive faith in predictability, the capacity to a priori identify a goal and chart a straight path to its attainment. In the case of Three-Mile Island, the failure of the sociotechnical system began with human error, the timing and type of which is only stochastically predictable. Once the error was introduced into the machine system, the closed feedback loops did not allow the human operator access to the emergent conditions to correct the mistake. The key design point is that error, defined here as the need to alter precreated assumptions, is inevitable and that all sources of error cannot be predicted. In Hirschhorn's (1984) words:

> Engineers may appeal to machine designs, but machines, as extensions of human communities are as vulnerable as ourselves. . . . The wishful utopianism of both the machine critics and the machine defenders reflects a shared desire to escape from the contingency and reality of evolving human communities. Machine systems inevitably fail, given the realities of materials and human behavior. Once we accept failure as a part of technological reality, we will gain a clearer perspective on postindustrial work. (p. 86)

The realization that reality is contingency-driven is foundational in FMS organizations that, while relying heavily on machines to carry out routine operations, invest as heavily in the human operators, locating in them the capability for homeostatic control.

THE INFLUENCE OF SOCIAL CONTEXT ON THE DESIGN PROCESS

To successfully contribute, technology must be designed as a component of the sociotechnical system. Taking account of the social context in which a technological system will be used is an essential feature of successful design. In this section, the social context of work is further developed.

Sharing Autonomy

Christie (1985, p. 32) observed: "the design of technology begins with the definition of work as a social process engaged in by people." At the social level, work imposes time structure, gives predictability, provides shared experience beyond the context of immediate family, links a person's goals to a larger community, confers status and identity, and offers an arena for acquiring and applying skill (Jahoda, 1979). The resulting goal for system design becomes making the work socially satisfying, self-fulfilling, and instilled with a user-centered rather than machine-centered locus of control (Schneiderman, 1987). This user-centered, organizationally contextualized perspective offers a good starting point for the design process. Brown and Newall (1985) call this the field of "social ergonomics."

Social ergonomics suggests that design must consider how work and other socially constituted activities fulfill human needs. In the case of work, motivations for performance go beyond the extrinsic reward of salary, posited by radical Taylorism. Margolis, Kroes, and Quinn (1974) conclude that the level of participation is the greatest source of motivation in one's work. Work develops meaning beyond the job itself. Huse (1980) describes the quality of work life (QWL) movement as explicitly recognizing that increased productivity requires that job experiences satisfy personal needs as well as organizational needs. These motivating influences embedded in the social context must be considered in the design process.

Christie (1985) suggests that work organizes the goals and volitions of individuals within the goals and volitions of organizations. For work to be successfully accomplished, these goals must be pursued in harmony. The need for this "co-orientation" of goal structures is heightened in teleological organizations that rely on the individual to react in emergent situations. These goals and their accomplishment are negotiated via communication channels.

A work context far removed from the daily office routine illustrates the importance of allowing individual and organizational goals to be co-obtainable. The setting was NASA's 1973 Apollo 3 flight during which the astronaut team was given a rigorous set of assignments to accomplish during their time in space (Cooper, 1976). In this work environment, telecommunications provided the only link between the management and performance of the job.

In part, the centralized management structure based in Houston mirrored the location of the computer power, a disequilibrium of technology. Because data were being fed to the ground-based computer banks for storage and analysis, it was assumed that the orders initiating the space research should also be dictated from the ground. However, direct access to the environment, and all of the uncertainties associated with space exploration, resided in the crew and in their technologically lesser-equipped (compared to Mission Control) space lab.

To assure that all tasks were accomplished, Mission Control set an agenda that they expected the astronauts could follow. As the inevitable unexpected delays mounted, the overall mission objectives fell further behind schedule. Rather than release authority to the astronauts to deal with the emergent environment, Mission Control further tightened the schedule, using voice and data communications as elements of control. Lunch was shortened, and the favorite leisure activities of watching the sun and earth were replaced by "mission oriented" activities (Cooper, 1976). Frustrated by the growing imbalance between organizational and personal objectives, the team of astronauts conducted the first space strike. For one day they "turned off" Mission Control to restore balance between personal and organizational needs. The cost to NASA of this 24-hour work stoppage was estimated at $2,520,000 (Schoonhoven, 1986).

The 1973 space strike is a dramatic example of the costs of divorcing organizational and individual goals and using communication technology to segregate the control and execution of work exclusively toward organizational ends. In this instance, communication technologies were used to sustain, at least in the short run, this imbalance between control and execution of work and between institutional and individual goals. This same imbalance is a contributing factor to the resistance with which new communication technologies are being introduced into other common work settings, such as the office (Leuder, 1986).

In spite of the promise of office technology, its diffusion into the office has been much slower than originally expected. Leuder (1986) associates much of the problem with the changes in work instituted by information technology. Among other factors, she argues that the new communication technologies decrease worker autonomy and at the same time increase individual accountability and job pressure. Several obvious examples of this technologically skewed relationship include word processing programs that count keystrokes per minute and electronic mail systems that automatically produce "paper trails" of interactions.

Not surprisingly, the response of workers to overly proscriptive technologies has ranged between slowed adoption and sabotage. The resultant cost to the organization is matched by equally damaging consequences in the form of job-related stress to users who cannot establish the autonomy to balance organizational and personal needs in the new office environment.

Smith, Colligan, and Hurrell (1977) found secretarial work, with its low autonomy, to rank second out of 130 occupations with respect to stress. However, technology-induced stress is distributed across organizational levels. New information systems have caused stress in senior management responsible for their implementation, and workers at midcareer concerned about being replaced by managers with greater computer literacy (Marks, 1985). Other stress-related issues associated with implementing new information technologies include reduced job security and increased job ambiguity and role conflict (Leuder, 1986).

Designs that induce stress have many negative consequences for workers. The relationship of stress to heart disease has been well established and well-publicized. Palmore (1969) found work satisfaction (inversely correlated to job-induced stress) to be the number-one predictor of life expectancy in the United States, a better predictor than ratings of happiness, results of medical examinations, or the use of tobacco. The sheer number of persons involved in office work underscores the importance of stress in the office. Since the turn of the century, clerical work has moved from the smallest (3% of the work force) to the largest (48% of the work force) occupational category (Braverman, 1974; Bureau of Labor Statistics, 1984). The point is that design that ignores social context and contributes to job-related stress has serious consequences for individuals and related high social costs.

Social Epicenter

In addition to its influence on autonomy, technology can impose problematic influences on social processes such as decision making. Increasingly, conditions arise in which the superior technology rather than the superior argument influences the outcomes of the negotiation process. An example of this occurred in a 1984 graduate class cosponsored by Ohio State University and Ohio University. In the course offering, a class at each institution was joined via audio, video, and computer channels for the purpose of negotiating a rewriting of the 1934 Communications Act within an "electronic decision making environment" (Acker, Clift, & Branco, 1985). Students met in mediated conferences as lobbyists representing broadcasting, cable, telephone, and the public interest, each with the expressed purpose of trying to influence the final legislation so that it reflected their constituencies' interests.

Although a subsequent analysis of audio-only transcripts indicated the positions taken by students at both sides were judged to be equally persuasive, when viewed as videotaped sessions, the lobbyists at one university were judged to be more persuasive. These students were imaged in a studio equipped with $70,000 cameras and presented by camera shots selected by a skilled director. The other group of students was shot in an "electronic classroom" equipped with a $3,000 camera set on a continuous medium long shot. Among the lessons learned from this encounter was that even when a situation was designed with the expressed purpose of creating equality of arguments, technical disparities interceded in the process. Superior equipment and its use created a host-remote relationship between the two videoconference sites. Only in later face-to-face meetings was the desired "epicenter communication environment" established between the two classes.

Action Language

The space station, electronic mail, and negotiation examples present circumstances in which the technological system was inconsistent with or distorted the healthy functioning and needs of the social system. In contrast, Winograd (1987-1988) describes how a designer can incorporate social context to produce a more useful technology. He describes an electronic mail system conceived on the role of conversational context and the flexibility it gives to the system.

Winograd (1987-1988) argues for a design perspective premised on language pragmatics, or the realization that language functions to achieve goals. Based on Austin's (1962) Speech Act Theory, as refined by Searle (1975), the language/action perspective suggests that language is exchanged between individuals in the global context of a *conversation* that ends in a state of *completion*. Completed conversations occur when neither party is awaiting further utterances on the topic of conversation. For example, a conversation might be initiated with a request for information. It is completed when the other person provides the information *or* indicates that they cannot answer the question. Either response tells the conversation initiator that the conversation is concluded.

By detailing the various transition points within a conversation, one can devise an electronic messaging system that tracks the social "contracts" between communicators, and that simultaneously conveys: (1) the context of an utterance, (2) whose turn it is to act, and (3) a set of possible response types. The power of the system is that it takes advantage of the interpretative skills of the users and requires the software designer to provide only the structure within which the conversation takes place (Winograd, 1987-1988). Such a system has been devised by Flores and his colleagues and released under the name of *The Coordinator* (Flores, Bell, Graves, & Ludlow, 1987; cf. Winograd, 1987-1888.)

The Coordinator is a menu-driven message exchange system. An opening menu initiates a conversation with a *request* or *offer* for action. When the message is received, the recipient's screen presents prompts that are available within which to contextualize the response. These prompts suggest such categories as *acknowledge, promise, counter-offer* and *decline*. The appropriately contextualized response is returned to the initiator for her next action, such as *interim report, cancel* or *report-completion*. Ultimately, the conversation is managed to a state of completed action. By extracting the current transition state from each of the conversations in which an individual is involved, a *commitment* list can be generated. This commitment list serves as a calendar to show the system user where she stands with respect to her obligations in completing social contracts. (The interested reader is referred to Winograd, 1987-1988, for a fuller discussion of the language-action perspective on system design).

While this application of social context demonstrates how the social system can be productively used by a designer, its application remains bound by the designer's assumptions about the social system into which it will be placed. For example, among persons who share power and are mutually benefited by completing social contracts, the advantages are clear. However, a dictatorial sales manager could misuse the system as a tool to consolidate power over a sales force.

In summary, social context plays an important role in communication system design. Three issues that must be considered are: (1) How can user autonomy be maintained through an appropriate balance between technological and user control? (2) How can distribution of the technology be accomplished as a "neutral" tool that equally empowers users brought together by the system? and (3) How can the tremendous associative and meaning generating capacities of the human users supplement the limited intelligence than can be made resident within a machine?

THE INDIVIDUAL USER

Social contexts are established among individuals. In the case of interactions mediated by communication technology, the interface between the user and the machine will influence the social context established. The designer's assumptions about the user interface are represented in her or his "mental model" of the user. At various levels of abstraction, mental models of the human-machine interface have been developed to guide the design process (Lansdale, 1985).

The designer's mental model has the difficult task of representing the multiple mental models brought to the technology by the individual users. Rich (1986) has argued that traditional system design has been premised on the idea of an "average" user, and that while such design will make the system accessible to many users, it will not be ideally suited for any one. "A much better system would be one in which the interface presented to each person was tailored to his [*sic*] own characteristics rather than to those of some abstract "typical person" (Rich, pp. 184-185).

It may be useful to compare the system designer's problems with individualization to those encountered by a conversationalist trying to "really communicate" in an interpersonal meeting. Both the designer and the conversationalist begin by inferring the needs, abilities, characteristics, and so on of their interacting partner. This is the process of constructing an *initial profile* of the conversational partner (system user). This initial profile establishes the basis on which the interaction session will begin and establishes constraints on where the interaction might lead. For example, an automatic teller machine (ATM) is designed to serve a very limited set of initial profiles: individuals needing to withdraw or deposit funds or those needing information on their current balance. To meet the needs of a larger set of initial profiles would require more complex system design.

Based on the initial profile, both the skilled conversationalist and competent designer will seek to structure dialogue that successfully keeps the session moving, and in such a way that both partners' needs are being met. In system design, this goal involves structuring the interaction patterns so that the system can respond to the queries of the user and the user knows how to request and convey information. This is the realm of *dialogue design* and identifies the problems in establishing the symbol systems (iconic or textual) and questioning protocols that guide interaction sessions.

Finally, a system designer would like to incorporate the skilled conversationalist's capacity to *dynamically reconfigure* the profile of the conversational partner (system user) so that the interaction can become more successful during the course of the dialogue. Incorporating this dynamic sensitivity is a major challenge of system design and underscores much of the research in artificial intelligence. If this "learning capacity" is not in the designer's repertoire, the success of the user-machine interactions will depend on how carefully the designer has "programmed in" useful conversational "scripts," or regular patterns that generally meet user needs. However, the trend is toward flexible system design for integrated work stations. Supporting this user preference, Bickson and Guteck (1983) found that technologies that assist in a broad range of activities are better accepted than are systems dedicated to a single need.

Usually, the designer operates from the desire to be the deferential conversational partner to the system user (but see Fredin, this volume, for arguments favoring more proactive assumptions). This desire to interpret and respond to the needs of the user has fostered the design perspective of *user-centered system design* (Norman & Draper, 1986). From a communication perspective, user-centered design can be approached as establishing a successful conversation based on the user's initial profile, responsive dialogue structures, and procedures of dynamically reconfiguring that profile.

Initial Profile

An early design issue involves assessing the level of knowledge with which a user comes to the technology-based interaction. The goal of the designer is to categorize the user and ideally adjust the interaction patterns to accommodate the level of expertise and conversational preferences of the individual. One approach to this issue is to use a taxonomy that defines a user's *semantic* and *syntactic* knowledge of machine-based communication systems (Cole, Lansdale, & Christie, 1985).

		Semantic Knowledge	
		No	Yes
Syntactic Knowledge	No	naive	casual expert
	Yes	associative experts	experienced pros

User initial profiles based on previous knowledge.

Figure 9.2 System users can be categorized into one of four groups based on their semantic and syntactic knowledge of machine-based communication systems (from Cole, Lansdale & Christie, 1985; p. 215).

Semantic knowledge refers to the user's *conceptual* information about how information systems might be organized to address problems. For example, a user's understanding of the sorting process by which a database might search along two dimensions and compile a list of "hits" is an example of semantic knowledge. Similarly, knowing that *delete* means that the system will purge information would be a representation of a user's semantic knowledge of information technologies.

Syntactic knowledge is *system specific* knowledge at the level of understanding the rules of a particular software system. For example, the Wylbur program implemented on an IBM 3081 system gets rid of files by "scratching" them. On the other hand, a Macintosh microcomputer deletes files by moving an icon representing the file into an icon of a trash can.

As Figure 9.2 indicates, four categories of users can be represented by this approach. *Naive users* know little of the general principles of how information technologies work or of specific commands related to a given system. *Casual users* understand how the technology works but know little of the specific language with which one interacts with the particular machine. *Associative experts* have memorized the particulars of a language, but have little underlying understanding of how the machine carries out their instructions. This group becomes very facile at routine work but has difficulty solving puzzles associated with new situations. The final group, *experienced pros,* understands the technology and has learned the exact syntax of the particular system. (See Figure 9.2).

From this initial profile, different dialogue structures can be developed to facilitate the human-machine interaction.

Dialogue Structure

The interaction pattern selected by the designer reflects the expected type of user and the task. Different approaches to mental modeling motivate different dialogue structures. Successful dialogue structures allow users to intuitively and easily interact with the machine (MacGregor & Slovic, 1986). Ideally, dialogue structures are matched to user groups and tasks. Cole, Lansdale, and Christie (1985) offer this taxonomy of dialogue structures:

question and answer	the system prompts for information provided by the user.
form filling-	the system displays a form that is filled in by the user.
query languages	the user initiates the dialogue with key words associated with specific functions.
menu selection	the system displays user options from which the user then selects.
function keys	the keyboard rather than the screen provides the options available to the user.
command language	similar to query language, but relies on "computerese" for efficiency.
graphic interaction	the user selects from a graphic menu rather than using verbal languages.
natural language	the user communicates with the system with little regard to specific word choice or syntax. Assumes very sophisticated, "interpretive" language used in system design.
hybrid dialogues	a dialogue structure that mixes interaction styles based on the specific transaction. While more powerful, may be more confusing.
parallel dialogues	the system offers several dialogue structures each operable at the preference of the user.

Each dialogue structure has applications in different situations. For novices, a system initiated session makes fewer demands on the user. For the professional, a user-initiated system often is more flexible and less time-consuming. Socially open systems allow different dialogue structures to be presented to different classes of users.

One highly developed form of hybrid system design incorporates visual imagery rather than text. It has been applied in many designs that avoid presenting the computer as a computer, but present the interaction environment as a surrogate for the office, or part of the user's environment. Spence and Apperley's (1982) Panorama Project demonstrates this approach. In their application, the needed information was presented as office icons projected onto the wall. When an icon was selected, it appeared on a screen before the user. The selected information was presented in "bifocal" vision: Whichever image was selected appeared in sharp focus, while perimeter objects were shown "blurred" to provide surrounding context for the object of focus. The Panorama Project illustrates the design principle of incompleteness in that the abstract icons are all given "custom" meanings by different users' representations of their own concrete office setting.

The Panorama Project and the earlier Spatial Data Management System (SDMS) project at MIT served as the basis for important developments in the microcomputer industry. Xerox's Star and Apple's Macintosh both refined ideas originally seen in Panorama and SDMS. All of these systems share a commitment to completing the technological system with references to the user's world.

Christie (1985, p. 143) offers a useful summary of serviceable dialogue structures. The interaction system should favor recognition over recall, deep processing, multiple prompts to facilitate incidental learning, context-rich imagery, high spatiality, concretization, familiarity, hierarchical nests, and personalization. Each of these characteristics draws the world knowledge of the user into the "ultimate" design of the system, one that assumes a complementary relationship between the social and technical system features.

Dynamic Reconfiguration

An important feature of mental models brought to a conversation is that they in fact are *not* static, but evolve through interaction of the system user and the machine (Norman, 1983). Usually these mental models that allow a person to act in their environment are not accurate in a technical sense, but are adequate in a functional sense. People intuit theories based on initial interactions and then modify them as needed through a trial-and-error process.

Besides allowing people to operate machine systems, an individual's mental models provide a greater or lesser feeling of security about the user's ability to interact with the technology. An individual's mental model assesses not only the technology but includes a user's beliefs about his or her own limitations. Individuals who feel insecure about their ability to use technology, often adopt suboptimum utilization strategies. For example, a person insecure about how to use a hand calculator might write down on paper intermediate results of a calculation rather than storing them in the calculator's internal memory. While this allows the user to successfully solve problems, it slows the process and introduces another step (transposing digits in the writing phase) of possible error into the calculation process.

A system designer creates a generalized conceptual model of the system that he or she tries to transfer as a mental model to be used by the end-users. The success of this transfer depends on the conceptual models' learnability, functionality, and usability (Norman 1983, p. 13). To be helpful, the designer's conceptual model must relate to the end-users world (learnability), help the user make decisions in situations they face (functionality), and be simple enough that they can be brought to bear on the problem at hand (usability).

Each feature of the conceptual model has ramifications for the design process. Learnability is important because early trials settle users into patterns that may or may not be efficient. This relates to Simon's (1982) assumption that people act on the first adequate rather than later optimum approach to a problem. Functionality implies the need for social grounding and usability suggests that the technology will be used only if it is easy to do so.

One popular approach to addressing the issue of learnability is to rely on analogy and metaphor. While this satisfies the condition of relating to the user's world, it can be limiting as well as adaptive. At some point, the new technology must function differently (better) than the operations that form the basis for the analogy, or there is no rationale for introducing it to the user. When analogies and metaphors are the basis for introducing users to technology, the limits of the analogy must be clearly expressed (Lansdale, 1985).

Bruner (1986) describes how individuals construct their worlds by invoking the highly inductive processes of *storytelling*. He differentiates storytelling as a way of thinking that is distinct from another system he calls *argument*. Both modes of thought can form the basis for learning. Argument derives understanding from valid statements, using formal logic as the transfer mechanism. Designers in the process of design often rely on argument to motivate their work. On the other hand, storytelling relies on verisimilitude, or lifelikeness to justify conclusions (Bruner, 1986).

In the area of communication technology, few users have the training to fathom the arguments of the system designers, so instead construct analogies or metaphors consistent with their own experiences. In other words, how machines operate are interpreted by a user, based on similarities with things he or she does understand.

DESIGNS OF INCOMPLETENESS

An overall goal of system design is to create technologies capable of adapting to the social contexts of individual users and their idiosyncratic mental models. Adaptability implies that the machine is *incomplete* without a social structure for form and function. A design principle of "incompleteness" requires the system designer to incorporate the user as a source of complementary resources and structure to "finish" the technology. Thus the design process, generating concrete realizations of conceptual problems, must await the catalytic properties of social context before it gels into a final form or "product." Five examples of system design informed by the principle of incompleteness follow.

REACH—The Bar-Coded Learning Environment[1]

REACH is a technology-based learning system developed along the lines of socially open architecture to teach audio production skills (Acker, 1985-1986). The learning system used a radio studio in which the production tools (e.g., cart machine, turntable, microphone) were labeled with bar codes similar to those found on items in grocery stores. A microcomputer equipped with a bar code wand was placed in the studio. By running the tip of the wand across one of the bar codes attached to each of 50 different pieces of equipment, the student could access information stored on a floppy disc about that piece of equipment. Passing the wand across a bar code triggered the computer's disc drive to find the material about the associated piece of audio equipment and present it on the computer's monitor.

Several socially open architecture characteristics distinguish this learning system. Most importantly, the dialogue structure, the process through which the student interacts with the computer, is invested in the user rather than the technology. Rather than responding to screen prompts, each query of the system is instigated by the user at the moment that he or she needs information.

The design principle of incompleteness is represented in that every user establishes the parameters of the interaction. Besides a very brief standardized direction set (pass the bar code reader attached to this computer across the labels attached to equipment to learn their function), the learning environment is fully customized by the learner through the series of question asked; the computer is not preprogrammed to sequence material in any particular way. This design assumes an active learner engaged in solving problems.

In addition to not containing a predefined learning path, the technology is incomplete in another important way. The material to be learned exists as the actual three-dimensional objects in the audio studio rather than as computer-generated text or graphics. To operate, this technology requires the user be in an environment to complete the learning system (local closure).

The features of local closure and user-centeredness relieve the designer from the complex tasks of creating graphic representations of the audio studio and surmising the knowledge gaps that may exist in different users. As an additional benefit, the system can be easily updated. When the studio changes, new descriptive screens are written and indexed to a new bar code attached to the new equipment. The intent of this design is to place the technology in the service of the user and to avoid restricting the user's interaction patterns to the system's software capabilities.

This approach has two potential limitations. First, the learner must visit an actual work environment in order to be trained. Second, the work environment must be customized with bar codes glued to equipment. Although it sacrifices some degree of concretization, the design principle of incompleteness can be extended to remote learning locations by using photographs of the studio rather than the actual equipment as the stimulus. To learn about a component of the audio lab, the user loads a database and calls particular screens by referencing the codes attached to the photographs. The virtues of relieving the designer from inferring the needs of the user and of preserving the user's autonomy remain.

MORE LIKE—A Group Decision-Making System

The work of Winograd and Flores (1986) informs the design of MORE LIKE, a decision-making system created to operate in highly ambiguous environments. This videodisc-based simulation serves the purpose of helping interrelated group members reach consensus under circumstances of a volatile decision-making environment characterized by incomplete information. Such a simulation has application in business, educational, and military environments (Acker & Debloois, 1986).

Ambiguity is another term for "cognitive distance" or the "chasm of inference" that a decision maker must span in dealing with uncertainty. Ambiguity has at least three dimensions: (1) the degree to which a decision maker is familiar with the environment, (2) the ratio of publicly shared knowledge to privately held knowledge among all individuals who must reach consensus in the decision-making process, and (3) the rate of change in the flow of events that define the problem.

As a general rule, we would expect the decision-making process to evolve as ambiguity was reduced. In a group process, discussion of an ambiguous situation could be viewed as a process of communication *breakdown* and *repair* (Winograd & Flores, 1986). Communication breakdowns do not necessarily mean failure of understanding, but refer to points in conversation at which interactants become aware of how language structures our understanding of a situation and will guide future action. Repair is the process by which interactants use this awareness to reach a consensus of intentions and negotiate their joint action.

This process of breakdown and repair succinctly describes how communication directs a group toward achieving goals. Through language use, individuals develop intention-driven, goal-directed action *in common*. Fostering a conscious awareness of this process is essential for effective action in nonroutine, rapidly changing environments since groups can act only in the representation of the environment created through language use. This is the key design point—in ambiguous environments the reality of the environment emerges in its representation by the group, it is not predetermined. Problem-solving actions have meaning and influence proportionate to the group's consensual understanding.

To train decision makers in how to operate under fast changing, ambiguous situations, a simulation environment can be helpful. For example, if the target learning group is entrepreneurs in charge of start-up companies, three vignettes could be designed: (1) a military command post, (2) a disaster relief agency and (3) a fictional high-tech start-up company. Each scenario poses the same problem: How can action be planned in the face of an ill-structured problem under rapidly evolving circumstances?

For each scenario, several levels of complexity can be established. At the lowest level of complexity, the characters of the simulations are represented on the videodisc as individuals with a finite menu of optional behaviors. The group of learners publicly discuss and then select the actions of the characters as the simulation moves toward completion of a task, such as transporting food from an airport to a relief shelter 30 miles away.

At this lowest level of complexity, the learning group acts in concert to control the activities of individual characters. This level of complexity is constituted by public debate of the intentions of each character in the interaction. Progress toward completion of the task in the simulation occurs as the group reaches agreement on what a character should do and why he or she would reasonably act in that particular way.

Complexity increases as the actors on the videodisc are replaced, one by one, with real persons from the learning group. With each replacement of a character by a live person, the group consensus process becomes more private and consequently more ambiguous. To allow group consensus to emerge, learners must explicitly argue the intentions of their individual characters. The skill developed is in foregrounding implicit, nonarticulated assumptions—a competency that describes the manager who is successful in operating under conditions of ambiguity. In the discussions, "breakdowns" in the group problem-solving strategies will emerge. The negotiations surrounding these breakdowns promote an understanding of how concerns appear to each member of the organization and how competent managers organize commitment to overcome these concerns.

By immersing learners in three more progressively novel settings, the invisible activities that constitute sense-making in an individual's day-to-day world will surface in the unfamiliar context. In other words, individuals often learn more from worlds in which they are not directly involved simply because they cannot take things for granted. For example, a university professor teaching in the "parallel world" of a business establishment will find that many taken-for-granted classroom strategies are challenged in the workplace. Implicit assumptions may fail to work in the changed teaching environment. The teacher learns precisely because corporate teaching is not routine and long-hidden assumptions become apparent and can be analyzed.

Through experience in the successively more distant simulated environments of the relief agency and the military command post, the entrepreneurs become progressively more self-analytic about their communication behavior. In the process, they may develop skill in resolving ambiguous problem-laden situations. This design can be seen as one in which the mediated components of the communication technology are progressively replaced with the social components of the decision-making process.

Looker—Using Visual Interest

Richard Bolt, of the MIT Media Lab group, has been experimenting with a unique system interface designed to meet the individual needs of users. In its current state of development, Looker uses a pupilometer to register the interest of users in a visual image presented on a screen. It does so by aggregating the record of eye fixations on different objects in the presented image. The areas of greatest interest suggest to the database developer where to put their efforts in the descriptive information that can be made available to the system user as output. The refinement of interest to Bolt is to allow Looker to operate interactively so that each person's individual preferences, as expressed through points of visual regard, can be used as an input device to access the database. The reciprocal system, Show-er, then dynamically reconstructs the database to "answer" questions responsive to the interests of the user as registered from their gaze patterns (MIT Media Laboratory Videodisc, 1987).

Grundy—A Personal Librarian

Rich (1986) offers an example of an "electronic reference librarian," whose task is to help patrons find interesting novels. The system, known as Grundy, operates on the basis of stereotypes. Grundy first asks a patron to input a few self-descriptive phrases. Grundy uses these "trigger" words to formulate a stereotype, or a "typical" set of interests associated with such a user-profile.

The books in Grundy's database are represented as values on a set of *facets* or attributes, such as *sports, romance, tolerate violence, gender of protagonist.* Based on a stereotype associated with the patron's self-described attributes, Grundy suggests a book that might interest the patron. If the patron indicates that the book is of interest, the stereotype is strengthened. If the patron rejects the selection, the stereotype is relaxed and a book from a different literary category (possessing a different mix of values on the facets) is offered. Grundy has a set of rules through which to resolve apparent contradictions in classifying the user. In the process, Grundy "learns" as it dynamically reconceptualizes the user during the session, and also uses each interaction to refine its stereotypic representation of males, females, sportsperson, and other defining categories (Rich, 1986).

ACCESS—Modern Visual Art Appreciation[2]

Among the things that limit access to modern visual arts may be the audience's unwillingness to invest in the unknown. To increase an audience's willingness to consider modern visual art, a videodisc-based museum "guide" was designed (Acker & Green, 1986). Rather than assume what to tell each individual museum patron, ACCESS was designed to be incomplete without the participation of the audience.

The videodisc's welcome screen presents an eight-by-five matrix of icons. The eight columns represent eight works of art and the five columns represent influences on the production of works of art. The influences are: (1) the artist's personal life or biography, (2) the sociopolitical milieu in which the artist worked (e.g., the Vietnam War), (3) the artistic culture of which the artist is a part, and preceding artistic movements that the work reacts against or advances, (4) the materials available (e.g., acrylic oils, spun aluminum, spray paint), and (5) the work's iconography or visual elements.

The guide works by allowing the user to touch the monitor at the intersection of any of the influences and works. Thus a user can make any of

40 selections per set of eight works of art. The pattern of selections permits the user to examine a work of art, or trace an influence across works of art. For example, if a user found him- or herself interested in the new forms of sculpture and dynamic balances made possible by new, stronger materials such as aircraft spun aluminum, the materials influence could be followed through a series of art works.

The videodisc's most complex design feature is the need to track the user's selections and then identify the common features among them. Through this process, the system constructs a profile of the user and can then "guess" as to the kind of interests that individual has. Acker and Fredin (1987) describe this process as constructing the user's "preference function." The preference function is used not to target the user's interests, but to move the system user "off center" by introducing a work of art that is related, but not identical to, the features of art pursued by the visitor. By selecting a work sufficiently different than the user's profile but not so different as to jar the user, the system can guide the user to an expanded set of accessible (interesting but not repelling) examples of art. Importantly, the user is essential to completing the system's design since the videodisc's purpose is to identify each individual's preferences and then elaborate on them.

Each of these five systems is an attempt to individualize rather than typify the human-machine interaction process. Modifications in creating the initial profile, structuring the dialogue, and dynamically reconfiguring the user profile are characteristics of each design. They represent possibly heuristic examples of socially open architecture and the design principle of incompleteness.

SUMMARY AND CONCLUSIONS

The design of information technologies has become increasingly important as the effectiveness of social and organizational systems grows more dependent on the communication among subsystems. Much of the work on information technologies has occurred as experimental or field evaluations of new technologies. While both are valuable sources of information, the contribution of each might best be realized from within a design orientation. Since both the social and technological systems are undergoing rapid evolution, there is little basis on which future action can be planned. However, taken together, field, experimental, and design studies can inform the process of implementing new communication technologies into various social contexts.

New communication technologies embody the philosophy of their designers. While these philosophies do not exist in a vacuum and certainly are partly formed by the organizational, social, and economic systems in which the designer works, the individual designer's expectations with respect to the purpose of the technology and the social and individual characteristics of the system's users contribute substantially to the technological system's final form and function. The technological system, the reification of the goal structures of designers, and the social system, an aggregate of individuals also pursuing goals, interact to produce social change.

The designer's value system operates because of the very nature of the design process. Design deals with the discovery process of action in which problems are formulated. Design can be grounded in action research that assumes that humans themselves structure situations and invent actions based on a principle of cognitive economy. Design structures emergent problems and then, based on that structure, presents to a user a set of possible actions. The design process must provide people a set of acceptable alternatives on which to premise their actions, or the system will not be adopted and used.

This chapter produced one set of values with respect to the sociotechnical system into which communication technology is embedded. The goals and assumptions were summarized with the phrase "socially open architecture," the purpose of which is to showcase the design principle of incompleteness. It was argued that a precursor to open architecture in the hardware sense assumes an essential complementary support structure will be provided by the user, not ultimately solved with a later generation of machines. The potential invested in the technology should be activated by the social system, characterized by autonomy, equal access, and a rich social organization that can be drawn on in such a way as to make the designer's role easier and the system configuration less complex. In contrast to this design orientation, much communication technology design has been premised on advanced Taylorism, or the expectation that cybernetics (feedback systems) can be conceived that will guide a system toward desired ends. As suggested by the Three-Mile Island nuclear accident, closed system design presents potentially serious dangers. Knowledge support systems defined so that machines provide only restrictive guidance can be equally self-limiting and destructive.

Values imply a process of choice and the goals associated with socially open architecture certainly are not the only available goal set, or even necessarily the best set. However, they are influential in that they result in concrete technologies, such as REACH, ACCESS, and Grundy. In turn, each of these technological systems influence how individuals will use them.

At the individual level, user-centered design is a dominant paradigm currently operating. In many respects, it borrows from communication competence by embodying the design process as relying on an initial profile, appropriately structured interchange mechanism and, ideally, the opportunity to adapt dynamically to the user in the course of interaction. While user-centered systems usually imply a deferential posture on the part of the technology, other situations, such as education, may be better served by an adversarial philosophy so that the initial desired ends are not achieved without some effort on the part of the user.

In conclusion, Christie (1985) has observed: "It will not be possible to program future systems to be entirely 'objective' or 'value free' in what information they decide to present to the user. It will be necessary for the designer to be very clear about the value judgments that are made in programming the system" (p. 169). This chapter has offered socially open architecture as one contributor to the necessary debate on this topic.

NOTES

1. The REACH project was supported by a grant from the Spencer Foundation.
2. ACCESS was supported in part by a grant from the Columbus Foundation.

REFERENCES

Acker, S. (1985-1986). Redesigning the human-machine interface for computer-mediated visual technologies. *Journal of Educational Technology Systems, 4*(1), 23-33.

Acker, S., Clift, C., & Branco, S. (1985). A two-way telecourse, interactive in both audio and video channels: A model for inter-institutional cooperation. *Issues in Higher Education, 14,* 16-23.

Acker, S., & Debloois, M. (1986). *Directing group action in highly ambiguous environments: Modeling organizational problem solving on videodisc.* Proposal to the Basic Research Office of the U.S. Army Research Institute.

Acker, S., & Fredin, E. (1987). *Designing interactive visual media: The issue of intelligibility.* Paper presented to the Visual Communication Conference, Alta, Utah.

Acker, S., & Green, J. (1986). *ACCESS: Introducing users to modern art.* Proposal to the Columbus Foundation.

Argyris, C., Putnam, R., & Smith, D. (1985). *Action science.* San Francisco: Jossey-Bass.

Argyris, C., & Schon, D. (1978). *Organizational learning.* Reading, MA: Addison-Wesley.

Austin, J. (1962). *How to do things with words.* Cambridge, MA: Harvard University Press.

Beniger, J. (1986). *The control revolution.* Cambridge, MA: Harvard University Press.

Bickson, T., & Gutek, B. (1983). *Advanced office systems: An empirical look at utilization and satisfaction* (N-1970-NSF). Rand Corporation.

Braverman, H. (1974). *Labor and monopoly capital: The degradation of work in the twentieth century.* New York: Monthly Press Review.

Brown, J., & Newall, S. (1985). Issues in cognitive and social ergonomics: From our house to Bauhaus. *Human-Computer Interaction, 1*(4), 359-391.

Bruner, J. (1986). *Actual minds, possible worlds.* Cambridge, MA: Harvard University Press.

Bureau of Labor Statistics, U.S. Department of Labor (1984). *Annual earnings by occupation and industry: U.S. labor force.* Washington, DC: Author.

Carnall, C., & Medland, A. (1984). Computer-aided design: Social and technical choices for Development. In M. Warner (Ed.), *Microprocessors, manpower and society.* Aldershot, England: Gower.

Christie, J. (Ed.). (1985). *Human factors of information technology in the office.* New York: John Wiley.

Cole, I., Lansdale, M., & Christie, B. (1985). Dialogue design guidelines. In B. Christie (Ed.), *Human factors of information technology in the office.* New York: John Wiley.

Cooper, H. (1976). *A house in space.* New York: Holt, Rinehart & Winston.

Dobos, J., & Grieve, S. (1985). Synchronous computer conferencing: Protocols and procedures for productive use of time. In. L. Parker & C. Olgren (Eds.), *Teleconferencing and electronic communication* (Vol. IV, p. 370-380). Madison, WI: University of Wisconsin-Extension, Center for Interactive Programs.

Eckholm, E. (1984, October 2). Computer conferences lose face. *New York Times*, p. C1, C5.

Flores, F., Bell, C., Graves, M., & Ludlow, J. (1987). *The coordinator workgroup productivity system I* [Computer program, Version 1.5P]. Emeryville, CA: Action Technologies.

Hiltz, R., & Turoff, M. (1978). *Network nation: Human communication via computer*. Reading, MA: Addison-Wesley.

Hirschhorn, L. (1984). *Beyond mechanization*. Cambridge, MA: MIT Press.

Huse, E. (1980). Quality of worklife and sociotechnical approaches. In E. Huse (Ed.), *Organization development and change*. St. Paul, MN: West.

Jahoda, M. (1979). The impact of unemployment in the thirties and the seventies. *Bulletin of the British Psychological Society, 32,* 309-314.

Jaikumar, R. (1986, November-December). Postindustrial manufacturing. *Harvard Business Review*, 69-76.

James, W. (1950). *The principles of psychology (Volume 1)*. New York: Dover. (Original work published in 1890)

Kiesler, S., Siegel, J., & McGuire, T. (1984). Social psychological aspects of computermediated communication. *American Psychologist, 39,* 1123-1134.

Lansdale, M. (1985). Beyond dialogue design: The role of mental models. In B. Christie (Ed.), *Human factors of information technology in the office*. New York: John Wiley.

Leuder, R. (1986). The office in context. In R. Leuder (Ed.), *The ergonomic payoff: Designing the electronic office*. New York: Nichols.

Lewin, K. (1948). *Resolving social conflicts*. New York: Harper & Row.

MacGregor, D., & Slovic, P. (1986). Graphic representation of judgmental information. *Human-Computer Interaction 2*(3), 179-200.

Margolis, B., Kroes, W., & Quinn, R. (1974). Job stress: An unlisted occupational hazard. *Journal of Occupational Medicine, 16*(10), 659-661.

Marks, S. (1985, April 15). High tech: High stress? *Datamation*, 97-100.

MIT Media Laboratory. (1987) [videodisc]. MIT Media Laboratory, Cambridge, MA.

Mooney, M. (1988). *The social-psychological effects of visually and aurally enhanced computer conferencing*. Unpublished masters thesis, Ohio State University.

Nadin, M. (1988, January 29). *Minds as configurations: Intelligence is process*. Graduate School Lecture Series, Ohio State University.

Newall, A., & Card, S. (1985). The prospects for psychological science in human-computer interaction. *Human-Computer Interaction, 1,* 209-242.

Norman, D. (1983). Some observations on mental models. In D. Gentner & A. Stevens (Eds.), *Mental models*. Hillsdale, NJ: Lawrence Erlbaum.

Norman, D., & Draper, S. (1986). *User centered system design: New perspectives on human-computer interaction*. Hillsdale, NJ: Lawrence Erlbaum.

Palmore, E. (1969). Predicting longevity: A follow-up controlling for age. *The Gerontologist, 9*(4), 247-250.

Pava, C. (1983). *Managing new office technology: An organizational strategy*. New York: Free Press.

Pava, C. (1986). Redesigning sociotechnical systems design: Concepts and methods for the 1990s. *Journal of Applied Behavioral Science, 22*(3), 201-222.

Peccei, R., & Guest, D. (1984). Evaluating the introduction of new technology: The case of word-processors in British Rail. In M. Warner (Ed.), *Microprocessors, manpower and society*. Aldershot, England: Gower.

Perez, R. (1985). *VMCO Documentation for Pre-release Version 1.2*. [Computer program]. Available as a text file in the Compuserve MACUS forum.

Phillips, A. (1983). Computer conferencing: Success or failure? In R. Bostrom (Ed.), *Communication yearbook 7* (pp. 837-856). Beverly Hills, CA: Sage.

Rich, E. (1986). Users are individuals: Individualizing user models. In R. Davies (Ed.), *Intelligent information systems*. New York: John Wiley.

Rogers, E. (1986). *Communication technology: The new media in society*. New York: Free Press.

Schneiderman, B. (1987). *Designing the user interface: Strategies of effective human-computer interaction*. Reading, MA: Addison-Wesley.

Schon, D. (1983). *The reflective practitioner: How professionals think in action*. New York: Basic Books.

Schon, D. (1985). *The design studio: An exploration of its traditions and potential*. London: RIBA.

Schoonhoven, C. (1986). Sociotechnical considerations for the development of the space station: Autonomy and the human element in space. *Journal of Applied Behavioral Science, 22*(3), 271-286.

Searle, J. (1975). A taxonomy of illocutionary acts. In K. Gunderson (Ed.), *Language, mind and knowledge* (pp. 344-369). Minneapolis: University of Minnesota Press.

Simon, H. (1982). Observation of a business decision. In H. Simon (Ed.), *Models of bounded rationality: Behavioral economics and business organization, Volume 2*. Cambridge, MA: MIT Press.

Smith, M., Colligan, M., & Hurrell, J. (1977). A review of NIOSH psychological stress research. *Proceedings of the 1977 NIOSH Conference on Occupational Stress*.

Spence, R., & Apperley, M. (1982). Data base navigation: An office environment for the professional. *Behavior and Information Technology, 1*(1), 43-45.

Trist, E., Higgens, G., Murray, H., & Pollock, A. (1963). *Organizational choice: Capabilities of groups at the coal face under changing technologies*. London: Tavistock.

Winograd, T. (1987-1988). A language/action perspective on the design of cooperative work. *Human-Computer Interaction, 3*(1), 3-30.

Winograd, T., & Flores, F. (1986). *Understanding computers and cognition: A new foundation for design*. Norwood, NJ: Ablex.

Interactive Communication Systems, Values, and the Requirement of Self-Reflection

ERIC S. FREDIN
Ohio State University

THIS commentary is an elaboration of points found in the Acker chapter and the Gagnon commentary, rather than a criticism of them. Basically, I am in agreement with the main points found in both works, and many of my points are complementary to theirs. I will start by developing a list of implications that can be drawn from an example Acker used to demonstrate that terms often fail to describe the state of new technology. The first implications explicate some of the difficulties involved in predicting the uses of a new technology. Additional implications lead to the question of whether the ultimate goal of a new communication system is being functionally equivalent to an older communication mode. I then discuss a new technology project—the development of a computer news system—in which we are attempting to go beyond the goal of functional equivalence. Moving beyond functional equivalence requires the socially open architecture proposed by Acker; new goals must emerge from interactions with the new technology. The aspect of socially open architecture I wish to elaborate upon is the kind of effort required by users. If individuals are to contribute significantly to the new goals, they must be self-reflective, else the locus of control lies in the technology. The emergence of new goals in turn raises methodological issues that become manifest during research done during the design stages of the technology. Verbalizing attempts at self-reflection can create data, the validity of which is most likely to be challenged within an experimental paradigm. Rather than pick sides, however, the designer and implementer should internalize any conflict.

AUTHOR'S NOTE: This work was funded in large part by a seed grant from Ohio State University.

Correspondence and requests for reprints: Eric S. Fredin, Department of Journalism, Ohio State University, Columbus, OH 43210.

Communication Yearbook 12, pp. 533-546

SOPHISTICATION, CONVENIENCE, AND SLIPPERY INFERENCES

Generalizations concerning the new technology must be made with reference to a particular system, and often with reference to a specific use of a particular system. Ways of systematically characterizing new technology and the contexts in which they are used are being developed (e.g., Heeter, 1985). At this point, however, both the communication technology and the contexts in which it is used should be considered unstable. The nature of some problems in designing, testing, and implementing new communication technology might be seen by elaborating upon Acker's notion of "lexical vestiges." Acker makes the important point that terms referring to new technology often evoke connotations associated with older versions of a technology. He argues that the term *computer conferencing* connotes a mode of communication that is weak in conveying nonverbal cues, and hence is a mode that reduces the social presence of the communicators. He then describes VCMO, computer-conferencing software, which runs on a Macintosh, and possesses very different qualities. (In the Apple system, discussants are represented by icons on the screen. Each discussant can control his or her icon. Using simple commands, discussants can make their icon show one of eight facial expressions, thus conveying nonverbal reactions.)

The issue is how can the generality of a statement or term be assessed when both the technologies and the contexts in which they are used are unstable? The points I am making purport to be general in that they indicate questions that can be addressed to many different kinds of systems and contexts. The bias in them is a bias toward more complex, interactive technologies that appear in contexts in which material or content is also complex. The points, in other words, do not pertain much to systems that are used for breaking tasks down into very simple units that can be done quickly and with little training.

Distractions of Simplistic and Sophisticated Features

Initial versions of new ideas can often have a simple, even childlike quality that can distract from assessing the importance of the underlying concepts. This characteristic is particularly true with graphics. It is hard to imagine, for example, that top executives would agree to use the VCMO personal icon system for conducting an important meeting. Conversely, sophisticated presentations can mask severe limitations in an underlying concept. A computer game, for example, might have fine resolution, fluid graphics, yet the game might quickly become boring because there is not enough variety and challenge to make the game intrinsically motivating (Malone, 1981). Simplistic graphics may be a symptom of inadequate hardware or low-level programming because simplistic graphics often can be traced to problems in computational speed or screen resolution. A simplistic game, on the other hand, is probably a symptom of excessively rigid higher-level software. If this is the case, then a key question is: Can the software be modified with reasonable ease?

The first point implies that a decision to accept or reject use of the technological system has not yet been made, but may be based on surface characteristics rather than on underlying system competencies.

Users Alter the Meaning of Technical Features

The second point is that once a system is implemented, users will seek ways to circumvent or overcome limitations in the technology in order to express themselves or better to achieve goals they deem important. Conventions to facilitate communication and to articulate what the system means to users will grow up around technologies (Hiemstra, 1983). For example, the Apple system allowed eight reactions, such as surprise, boredom, and anger, but did not allow for combinations, such as both surprise and anger, or both surprise and happiness. In many meetings it is necessary to express combinations of reactions. Conventions for expressing combinations of reactions could arise, which would circumvent this limitation. Combinations of reactions, for example, might be shown by toggling quickly between two reactions. This might have the initial effect of looking even more childlike than does just a single facial expression. However, if the need to express combinations of reactions were strong enough, the participants could learn to concentrate upon the intent of the others in the meeting rather than upon the style of expression. It should be noted that this scenario, which was speculation, did in fact happen (Perez, 1985).

The redefining of the purposes to which a technology is put may not simply elaborate the meaning originally assigned by the implementers. That users find new purposes that are far different than was the intent of the implementers is a recurrent theme in the study of communication technology (Rogers, 1983). In one research project that combined both experimental techniques and naturalistic observation, middle-school students used a videotext encyclopedia to gather information for a science term paper (Krendl & Fredin, 1985; Fredin & Krendl, 1987). The videotext encyclopedia presumably gave students more flexibility in searching for different articles related to the same topic. It was assumed that students would take notes as they used the encyclopedia, just as students using a regular encyclopedia would. However, many students used the videotext system to avoid taking notes. They simply found an article, then had the system print it, and took the copy home to write the paper. Often, these students spent little time looking at the article while they were using the computer system. Conversations students had while using the systems also revealed other meanings that students constructed about the system and how it worked (Anderson & Eastman, 1983).

The Principle of Slippery Inferences

The third point assumes that one is coping with a situation in which limiting features of the system can be changed. In this situation, the contexts in which the system might be embedded must be conceptualized in some detail. Specific properties of the presumed context must be identified, then considered in relation to the communication technology. There are no simplifying rules for identifying properties that may be important; if such rules existed, then the potential of new communication technology would be far more clear. With new communication technologies, the opportunity for change brings with it a peculiar set of difficulties.

A suggested solution to a problem often raises a long series of new potential opportunities and difficulties. From the perspective of the designer or implementer, the seriousness of the problems and the power of the opportunities are difficult to assess. From the perspective of the user, the novel problems may be difficult to keep in mind and tedious to correct. To illustrate these generalities, the specific properties of the context of use must first be identified. As an example, I have selected a personality trait that would seem to be relevant to the conduct of individuals during meetings. It also is a trait that may be relevant to the means by which the VCMO system might overcome the difficulties of nonverbal expression in computer conferencing.

It is plausible that the VCMO system could have several effects on self-monitoring (Snyder, 1974). Self-monitoring is the extent to which one observes and adjusts one's social presence in order to achieve one's goals. A person high in self-monitoring will often decide how to behave by attending carefully to others. A person high in self-monitoring may express more or less emotion than he or she feels or may express a different emotion. A person high in self-monitoring does not necessarily hide his or her feelings in order to be liked, but does so to achieve goals. The self-monitoring scale does not correlate strongly with scales tapping cynicism (Machiavellianism) because the self-monitor does not necessarily assume that the actions and motives of others are selfish and amoral. Also, self-monitoring does not correlate strongly with scales tapping the desire to act in socially appropriate ways because individuals high on such scales often are socially awkward (Fenigstein, 1979; Berger & Roloff, 1980).

Using icons to communicate reactions means that self-monitoring must in part operate through a new medium. (Self-monitoring also works through verbal communication, an aspect that is not addressed here.) Instead of communicating through gesture and facial expression, the user must decide which of the eight faces best matches what he or she wants to show. Further, the largely unconscious processes of setting gesture and facial expression while listening to others speak must be replaced by conscious processes. Thus, for the user, the new system would intrude, perhaps frequently, in a novel and potentially annoying manner. In general, new communication technologies can create problems that are difficult to keep in mind, and tedious as well. The problems may be overcome by practice, of course. They are not necessarily permanent any more than are numerous other properties of a system and its uses. But their impermanence does not distract from their importance. Users may treat the problem as more permanent than it need be, or the problem may be used as a reason for abandoning the technology altogether.

The possibility that self-monitoring will be disrupted could have group-level effects as well. Differences between high and low self-monitors may be altered. Low self-monitors may increase their self-monitoring, while high self-monitors may sense some loss of control. Further, each participant would be aware that the changes in self-monitoring are occurring, and the very awareness of the consciousness of the process might further alter, and confuse, interpretation of the reactions shown through the icons. Beyond this, any notions about using and interpreting the icons may need to shift as participants became more expert at manipulating the system and as conventions are established.

From the intersection of certain system features and certain features of users, inferences concerning potential problems can be drawn. One of the main reasons such inferences are slippery is that what are initially identified as problems often turn out not to be. The phenomenon may not be important. It may also be that the new system is readily learned, and a feature of the system becomes almost automatically used as the functional equivalent of a feature in older communication modes. In the case of the VCMO system, manipulating and watching icons may quickly become the functional equivalent of the control and reading of facial expression. This equivalence, of course, is what the system invites us to consider. Aspects of a system, which from one perspective are definitely novel, may be unimportant from another perspective because they are readily made the functional equivalent of some other process or phenomenon.

The points so far have made reference chiefly to implementation and early use. The focus also has been on cognitive and affective processes rather than on actual interaction with the technology. The response to the kinds of issues raised may, of course, be more technological than psychological or social. This possibility leads to the fourth point.

Initial Solutions May Lie in More Sophisticated Technology

Problems encountered can lead to the design of systems that are more sophisticated, particularly regarding the ways in which users input information. In the case of the Apple system, more sophisticated technology could lead to a way to manipulate the icons that in certain respects is more natural. Sensors could be placed on the faces of each participant. The sensors could pick up changes in facial expression that could lead to similar changes in the icons. Of course, wearing a kind of mask with sensors could be novel and distracting, to say the least. However, in one sense, the sensors could make control of the icons less intrusive because the same means people use to control facial expression would also be used to control the icons. The icons themselves could also be made more flexible so that more subtle and ambiguous reactions could be communicated. These proposed solutions should be considered as initial solutions only. The invention of a new technical solution should also initiate the construction and consideration of a new set of slippery inferences regarding potential problems and opportunities.

For example, the more sophisticated system might make the icons too sensitive to the reactions of users. Emotions expressed very briefly in face-to-face meetings might be more readily noticed on the screen, where all icons can be seen at once. Thus the highly sophisticated system, like the original primitive one, might alter the relations between low and high self-monitors by taking away some of the control that those high in self-monitoring have during face-to-face meetings. And once again, participants might find the communication technology intruding in annoying ways. And it may be that the revealing sensitivity of the system cannot be overcome as a practical matter.

This particular slippery inference also illustrates, at least in part, another principle: the grand-piano fallacy. The grand-piano fallacy states that great classical keyboard music is best when played on a grand piano, an instrument that did not exist during the lives of J. S. Bach, Scarlatti, Mozart, or Beethoven. The fallacy is meant here to suggest that a communication system that is more sophisticated or more sensitive to certain nuances is not necessarily a better means of communicating. Constraints along some dimensions may provide users needed control. The constraints on some dimensions may also focus attention on other dimensions. In some instances this may increase the effort involved, forcing greater clarity or understanding.

Designing more sophisticated input and output devices generally appears to move this particular communication technology toward a more complete replication of a face-to-face meeting. But this leads to questions about the goals of using the communication technology.

Goals: What Mix of Equivalence, Convenience, and Potential for Novelty?

Is designing a new communication technology ultimately worth the enormous effort if it primarily replicates an older communication mode? In the case of replication, the goal might be said to be complete functional equivalence. Functional equivalence, however important, does not really exploit the potential of new technologies. Yet even a system that appears to be functionally equivalent to some other may have the potential for spawning considerable change because it may make particular uses more convenient or less convenient. Changes in convenience may be powerful. The sweeping effects Innis (1977) attributes to changes in communication technology often stem from some technological aspect that makes certain activities—such as locating a quote or transporting written material—far more convenient (Krendl & Fredin, 1985). One need not be a technological determinist to appreciate changes that can begin by making an action more practical or simply more convenient. When designing and implementing new communication technology, the identification of convenience is another manifestation of the principle of slippery inferences: many conveniences may not be important, others may emerge as important only within contexts that develop around new technology, and some conveniences may emerge only with effort.

The issues of equivalence and convenience can be drawn out of the example of the VCMO system. Novelty of goals is more distant, however. A new technology project that moves toward fostering new goals, though it may not actually reach that point, is the computer news system I have been developing with others. A description of that system is needed to ground points about the novelty of goals and the requirements they may place upon users. The example will also serve to ground points about methodological issues involved in research into new technology.

THE COMPUTER NEWS PROJECT: CONSTRUCTING ONE'S OWN VERSION OF A STORY

In terms of a tangible product, the goal of the project is a prototype format for the presentation of news through the computer. It is assumed that if the computer is to become a medium for news, it must hold out the possibility of being substantially different from existing media in some respects. Functional equivalence with an existing medium is not enough, partly because the convenience of existing media in various contexts is difficult to beat. Parallels to existing media are inevitable, however, and in this regard, the new system is seen as being closest to a news and opinion magazine.

The basic strategy for developing the prototype is to place a wide range of choices about the amount and type of material seen *within* news stories and not simply *between* stories. This simple change raises fundamental questions about the construction of news articles because many of the forms and processes used are based in large measure upon the idea that one article is delivered to all users. It is clear that the notion of simply exploring a new medium is not enough to provide further direction, for it does not provide any standard against which to measure a design. One approach would be to devise statements about the needs of potential audiences, and to test them through empirical means. Our approach has been different. It has been to ask in what ways the computer system might address some of the perennial problems in journalism, particularly those concerning the idea of completeness (Klaidman & Beauchamp, 1987). Providing choice should offer the possibility of thorough explanations of terms and concepts, and of legal and organizational procedures that often underlie the news. Providing choice should also allow for fairly complete explication of differing viewpoints, and in general a more complete description of the contexts of events.

The format developed thus far is complex. It is based on the idea of hypertext. In hypertext, blocks of text are linked in a variety of ways. The overall organization is a flexible, complex network that allows each user to pursue and associate ideas and information in his or her own way (Conklin, 1987). A single story or "hyperstory" covers a large topic and consists of information from an extremely wide range of printed sources. It includes analysis, opinion, and background data as well as news reports. The content is divided into text panels of moderate length, each with its own headline. The panels are linked in a rather dense network that is established by the journalist. (As a start, there are about 100 text panels in a single story.) The structural context forces an emphasis on devising ways of organizing and presenting the material. Sets of links connect panels. Links include keywords as well as markers indicating whether material is news or opinion. Syntactic links are also important. Types of syntactic links include consequence, context, proposed solution, and evaluation. Panels of text appear in windows, and other windows carry headlines and linkage information about panels the reader can choose next. Multiple pathways between key panels the reader might follow are constructed by the journalists. Readers may stay on these paths, compare them, or make their own paths. Thus the amount of choice presented readers varies (Fredin & Acker, 1987).

This range of choices leads to the issue of goals, of what purpose the system serves. The overall goal that has emerged is that readers should put more emphasis on constructing their own understanding of the topic and less emphasis on absorbing another person's reported understanding of the topic. Stated somewhat differently, the overall goal of using the system is for a reader to construct his or her own version of a story from the various panels rather than to absorb and react to someone else's version. Details on the ways of using the system can be seen basically as tools for accomplishing the overall goal.

The computer news stories are not being developed on-line, that is, they are not being developed to deliver to customers that have already been lined up. The system is not being developed within a specific commercial context or with a specific commercial intent. And this raises another point that can be addressed to complex, new technologies.

Pressing Practical Concerns May Lead to Conservative Systems

The demands that a system operate smoothly from the start, and that a system be relatively easy to learn can often lead to conservative systems. Systems that are easier to learn often will be those most like other communication technologies, hence the emphasis would be on convenience and functional equivalence. This emphasis is not necessarily wrong, but it is worth noting because of some of its implications. A conservative system may involve use of hardware or software packages that are not flexible. Hence even if there are people and resources available for exploring more innovative uses, it may not be feasible. For example, the presentation of news is severely limited if the 25 lines of text on the monitor can be only 40 columns wide. In this case, too little material appears on the screen at once. Reading is often interrupted within sentences because another screen of text must be called up (Fredin & Becker, 1986). This simple, and not uncommon, limitation also shows how a complex relationship can exist between the content and the way the system allows content to be structured. To continue with the news example, the lack of screen space can lead to terse writing, and to short articles. Hence the computer system becomes a rather cumbersome means of acquiring a radio-format version of news.

This is not to say that a journalistic format or any other development in new technology does not ultimately have to be commercially viable. However, new communication technology is sufficiently complex that less context-bound explorations are important, and may be the route to producing innovative results that eventually could have effects in the marketplace.

If some communication technologies should lead to more than functional equivalence and convenience, precisely where should they lead? Unfortunately that question cannot be answered in specifics; rather, as with the example of the computer news system, it can be answered only by pointing to the direction that must be taken. Basically, new systems should lead to new goals that emerge through use of the system.

It should be noted that this conclusion does not emerge solely from optimistic views of new technology. For example, Olson (1974) noted that there is little hard evidence to support the hypothesis that new technology has had a beneficial effect in education. A more recent review is no more optimistic (Clark, 1983). Olson (1974) suggested, however, that much of the research may be limited because it involved the application of new media to conventional goals and conventional methods. He then suggested a different approach.

> Perhaps the function of the new media is *not* primarily that of providing more effective means for conveying the kinds of information evolved in the last five hundred years of a book or literate culture, but rather that of using the new media as a means of exploring and representing our experience in ways that parallel those involved in that literate culture. In this sense, media are not to be considered exclusively as a means to preset ends, but rather as means for reconstruing those ends in the light of the media of expression and communication. (p. 8)

The potential of new goals emerging from the system implies that, despite their importance, the goals cannot be really identified outside of the communication system. They must emerge through its use. New goals will emerge only if the systems involved have what Acker calls a socially open architecture. Their design is essentially incomplete until individuals are working with them. Such systems must permit sophisticated interaction, and must permit design changes, such as the implementation of more intelligent software. Most importantly, system and user are complementary; control over uses and results must be shared. What requirements might such systems make of their users? If goals are to emerge, then the systems alone cannot be novel; the users will need to change as well.

GUESSING WHERE THE NOVELTY WILL TURN OUT TO BE: THE NEED FOR A DIFFERENT KIND OF SELF-REFLECTION

The changes that may be required of individuals might best be approached by noting first a characteristic of individuals that I assume no system can change. Communication technologies cannot alter the very limited capacity of short-term memory. As a result, a crucial issue becomes the organization of additional material that is readily available for use in the processing of the material that is in the short-term memory store. This readily available material is in the individual's mind already, and has presumably been activated in long-term memory (see van Dijk & Kintsch, 1983, for one model). One conclusion from this circumstance is that it is extremely important to organize carefully any material that is presented to the individual. Good organization is necessary for efficient processing and storage (Craik & Lockhart, 1972). This line of reasoning leads to a call for better organized content; and new technology, including the computer-news system, may assist in generating the best organization for each individual. But there is a twist.

Many new communication technologies place in the hands of the user important aspects of organizing the very material that is presented. By making choices and decisions, that is, by interacting with the communication system, the user takes on an editing function. But the user is not simply editing, for the editing must occur simultaneously with the acquisition or learning of the material. Therefore, the editing function means that the individual must be or become more directly aware of what he or she *lacks* in knowledge or understanding. Further, the individual must be able to translate the lack into commands or requests that are meaningful in the communication system. In some respects, this process parallels the speculations about how the VCMO system might disrupt self-monitoring. In both instances, the individuals must increase self-awareness in selected areas that are relevant to the communication system. And as with self-monitoring, levels of understanding must frequently be reassessed.

An interactive system, such as the computer news system, can itself make various kinds of suggestions for organization of material, and the user could take these as suggestions for ways of understanding material. The system may also help the individual in cultivating mental skills (Salomon, 1979). The system may help in detecting weaknesses in an individual's understanding, and may demonstrate ways of both identifying weaknesses and strengthening them. Preferences of individuals can be detected and used to determine, at least in part, what options the system later suggests. These suggestions do not have to consist solely of items the individual would presumably most prefer. For example, Singletary (1985) created a simple program designed to broaden taste for a particular type of story by moving people slowly away from their greater preferences, but moving them back toward their greater preferences if they reacted too strongly against a selection. Systems can be individualized in numerous, more sophisticated ways. Cognitive and affective styles could be detected and used in determining what material to present to users. All these are areas, as Gagnon (this volume) notes, in which important and exciting work will be done, and areas in which work must be done if new systems are to be disseminated widely.

However, if the system takes over the editing and performs the task through a series of very general rules—even rules that include preferences and styles of each user—then the goals lie primarily in the system itself. If goals are to *emerge* from interaction with the system, the user must participate in more active ways than simply revealing styles and preferences within even a broad set of alternatives. The forms of individualization can make effort on the part of the individual more efficient and sometimes more effective. If the forms of individualization merely make matters easy, however, novel goals will not emerge. And systems seeking only to make matters easy may run into different kinds of problems, taking on some of the characteristics Adorno (1941) found in some popular music: "The composition hears for the listener. This is how popular music divests the listener of his spontaneity" (p. 32). Adorno's observation can be taken as a warning that is particularly applicable to interactive media because of interacting with the system. Interaction without spontaneity or surprise would not lead to emergence of goals, and, sooner or later, would also be dull. Adorno states a related hypothesis that is also applicable to a highly interactive communication system such as the hypertext-based computer news system: "To escape boredom and avoid effort is incompatible" (p. 30). The hypothesis alone is important for the design of new communication technologies. On an interactive system, frequent communication of mechanical decisions to a system is monotonous. Sometimes, perhaps with some frequency, interactions must involve some challenge and some effort. As part of the challenge, the user must reflect upon his or her understanding, draw conclusions about where the understanding might lead, and try to formulate goals about where changing understanding should lead.

NOVELTY AND ACTION SCIENCE

The second source for the notion that goals emerge through the interactions with the system is action science, a methodological approach that Acker argues should be incorporated into the design and implementation of new technology. "Action scientists engage with participants in a collaborative process of critical inquiry into problems of social practice. . . . The core feature of this inquiry is that it is expressly designed to foster learning about one's practice and about alternative ways of constructing it. It therefore pushes back some of the constraints inherent in real-life contexts in order to enable participants to come to know their practice as they have defined it and to experiment with the new moves and competencies characteristic of a new definition" (Argyris, Putnam, & Smith, 1985, p. 237).

At the core of action science, then, lie the assessment of goals and the forming of new goals and intentions. Further, a concern with questions of value is implicit in the forming of purposes and goals. Another crucial aspect of the critical study of action is the process of making tacit knowledge explicit, that is, making explicit the rules we actually follow in our actions even though we cannot articulate those rules under normal circumstances. The action scientist is an interventionist seeking to help clients by creating conditions in the world of the client that are conducive to the necessary inquiry and learning. Lasting improvement requires that clients change themselves such that their own interactions can create the same conditions needed for learning (Argyris, Putnam, & Smith, 1985).

Communication systems embodying Acker's notion of socially open architecture may serve as one part of the implementation of action science. The systems could in effect be one recursion behind the action scientist. Such systems should be designed to foster the development of new goals, new means of achieving those goals, and concern for the values expressed. Design of such systems would rest on the principle of incompleteness proposed by Acker. Such interactive systems would be tools that could be used to continue interpreting the methods of action science, and the rules evolved from the application of action science in specific situations. This, then, is one direction in which systems should move if new goals are to emerge.

The role of the individual within any systems exhibiting the principle of incompleteness may be summed up as follows: The price of individuality is self-reflection much as the price of freedom is vigilance. Like vigilance, self-reflection need not be practiced at all times by everyone using a system. But self-reflection must be recurrent. It is not a learning phase in system adaptation. The individuality implied by self-reflection goes beyond a unique location in a multidimensional space in which preferences and other attributes form the dimensions. The system may be able to calculate this location and may relay it to the individual. Then the individual must go further; he or she must understand this location, why he or she is there, and what it might mean. He or she must also ponder the implications of trying to change this location, and even of trying to change the dimensions by which the space is defined (Anderson, 1987).

Work on self-reflection and the emergence of goals does not begin after a system is in place. It must begin within the design phase, and it is intimately linked to methodological issues central to the research into the design of new systems.

REFERENCES

Adorno, T. (1941). On popular music. *Studies in Philosophy and Social Science, 9,* 17-48.

Anderson, J. (1987). *Communication research: Issues and methods.* New York: McGraw-Hill.

Anderson, J., & Eastman, S. with Agostino, D., Daugherty, T., Fredin, E., Galloway, N., Halvorson, J., Hollingswoth, H., Krendl, K., Lacy L., Shields, J., & Zager, C. (1983, November). *Conversations occurring during the use of videotext resources in writing 8th grade science themes.* Paper presented at the annual convention of the Speech Communication Association, Washington DC.

Argyris, C., Putnam, R., & Smith, D. (1985). *Action science.* San Francisco: Jossey-Bass.

Berger, C., & Roloff, M. (1980). Social cognition, self-awareness and interpersonal communication. In B. Dervin & M. Voight (Eds.), *Progress in communication sciences* (Vol. 2, pp. 2-49). Norwood, NJ: Ablex.

Clark, R. (1983). Reconsidering research on learning from media. *Review of Educational Research, 54,* 445-459.

Conklin, J. (1987, September). Hypertext: An introduction and survey. *Computer,* 17-41.

Craik, F., & Lockhart, R. (1972). Levels of processing: A framework for memory research. *Journal of Verbal Learning and Verbal Behavior, 11,* 671-684.

Fenigstein, A. (1979). Self-consciousness, self-attention and social interaction. *Journal of Personality and Social Psychology, 37,* 75-86.

Fredin, E., & Acker, S. (1987). *Metaphors from architecture and music in the design and conceptualization of interactive news and art systems.* Paper presented to the Visual Communication Conference, Alta, Utah.

Fredin, E., & Becker, L. (1986). *Initial reactions to two forms of videotext: Learning to use a new medium.* Paper presented at the annual conference of the Midwest Association for Public Opinion Research, Chicago.

Fredin, E., & Krendl, K. (1987). Media frames, media characteristics, and knowledge structures: A theoretical exploration of young adolescents' use of a videotex encyclopedia, Part II: Analysis and results. *International Journal of Instructional Media, 14,* 273-280.

Heeter, C. (1985). *Perspectives for the development of research on media systems.* Unpublished doctoral dissertation, Michigan State University.

Hiemstra, G. (1983). You say you want a revolution? "Information technology" in organizations. In R. Bostrom (Ed.), *Communication yearbook 7.* Beverly Hills, CA: Sage.

Innis, H. (1977). *The bias of communication.* Toronto: University of Toronto Press.

Klaidman, S., & Beauchamp, T. L. (1987). *The virtuous journalist.* Oxford: Oxford University Press.

Krendl, K., & Fredin, E. (1985). Knowledge structures and instructional design characteristics: An examination of two communication systems. *Journal of Educational Technology Systems, 14,* 75-86.

Malone, T. (1981). Toward a theory of intrinsically motivating instruction. *Cognitive Science, 4,* 333-369.

Olson, D. (1974). Introduction. In D. Olson (Ed.), *Media and symbols: The forms of expression, communication and education* (seventy-third yearbook of the National Society for the Study of Education). Chicago: University of Chicago Press.

Perez, R. (1985). *VCMO documentation for pre-release version 1.2 [computer program].* Available as a text file in the Compuserve MACUS forum.

Rogers, E. (1983). *Diffusion of innovations* (3rd ed.). New York: Free Press.

Salomon, G. (1979). *Interaction of media, cognition, and learning*. San Francisco: Jossey-Bass.
Singletary, A. (1985). *Giving them what they want: An interactive videotex program.* Unpublished master's thesis, Indiana University, Bloomington.
Snyder, M. (1974). The self-monitoring of expressive behavior. *Journal of Personality and Social Psychology, 30*, 526-537.
van Dijk, T., & Kintsch, W. (1983). *Strategies of discourse comprehension*. Orlando, FL: Academic Press.

Toward an Open Architecture and User-Centered Approach to Media Design

DIANA GAGNON
Massachusetts Institute of Technology

ALTHOUGH interactive media have existed for some time in institutional environments (such as the office, training centers, and schools), they may soon be expanded to reach the broader, mass audience. Many new technologies, such as CDI (compact disc interactive), DVI (digital video interactive), add-on devices for VCRs, devices that respond to TV signals, hybrid telecommunication technologies, interactive cable channels, and broadband fiber optics services, promise to introduce some form of interactive media into the home. As "interactive media" become "mass media" the need for a coherent philosophy of design becomes increasingly important.

Acker proposed an open architecture approach to media design. This design philosophy, which he calls "socially open architecture," has at its base the principle of incompleteness. The technology does not solely determine its function, instead the user participates with the technology to determine the function. The system acts as a partner in problem solving. Such systems can easily adapt to changes in both the environment and user.

How well technologies are able to adapt to various environmental contexts and users becomes an important consideration when transferring interactive media out of the institutional environments and into the home. The home environment varies significantly from institutional environments both in physical layout and in the motivations and orientations of the user. Unlike the often homogeneous groups that encounter interactive media in institutions, the home audience varies drastically in skill level, prior knowledge, and age. The use of the media in the home is also driven by different motivations.

Correspondence and requests for reprints: Diana Gagnon, MIT Audience Research Center, Massachusetts Institute of Technology, Cambridge, MA 02139.

Communication Yearbook 12, 547-555

Consumers approach the problem of receiving information very differently in a home setting than in an institutional setting. In an institutional setting, people may approach information in a more task-oriented manner, based on an information need that arises from the work or learning environment. In the home, the use of media is a voluntary act and as such must be intrinsically motivating. Home consumers may seek, or in many cases, browse through information for entertainment, to meet some generalized need to be informed, or for any of a number of idiosyncratic reasons that may not enter into the workplace information search. Furthermore, the search for information in the home may often be only halfhearted and fraught with competition from a range of other distracting inputs. When designing media for this heterogeneous mass audience, the issues of social context and user adaptability become harder to predetermine into the media design.

Given the often undirected and half-attentive nature of information acquisition in the home, the concept of designing application software, which requires the user to participate, also presents a unique set of problems. For the past 20 years, the mass audience has developed a set of passive patterns for receiving information through television. Such patterns may be slow to change, especially among older consumers who have had little exposure to interactive media, such as computers and video games (Gagnon, 1988). Recent changes in television viewing patterns do suggest that consumers may be taking more control over their television viewing through the use of remote control devices and VCRs. These devices are used for time shifting and program choice, as well as content manipulation and nonlinear viewing of multiple programs (Gagnon, 1988).

Even though consumers do appear to be exercising more control, preliminary research suggests that consumers may not always want to be an active partner in the information process (Gagnon, 1986, 1988). Traditional interactive media designs require the user to respond before the program will continue. At points where the user must choose, the program stops and waits for the user to respond. Like an automatic bank machine, it will not continue without an input. Unlike traditional interactive branching designs, interactive applications in the home may be forced to allow for the often inattentive or interrupted nature of media use.

This requirement inspired designers to develop media designs that allow consumers the choice of interacting or moving the system to proceed in a linear fashion. These "optional interactivity" designs contain default modes that allow the program to pick a choice and continue if the consumer decides not to give a response. An example of this design is a video game that will play on to completion if the user stops actively playing, or an interactive information program that selects its own topic if the user does not respond.

In both cases, the content has a strict structure. Although such designs could be considered to be minimally adaptive because they do allow users to select content and an active or passive usage pattern, they are a far cry from an open architecture environment. The content is explicitly designed to accommodate a predefined set of choices. In this case, the technology does determine its function. It presents only the illusion of incompleteness and user control. Databases may come somewhat closer to the user/machine partnership proposed by Acker; however, these types of applications have not yet found a significant place in the home environment.

How much structure and control should be designed into the media is a central issue underlying an open architecture approach. How much structure or lack of structure is necessary and preferred? What is the appropriate balance of control between media and user? The answers or lack of answers to these questions lie at the heart of an open architecture approach to media design.

HOW MUCH STRUCTURE SHOULD INFORMATION SOFTWARE IMPOSE?

Many early computer-based instruction (CBI) programs included in metaanalysis studies (e.g., Kulik, Kulik, & Cohen, 1980) featured highly defined lesson designs. The philosophy behind this approach is that the media designer has the knowledge and can best prescribe an effective form of information presentation. This approach has been criticized for being insensitive to the users, not encouraging users to assume responsibility for their own learning, and not promoting user self-sufficiency (e.g., Tennyson, 1984).

It has also been found that learning structures and strategies are not universal. Lesson or program structures that benefit one group may actually hinder the performance of others (Bouy, 1981; Cronback & Snow, 1977; Salomon, 1987). Research suggests that excessively structured activities may conflict with individuals' schema-driven needs for knowledge (Derry, 1984). Salomon (1987) found that using a tool called Writing Aid, which provided metacognitions about the writing process, had a negative effect on users with a tendency to be "mindful." In this case, the metacognitive guidance provided by the tool conflicted with their own effortful processing. Saloman concludes that such guidance is best, if it is optional. This conclusion again points to another type of optional structuring: in this case, pedagogical feedback on writing style. Unlike the interactive home entertainment formats, this design implies an interactive structure or tool environment with a second layer of embedded instruction that can be accessed upon demand.

The idea of providing a structure that users have the option of accessing can be seen as a part of a hypermedia approach to open architecture. Hypermedia is a database method that provides a new way of accessing information. Pieces of data are connected by a dynamic nonlinear linking structure. Users can choose their own path through the material by selecting which links to follow (see Conklin, 1987). For example, when looking at a series of images of houses a user may select the roof and access further information on indigenous building materials or architectural styles common to the period. Each user's path through the material is unique and self directed. Thus hypermedia systems rely on the users having the option to develop their own path through the system.

One of the problems inherent in the hypermedia approach is that users may get lost or disoriented in the structure (Conklin, 1987). In larger hypermedia databases, the numbers of documents and spiderweb connections between items may become confusing. Conklin (1987) suggests that graphical representations (using color, size, and shape) and query research mechanisms may be used to help users. Even graphical representations that create virtual spatial environments that the user can walk through can become confusing if they are large. As Conklin (1987) points out, there is no natural typology for an information space, so until the user is familiar with the structure, he or she may become disoriented.

The second difficulty with the hypermedia approach is what Conklin calls "cognitive overhead," which is the added difficulty of naming every piece of information and every link between pieces of information. This naming also becomes a problem when looking for information in a large hyperdocument. Often the only information about a link is the short name, which may not provide enough information to make a decision. These names may also be very similar in concept in a highly related database, making it even harder to distinguish and select related documents.

Pictural analogies have also been used to help users know what is available, and to give the information a tangible and understandable structure. For example, in the interactive hypercard version of Donald in Math Land, the designers used a classroom as the organizing structure. Each item in the classroom represents a function or database of information. In another prototype application simulating CDI, an image of Frank Sinatra's office is used as an analogy menu for a database on his life and work. For example, if users select the scrapbook on the desk, they will receive pictures of Sinatra's life accompanied by voice-over narration by his daughter, Nancy Sinatra. If users should choose the Oscar located on the shelf in the office, they could receive information about the movies Sinatra has made.

In this design approach, the pictural environment of the office or classroom acts as an organizer or icon menu that contains information about both the individual database available and the relationship between the different databases. Finding an effective visual analogy, however, may not always be possible. Some types of information and collections of unrelated pieces of information do not easily fit into this model. Furthermore, in the pictural analogy approach, what function or database an image represents may not always be clear.

Overall, hypertext systems rely on the users having a "schema-driven need for knowledge" and an information goal. Users must also be able to develop their own strategies for reaching these goals. As Fredin points out in his chapter (this volume), users must be aware of their lack of knowledge, develop an individual goal and then translate this lack of knowledge into commands or requests that are meaningful to the communication system.

Unfortunately, some research has found that learners are often poor judges of their own understanding or lack of understanding (e.g., August, Flavell, & Cliff, 1984). In many cases, users lack effective cognitive monitoring techniques. Adaptive media designs could be used that are sensitive to these limitations in the user. The computer's power could be used to present information that is customized to the needs of the individual user. This customizing can range from simple modifications based on the inputs of the user to artificial intelligence-driven systems that make assumptions about how the user is behaving.

Many computer programs and databases are now being designed to accommodate different groups and types of users. Computer-based instruction has also shown a clear trend away from the formal behaviorist approach of traditional computer aided instruction (CAI) toward a more learner-oriented, cognitive approach in current intelligent computer aided instruction (ICAI).

Early CAI programs used stereotypic models of the student to induce learning strategies. With the use of artificial intelligence (AI) techniques, student modeling has come to include prediction of individual user behavior and diagnosis of errors. For example, some systems may diagnose the logic underlying a set of mistakes a student is making in answering math problems. The system could then remember this logic and use it to predict problems the student may have with other types of tasks that require the same logic. These sophisticated student models require increased understanding of the influences of individual affective and cognitive style variables on the learning process.

ADAPTIVE DESIGNS

Adaptive designs can be based upon a variety of variables, such as prior knowledge, skill level, cognitive ability, or ongoing performance (e.g., Goetzfried & Hannafrin, 1988; Ross, McCormick, Krisak, & Anand, 1987). Several adaptive designs have been proposed including response sensitive sequencing (Park, 1987); adapting amount of instruction, instructional sequence, and presentation display time (Tennyson, Christensen, & Park, 1984), varying information based on interests or preferences (Lippman & Bender, 1987), embedding individual learner information within lessons (Ross, 1984), and varying formal features, format, style, and media of presentation (McComb & McDaniel, 1981).

The most simple and common adaptive designs are those that modify the sequence, length, and amount of information presented based on the learner's response. These modifications could be based upon learner performance or choice. For example, if the learner failed to answer a set of questions, the system could give them appropriate sections to review. The sequence and amount of information could also be determined by the user through selections made from menus.

Prefilter systems could also be used to organize information presentation. On the lowest level, the system could inquire whether the user is a novice, intermediate, or expert user, and present the information and instructions accordingly. Such systems may provide a scaffold approach that presents the novice users with a tutorial; intermediate users with minimal menu structure; and experts, who have knowledge of the systems, with the option of using commands.

More sophisticated AI driven prefilters have also been proposed. Lippman and Bender (1987) developed an interactive news system that prefilters a broad stream of news sources and assembles a customized newspaper. Users initialize the system by feeding in their interests. The system then assembles a customized newspaper based on their interests and preferences. The system also has an AI component that monitors the selections made by the user and intelligently adds and deletes topics from its filter. This type prefilter is dynamic and actively changes, based upon the user.

Another simple adaptive design principle is the idea of embedding individual user information within the presentation. This information could be as simple as referring to the user by name or appropriate gender. The system could also hold information about what the user has already seen and refer to this established base of knowledge. A more sophisticated version may actually take the individual thinking of the user into account and present the information in a way that matches the user's thinking style. For example McComb and McDaniels (1981) varied the formal features of the media presentation based upon the user's learning efficiencies. Using a multiple stepwise regression approach, various cognitive and affective characteristics of the students were used to predict the students' performance and completion time for a number of courses. The factors that appeared to affect performance were reading, reasoning, memory abilities, and anxiety. These predictor variables were then used as the basis for designing alternative class modules that compensated for these individual differences.

For many years, it has been theoretically proposed that learners perform best with media that match their preexisting style of learning (Salomon, 1979). Ausburn (1978) further suggests that media can be used as a tool for "compensatory" or "conciliatory" supplantation. That is, the media can be used to perform the cognitive transformations for the learner whose cognitive style is incompatible with the learning task. Alternatively, media can be used that will allow learners to use their preferred cognitive skills to extract the information.

Such a theory suggests that media can be designed to accommodate the preexisting thinking styles of the learner. This accommodation could allow for both educational goals (by exercising and advancing the user's underdeveloped cognitive skills) and traditional training goals (by compensating for weaknesses and allowing all users to perform essential tasks).

In the future, a fully customized cognitive interface could be developed based upon complete academic history, as well as cognitive and affective thinking styles. This cognitive interface could include an AI component with a dynamic student model that would monitor the user, interpret his or her behavior, and adjust for learning and behavior changes. Thus the system becomes a dynamic media designer, actively designing information presentations based on individual differences and user inputs matched to a set of concrete design heuristics.

Such a system would require the user to answer initially a battery of cognitive and affective tests. The system would also include an AI component that would actively modify its model of the user based upon his or her behavior. This dynamic model would allow for learning and changes in the individual. Thus the user model from which the system makes its assumptions varies and grows with the user. These assumptions about the user could be used to guide the presentation of content, as well as formal media features and style of presentation. Like a tutor who knows the student very well, the system could customize the presentation with examples based upon a collective knowledge of the user, and anticipate areas of difficulty.

This type of application would require a great deal of system intelligence. Before such a system could be implemented, a great deal of research is needed to determine which individual differences influence effective learning from media, which media design techniques can be used to accommodate them (Gagnon, 1985), what relevant cognitive and affective variables should be taken into account, and what media design features, formats, and styles of presentation best accommodate these individual differences.

MACHINE CONTROL VERSUS USER CONTROL

One caveat to these adaptive designs is that they take control away from the user and invest it back into the system. Fredin suggests that if the system takes over the editing of information, then the goals lie primarily with the system. Even if the system is intelligent in its selections, it is still making choices for the user. The question then remains: How much control should the system have?

Acker warns us of the dangers inherent in systems that are disconnected from the social context. Interactive and adaptive systems that prefilter information could make decisions that are blind to the users. In a complex, dynamic, adaptive model, it could become impossible to trace the assumptions made by the system in designing its presentation. After the initial imputs of the user, the system would continue to modify its model of the user, based upon observations of his or her usage behavior. After a series of these modifications, it may no longer be obvious what assumptions the system is acting upon when it makes a response or assembles a presentation. This system takes the design decisions away from the human media designer.

If this system also selects the information that is presented, then it also takes the learning control away from the end user and becomes a sophisticated example of the closed cybernetic systems Acker warns of. As Fredin and Acker both contend, the goals must come from the user, not from the technology. However, placing the goals of the learning with the user assumes that users will be motivated to develop goals and acquire the prerequisite skills necessary for achieving these goals.

TEACHING USERS TO TAKE CONTROL

Through the years, many theorists have advocated methods that promote greater user self-direction or control over the information process (e.g., Dewey, 1959). As Fredin (this volume) states, "The role of the individual within such a system may be summed up as follows: The price of individuality is self-reflection much as the price of freedom is vigilance." Although the media may aid the learning process, users of systems must continue to explore and guide their own understanding.

Fredin further contends that communication technology should lead to more than the simple functional equivalency and convenience. New technologies should not simply replace the same functions of older technologies. New systems should lead to new goals that emerge through the use of the system. One such goal should be to teach users how to take control of the media.

As interactive media enter the home, the traditionally passive media consumers could be faced with the option of controlling television and television content. These new interactive, television technologies could be designed to support a socially open architecture and a hypermedia design approach. These systems could provide users with unprecedented control over their information selection and consumption. Given some guidance, users could be taught to take this control and structure their own understanding of the world's knowledge. One might even imagine a future world in which the once-passive media consumers are empowered and entertained by the search for knowledge.

Until that day, media designers should begin to work toward designs that are driven by AI prefilters and individually adaptive designs that are under the control of the user. Much like a sensitive conversationalist, these systems should be thinking, observing, and formulating their responses while still remaining open to the requests of the user. Systems should also be designed with open structures that allow users to direct their own information acquisition. However, these systems should also provide a prestructured path when requested. These simple design principles move us one step closer to a truly open architecture and user centered approach to media design.

REFERENCES

August, D. L., Flavell, J. H., & Clift, R. (1984). Comparison of comprehension monitoring of skills and less skilled readers. *Reading Research Quarterly, 20,* 39-53.

Ausburn, L. J., & Ausburn, F. B. (1978). Cognitive styles: some information and design implications for instructional designs. *Educational Communication and Technology Journal, 26.*

Buoy, R. C. (1981). Successful instructional methods: A cognitive information processing approach. *Educational Communication and Technology Journal, 29,* 203-217.

Cronback, L. J., & Snow, R. E. (1977). *Aptitude and instructional methods: A handbook for research on interactions.* New York: Irvington.

Derry, S. J. (1984). Effects of an organizer on memory for prose. *Journal of Educational Psychology, 76,* 98-107.

Dewey, J. (1959). *Experience and education.* New York: Macmillan.

Gagnon, D. (1985). *Interactive vs observational media: The influence of user control and cognitive styles on spatial learning.* Unpublished doctoral dissertation, Harvard University.

Gagnon, D. (1986). *Focus groups on interactive* Dallas *and interactive* CBS Evening News. Danvers, MA: MIT Audience Research Facility.

Gagnon, D. (1988). *Focus groups on interactive shopping.* Danvers, MA: MIT Audience Research Facility.

Goetzfried, L., & Hannafrin, M. J. (1988). The effects of embedded CAI instruction control strategies on the learning and application of mathematic rules. *American Educational Research Journal, 22,* 273-278.

Kulik, J. A., Kulik, C., & Cohen, P. (1980). Effectiveness of computer-based college teaching. *Review of Educational Research, 50,* 525-544.

Lippman, A., & Bender (1987). *News and movies in the 80 megabit living room.* Tokyo: Globecon, IEEE.

McComb, B., & McDaniels, M. (1981). On the design of adaptive treatments for individualized instruction systems. *Educational Psychologist, 16,* 11-22.

Park, O. (1987). Empirically based procedures for designing a response sensitive sequence in computer-based instruction. An example for concept teaching strategies. *Journal of Computer-Based Instruction, 11,* 14-18.

Ross, S. M. (1984). Matching the lesson to the student: Alternatively adaptive designs for individualized learning systems. *Journal of Computer-Based Instruction, 11,* 42-48.

Ross, S. M., McCormick, D., Krisak, W., & Anand P. (1987). Personalizing content in teaching mathematical concepts: Teacher managed and computer assisted models. *Educational Communication and Technology Journal, 33,* 169-178.

Salomon, G. (1979). *Computer tools for learning and for thinking.* Tel Aviv University and the University of Arizona.

Salomon, G. (1979). *Interaction of media cognition and learning.* San Francisco, CA: Jossey Bass.

Tennyson, R. D. (1984). Artificial intelligence methods in computer based instructional design: The Minnesota adaptive instructional system. *Journal of Instructional Development, 7,* 17-22.

Tennyson, R. D., Christensen, D. L., & Park, S. I. (1984). The Minnesota adaptive instructional system. *Journal of Instructional Development, 11,* 2-13.

SECTION 4

MEDIA CULTURAL STUDIES

10 The Return of the "Critical" and the Challenge of Radical Dissent: Critical Theory, Cultural Studies, and American Mass Communication Research

HANNO HARDT
University of Iowa

This chapter outlines the development of a critical approach to the problems of communication and media in American social science scholarship. It traces the understanding of a "critical" position through four successive periods and their contribution to an intellectual history of the field: the pragmatism of the Chicago School, the empirical sociology of the Lazarsfeld tradition, the critical theory of the Frankfurt School, and the cultural studies movement in Great Britain. The essay argues that communication and media theorists in the United States have embraced a notion of critical research that emerged from a reformist environment and was based upon a sense of social responsibility among social scientists that operated well within the dominant ideology. Thus the introduction of radical social theories, including a critical, Marxist perspective since the 1940s, has been either ignored or considered a peripheral intellectual activity by communication and media scholarship, the most recent analyses of media and society offered by Critical Theory and Cultural Studies notwithstanding.

> The question is not whether we should take sides, since we invariably will, but rather whose side we are on.
>
> —Howard S. Becker (1967)

> The intellectual as ideologist is an object of unqualified suspicion, resentment, and distrust.
>
> —Richard Hofstadter (1962)

AUTHOR'S NOTE: Parts of this chapter appeared as "British Cultural Studies and the Return of the 'Critical' in American Mass Communication Research: Accommodation or Radical Change?" in *Journal of Communication Inquiry* (Vol. 10, Summer, 1986, pp. 117-125).

Correspondence and requests for reprints: Hanno Hardt, School of Journalism and Mass Communication, University of Iowa, 205 Communications Center, Iowa City, IA 52242.

Communication Yearbook 12, 558-600

> Criticism by definition implies judgment, and historically it has been effective through the fervor of its bias more often than by its impartiality.
>
> —Robert Morss Lovett (1973)

This chapter will explore the development of mass communication research as a problem of adapting and integrating theoretical constructs as they emerge from a continuing intellectual exchange of social and political ideas located within the specific historical context of American social theories and the renewed challenge of a Marxist perspective. In this context, the chapter will focus upon the idea of the "critical" as it emerged from the literature of mass communication research in the United States, informed by pragmatism and the practice of a positivistic social science and more recently, expressed elsewhere under the influence of Marxism, particularly by Critical Theory and British Cultural Studies.[1] Thus the term "critical" refers to the rise of social criticism as it emerged from the 19th century with the advancement of science and the effects of industrialization. Although frequently linked to socialism and Marx's critique of political economy, social criticism as a scientific approach to the solution of social problems should be considered in the social and cultural context of different theories which have as their determinate goal the improvement of society. Similarly, the idea of culture should be broadly interpreted to refer to the social context of human existence.

Thus the study of culture has been a concern of many disciplines, including the field of communication and mass communication studies, most recently expressed through an exploration of ideological representations and the process of ideological struggle with and within the media, and with an emphasis upon the relationship between media, power, and the maintenance of social order. This perceived need for an alternative explanation of media and communication in society stresses the importance of culture and cultural expressions and has focused on the work of British Cultural Studies[2] as an appropriate alternative, although there have been earlier encounters with a critical, cultural tradition in the American social sciences.

THE RISE OF COMMUNICATION IN THE STUDY OF SOCIETY

Throughout the intellectual history of the United States there has been a continuous influence of European thought, particularly British and Continental philosophy, upon the development of the American mind. In fact, the rise of pragmatism as an American philosophy provides a vivid example that "the conglomerate manifestations of the American mind are the result of local adaptions, graftings, and crossings of the older loyalties and ideas that migrated from Europe" (Thayer, 1973, pp. 228-229). The theoretical discourse at the beginning of this century involved a critique of the existing philosophical tradition; it coincided with the breakup of the old orthodoxies and replaced the domination of a classical-religious perspective with a reformist-scientific position.

Pragmatism

In fact, American pragmatism sought a reconciliation between morals and science (James), the adoption of a scientific practice based upon the primacy of the community of inquirers (Peirce), and an understanding of the practical character of thought and reality based upon a behavioral interpretation of the mind (Dewey, Mead). The appeal of pragmatism as a new foundation of social and scientific knowledge, however, rested in Dewey's (1931) "almost revolutionary" suggestion that "Pragmatism . . . presents itself as an extension of historical empiricism but with this fundamental difference, that it does not insist upon antecedent phenomena but consequent phenomena; not upon the precedents but upon the possibilities of action. And this change in point of view is almost revolutionary in its consequences" (p. 24). When the idea of communication produced by such "adaptions and crossings" surfaced in the literature of the social sciences, it reflected a philosophical movement that struggled against Cartesianism in modern philosophy to develop a new position in which the social became "*the* inclusive philosophic category" (Bernstein, 1967 p. 133).

Among the pragmatists, Dewey's prolific writings on societal questions based upon his interest in the social, his belief in the centrality of community, and his faith in the workings of democracy, supplied a theoretical context for the growing interest among social scientists in the social problems of society. Their activities grew out of the realization that with an increasing concentration of political and economic power, the study of institutions and collective activities was an appropriate and necessary direction for social scientific inquiry. They resulted in efforts to disclose the predatory nature of American industry (Veblen), to render an economic interpretation of history (Beard), and to offer a sociological critique of traditional thoughts of individuality and morality (Small, Ross, Park), in an effort to expose and share with others their understanding of the harsh reality of American life. The emphasis in these inquiries was on the social process and the prospects for a perfect society that would be identical with a perfect democracy.

The notion of communication became a major theoretical issue and a measure of the success of a democratic society, since there was an understanding of culture or society that was based upon the process of communication. In fact, George Herbert Mead (1967) had described an ideal society as one "which does bring people so closely together in their interrelationships, so fully develops the necessary system of communication, that the individuals who exercise their own peculiar functions can take the attitude of those whom they affect" (p. 327). For Mead, who proceeded to demonstrate in his own work how the self emerges through communication, it seemed plausible that under such perfect and ideal conditions "there would exist the kind of democracy. . . in which each individual would carry just the response in himself that he knows he calls out in the community" (p. 327). Since communication always involved "participation in the other" (p. 253), its problems and, in a sense the problems of democracy, remained a question of "organizing a community which makes this possible" (p. 327). These notions were related to Dewey's (1925) appreciation of communication as being "uniquely instrumental and uniquely final. It is instrumental as liberating us from the otherwise overwhelming pressure of events and enabling us to live in a world of things that have meaning. It is final as a sharing in the objects and arts precious to a community, a sharing whereby meanings are enhanced, deepened, and solidified in the sense of communion" (p. 169). Such mystical and powerful explanation of communication also involved the idea of democracy; for Dewey (1966) it was "more than a form of government," it represented "a mode of associated life, of conjoint communicated experience" (p. 87).

Thus communication as the foundation of society and a necessary condition for the working of democracy became the nexus of a critical perspective on American culture. The evolving critique of society was also a critique of an atomistic view of the individual that had become incompatible with the ideas of democracy when it disregarded the collective interests under the technological and economic consequences of a new era in American life. At the same time, industrialization and the rapid growth of society had also led to the creation of a "public" that was disoriented and unable to identify itself. Dewey (1954) lamented the fact that "the machine age in developing the Great Society has invaded and partially disintegrated the small communities of former times without generating a Great Community" (pp. 26-27). His goal, and that of others, was the perfection of the "machine age" that would eventually lead to a democratic way of life. They "saw the new machinery as a means to scale the obstacles to moral unity—ignorance, parochialism, and antagonism between classes. They believed that the new technology would encourage the growth of a mutual sympathy and a rational public opinion that transcended the boundaries of class and locality" (Quandt, 1970, p. 34). Dewey (1954) thought that such development would be aided by and through a process of expert inquiry by social scientists, whose participation would confer upon them a special status in society. He proposed that "it is not necessary that the many should have the knowledge and skill to carry on the needed investigations; what is required is that they have the ability to judge the bearing of the knowledge supplied by others upon common concerns" (p. 209). A similar position was expressed by Albion Small (1910), who felt that consensus in society should be reached by "scientists representing the largest possible variety of human interests" (p. 242). Thus within the critique of society at that time, there was an emerging sense of the importance of intellectual leadership, specifically of the political role of social scientists as expert representatives of a variety of societal interests. It would dramatically increase in later years, when mass communication research became entrenched in the academic environment that catered to specific political and economic interests.

But regardless of the location of political or economic control over social research, a critical position vis-à-vis the process of communication and the role of societal institutions contained the notion of change. Pragmatism projected a definition of evolution (under the influence of Darwinism) that emphasized the processes of gradual change, adjustment, and continuity. In contrast, a dialectical definition recognized discontinuity, abrupt changes of existing structures, or even the prospects of regression, as Trent Schroyer (1975b, pp. 108-109) has suggested. Its practitioners, who had acknowledged the problems of existing social structures, were ideologically committed to support continuity, and they responded to the needs and requirements of an urban, industrialized society by advocating various measures of adjustment. Among them were members of the Chicago School who shared in the criticism of economic and social injustices of society and provided theoretical and moral support for the just and humane distribution of material resources. For instance, Simon Patten, speaking in the language of a new economics around the turn of the century about the "surfeited and exploited," stressed the importance of communication in an effort to help large numbers of Americans to adapt to abundance.

> His social concerns and the expressed need to decrease social and economic differences through communication and cooperation resulted in the development of economic rights that extended traditional political rights and were designed to protect individuals who were adjusting to the new American environment. (Hardt, 1988, p. 151)

Such positions were developed with a growing appreciation of the cultural context of political and economic decisions and their effect upon the survival of the community as a cultural and spiritual resource. In the past, the American perspective on culture had been more closely related to a biological approach toward man and was less committed to emphasizing the differences between natural and cultural disciplines than the German tradition, which began to influence American social sciences after the turn of the century. This position was reflected in the struggle against the biological bias of Spencer's sociological methods that had occupied a generation of social scientists and continued while the trend toward a cultural analysis of social phenomena gained ground with the coming of the Progressive era in American social history.

The context of culture had become a significant feature of the sociological enterprise, particularly with the rising spirit of collectivism in American thought before World War I, when its theoretical position was a reflection of

European and American influences. Similarly, a cultural-historical approach emerged from the writings of political economists, such as Patten (1924), who described the common ground of social research by insisting that

> pragmatism, sociology, economics, and history are not distinct sciences, but merely different ways of looking at the same facts. . . . They all must accept consequences as the ultimate test of truth, and these consequences are measured in the same broad field of social endeavor. (p. 264)

Similarly, Ogburn (1964) observed about 10 years later that although the "trend toward specialization and that toward the solution of practical problems are at times in conflict . . . a trend toward fluidity in boundary lines" had become quite noticeable because of the changing conditions of society and the nature of the search for knowledge (pp. 213-214). Thus the study of communication as a social phenomenon and a potential source of social problems defied disciplinary boundaries and invited investigations from a number of perspectives, including sociology, economics, political science, psychology, as well as philosophy.

The Critical Perspective and Social Reform

The critical perspective of social science scholarship emerged most clearly with an extended analysis of the American press, which had become a frequent target of criticism for social activists and critics within the social science enterprise. Indeed, the concern about the proper role of the press became widespread and was reflected in the *American Journal of Sociology*, which served as an important forum for articles ranging from journalism education to press ethics and the effects of press coverage (Yarros, 1889-1900; 1916-1917; Fenton, 1910-1911; Vincent, 1905-1906). As a result, a diverse and critical literature of the media of public communication emerged that reflected scholarly interests and an articulated, reformist desire for a regular and systematic treatment of questions concerning the position of the media in American society. Although published 70 or 80 years ago, these contributions to a critique of the media "remind contemporary readers of the universality of the problem and the number of issues still unresolved despite enormous efforts throughout the last thirty years to understand the workings of the communication process" (Hardt, 1979, p. 192).

The strength of the critique arose from an alliance between social reformers and social scientists that was based upon a need to justify scientifically the reform activities. More specifically, reformers had "faith in the capacity of social science to translate ethics into action. They hoped to find in social science not merely a description of society but the means of social change for democratic ends" (Oberschall, 1972, p. 206). A critical position vis-à-vis the development of society also emerged with the rise of intellectuals in American society and their potential threat as an oppositional force to the established institutions of society. Commenting upon the role of American intellectuals, William James (1920) suggested that "Every great institution is perforce a means of corruption—whatever good it may also do. Only in the free personal relation is full ideality to be found" (p. 101).

This was the historical context for the contribution by members of the Chicago School, particularly the work of Albion Small as an organizer of sociological research at Chicago, Edward Ross, who wrote extensively about the media, and Robert Park, whose humanistic perspective brought a strong cultural bias into the social sciences. Both Small and Ross had been influenced by the activist sociology of Lester Ward, his distinction between physical and human evolution, and his development of a social theory that led to social reform. Ward had advocated collectivism at a time of laissez faire individualism and a planned society, when government interference had become commonplace. Under the influence of Georg Simmel and John Dewey, Park was interested in the problems of social process rather than structure, and the potential of an enlightened public. Together, these contributions reflected the concerns of a generation of American social scientists who had been witnesses to decisive social and economic changes in their society.

Small had been influenced by the writings of Spencer and Schäffle that committed him to an organismic view of society. In fact, he advanced an idea of society as

> a plexus of personal reactions mediated through institutions or groups. One among these reaction-exchanges was the state; but the state was no longer presumed to be in the last analysis of a radically different origin, office, or essence from any other group in the system. (Small 1912, p. 206)

Such a theoretical perspective was the basis for an extensive, contemporary critique of the social system, including communication and the media.

In his 1984 *Introduction to the Study of Society* (with George Vincent), Small developed a communication model that appeared to be based upon the biological analogies of Schäffle's theory of communication in which the press, among other systems, was "incorporated in nearly every division of the psycho-physical communicating apparatus" (Hardt, 1979, p. 199). The authors recognized the role and influence of the press as an instrument of communication between levels of authority and, given the pervasive nature of the press in modern society, they criticized content and conduct of the press, while placing the burden of responsibility on society. Their writings anticipated major areas of mass communication research devoted to gatekeeping and two-step flow phenomena of the media (Hardt, 1979, p. 203).

Ross combined his scholarship with an intense engagement in the social issues of the day. He identified communication as an important social process and remained highly sensitive to the power of the press as a potential instrument of public manipulation. In particular, he deplored the influence on the press of economic interests through advertisers and, consequently, the commercialization of the newspaper. He staked his hopes on the alertness and intelligence of the reading public to control the excesses of the press and on the strengthening of corrective influences that had to be provided by society (Ross, 1910, pp. 303-311; 1918, pp. 620-632).

Park's theory of communication was built upon Dewey's notion that "society exists in and through communication" and the suggestion that communication also produces conflict, and potentially, collision with another mind or culture. This argument was a reflection of Georg Simmel's subjectivist perspective that had appealed to Park (as did the idea of "social distance," which influenced his extensive work on racial problems). Park's sensitivity to the role of the individual in society (also expressed through his work on the marginal man) shaped his definition of communication as a confrontational process. In his "Reflections on Communication and Culture," Park (1938) offered the view that communication also fosters competition and conflict, but that

> it is always possible to come to terms with an enemy . . . with whom one can communicate, and, in the long run, greater intimacy inevitably brings with it more profound understanding, the result of which is to humanize social relations and to substitute a moral order for one that is fundamentally symbiotic rather than social. (pp. 195-196)

Communication as a process of transformation involves a confrontation of individual, cultural differences, and implies movement or change as a consequence of such exposure to communication when competition and conflict become conscious. Park's discussion of the foreign language press was an example of how minorities gain knowledge and understanding of their environment, but more importantly, of themselves. The desire to know created unrest, even conflict, between generations, and changed goals and perspectives. For instance, talking about the foreign language press, Park (1967) concluded that the Yiddish socialist press, which made people think, "ceased to be a mere organ of the doctrinaires, and became an instrument of general culture. All the intimate, human, and practical problems of life found place in its columns. It founded a new literature and a new culture, based on the life of the common man" (p. 143). In short, a return to community was essential for retaining the stability of social relationships, and he warned against the potentially destructive power of technological society. The media were means of creating fictitious communities and a false sense of proximity. It was sociology for Park that was "a humanistic and healing study, a 'science' in the older sense, a body of knowledge and insight that made man more at home in the world" (Matthews, 1977, p. 193).

The Notion of Communication

From these early sociological considerations emerged a pluralistic model of society that offered an alternative to the potential excesses of individualism and socialism in *laissez faire* and Marxist doctrines of the times. Indeed, the articulation of socialization, cooperation, and balance described a process of change toward the accomplishment of democracy in the United States. Throughout these writings, from the theoretical propositions of John Dewey to the social scientific inquiries into the conditions of American society by Chicago sociologists, communication remained an abstract idea, though the critical stance suggested concrete analyses of the media as a problematic in the context of exploring the notion of democracy. Such an idea of communication described a process that differentiated between those in control of the technology (the operators of the press) and those receiving the messages (the public), but failed to recognize the effects of cultural or economic differences of the communication process on the workings of society. Thus the "Great Community," or the ideal democracy in the minds of these critics, was populated by individuals whose interests, capabilities, and understandings coincided with the essence of the community. Communication became the vital, integrating and socializing force in the process of democratization and, as such, remained a major concept in social theory and research.

A late attempt to offer an extensive and qualitative critique of the media and their failure in American society to participate in the search for the "great community" was the report by the Commission on Freedom of the Press in 1947. Although published after the war, its reformist spirit and recommendations reflect the critical position of earlier writings and signal the end of an era of critical discourse in American social sciences. In fact, the Commission report summarized the critique of previous decades; it reaffirmed a belief in the free flow of information and the diversity of ideas, and it reiterated the dangers of a press dominated by the ideas of owners and those who control the press through economic or political means. As an indictment of the contemporary media, the report was a remarkable document; based upon broad principles and general truths, it called for an "accountable freedom" of the press. McIntyre (1987) has suggested that the "most enduring legacy of the Commission is that it draws attention to the connection between the continuing problems of mass communication in a modern democratic society and some of the most fundamental and enduring questions of modern political thought" (p. 153). But the report also reflected an appreciation of human values and a sensitivity to the interdependence of human affairs that Haskell (1977) has identified with Dewey and his generation as a product of social experience. He found that

> they experienced society not only in the vicarious, deliberate, rational manner of the social researcher—presumably always master of his data, holding society at arm's length as a mere object of examination—but also in the immediate,

> haphazard, unaware manner of the voter, lover, consumer, and job-seeker who is himself an object and onrushing element of the social process. Both kinds of experience prompted their recognition of interdependence. (p. 16)

Nevertheless, the report failed to persuade the media; instead, it remained a thoughtful and eloquent appeal by a group of scholars who were unable to overcome the political reality of their own positions vis-à-vis the commercial interests of the culture industry. If anything, the report continues to serve as a reminder that social institutions, like the media and the economic interests that hold their future, will not be moved by the intelligence or conviction of theoretical propositions. Instead, the fate of the Commission report demonstrates the existing gap between intellectual positions and political practice, that is, the isolation of informed judgment from the public sphere and the inability of the media to consider the ethical dimensions of their professional practice.

Throughout the over 40 years of critical writings about communication, there was hardly any disagreement over the suggestion that there can be no human nature independent of culture. The question was rather how to deal conceptually with the historical components in the examination of social and cultural processes. Indeed, there was a strong movement among the first generation of American social scientists at the beginning of the twentieth century that reflected a sophisticated understanding and appreciation of the German historical school, including socialist writings. As exponents of a cultural-historical tradition in social science scholarship, its most prominent representatives provided academic leadership in the critique of social and political conditions of society with works that were a direct response to the reality of their own age. However, in their writings they sought to reach an accommodation with existing economic structures and political power, and their solutions to the problems of modern capitalism were based upon the conviction that despite its failures, capitalism offered an appropriate context for the growth and success of a great society.

Thus the first encounter with a critical perspective in the social sciences, and specifically in the study of mass communication as a concern of modern American sociology, reflected more accurately the tolerance for dissent within the academic establishment, and therefore within the dominant theoretical paradigm, than the emergence of an alternative, let alone Marxist, theory of society.

THE AGE OF SCIENTISM

By the 1940s the decline of the critical approach to the study of society and communication led by the Chicago School was complete. It had been a result of "an increasing concern with the scientific status of the field, reflected in the preoccupation with methodology; the rise of other sociology departments as centers of research and graduate instruction; the absorption of major European sociological theories; and changing concepts of the proper role of the sociologist in relation to the society he studied" (Matthews, 1977, p. 179). Thus a generation later, traditional sociology had rediscovered nature and, under the influence of Talcott Parsons, embraced structural functionalism with its claim to move steadily in the direction of a theoretical system, not unlike classical mechanics (Parsons & Shils, 1951, p. 51). For instance, under the influence of Parsons (and Clyde Kluckhohn), A. L. Kroeber's concept of culture was significantly modified to restrict its definition to behavior shaped by "patterns of values, ideas, and other symbolic-meaningful systems" (Harris, 1979, p. 281), reflecting an idealist notion of culture and an attempt to accommodate a structural functionalist explanation of society. Such emerging idealist cultural anthropology not only fulfilled "the conservative bias inherent in institutionalized social science," it was prone to follow Parsonians who "accept the system as a given and seek to account for its stability" (Harris, 1979, pp. 284-285).

Furthermore, the continuing problems caused by the depression, the increasing importance of the media as political and economic institutions, and the rise of fascism and communism in Europe helped shift the focus of social scientific research. There was a loss of confidence in American society and the promise of a rediscovery of the self through the work of J. B. Watson and Sigmund Freud and the help of psychoanalysis. This was also the time when modern science became a social and political force and a source of social knowledge, constituting a significant departure from the historical scholarship of the early twentieth century. These changes were accompanied by the decline of common sense and the rise of expert opinion by social scientists for whom society had become an object of study. Robert Park observed at the time that "scholars were being replaced by intellectuals, men of wisdom, knowledge, and balance, by men with a drive for maximum conceptual abstraction and an outcaste sensibility" (Matthews, 1977, p. 186).

In this context, the field of mass communication theory and research turned from a cultural/historical interpretation of communication offered by pragmatism and the work of the Chicago School, to a social scientific explanation. An emergent series of scientific models of communication and mass communication, particularly since the late 1940s and throughout the 1950s, represented a decisive shift to a scientific/empirical definition of the field. It also served a number of immediate goals, specifically the definition of the field, the demonstration of its scientific nature, and its legitimation as a social scientific enterprise.

Thus when Harold D. Lasswell (1948) offered a "convenient way to describe an act of communication" (p. 37), he proposed what became an influential and considerably powerful formula for understanding communication. He proceeded to identify not only the elements of the communication process—communicator, message, medium, receiver, and effects—but he labeled the corresponding fields of media analysis, audience analysis, and effect analysis (p. 37). While such description revealed Lasswell's primary interest in persuasive (political) communication, it referred to organismic equivalencies within an approach dominated by the intent of the communicator and the effect of messages (p. 41). As such, his description of communication is reminiscent of the stimulus-response model, rooted in learning theory, which became a significant force in mass communication theory. Focused upon effects, this approach implied a concept of society as an aggregate of anonymous, isolated individuals exposed to powerful media institutions engaged in reinforcing or changing social behavior.

Equally important and quite persuasive in its scientific (mathematical) intent was the work of Claude Shannon and Warren Weaver (1949), whose model described communication as a linear, one-way process. Their efforts can be traced to a series of subsequent constructions of behavioral and linguistic models of communication. As Johnson and Klare (1961) concluded, "Of all single contributions to the widespread interest in models today, Shannon's is the most important. For the technical side of communication research, Shannon's mathematical formulations were the stimulus to much of the later effort in this area" (p. 15).

In the following years, mass communication research was informed by a variety of communication and mass communication models (McQuail & Windahl, 1981). Stimulated by earlier efforts and by the rise of psychological models that included aspects of balance theory and coorientation (Heider, 1946; Newcomb, 1953; Festinger, 1957), they provided an attempt to order and systematize the study of mass communication phenomena (Schramm, 1954; Gerbner, 1956; Westley & MacLean, 1957). Their authors shared an understanding of the complexity of mass communication and its integration in society. At the same time, the impact of these models directed mass communication research toward an investigation of specific components and encouraged or reinforced a preoccupation with questions of communication effects. Furthermore, it accommodated the development and critique of research methodologies based upon a theory of society that had been firmly established with the creation of mass communication models. Consequently, the field sought to offer explanations for the stability of the social, political, and commercial system without developing a critical perspective of its own communication-and-society paradigm. Indeed, it was not until a widespread paradigm crisis had reached the social science establishment, particularly in the 1970s and 1980s, when British Cultural Studies presented an alternative position.

Administrative and Critical Perspectives

Instead, the field of mass communication studies remained identified with the mainstream perspective of social science research. Both shared the implications of a pragmatic model of society. Their research related to the values of individualism and operated on the strength of efficiency and instrumental values in their pursuit of democracy as the goal of individual members of a large-scale, consensual society.

The work of Paul Lazarsfeld emerged at this point as a definitive contribution to the field of mass communication research with his display of professional ingenuity and political astuteness. His interest in methodological problems, combined with the study of effects, resulted in a number of media studies that had a significant modeling effect upon the development of the field. At the same time, Lazarsfeld (1969) recognized the marketing potential of mass communication research, and in his attempts to secure the position of his research activities between academic pursuits and commercial interests, he became particularly sensitive to the reaction from media industries to communication research. He realized that

> we academic people always have a certain sense of tightrope walking: at what point will the commercial partners find some necessary conclusion too hard to take and at what point will they shut us off from the indispensible sources of funds and data. (p. 314)

Lazarsfeld considered contemporary criticism of the media as "part of the liberal creed" and thought that the media were overly sensitive to such criticism while intellectuals were too strict in their indictment of the media (p. 315). His solution to avert a possible disenchantment of "commercial partners" was to suggest raising criticism to a legitimate activity, using journalism schools as training grounds for media personnel.

From his historical analysis of American society Lazarsfeld had come to the conclusion that political power was the result of relationships formed between citizens, government, and, most recently, mass media. He argued that such a "'three-cornered' relationship" produced "complicated and sometimes surprising alliances" (p. 321). His model assumed a separation of power and proposed that individuals were actually in control of their political or economic destiny, which would make them viable partners in any alliance of power. Specifically, Lazarsfeld's research strategy was built upon the idea that such alliances shift, depending upon the issues and their varying implications; consequently he intended to "keep the Bureau [of Applied Social Research] maneuvering between the intellectual and political purist and an industry from which I wanted cooperation without having to 'sell out'" (p. 321). His sense of criticism was fueled by his own intellectual curiosity and supported and justified by his belief in the function of criticism within the liberal-pluralist system.

The beginning of World War II brought the arrival of a number of German philosophers and social scientists in the United States, which enriched the intellectual climate at American universities by two traditions, logical positivism and Marxism. Paul Lazarsfeld, as a "European positivist" who had been influenced by Ernst Mach, Henri Poincare, and Albert Einstein, and who felt intellectually close to members of the Vienna Circle (Lazarsfeld, 1969, p. 273), encountered members of the Frankfurt School, particularly Theodor Adorno and Max Horkheimer, within the first years of their exile. Lazarsfeld was not particularly familiar with Critical Theory, but shared an interest in the problems of mass culture and the investigation of media content. The presence of Adorno in the Princeton Office of Radio Research was based upon a hope to "develop a convergence of European theory and American empiricism" (Lazarsfeld, 1969, p. 323), but the proposed vehicle for such undertaking, the music project, failed when Adorno gave instructions that "could hardly be translated into empirical terms" and the funding by the Rockefeller foundation was terminated (Lazarsfeld, 1969, p. 324). In his memoirs, Lazarsfeld characterized Adorno as a "major figure in German sociology" who "represents one side in a continuing debate between two positions, often distinguished as critical and positivistic sociology" (Lazarsfeld, 1969, p. 322).

The encounter with Adorno and Horkheimer was fruitful only in that it led to a collaborative effort between the Institute of Social Research and Columbia University's Office of Radio Research with the publication of a special issue of *Studies in Philosophy and Social Science* in 1941 on the problems of mass communication. It included Lazarsfeld's frequently cited "Remarks on Administrative and Critical Communications Research"; other contributors were Theodor Adorno ("On Popular Music"), Harold Lasswell ("Radio as an Instrument of Reducing Personal Insecurity"), Herta Herzog ("On Borrowed Experience. An Analysis of Listening to Daytime Sketches"), William Dieterle ("Hollywood and the European Crisis"), and Charles Siepmann ("Radio and Education"). Horkheimer (1941a) stressed in a brief, introductory remark that "some of our ideas have been applied to specifically American subject matters and introduced into the American methodological debate" (p. 1).

In his contribution to this issue, Lazarsfeld developed his understanding of the mass communication research establishment in the United States. According to Lazarsfeld (1941) "*administrative research*... is carried through in the service of some kind of administrative agency of public or private character," while "*critical research* is posed against the practice of administrative research, requiring that, prior and in addition to whatever special purpose is to be served, the general role of our media of communication in the present social system should be studied" (pp. 8-9). Lazarsfeld credited Horkheimer with the idea of critical research, but he did not pursue the philosophical or theoretical implications of Critical Theory for media research. Consistent with his own ideological position, Lazarsfeld's definition of critical research ignored the historical nature of critical research in the tradition of the Frankfurt School and failed to consider the role of culture in the positioning of the media in society. Indeed, Lazarsfeld and many of his contemporaries saw the problems of the media in technological terms, dealing with the inevitability of industrialization, the massification of audiences, and the effects of the "mass" media on people. In their activities, they adopted a technological rationale that Horkheimer and Adorno (1972) once defined as "the rationale of domination itself" (p. 121), and that could provide only solutions consistent with the prevailing theory of society. Furthermore, over time, American mass communication research has remained insensitive to changing historical conditions that effectively defined the problems of communication in society. Instead, the research activities projected an ideological position that identified the major proponents of mass communication research with the power structure of a society, which Horkheimer and Adorno had exposed and continued to attack for its communication practice.

Reviews of his work (Gitlin, 1981; Morrison, 1978; McLuskie, 1975; Mills, 1970) and Lazarsfeld's own discussion of his involvement in the definition and organization of empirical social research, support the conclusion that mass communication research under the intellectual leadership of Lazarsfeld was concentrated upon the existing conditions of the media and society. He was engaged in a search "for models of mass media effects that are *predictive,* which in the context can mean only that results can be predicted from, or for, the commanding heights of the media" (Gitlin, 1981, p. 93). The role of the critical in this context of Lazarsfeld's writings was still one of providing a scientific rationale for an adjustment to the dominant forces in American society. It was not a critique of the political-economic system or a challenge of positivism as a foundation of mass media research at that time, or an attempt to impose a new vision of a (social) democratic society upon the political system, his Austrian experience with socialist ideas notwithstanding. Instead, critical research in Lazarsfeld's view was identical with participating in the traditional pattern of domination and control, in which "three-cornered" relationships could be analyzed in terms of influences and effects to produce a sense of real and potential imbalances. Lazarsfeld's arguments represented an administrative research perspective, as Gitlin (1981) has argued in his critique of the dominant paradigm in mass communication research (p. 93). Elsewhere, McLuskie (1977) has concluded that "Lazarsfeld's idea was to institutionalize critical research, make it a tradition—in part to sensitize clients to criticism. But behind this heuristic role was Lazarsfeld's agenda to force the critical theorist "to separate clearly fact from judgment" (p. 25). By doing so, Lazarsfeld retained the hegemony of administrative research.

Mass communication research of this period, with its intensive effort to produce a variety of mass communication models since the 1950s, had also sought theoretical unity and strength of the field as it moved from a purely sociological concern to a multidisciplinary area of communication and mass communication studies that offered new opportunities for critical research. Lazarsfeld had recognized this trend, but he was unable to forge his critical research perspective into a major, theoretical statement. Indeed, when Paul Lazarsfeld began to formulate his position vis-à-vis the reality of economic and political authority in mass communication research, he offered a reading of critical theory and the Frankfurt School that ignored the theoretical premises and their practical consequences (particularly as suggested in the work of Horkheimer & Adorno), while his own claims for critical research never left, theoretically or practically (politically), the traditional bourgeois context of the social science enterprise. The notion of a critical position ultimately meant a recognition of authority and a reconciliation with power; it also meant working with the necessity for change within the dominant paradigm and arguing for the convergence of existing theoretical or practical perspectives. Thus the critical research of Lazarsfeld was neither based upon a critique of society nor engaged in a questioning of authority in the populist, reformist sense of traditional social criticism in the United States.

Consequently, Lazarsfeld's remarks about critical research represented the respositioning of traditional social science research *within* the practice of what C. Wright Mills (1970) has called abstracted empiricism (p. 60). The notion of critical research (as opposed to administrative research) became a point of legitimation in the development of mass communication studies. It asserted the neutral, independent position of mass communication research in the study of society and established mass communication research not only as a field (and therefore, as an administrative unit within universities), but as a relevant and important *methodological* specialization of a branch of sociology, in which the priorities of the method became the determinants of social research and the source of research agendas.

In this form, the accommodation of a critical position within mass communication research, as suggested by Lazarsfeld, may have served as a convenient strategy for defusing potentially controversial (since ideologically unacceptable) and challenging threats to the authority of the sociological enterprise in mass communication studies, including public opinion research. These threats arose from two directions: traditional social criticism, latent in American social scientific scholarship since the turn of the century, and post-World War II Western European Marxism, engaged as a theoretical force in the explanation of social changes and the historical conditions in Western Europe since the end of the war.

Lazarsfeld's contributions to media studies also created a sense of urgency in the search for knowledge about the process of mass communication and its effects upon society. Society needed explanations and solutions to a variety of social, political, and economic problems during World War II and later, with its anticipated return to normalcy. Combined with the persistent growth of mass communication research agendas involving conspicuous topics, like children, advertising, pornography, violence, crime, and the media, Lazarsfeld and others produced spontaneous definitions and an extensive compilation of social problems.

In his reaction to Lazarsfeld's notion of critical research, George Gerbner (1964) summarized social scientific contributions to the identification of social problems (through content analysis) and came to the conclusion that the liberal-pluralist system, founded upon a "community of publics" (p. 498) was endangered by the creation of mass markets and mass market research. Echoing C. Wright Mills, Gerbner (1964) observed that the

> dissolution of publics into markets for mass media conceived and conducted in the increasingly demanding framework of commodity merchandizing is the cultural (and political) specter of our age. This fear is now joined by a growing concern over the trend of social science research, especially in the field of communications. More and more of this research is seen to succumb to the fate of mass media content itself in being implicitly tailored to the specifications of industrial and market operations. (p. 498)

In his review of the "consequential meaning of media content," however, Gerbner failed to clarify the fundamental ideological differences between the cultural criticism based upon a Marxist critique of capitalist society, which he cited, and the critical position of (some) American social scientific inquiries into media content.

Mass communication research in this era typically reduced its inquiry by isolating specific conditions of the environment. It delved into relationships among people, investigated questions of social identity, and, generally speaking, raised some doubts about the stability of individuals in their social relations. At the same time, however, there was a marked absence of questions being raised about the role of the media in the process of cultural expressions and ideological struggles and of investigating the structure of society, including the location of authority and the distribution of power. Thus Gerbner's (1964) "challenge for mass communications research" reflected his own commitment to a liberal-pluralist vision of society, based upon the participation of individuals in a "genuine" public. He asked media scholars

> to combine the empirical methods with the critical aims of social science, to join rigorous practice with value-conscious theory, and thus to gather the insight the knowledgeable individual in a genuine public must have if he is to come to grips (and not unconsciously to terms) with the sweeping undercurrents of his culture. (p. 499)

Such a challenge was a confirmation of Lazarsfeld's call for critical research and a reflection of a democratic ideal that had characterized earlier reformist notions in American social science research. Although reform minded in the sense of understanding itself as contributing to the betterment of society, mass communication research remained committed to a traditionally conservative approach to the study of social and cultural phenomena, in which instrumental values merged and identified with moral values. Almost 30 years after the Lazarsfeld's initial writings, Dallas Smythe (1969) commented upon the "oversupply" of administrative research at the expense of critical inquiry (p. vii).

Under Lazarsfeld's leadership, mass communication research in the United States had become a formidable enterprise that was deeply committed to the commercial interests of the culture industry and the political concerns of government. Some time ago, Robert Merton (1957) had summarized the major intellectual and theoretical conditions of the field, including the potential consequences of applied social research whose categories were shaped by "market and the military demands" (p. 451). He acknowledged that "in the field of mass communications research, industry and government have largely supplied the venture-capital in support of social research needed for their own ends" and wondered whether such administrative research had "been too closely harnessed to the immediate pressing problems, providing too little occasion for dealing with more nearly fundamental questions of social science?" (p. 452).

Lazarsfeld's suggestion of critical research as a socially desirable goal within the limits of the dominant perspective of democratic practice was an anachronism. It appealed to a commonsense notion of criticism at a time when common sense had been replaced by expert opinion. In addition, by arguing the primacy of empiricism as the basis of social theory, Lazarsfeld successfully excluded Critical Theory from social theory (McLuskie, 1977, pp. 26-33). His introduction of critical research represented a successful attempt to create a pseudoconfrontation of research practices, which, in fact, occupied the same theoretical (and political) premises. It reflected an unwillingness to explore alternative explanations that was not a particularly unique characteristic of American mass communication research at that time. For instance, Robert Sklar (1975) found that American Studies was similarly disadvantaged with its "reluctance to utilize one of the most extensive literatures of cultural theory in modern scholarship, coming out of the Marxist intellectual tradition." He concluded his assessment of that field with the suggestions that "to have left untouched such a potential resource exposes one of the essential causes of the problem of theory in American Studies" (p. 260).

Ultimately, however, such "reluctance" to use a Marxist approach for an analysis of culture and communication has its roots in the conservative tradition of the social sciences, including the field of mass communication theory and research, whose practitioners have been occupied with a search for causes underlying the decline of political authority in American society. In a variety of ways, they had established the media as indicators of social integration in their efforts to explain and reaffirm the workings of the democratic system, particularly with the emergence of new social movements and the pressures of a society with increasing material needs. In fact, media research has claimed a significant share of the attempt to preserve and support the ideological status quo with its explorations of the decline of credibility and legitimacy of the system, or the threats to populism.

Consequently, the prevailing theory of anticommunism would continue to identify a Marxist critique of culture and society as constituting an adversary, if not hostile position on questions of media and communication, which could only aggravate the crisis of democracy.

CRITICAL PERSPECTIVE

Under these confining intellectual circumstances, there was no room for the type of critical research proposed by Horkheimer and Adorno and suggested by the introduction of Critical Theory. Indeed, the differences between German *Sozialforschung* and American social science research methodology remained profound enough, and often surfaced with the question of empirical verification, which preoccupied American social scientists and against which Horkheimer (1941b) had insisted upon the critical nature of societal concepts by pointing to the problem of value judgments.

> The media of public communication . . . constantly profess their adherence to the individual's ultimate value and his inalienable freedom, but they operate in such a way that they tend to forswear such values by fettering the individual to prescribed attitudes, thoughts, and buying habits. The ambivalent relation between prevailing values and the social context forces the categories of social theory to become critical and thus to reflect the actual rift between the social reality and the values it posits. (p. 122)

Such a historical approach to mass communication research methodology reflected the fundamental differences between two intellectual traditions and their approaches to culture and media phenomena. Merton (1957) once referred to this difference in terms of a concern about knowledge and information. He suggested that knowledge "implies a body of facts or ideas, whereas information carries no such implication of *systematically connected* facts or ideas. The American variant accordingly studies the isolated fragments of information available to masses of people; the European variant typically *thinks about a total structure of knowledge* available to a few." (p. 441). Consequently, the approach to the study of culture by members of the Frankfurt School (and their development of an aesthetic theory that had originated during the early days of the Institute of Social Research) would be significantly different from American concerns with mass society and mass culture. The view that "the term 'critical' did not so much describe a position as a cover under which Marxism might hide during a hostile period in exile" (Carey, 1982, p. 22) alludes to the problems of Marxist scholarship as an alien phenomenon in this country. But it disregards the historical development of

Critical Theory as a series of distinct philosophical perspectives by a number of German emigres who were united in their position as critics of contemporary bourgeois society.

Indeed, in *Dialectic of Enlightenment* (1972), Horkheimer and Adorno presented their theory of mass culture that has become a classic statement of their theoretical position. Its impact upon the American mass society debate, however, was felt much later than at the moment of its original German publication in 1944. As a direct attack upon the political values of American society, perpetuated by the media, the authors suggested that

> in the culture industry the individual is an illusion not merely because of the standardization of the means of production. He is tolerated only so long as his complete identification with the generality is unquestioned. . . . The peculiarity of the self is a monopoly commodity determined by society; it is falsely represented as natural. (p. 154)

It questioned not only the contemporary manifestations of the media industry, but raised doubts about the values perpetuated in defense of the prevailing ideology. While critical research (in the tradition of Critical Theory) with its speculative approach to contemporary culture and society sought to challenge the theoretical basis of traditional, social research, critical-administrative research was driven by methodological considerations and the immediacy (and potential threat) of mass culture phenomena.

This was the time when American mass communication research began to expand upon the pioneering work of Lazarsfeld, Carl Hovland, Harold Lasswell, and others, launching with an increasing sophistication of its empirical methodology into what Lazarsfeld had called administrative research and what members of the Frankfurt School identified as a market research approach that could reflect only "reified unmediated reactions rather than the underlying social and psychological function of the cultural phenomena under scrutiny," according to Leo Lowenthal (Jay, 1985, p. 50). The problems of mass society with its feared cultural and political consequences (particularly in the face of fascist and communist threats from Europe) encouraged research into questions of collective behavior (Blumer), media and diffusion (Lazarsfeld), persuasion (Hovland) and propaganda (Lasswell), which sought empirical evidence to demonstrate the workings of a pluralist society in the United States. However, there were others, like David Riesman, with a critical view of American public life and influenced by the work of Erich Fromm and psychoanalytic analyses of culture, who dealt with the problem of historical change (*The Lonely Crowd,* 1950) in industrial middle-America; while C. Wright Mills, who railed against the "abstract empiricism" of the social sciences and the dogma of methodology, provided a scathing critique of advanced urban society (*New Men of Power,* 1948; *White Collar,* 1951; *The Power Elite,* 1956). These and similar studies understood the importance of "power" and "domination" and sought to locate their basis in the socioeconomic distribution of property or influence. But their contributions seemed to be of peripheral interest to the field of mass communication research that had managed to retain a singularly narrow, theoretical, and historical base in its endeavor as a scientific enterprise. Publications like *Journalism Quarterly, Public Opinion Quarterly, Journal of Broadcasting,* or *Journal of Communication,* in particular, did not participate in any assessment of American media research and social theory as the field was confronted with the writings of the Frankfurt School.

The 1970s, however, saw the emergence of a brand of social criticism strongly related to an earlier critique of American society. These expressions had ranged from the socialist writings of political economists and sociologists during the turn of the century, to populist criticism of political and economic authority by publicists and muckraking journalists in the late 1920s, and to the social criticism of social scientists since the 1950s.

Critical Theory

The introduction of Critical Theory as a competing social (and political) theory of society constituted a significant development in American social thought. It rekindled a debate of Marxism and radical criticism and signaled the beginning of substantial Marxist scholarship after World War II, though not in American mass communication research. The ensuing critique of contemporary American social theory and research practice also established the intellectual leadership of British, French, and German social theorists. Thus the encounter with critical theorists provided a solid opportunity to examine form and substance of an ideological critique of society. Specifically, the cultural pessimism of Theodor Adorno and Max Horkheimer, together with the political critique of Herbert Marcuse and the theoretical inquiries of Jürgen Habermas concerning the role of communication in the struggle against bureaucracies and authority, provided American social theorists with an alternative approach to the questions of power, change, and the future of society. Throughout, this body of critical writings exemplified an abiding commitment to the study of culture, including the complicity of the media industry in the ideological struggle, and to an analysis of the cultural process. The cultural critique of contemporary society stressed

> sociocultural consequences of stimulated economic growth that . . . transforms the human milieu into a technologically determined system, and systematically blocks symbolic communication by the superimposition of more and more technical rules and constraints deriving from rationalizing processes. (Schroyer, 1975a, p. 223)

These were continuing concerns among cultural critics and Alvin Gouldner (1976), in particular, has traced similarities and differences between pragmatism

(Chicago School) and Critical Theory in their analysis of the "cultural apparatus" and the "consciousness industry" (pp. 118-178.).

When Critical Theory reached the representatives of mainstream mass communication research in the 1970s, it had been a major theoretical event for over four decades, constituting a considerable body of literature that reflected the extent and quality of the modernist debate in a number of disciplines. Beginning with Martin Jay's *The Dialectical Imagination: A History of the Frankfurt School and the Institute of Social Research, 1923-1950* (1973), the volume of original works by Adorno, Horkheimer, Herbert Marcuse and Jürgen Habermas, together with translations of German contemporaries and secondary sources about the Frankfurt School increased dramatically,[3] although the subsequent readings and interpretations of Critical Theory by mass communication research remained a peripheral intellectual enterprise.

The marginal role of Critical Theory, or any other radical challenge of traditional social theories, was revealed in the frequently cited 1959 *Public Opinion Quarterly* review of the "state of communication research." Berelson's (1959) pessimistic statement included no reference to Critical Theory as a potential source of theoretical stimulation; his consideration of "minor" approaches referred to David Riesman and Harold Innis as well as the "reformist" appproach of the Commission on the Freedom of the Press; in those cases, Berelson questioned their legitimacy as scientific inquiries (p. 4). Implicit in his general observations about the demise of the field was an accurate description of mass communication research as a passing interest among social scientists (e.g., Hovland, Lasswell, even Lazarsfeld, who turned toward theoretical issues later in his career). Unlike other fields, mass communication studies have not specifically attracted the work of social theorists, but provided opportunities for specific research interests that were widely accepted, imitated, and published. The theoretical debates in other disciplines, however, were not as readily reflected in the mass communication literature. This failure to respond to the interdisciplinary nature of the theoretical discourse serves as an additional indication that the field of mass communication research had been project-oriented and dedicated to the practical application of research methodologies.

In the same issue of *Public Opinion Quarterly,* however, David Riesman (1959) referred to a critique of society with the publication of *The Authoritarian Personality* (1950). He raised some questions concerning research on broader cultural and societal issues and mentioned the creative work of Leo Lowenthal, while accusing the "scientific superego" as "particularly effective in intimidating adventurous research, because the young were learning more about methodological pitfalls than had their elders—from precisely such mentors as Mr. Berelson" (p. 11). Indeed, Lowenthal, who had established himself as an early member of the Frankfurt School with his application of Critical Theory to literature, was its most visible representative in American mass communication research circles. He had collaborated with Joseph Klapper (opinion research and psychological warfare) and Marjorie Fiske (popular culture) and had contributed to a number of collected works, edited by Lazarsfeld and Frank Stanton, Wilbur Schramm, and Norman Jacobs.

A more recent review of mass communication research was equally absorbed in the narrow, administrative research tradition to assess or reassess after several decades the influence of other theoretical writings on the field. Its editors regretted the "lack of broad theorizing," wondering where the "elder statesmen, the philosophers of the communication field" were and why no names besides "Innis, McLuhan, Lasswell and a few others" had been added to the roster (Davison & Yu, 1974, pp. 200-201). A few years later, the editors of *Communication Research—A Half-Century Appraisal* suggested that the "story of communication research begins with the publication in 1927 of Lasswell's *Propaganda Technique in the World War* and proceeded with contributions by communication researchers representing the traditional approach to the field. There is no attempt to provide a theoretical context or a historical account of the last 50 years (Lerner & Nelson, 1977, p. 1).

An acknowledgment of a much broader context of social theoretical work appeared more recently with Rogers's rather abbreviated and incomplete presentation of Critical Theory. The author attempted to dichotomize "empirical and critical schools of communication" (Rogers & Balle, 1985), but managed to obscure the differences between Lazarsfeld's use of critical research (with which he sympathizes) and the concept of critical research in the spirit of the Frankfurt School and other Marxist positions. This lack of differentiation (even among members of the "empirical" school) weakened his assertions about the theoretical premises of the "schools." The article made no substantive contribution to clarify the positions of Critical Theory vis-à-vis traditional theories of mass communication research, it merely pleaded for a dialogue. Indeed, for Rogers the "Critical School" had "its Marxist beginnings as the Institute for Social Research in Frankfurt, Germany, in the early 1930's," while "critical scholars set themselves off from empirical scholars by objecting to the effects-oriented, empirically minded nature of most communication research" (p. 115).

The issue, however, is not a polarization of "schools," but the reaction to a necessary, critical reexamination and assessment of the field. The emergence of critical scholarship is the result of such self-reflection about the conditions of a theoretical premise that does not reflect social (and political) realities of everyday life. The problem of empirical research, at least in this context, remains a secondary issue.

The question of critical research emerged more substantively with the most recent debates concerning Critical Theory and other Marxist approaches to mass communication research in "Ferment in the Field," a special issue of the *Journal of Communication* (1983). Despite its ambitious goals, the publication barely moved beyond an acknowledgment of Critical Theory or neo-Marxist perspectives on communication to engage the field in an epistemological debate of any significance. Nevertheless, Jennifer Daryl Slack and Martin Allor offered a particularly useful contribution to the debate. The authors acknowledged that "critical mass communication research is not a single entity, but rather a range of developing alternative approaches to the study of communication," and they provided a decription of the *critical* as an "appropriation of the term" from the Frankfurt School (Slack & Allor, 1983, pp. 208-209). Other authors were vague in their use of the term *critical research* or *European-style* research (Haight, 1983, p. 232; Schiller, 1983, p. 255; Mosco, 1983, p. 237; Stevenson, 1983, p. 262), although the implications were that such research activities involve questions of power and control, since, as Slack and Allor (1983) suggested, the "central concern of all critical positions is the effectivity of communication in the exercise of social power" (p. 215). Dallas Smythe and Tran Van Dinh (1983), while commenting upon the conditions of Marxist scholarship in communication studies, advanced a definition of critical theory that "requires that there be criticism of the contradictory aspects of the phenomena in their systems context" (p. 123). George Gerbner (1983), in his summary of the discussions, extended the notion of "critical scholar" to include those "who search and struggle" in order "to address the terms of discourse and the structure of knowledge and power in its domain and thus to make its contribution to human and social development" (p. 362).

The presentation of critical alternatives to the traditional approach to mass communication research revealed that the choice is not between ideology and social science, but that social science practice remains embedded in an ideological context. Although the language of orthodox Marxism, Critical Theory, or Cultural Studies is reflected throughout the discussion of "ferment in the field," providing a vocabulary and a focus for a critique of contemporary societal practices, it was reproduced by many authors without further discussion of the consequences for the ideological perspective of mainstream American mass communication research.

The practice of collecting and adapting theoretical propositions and practical applications for the betterment of society, disregarding cultural or political origins and ideological foundations reflects an intellectual process of Americanizing ideas. It has occurred in the social sciences with the influence of European knowledge on American scholarship since the beginning of academic institutions in the United States, and is most clearly visible since American pragmatism (particularly in Dewey's instrumentalism), which seemed to acquire and apply suitable theoretical propositions according to the interests they served at the time. For instance, Georg Novack's (1975) confrontation of Dewey's liberal position vis-à-vis the political reality of his days is an appropriate example of a Marxist critique of pragmatism as a philosophical and political power in American society.

Thus, to realize the potential contribution of Critical Theory to a critique of contemporary society, mass communication research needed to explore the rise of Critical Theory in the cultural and political context of Weimar Germany. Specifically, its attempts to replace the preoccupation of traditional philosophy with science and nature by shifting to an emphasis upon history and culture, and its acute awareness of the relationship between epistemology and politics, were decisive elements for such analysis.

Habermas

The writings of Critical Theorists offered the basis for an intensive examination of the critique of modern society, including a discussion of its philosophical (and political) consequences for mass communication research. Such inquiry, however, remains uncompleted, and a debate of Critical Theory as the foundation of a critical theory of communication has been limited to the literature of social theory, particularly to the work of Jürgen Habermas (1981), who offers an epistemological justification for human emancipation. Indeed, taken as a critical position rather than as a theory, Critical Theory embarks upon a critique of the present and points to the potential of the future. For Habermas it involves an emancipatory interest with the potentiality of the human being at its center.

Communication is a central idea in Habermas's theoretical project. It surfaced with *Knowledge and Human Interest* (1971), in which he presented his approach to language in the context of the development of a critical social science, and culminated with the publication of *The Theory of Communicative Action*, (1984a), which contains the normative basis of his social theory. In it he asserts:

> If we assume that the human species maintains itself through the socially coordinated activities of its members and that this coordination has to be established through communication—and in certain central spheres through communication aimed at reaching agreement—then the reproduction of the species *also* requires satisfying the conditions of a rationality that is inherent in communicative action. (p. 397)

Specifically, Habermas (1984a) constructs the concept of communicative action from three "intertwined topic complexes": (a) a communicative rationality freed from the limitations of individualistic approaches of social theory, (b) a two-level concept that "connects the lifeworld and systems" paradigms, and (c) a theory of modernity that accounts for "social pathologies." He adds "thus the theory of communicative action is intended to make possible a conceptualization of the social-life context that is tailored to the paradoxes of modernity" (p. xi).

The route towards such theoretical position leads through the application of a reconstructive science. In *Communication and the Evolution of Society*, Habermas (1979) already asserted that the

> task of universal pragmatics is to identify and reconstruct universal conditions of possible understanding (*Verständigung*). In other contexts we also speak of "general presuppositions of communication," but I prefer to speak of general presuppositions of communicative action because I take the type of action aimed at reaching understanding to be fundamental. (p. 1)

Indeed, for Habermas (1979) the

> goal of coming to an understanding (*Verständnis*) is to bring about agreement (*Einverstandnis*) that terminates in the intersubjective mutuality of reciprocal understanding, shared knowledge, mutual trust, and accord with each other. Agreement is based on recognition of the corresponding validity claims of comprehensibility, truth, truthfulness, and rightness. (p. 3)

Such conditions underlying communicative practice are based upon a rationality that is determined by whether the participants "could, *under suitable circumstances,* provide reasons for their expressions." Habermas (1984a) explained that

> the rationality proper to the communicative practice of everyday life points to the practice of argumentation as a court of appeal that makes it possible to continue communicative action with other means when disagreements can no longer be repaired with everday routines and yet are not to be settled by the direct or strategic use of force. (pp. 17-18)

Since communicative practice occurs in the context of social and cultural structures, Habermas (1984a) directs attention to the importance of the "lifeworld" as the context for symbolic reproduction. He identified and described three structural components.

> In coming to an understanding with one another about their situation, participants in communication stand in a cultural tradition which they use and at the same time renew; in coordinating their actions via intersubjective recognition of criticizable validity claims, they rely on memberships in social groups and at the same time reinforce the integration of the latter; through participating in interaction with competent reference persons, growing children internalize the value orientations of their social groups and acquire generalized capabilities for action. (p. xxiv)

And he continued to suggest that communicative action serves three functions: the transmission and renewal of cultural knowledge, social integration and group solidarity, and personal identification.

Habermas (1984a) defined the cultural context of the participants in communication, the "world" of the actors, in terms of the relations between the speech act and three worlds. They are the "objective world (as the totality of all entities about which true statements are possible)," the "social world (as the totality of all legitimately regulated interpersonal relations)," and the "subjective world (as the totality of the experiences of the speaker to which he has privileged access)" (p. 100).

Communication becomes a process of negotiation against the background of a shared culture, a "lifeworld" that offers the presuppositional condition for any meaningful participation. Indeed, culture, society, and the individual are structural components of the "lifeworld," in which communicative action serves to reproduce cultural knowledge, to integrate individuals, and to shape personalities. Habermas (1984b) sees *culture* as the reservoir of knowledge from which participants in communication about the world take their interpretations; *society* represents the legitimate order, through which participants secure their membership in social groups and affirm their solidarity; and *personality* refers to the competencies that enable a subject to participate in the processes of understanding while maintaining its own identity. In the semantic field of symbolic contents, the social space and historical time form the *dimensions* in which communicative actions take place (pp. 594-595).

The media as part of the everyday activities of the "lifeworld" function as "generalized forms of communication." Thus the press, radio, and television, for instance, have an enabling function. They free participants from their spatial-temporal limitations, provide availability of multiple contexts, and become instrumental in the creation of public spheres capable of serving authoritarian or emancipatory interests (Habermas, 1984a, p. 406).

This perspective on communication and media suggests that "mass communication" theory and research are invariably tied to the analysis of communicative practices, that is, issues of communicative competence, understanding, and participation of individuals in their lifeworld. Daniel Hallin (1985) has observed, that "For Habermas, all forms of human communication, even under conditions of mass dissemination, are essentially relationships between human subjects, derived ultimately from the elementary structure of dialogue" (p. 142). Habermas proposes that the study of the media must be a study of culture, the conditions of the lifeworld, and, indeed, the prospects of a public sphere that serves the emancipatory interests. It is based upon a perspective on knowledge that is committed to openness (truth) and the process of self-reflection. As Richard Bernstein (1985) argues:

> An emancipatory interest is basic in the sense that the interest of reason is in furthering the conditions for its full development; the demand for non-distorted communication becomes fully explicit. . . . Non-distorted, reciprocal communication cannot exist unless we realize and institute the material social conditions that are required for mutual communication. (p. 11)

With his latest work, Habermas has outlined a broad theoretical framework and provided a formidable agenda for communication research. The complexity of his work and the encyclopedic range of his intellectual effort offer a major challenge to the practitioners of communication theory and research in the United States. Indeed, the problems of theoretical complexities and intellectual accessibility may have contributed to the failure of the field to participate in the critical assessment of Habermas's work. More likely, however, is the (intuitive) rejection of a theory of communicative action, because, as Rorty (1985) has suggested,

> The desire for communication, harmony, interchange, conversation, social solidarity, and the merely beautiful wants to bring the philosophical tradition to an end because it sees the attempt to provide metanarratives, even metanarratives of emancipation, as an unhelpful distraction from what Dewey calls "the meaning of the daily detail." (p. 175)

The Persistence of Pragmatism

In fact, the field of communication theory and research is most likely to support and follow Rorty, whose criticism of Habermas reveals a strong commitment to the writings of American pragmatism. Rorty's (1985) argument is based on the notion that the "progressive changes" in society may tell the story

> without much reference to the kinds of theoretical backup that philosophers have provided for such politics. It is, after all, things like the formation of trade unions, the meritocratization of education, the expansion of the franchise, and cheap newspapers, which have figured most largely in the willingness of the citizens of the democracies to see themselves as part of a "communicative community"—their continued willingness to say "us" rather than "them" when they speak of their respective countries. (p. 169)

Such perspective reflects not only the compelling influence of the pragmatist tradition, but also reveals its continuing theoretical appeal. As Habermas (1985) concluded in his reply, Rorty

> wants to destroy the tradition of the philosophy of consciousness, from its Cartesian beginnings, with the aim of showing the pointlessness of the entire discussion of the foundations and limits of knowledge. . . . The stubbornness with which philosophy clings to the role of the "guardian of reason" can hardly be dismissed as an idiosyncrasy of self-absorbed intellectuals, especially in a period in which basic irrationalist undercurrents are transmuted once again into a dubious form of politics . . . and it is precisely the neoconservatives who articulate, intensify and spread this mood via the mass media. (pp. 193-195)

This conclusion may very well describe the position of the field of communication and mass communication theory and research toward the Habermasian struggle to forge a path for the position of an emancipatory social science in a world in which the problems of cultural reproduction create tensions and social conflicts.

BRITISH CULTURAL STUDIES

Not unlike Critical Theory a few years earlier, the introduction of British Cultural Studies as a European critique of contemporary society is a political challenge and a direct confrontation between liberal pluralism and Marxism as competing theories of society. Such critique not only reflects a specific British interpretation of contemporary Western Marxism, but indicates the quality and intensity of an intellectual commitment to a critique of ideological domination and political power. The question of adapting Cultural Studies to an analysis of social and political conditions of American society is not only a commitment to the uses of history, it requires an emphasis upon ideological practice in the review of those intentions, interests, and actions that intersect in the spheres of cultural, economic, and political power, thus rendering a fundamental critique of the dominant model of society. This stance means an understanding of "the 'subject' positioning himself [*sic*] in the specific complex, the objectivated field of discourses and codes which are available to him in language and culture at a particular historical conjuncture" (Hall, 1979, p. 330). Implicit in this approach is the consideration of authority, that is, of people living and thinking an existence under specific conditions of domination that organize the ideas and beliefs of individuals through social institutions, including the media.

Culture and Ideologies

The rise of Cultural Studies has been documented by Hall (1980a, pp. 15-47) as it broke with mainstream British sociology and established itself as an integrative academic field of study that retraced its roots through the Weberian, interpretative branch of sociology to the ethnographic discourse of subcultural theorists (Howard Becker). Similarly important was the impact of Western Marxist writings, from George Lukacs to the works of Lucien Goldmann, Walter Benjamin, and the Frankfurt School, particularly Horkheimer, Adorno, and Marcuse. According to Hall (1980a) these texts "restored to the debate about culture a set of theorizations around the classical problem of ideologies. They returned to the agenda the key question of the determinate character of culture and ideologies—their material, social and historical conditions of existence" (p. 25). They also reaffirmed the importance of a holistic perspective and confirmed the critique of empiricism and its insistence upon isolated facts. More recently, the impact of Louis Althusser's (1971) "ideological state apparatuses," and Antonio Gramsci's concept of "hegemony," on Cultural Studies have helped build a rationale for the study of social practices within societies "as complex formations, necessarily contradictory, always historically specific" (Hall, 1980a, p. 36).

Cultural Studies employs but one of several strategies of cultural interpretation that have emerged from contemporary Marxist theory in recent times (Curran, Gurevitch, & Woollacott, 1982; Grossberg, 1984). It occupies a position opposed to economic reductionism, as exemplified in the cultural tradition of Raymond Williams and Richard Hoggart, in particular, while stressing experience as the product of cultural practices. Thus the "problematic of cultural studies is transformed, concerned with how a particular practice—signifying or social—is located in a network of other practices, at a particular point, in particular relations" (Grossberg, 1984, p. 412). This means that Cultural Studies locates the media and media practices "within a society conceived of as a complex expressive totality" (Curran, Gurevitch, Woollacott, 1982, p. 27). The media have become a major field of critical analysis, since they dominate the cultural sphere in urban, industrialized societies. They are important, because they help produce the understanding of a social totality by bringing together and, if necessary, reconciling conflicting and confusing fragments of reality. The study of media, and with it the question of power, constitute an ideological issue, which is raised in an analysis of cultural practices within the larger, "complex expressive totality." That is to say, media studies are involved in the issue of human practice. Raymond Williams (1977) stressed such a holistic perspective as the underlying condition of a Marxist sociology of culture when he stated that "the most basic task of the sociology of culture is analysis of the interrelationships within this complex unity . . . [of] institutions, formations, and communicative relationships . . . insisting on what is always a whole and connected social material process" (pp. 139-140).

The discursive approach to culture views ideology as "the power of a particular system to represent its own representations as a direct reflection of the real, to produce its own meanings as experience" (Grossberg, 1984, p. 409). Consequently, the conditions for individuals in their social and political environments are defined within the sphere of the media. Grossberg (1984) argued that the "issue is not so much the particular knowledge of reality (true or false, mystified or utopian) which is made available, but the way in which the individual is given access to that knowledge and consequently, empowered or de-powered" (p. 409). The media function in several ways to maintain their cultural and ideological position: they provide and selectively construct social knowledge; they classify and reflect upon the plurality of social life; and they construct a complex, acknowledged order (Hall, 1979, pp. 340-342). The implications of this perspective for an analysis of cultural processes are twofold; they suggest a return to the subject of experience and the struggle over the power of the text within a cultural and historical moment, and a consideration of the ideological effect of the media as they necessarily and incessantly intersect with the social practices of groups and individuals in society.

The Rise of the Audience

The intervention of Cultural Studies in the traditional approach to media studies may serve as a measure of the fundamental changes involved in turning from an American mass communication research perspective to a critical, cultural focus on the media and society. Specifically, by the 1970s American mass communication research had shifted its focus to audiences. However, the uses and gratification approach of this period (Katz, Blumler, & Gurevitch, 1974) retained its functionalist character regarding the presence of an active (e.g., consuming, need-fulfilling) audience, while struggling with the notion of the effects of texts and producers upon audiences under specific cultural, social, or economic conditions. Similarly, the agenda-setting model (McCombs & Shaw, 1972, 1976) continued to perpetuate an effects model of the media while identifying itself with the traditional, theoretical assumptions of the uses and gratification approach (Shaw, 1979).

Cultural Studies "broke with the models of 'direct influence' . . . into a framework which drew much more on what can broadly be defined as the 'ideological' role of the media"; it "challenged the notions of media texts as 'transparent' bearers of meaning . . . and gave much greater attention . . . to their linguistic and ideological structuration"; it replaced the passive conception of the audience with a "more active conception of the 'audience,' of 'reading' and of the relation between how media messages were encoded, the 'moment' of the encoded text and the variation of audience 'decodings'"; and finally, it engaged in the study of the role "which media play in the circulation and securing of *dominant* ideological definitions and representations." (Hall, 1980, pp. 118-119). Thus the approach of Cultural Studies is based upon an understanding of communication as related to the historical process of which it is also an "indissoluble" part. This vision is quite removed from the conceptualization in the American mass communication literature on popular culture and mass society that preferred the analysis of culture as an investigation of a series of empirical facts about media, contents and the effects on audiences. Indeed, such a position led to the Cultural Studies critique of the prevailing models of communication and society in the field.

Specifically, the British Cultural Studies tradition emerged from an intellectual climate created and sustained by a political discourse (as represented in the *New Left Review*) that operates on the assumption that Marxism as a social theory is quite capable of producing a change of the social and economic conditions of British society. These debates, informed by the contributions of Western European Marxism, French structuralism, and the work of Althusser in particular, continue to serve as the intellectual resources for alternative, political responses to the problems of British society, including the distribution of economic and political power and the role of the media.

Influence on American Cultural Studies

British Cultural Studies has appealed to the critics of American mass communication research with its provocative investigations of contemporary social problems, demonstrating a sense of engagement between political practice and theoretical consideration within the public sphere. This is a qualitatively decisive difference from a system in which the nature and extent of social research depend upon the relationship between academic organizations, economic interests, and the political system. Hence, mass communication research in the United States, with its primary location within the organization of universities, encounters the practical effects of politicizing research (for instance, through the policies of funding social scientific inquiries). In seeking alternative paths, American mass communication research may find the organizational aspects of the British Cultural Studies perspective in a climate of political engagement equally appropriate and useful for producing its own answers to socially important and politically relevant problems. At a different level, the reception and assimilation of such distinct theoretical propositions and research practices raise a number of questions concerning the ways in which they are transformed into a problematic that can be accommodated by a rather distinct, if limiting, system of academic disciplines in the United States. Although this is an issue that has been underlying the study of communication and media practice in American universities for many years, the advent of British Cultural Studies on the American academic scene has dramatized this question of disciplinary boundaries and academic compartmentalization of knowledge, including the construction and administration of appropriate social research agendas. Speaking of the study of culture, Ernest Gombrich (1969) once concluded that the "so-called disciplines on which our academic organisation is founded are no more than techniques; they are means to an end but no more than that" (p. 46). The arrival of Cultural Studies in the research literature of American mass communication studies has been a promising change since the earlier encounter with Critical Theory and the subsequent critique and exposure of the field to the work of Dallas Smythe, Herbert Schiller, Todd Gitlin, Stuart Ewen, and others, including critical European reactions to American mass communication scholarship.[4]

British Cultural Studies belong to an intellectual tradition in Western Europe, for which the matrix of literature, literary criticism and Marxism produced a convenient context for the questioning of cultural activities, including social communication. Such contextualization and the location of the problematic in the cultural process, specifically among cultural, political and economic phenomena, restored theoretical complexity and descriptive power to the analysis of communication and media practice. Notably the field of literary studies with its curiosity about the process of social communication, including the role of the media, has moved freely among leading intellectual currents and created an awareness of British and Continental European thought and its contribution to the modernist and postmodernist debates. In the meantime, mass communication research, which proceeded with its narrowly defined, atomistic vision of communication and media, has revealed its own definitive and irreconcilable differences with the exponents of an ideological approach to the processes of culture and communication.

But the attraction of Cultural Studies as an alternative in the discourse about communication and media studies cannot alleviate a number of problems beginning with the accessibility of these ideas for the development of a type of research that is conceptually rooted in the traditional, sociological model of mass communication research. This problem is exacerbated by the atheoretical nature of the majority of mass communication studies, the continuing isolation of this scholarship from other disciplines that are engaged in an exchange with Critical Theory and Cultural Studies, and, possibly, by an identification of Cultural Studies with a Marxist critique of society, and thus with a devastating critique of the culture industry, which threatens the traditional relationship between media research and commerce, and effectively precludes the accommodation of radical criticism. Suggestions for compromises, however, presented in terms of cooperation or merger of theoretical or methodological traditions, persevere (Gerbner, 1983, pp. 355-362). They are also offered as a "return to the bridge building between the social sciences and the humanities" or as a "cultural-empirical approach" (McQuail, 1984, p. 186), without specific references to the ideological problematic—the conflicts of theory. Indeed, there is a noticeable tendency to search for an underlying intellectual consensus. In his discussion of the development of sociological theories, Alvin Gouldner (1970) referred to this process of discovering a common ground as an "Americanized version of Hegelianism, in which historical development presumably occurs not through polemic, struggle, and conflict, but through consensus" (p. 17). On the other hand, the approval of a pluralism of critical approaches to the problems of media and communication also continues to be couched in terms of methodological diversity, preferably as long as it excludes "an ideological approach" (Halloran, 1983, p. 272). Such a position is reminiscent of the arguments by Howard Becker and Irving Louis Horowitz (1972) in the 1970s that "radical sociology" can be "good sociology," if it is purged of an ideological bias (pp. 48-66). There are valid reasons to suspect that "good" mass communication research would operate on principles derived from the traditional epistemology of media studies that would also emphasize—to use the vocabulary of Becker and Horowitz—"meaningful descriptions" and "valid explanations" of social phenomena, while an accomodation of radical criticism would be "a full exploration of possibilites" within the range of a dominant, liberal-pluralist theory of society (pp. 50-51).

Similarly, American cultural studies may have gained from Carey's (1975) reconceptualization of the "transmission" view of communication with its roots "in essentially religious attitudes" of American society (p. 3) into a "ritual" perspective on communication, based upon predominantly European sources, as an opportunity "to rebuild a model of and for communication of some restorative value in reshaping our common culture" (p. 21). Carey's explanation documents a historical condition of the American social sciences and indicates a realization of an alternative perspective, that is to say, a cultural concept of communication identified with the tradition of pragmatism and the Chicago School. Specifically, for Carey (1982), an approach to cultural studies involves a definition of communication that "constitutes a set of historically varying practices and reflections upon them. These practices bring together human conceptions and purposes with technological forms in sedimented social relations." He identified the central problem of this approach as "that of meaning in order to contrast it with versions of communication that search for laws and functions and to focus on the hermeneutic side of the task" (p. 30). Such a perspective, however, still operates within the dominant system of meanings and values and can offer only a nostalgic vision of the potential of communication and the power of the community as long as it fails to generate a critique of its own tradition and an alternative cultural perspective that overcomes the ideological conditions of the prevailing theory of democracy.

Although it seems quite appropriate for American cultural studies to begin addressing questions of contemporary culture (instead of problems of mass communication), there is a need to develop theoretical propositions, under which the idea of "culture as a total way of life" (Carey, 1979, p. 424-425) becomes a necessary and appropriate context for the study of individual practice and collective action. Most recently, Carey (1983) has characterized the conditions of American cultural studies as being in a ferment concerning "its ability to retain enough of the origins, insights, and tone of pragmatism while it squarely faces the fact that societies are structured not only in and by communications but also by its relations of power and dominance"(p. 312). To be sure, the discussion of "power" and "domination," and the consideration of "process" and "change" as important principles of a cultural theory are not a commitment to Marxist theory, but a reflection of their usefulness for the analysis of contemporary culture. In fact, if Marxist theory helps stimulate a search for alternative theoretical positions, there is a need to clarify its relationship to pragmatism or to any other theoretical foundation of American cultural studies. While certain conceptualizations of culture and cultural processes, like the treatment of language (Peirce) and the role of communication (Dewey), are useful elements in a theory of communication (and media practice) as they evolved from American pragmatism. Other considerations, like the relationship among social, economic, and cultural practices and the role of the media, the power of institutions, and the concepts of freedom and participation, continue to be problematic, because they are defined in terms of dominant social and economic interests and, therefore, remain outside the reach of radical change. As Bernstein (1971) suggested in his sympathetic review of pragmatism, Dewey failed to be genuinely radical, because "he underestimates the powerful social, political, and economic forces that distort and corrupt" and despite his intentions, "the consequence of his own philosophy is to perpetuate the social evils that it seeks to overcome" (p. 228). These forces are also grounded in an empirical-analytic approach to the social and natural environment, which is interested in technical control and differs from hermeneutic or critical "knowledge-constitutive" interests (Habermas, 1971, pp. 195-197). American cultural studies, following Carey's argument in favor of pragmatism as a useful theoretical context, needs to resurrect a theory of inquiry that develops and supports a notion of radical thinking linked to an understanding of the constitution of social life.

In the meantime, the emergence of a theoretical position and its domination is also a condition of intellectual leadership; particularly in its return to an understanding of intellectual work (based upon Gramsci's writings) as involved in the collective practice of producing and sharing knowledge. Thus the diversity and quality of theoretical insights gained through retracing the hermeneutic tradition of European thought, and the impact of Western Marxism and feminism on contemporary social theory, have influenced these joint intellectual tasks of formulating theoretical propositions and research projects under a Cultural Studies approach in Britain. In the past, the behavioral sciences have provided such guidance in the field of mass communication research on both sides of the Atlantic. More recently, the application of Western Marxism has gained strength, and an extensive body of Marxist literature available in English translation added a considerable voice to the theoretical discourse. Perhaps more importantly, however, are the political conditions of societies, derived from racist governments that threaten the lives of millions with the prospects of nuclear holocaust, which continue to draw social scientists and their professional concerns to the reality of human misery and global disaster with the realization that generations of scholarship and research have been unable to effect the political and economic destiny of people. Consequently, there has been a willingness to reconsider theoretical (and methodological) issues, testifying to the domination of a particular ("American") position and resulting in critical reflections and possibly changes in the theoretical assumptions governing mass communication research.

As a matter of fact, there is considerable power in the role of mass communication researchers as intellectuals engaged in the creation and defense of theoretical positions. They maintain not only the prevailing traditional values, providing an ideological defense of particular (class) interests, but they are also indispensible in the struggle for alternative expressions. In recent years, the proponents of Critical Theory and Cultural Studies have been deeply committed to the task of "breaking" with traditional notions of communication in society. They have redefined the realm of academic scholarship and professional specialization to engage in a pedagogical project through the selection of problems and the type of research that deals with the daily existence of people, but also through a conscious intellectual engagement within the political structure of their societies. There is a continuing need for such involvement, as Trent Schroyer (1975a) pointed out several years ago, because

> the real process of enlightenment refers to the reinterpretation of their needs by the many people who are currently unable to do so. Thinking about ways in which communicative processes can be stimulated is crucial. Critical theorists must construct models for the activation of communication about human requirements and the ways in which institutions can be changed to meet them. (pp. 248-249)

CONCLUSIONS

Under the leadership of American pragmatism, social theorists had focused upon the importance of culture and the idea that communication as a life process leads to democratic practice. This conclusion constituted the beginning of a critical position in social science theory and research within a liberal pluralist tradition. When the Frankfurt School offered a comprehensive modernist view of the cultural and political crisis of Western society, its Critical Theory evoked a modest and eclectic response among communication and media scholars in the United States. The success of British Cultural Studies at this time has been a reminder that a cultural approach to the problems of communication and media has remained a consistent and recognized theme in the literature of the field. There can be no doubt that the problems of communication, including the operation of the media, are embedded in the history of a culture. For this reason there is also an affinity with those mass communication studies in the United States that have had a strong cultural tradition. After all, the idea of culture and society in the context of mass communication research in the United States is defined through its assimilation of nineteenth-century European social thought into American practice; that is to say, by the effects of American pragmatism on the development of academic disciplines and their particular social concerns. Thus the evolutionary concept of society with its own social dynamic, the emphasis upon social forces, and the recognition that individuals may need the assistance and protection of the state in their encounters with the modern world, were not only characteristics of the German historical school or of nineteenth-century European socialism, they also described the theoretical thrust of American political economy after the turn of this century. Pragmatism added a dynamic vision of the new world to this perspective and provided the social context for the study of media and communication.

Consequently, mass communication studies rose to academic prominence and political importance with the recognition of commercial and political propaganda as essential aspects of mass persuasion vis-à-vis an increasing need for the mediation of knowledge in a complex urban society. But the cultural approach of the field also shared the basic tenets of the social sciences of the time, namely the belief in a world that is knowable through the application of scientific techniques that stressed the plurality and equality of facts, through the belief in the objectivity of expert observations and the power of empirical explanations. Mass communication was treated as a series of specific, isolated social phenomena, that resulted in a narrow understanding of communication and culture and in a conduct of media studies that lacked historicity.

This approach to communication and culture in the United States depended upon a firm belief in a utopian model of society. It was based upon a vision of consensual participation as democratic practice and an understanding of the exercise of political and economic power as acts of progressive intervention in the advancement of people. Radical dissent, including Marxist criticism of American society, remained outside the mainstream of mass communication research. When it arose, it belonged to the literature of social criticism rooted in rhetorical studies, literature, political economy, and sociology, in particular, from which it was unable to engage the field in an extensive and prolonged debate concerning the foundations of social theory and the false optimism of social inquiries into the role and function of communication and media.

At the same time, the enthusiasm for an alternative explanation of communication in society, if sustained, cannot rest upon the good will toward Cultural Studies and a calculated indifference toward the dominant interpretation of the social structure. Instead, a commitment to a critical approach, in the sense of a Marxist critique of society, will lead to a number of significant changes in the definition of society, social problems, and the media as well as in the organization and execution of research projects. They are changes rooted in radical ideas, uncompromising in their demands for rethinking the theoretical basis of mass communication studies and innovative in their creation of appropriate methodologies. Thus Cultural Studies, not unlike radical sociology of the late 1960s and early 1970s, "finds itself providing the facts, theories, and understandings that a radical politics requires for its implementation" (Becker & Horowitz, 1972, p. 54). It also reflects the emancipatory power of a social theory that is grounded in the potential of individuals to rise above their social and economic conditions. Since the traditional literature of mass communication theory and research restricts the imagination by its refusal to engage in critical reflections on human ideals as normative (or unscientific) issues and by its denial of the historical process in the presentation of mass communication phenomena, it must be replaced by an emancipatory social theory that locates the inquiry about mass communication in the realm of the ideological and explains the role of communication and the place of the media through an examination of the cultural process. The result will also be a reconceptualization of disciplinary (and administrative) boundaries, which has theoretical (and political) implications for the definition of a field in which culture as a way of life will become the framework for an interpretation of communication in society. Similarly, Robert Sklar (1975) argued over 10 years ago that American Studies, by turning to the works of Roland Barthes, E. P. Thompson, Eric Hobsbawm, Antonio Gramsci, Theodor Adorno, Walter Benjamin, Raymond Williams, and George Lukacs, would discover "an untapped powerful resource for the essential task of linking the forms of consciousness and expression with the forms of social organization" (pp. 260-261).

But the "discovery" of Cultural Studies through the exposure to a specific type of media studies in the United Kingdom, and the current preoccupation with "critical" research should not obscure the fact that there is no history of a systematic acknowledgment of Marxist scholarship by traditional mass communication research in the United States. Subsequently, the reception of individual Marxist scholars throughout various periods by mainstream mass communication research has remained questionable, and their influence upon the development of the field has continued to be negligible. In general, mass communication studies have followed the path of American social science in the rejection of a critical, Marxist approach to questions of media and society. In light of these experiences and the history of social criticism and radical critique in the field, the Cultural Studies perspective remains a temporary phenomenon, while the notion of "critical" research will be defined by and identified with "liberal" mass communication scholarship and its own critical position vis-à-vis society.

Indeed, there is always a chance for the return of the "critical" as an accommodation of liberal dissent, while Marxist thought retreats again into the shadow of the dominant ideology. In any case, British Cultural Studies, as a cultural phenomenon, holds its own interpretation; its language and practice are contained in the specific historical moment, which may become accessible to American mass communication research, though it cannot be appropriated, adapted, or co-opted without losing its meaning. The dilemma of American mass communication studies continues to lie in the failure to comprehend and overcome the limitations of its own intellectual history, not only by failing to address the problems of an established (and politically powerful) academic discipline with its specific theoretical and methodological requirements, but also by failing to recognize the potential of radical thought.

NOTES

1. In this chapter, British Cultural Studies and Critical Theory are capitalized as references to specific schools of thought.

2. In addition to the cited material, the following sources are particularly useful for a perspective on Cultural Studies: Colin Sparks (1977, 1987), Stuart Hall (1979, 1980b, 1980c, 1982), Raymond Williams (1980), Larry Grossberg (1983), and Richard Johnson (1983). The influence of Cultural Studies upon cultural and historical studies in the United States has been

documented in a special issue of the *The Radical History Review* (Vol. 19, Winter 1978/1979), titled: "Marxism and History: The British Contribution." More recently, the *Journal of Communication Inquiry* (1986, Vol. 10, p. 2) devoted a special issue to Stuart Hall that contains a working bibliography of Hall's publications. For a historical overview of the concept of *totality* and contemporary Western Marxism, see Martin Jay (1984).

3. A historical treatment of Critical Theory is provided by Martin Jay (1973). Recent literature on Critical Theory, which should be of particular interest to communication scholarship, contains the following monographs: Phil Slater (1977), Zoltan Tar (1977), Susan Buck-Morss (1977), Andrew Arato and Eike Gebhardt (1978) Thomas McCarthy (1978), Paul Connerton (1980), David Held (1980), George Friedman (1981), John Thompson and David Held (1982), Helmut Dubiel (1985), and John Forester (1985). An indispensable source for an ongoing discussion of issues in Critical Theory is the *New German Critique*.

4. Among the critical contributions at that time were Dallas W. Smythe (1954), Kaarle Nordenstreng (1968), Herbert Gans (1972), Herbert I. Schiller (1974), and Veikko Pietila (1975).

REFERENCES

Althusser, L. (1971). *Lenin and philosophy and other essays*. London: New Left.

Arato, A., & Gebhardt, E. (Eds.). (1978). *The essential Frankfurt School reader*. New York: Urizen.

Becker, H. S. (1967). Whose side are we on? *Social Problems, 14*(3), 239-247.

Becker, H. S., & Horowitz, I. L. (1972, July). Radical politics and sociological research: Observations on methodology and ideology. *American Journal of Sociology, 78*(1), 48-66.

Berelson, B. (1959). The state of communication research. *Public Opinion Quarterly, 23*(1), 1-6.

Bernstein, R. J. (1967). *John Dewey*. New York: Washington Square Press.

Bernstein, R. J. (1971). *Praxis and action: Contemporary philosophies of human activity*. Philadelphia: University of Pennsylvania Press.

Bernstein, R. J. (Ed.). (1985). *Habermas and modernity*. Cambridge, MA: Polity Press.

Buck-Morss, S. (1977). *The origin of negative dialectics*. New York: Free Press.

Carey, J. W. (1975). A cultural approach to communication. *Communication, 2*(1), 1-22.

Carey, J. W. (1979). Mass communication research and cultural studies: An American view. In J. Curran, M. Gurevitch, & J. Woollacott (Eds.), *Mass communication and society* (pp. 409-425). Beverly Hills, CA: Sage.

Carey, J. W. (1982). The mass media and critical theory: An American view. In M. Burgoon (Ed.), *Communication yearbook 6* (pp. 18-33). Beverly Hills, CA: Sage.

Carey, J. W. (1983). The origins of the radical discourse on cultural studies in the United States. *Journal of Communication, 33*(3), 311-313.

Connerton, P. (1980). *The tragedy of enlightenment: An essay on the Frankfurt School*. New York: Cambridge University Press.

Curran, J., Gurevitch, M., & Woollacott, J. (1982). The study of the media: Theoretical approaches. In M. Gurevitch, T. Bennett, J. Curran, & J. Woollacott (Eds.), *Culture, society and the media* (pp. 11-29). London: Methuen.

Davison, W. P., & Frederick, T.C.Y. (Eds). (1974). *Mass communication research: Major issues and future directions*. New York: Praeger.

Dewey, J. (1925). Nature, communication and meaning. In *Experience and Nature* (pp. 138-170). Chicago: Open Court.

Dewey, J. (1931). The development of American pragmatism. In *Philosophy and civilization* (pp. 13-35). New York: Minton, Balch.

Dewey, J. (1954). *The public and its problems*. Chicago: Swallow.

Dewey, J. (1960). *Quest for certainty: A study in the relation of knowledge and action*. New York: Capricorn.

Dewey, J. (1966). *Democracy and education.* New York: Macmillan.
Dubiel, H. (1985). *Theory and politics: The development of Critical Theory.* Cambridge: MIT Press.
Festinger, L. A. (1957). *A theory of cognitive dissonance.* Evanston, IL: Row & Peterson.
Forester, J. (Ed.). (1985). *Critical theory and public life.* Cambridge: MIT Press.
Friedman, G. (1981). *The political philosophy of the Frankfurt School.* Ithaca, NY: Cornell University Press.
Gans, H. (1972). The famine in American mass communications research. *American Journal of Sociology, 77,* 697-705.
Gerbner, G. (1956). Toward a general model of communication. *Audio-Visual Communication Review, 4*(2), 171-199.
Gerbner, G. (1964). On content analysis and critical research in mass communication. In L. A. Dexter & D. M. White (Eds.), *People, society and mass communication* (pp. 476-500). New York: Free Press.
Gerbner, G. (1983). The importance of being critical—in one's own fashion. *Journal of Communication, 33*(3), 355-362.
Gitlin, T. (1981). Media sociology: The dominant paradigm. In G. C. Wilhoit & H. de Bock (Eds.), *Mass communication review yearbook* (Vol. 2, pp. 73-121). Beverly Hills, CA: Sage.
Gombrich, E. H. (1969). *In search of cultural history.* Oxford: University of Oxford Press.
Gouldner, A. (1970). *The coming crisis of Western sociology.* New York: Basic Books.
Gouldner, A. (1976). *The dialectic of ideology and technology. The origins, grammar, and future of ideology.* New York: Seabury Press.
Grossberg, L. (1977). Cultural interpretation and mass communication. *Communication Research, 4,* 339-360.
Grossberg, L. (1983). Cultural studies revisited and revised. In Mary S. Mander (Ed.), *Communications in transition* (pp. 39-70). New York: Praeger.
Grossberg, L. (1984). Strategies of Marxist cultural interpretation. *Critical Studies in Mass Communication, 1*(4), 392-421.
Habermas, J. (1971). *Knowledge and human interests.* Boston: Beacon.
Habermas, J. (1979). *Communication and the evolution of society.* Boston: Beacon.
Habermas, J. (1981). *Theorie des kommunikativen Handelns* (2 vols.). Frankfurt: Suhrkamp Verlag.
Habermas, J. (1984a). *The theory of communicative action: Volume I. Reason and the Rationalization of Society.* Boston: Beacon.
Habermas, J. (1984b). *Vorstudien und Erganzungen zur Theorie des kommunikativen Handelns.* Frankfurt: Suhrkamp Verlag.
Habermas, J. (1985). Questions and counterquestions. In R. J. Bernstein (Ed.), *Habermas and modernity* (pp. 192-216). Cambridge, MA: Polity Press.
Haight, T. R. (1983). The critical researcher's dilemma. *Journal of Communication, 33*(3), 226-236.
Hall, S. (1979). Culture, the media, and the "ideological effect." In J. Curran, M. Gurevitch, & J. Woollacott (Eds.), *Mass communication and society* (pp. 315-348). Beverly Hills, CA: Sage.
Hall, S. (1980a). Cultural studies and the Centre: Some problematics and problems. In S. Hall, D. Hobson, A. Lowe, & P. Willis (Eds.), *Culture, media, language* (pp. 15-47). London: Hutchinson.
Hall, S. (1980b). Cultural studies: Two paradigms. *Media, Culture and Society, 2,* 57-72.
Hall, S. (1980c). Encoding/decoding. In S. Hall, D. Hobson, A. Lowe, & P. Willis (Eds.), *Culture, media, language* (pp. 128-138). London: Hutchinson.
Hall, S. (1980d). Introduction to media studies at the Centre. In S. Hall, D. Hobson, A. Lowe, & P. Willis (Eds.), *Culture, media, language* (pp. 117-121). London: Hutchinson.
Hall, S. (1982). The rediscovery of "ideology": Return of the repressed in media studies. In M. Gurevitch, T. Bennett, J. Curran, & J. Woollacott (Eds.), *Culture, society and the media* (pp. 56-90). London: Methuen.

Hallin, D. C. (1985). The American news media: A critical theory perspective. In J. Forester (Ed.), *Critical theory and public life* (pp. 122-146). Cambridge: MIT Press.
Halloran, J. D. (1983). A case for critical eclecticism. *Journal of Communication, 33*(3), 270-278.
Hardt, H. (1979). *Social theories of the press: Early German and American perspectives.* Beverly Hills, CA: Sage.
Hardt, H. (1987). Communication and economic thought: Cultural imagination in German and American scholarship. *Communication.*
Harris, M. (1979). *Cultural materialism: The struggle for a science of culture.* New York: Random House.
Haskell, T. (1977). *The emergence of professional social science.* Urbana: University of Illinois Press.
Heider, F. (1946). Attitudes and cognitive information. *Journal of Psychology, 21,* 107-112.
Held, E. (1980). *Introduction to critical theory: Horkheimer to Habermas.* Berkeley: University of California Press.
Hofstadter, R. (1962). *Anti-intellectualism in American life.* New York: Vintage.
Horkheimer, M. (1941a). Preface. *Studies in philosophy and social science, IX*(1), 1.
Horkheimer, M. (1941b). Notes on Institute activities. *Studies in Philosophy and Social Science. IX*(1), 121-123.
Horkheimer, M., & Adorno T. W. (1972). *Dialectic of enlightenment.* New York: Herder & Herder.
James, H. (Ed.). (1920). *The letters of William James* (Vol. 2). Boston: Atlantic Monthly Press.
Jay, M. (1973). *The dialectical imagination: A history of the Frankfurt School and the Institute of Social Research, 1923-1950.* Boston: Little, Brown.
Jay, M. (1984). *Marxism and totality. The adventures of a concept from Lukacs to Habermas.* Berkeley: University of California Press.
Jay, M. (1985). *Permanent exiles: Essays on the intellectual migration from Germany to America.* New York: Columbia University Press.
Johnson, F. C., & Klare, G. R. (1961). General models of communication research: A survey of the developments of a decade. *Journal of Communication, 11*(1), 13-26.
Johnson, R. (1983, September). *What is cultural studies anyway?* Stencilled Occasional Paper (General Series: SP No. 74). Centre for Contemporary Cultural Studies, University of Birmingham.
Katz, E., Blumler J. G., & Gurevitch, M. (1974). Utilization of mass communication by the individual. In J. G. Blumler & E. Katz (Eds.), *The uses of mass communications* (pp. 19-32). Beverly Hills, CA: Sage.
Lasswell, H. D. (1948). The structure and function of communication in society. In L. Bryson (Ed.). *The communication of ideas* (pp. 37-51). New York: Harper & Row.
Lazarsfeld, P. F. (1941). Remarks on administrative and critical communications research. *Studies in Philosophy and Social Science IX*(1), 2-16.
Lazarsfeld, P. F. (1969). An episode in the history of social research: A memoir. In D. Fleming & B. Bailyn (Eds.), *The intellectual migration, Europe and America, 1930-1960* (pp. 270-337). Cambridge: Harvard University Press (Belknap Press).
Lerner, D., & L. M. Nelson (Eds.). (1977). *Communication research—A half-century appraisal.* Honolulu: University of Hawaii Press.
Lovett, R. M. (1937). Social criticism. In *Encyclopedia of the social sciences* (Vols. III-IV, pp. 599-602). New York: Macmillan.
Matthews, F. H. (1977). *Quest for an American sociology: Robert E. Park and the Chicago School.* Montreal: McGill-Queens University Press.
McCarthy, T. (1978). *The critical theory of Jurgen Habermas.* Cambridge: MIT Press.
McCombs, M. E., & Shaw, D. L. (1972). The agenda-setting function of mass media. *Public Opinion Quarterly, 36*(2), 76-87.
McCombs, M. E., & Shaw, D. L. (1976). Structuring the "unseen environment." *Journal of Communication, 26*(2), 18-22.

McIntyre, J. S. (1987). Repositioning a landmark: The Hutchins Commission on Freedom of the Press. *Critical Studies in Mass Communication,* 4(2), 136-160.
McLuskie, E. (1975). *A critical epistemology of Paul Lazarsfeld's administrative communication inquiry.* Unpublished doctoral dissertation, University of Iowa.
McLuskie, E. (1977). *Integration of critical theory with North American communication study: Barriers and prospects.* Paper presented at the ICA convention, Berlin, West Germany.
McQuail, D. (1984). With the benefit of hindsight: Reflections on uses and gratification research. *Critical Studies in Mass Communication, 1*(2), 177-193.
McQuail, D., & S. Windahl (1981). *Communication models for the study of mass communications.* New York: Longman.
Mead, H. G. (1967). *Mind, self and society.* Chicago: University of Chicago Press (Phoenix Books).
Merton, R. (1957). *Social theory and social structure.* New York: Free Press.
Mills, C. W. (1970). *The sociological imagination.* Harmondsworth: Penguin.
Morrison, D. E. (1978). Kultur and culture: The case of Theodor W. Adorno and Paul F. Lazarsfeld. *Social Research, 45*(2), 331-355.
Mosco, V. (1983). Critical research and the role of labor. *Journal of Communication, 33*(3), 237-248.
Newcomb, Theodore M. (1953). An approach to the study of communicative acts. *Psychological Review, 60*(6), 393-404.
Nordenstreng, K. (1968). Communication research in the United States. *Gazette, 14*(3), 207-216.
Novack, G. (1975). *Pragmatism versus Marxism. An appraisal of John Dewey's philosophy.* New York: Pathfinder.
Oberschall, A. (Ed.). (1972). *The establishment of empirical sociology.* New York: Harper & Row.
Ogburn, W. F. (1964). Trends in social science. In O. D. Duncan (Ed.), *William F. Ogburn on culture and social change* (pp. 207-220). Chicago: University of Chicago Press.
Park, R. E. (1938). Reflections on communication and culture. *American Journal of Sociology, 44*(2), 187-205.
Park, R. E. (1967). Foreign language press and progress. In R. H. Turner, (Ed.), *Robert E. Park on social control and collective behavior* (pp. 133-144). Chicago: University of Chicago Press,
Parsons, T., & Shills, E. A., (Eds.). (1951). *Toward a general theory of action: Theoretical foundations of the social sciences.* New York: Harper Torchbooks.
Patten, S. N. (1924). In R. G. Tugwell (Ed.), *Essays in economic theory.* New York: Knopf.
Pietila, V. (1975). *On the scientific status and position of communication research* (Report No. 35). Institute of Journalism and Mass Communication, University of Tampere, Finland.
Quandt, J. B. (1970). *From the small town to the great community.* New Brunswick, NJ: Rutgers University Press.
Riesman, D. (1959). The state of communication research: Comments. *Public Opinion Quarterly, 23*(1), 10-13.
Rogers, E. M. (1986). *Communication technology: The new media in society.* New York: Free Press.
Rogers, E. M., & Balle, F. (Eds.). (1985). *The media revolution in America and Western Europe.* Norwood, NJ: Ablex.
Rorty, R. (1985). Habermas and Lyotard on postmodernity. In R. J. Bernstein (Ed.), *Habermas and modernity* (pp. 161-175). Cambridge, MA: Polity Press.
Ross, E. A. (1910, March). The suppression of important news. *Atlantic Monthly,* pp. 303-311.
Ross, E. A. (1918). Social decadence. *American Journal of Sociology, 23*(5), 620-632.
Schiller, H. I. (1974). Waiting for orders—Current trends in mass communication research in the United States. *Gazette, 20*(1), 11-21.
Schiller, H. I. (1983). Critical research in the information age. *Journal of Communication, 33*(3), 249-257.

Schramm, W. (1954). How communication works. In W. Schramm (Ed.), *The process and effects of mass communication* (pp. 3-26). Urbana: University of Illinois Press.

Schroyer, T. (1975a). *The critique of domination: The origins and development of critical theory.* Boston: Beacon Press.

Schroyer, T. (1975b). The re-politicization of the relations of production: An interpretation of Jürgen Habermas' analytic theory of capitalist development. *New German Critique, 5,* 107-128.

Shannon, C., & Weaver, W. (1949). *The mathematical theory of communication.* Urbana: University of Illinois Press.

Shaw, E. F. (1979). Agenda-setting and mass communication theory. *Gazette, 25*(2), 96-105.

Sklar, R. (1975). The problem of an American studies philosophy: A bibliography of new directions. *American Quarterly, 27*(3), 245-262.

Slack, J. D., & Allor, M. (1983). The political and epistemological constituents of critical communication research. *Journal of Communication, 33*(3), 208-218.

Slater, P. (1977). *Origin and significance of the Frankfurt School: A Marxist perspective.* London: Routledge & Kegan Paul.

Small, A. (1910). *The meaning of social science.* Chicago: University of Chicago Press.

Small, A. (1912). General sociology. *American Journal of Sociology, 18*(2), 200-214.

Small, A., & Vincent, G. (1894). *An introduction to the study of society.* New York: American Books.

Smythe, D. W. (1954). Some observations on communications theory. *Audio-Visual Communication Review, 2*(1), 24-37.

Smythe, D. W. (1969). Preface. In H. I. Schiller, *Mass communications and American empire* (pp. vii-viii). New York: Augustus M. Kelly.

Smythe, D. W., & Dinh, T. V. (1983). On critical and administrative research: A new critical analysis. *Journal of Communication, 33*(3), 117-127.

Sparks, C. (1977). The evolution of cultural studies. *Screen Education, 22,* 16-30.

Sparks, C. (1987, September). *The strengths and limits of the "cultural" approach to communication.* Paper presented at the Communication and Culture Colloquium, Dubrovnik, Yugoslavia.

Stevenson, R. L. (1983). A critical look at critical analysis. *Journal of Communication, 33*(3), 262-269.

Tar, Z. (1977). *The Frankfurt School: The critical theories of Max Horkheimer and Theodor W. Adorno.* New York: Wiley-Interscience.

Thayer, H. S. (1973). *Meaning and action: A study of American pragmatism.* Indianapolis: Bobbs-Merrill.

Thompson, J., & Held, D. (Eds.). (1982). *Habermas: Critical debates.* Cambridge: MIT Press.

Westley, B., & MacLean, M. S. (1957). A conceptual model for mass communication research. *Journalism Quarterly, 34*(1), 31-38.

Williams, R. (1977). *Marxism and literature.* New York: Oxford University Press.

Williams, R. (1980). *Problems in materialism and culture.* London: Verso.

Cultural Studies: From Old World to New World

FARRELL CORCORAN
National Institute for Higher Education, Dublin, Ireland

CULTURAL Studies differs from most American approaches to mass communication research by addressing awkward issues about culture that have been ignored in mainstream thinking because they involve adopting a political perspective sensitive to the matrices of power in contemporary society. From its emergence two decades ago, Cultural Studies has placed at the center of its agenda the analysis of the processes through which a particular hegemonic worldview is consistently privileged in contemporary culture, and thus the existing structure of power and domination reproduced. It is also different from most American research paradigms because of its genealogical connections with a particular mix of disciplines—the seemingly disparate traditions of literary criticism, social history, semiotics, political economy, psychoanalysis, and ethnography.

This commentary will amplify Hardt's exploration of the American encounter with approaches to cultural interpretation already well established in anglophone Europe, first, by describing the commonalities that allow different approaches to be grouped under one label. Then it will try to open out that range of approaches so that important distinctions and disagreements become apparent and Cultural Studies is prevented from being collapsed into a dense theoretical mass that can be co-opted into the panoply of American communication theories rather than made to challenge them. And if, as seems likely, we are now in the middle of the second epoch of this century in which a rare window is opened in American academia onto the main currents of thinking in the European left, it is important not only that we understand what

Correspondence and requests for reprints: Farrell Corcoran, Communication and Human Studies, National Institute for Higher Education, Dublin, Ireland.

Communication Yearbook 12, pp. 601-617

happened to the first epoch (in the postwar years) but also that we reflect on the possible fate of the second.

ROOTS

Theoretical approaches that stress the connections between cultural practices or institutions and social change or stability have greatly expanded over the last 10 years in communication studies curricula and research programs. A unifying concern is the role played by contemporary culture in general, but particularly the mass media, in defining social relations and political problems while seeming to function as a "transparent" bearer of meanings "found" in society.

The Cultural Studies paradigm, rejecting the view that media organizations enjoy an important degree of autonomy from the state and the power of monopoly capital, began to seek a materialist explanation for the problem of how the powerless majority in contemporary societies give "free consent" to the rule of powerful minorities, organized in Western democracies through the form of interlocking webs of mutual interest embedded in national and transnational corporations, coordinated by the state. It suggested that media professionals, while enjoying the illusion of autonomy, relay interpretive frameworks that are consonant with the interests of the dominant culture. It questioned how audiences are prevented from having access to alternative or oppositional frameworks and how they can be said to accept, reject, or construct for themselves negotiated readings of the dominant definitions of social reality being offered, and how they do all this within an ideological environment that stresses the "freedoms" that prevail: of choice, of the press, of artistic creation, of professional norms, and so on.

The Cultural Studies paradigm is squarely in the intellectual tradition that draws its inspiration from Marx and Engels's (1962, pp. 272-273) assertion that the propertied classes of nineteenth-century Europe and America created "an entire superstructure of distinct and peculiarly formed sentiments, illusions, modes of thought and views of life," so pervasive that the individual members of society internalized them "through tradition and upbringing" to the point that they "imagine that they form the real motives and the starting point" of their activity. All of the contemporary approaches to understanding culture that could be labeled Cultural Studies—whether interested in the way texts construct meanings, or the political economy determining the production of those texts, or the way people interact with them—derive from this situating of the notion of culture firmly in the dialectic between social being and social consciousness. Although the Marxian formulation gives coherence to the field, it also opens up many significantly divergent views on the way the superstructure is related to its base and the way individuals can be said to internalize that superstructure.

It may well be asked why such a direction of inquiry has taken so long to emerge. The attempt to answer this would take us far outside the limited scope of this essay, but it is relevant to note that it emerged in the British tradition primarily through literary studies and social history rather than through sociology, dominated as that was in the postwar period by a distinctly American theoretical framework that celebrated the "pluralist" society (as opposed to the "totalitarian" society) as an unproblematic scientific fact rather than as an ideological construct. Most accounts of the roots of Cultural Studies (e.g., Hall, 1980) look to the literary and historical work of Richard Hoggart, Raymond Williams, and E. P. Thomson in the 1950s for the originating texts of the field. This body of work departed from the dominant perspective of pre-War elitist definitions of "culture" forcefully presented in the work of T. S. Eliot, F. R. Leavis, and the *Scrutiny* group, which were polarized around the high/low culture distinction driven by the search for an essential "organic culture" of the past, an ideal order against which "mass culture" could be (moralistically) measured. Leavisite criticism remained ascendant in British intellectual life until the 1950s, easily predominating over earlier Marxist thinking on the connections between culture and society, thinking that had failed to mount a successful rival theoretical approach that could escape from the tendency to explain cultural texts solely by reducing them to reflections of the economic structure of society. It can be argued plausibly that very many of the most important questions in the theory of culture today are posed between those working within a much more complex Marxism, rather than between Marxist and non-Marxist paradigms. The history of the shift from the heyday of Leavisite criticism 30 years ago is the history of Cultural Studies. Hoggart, Williams, and Thomson, each in a different way, widened the focus of cultural criticism to include the traditional cultures of the urban working class, in the process transforming the methods of literary criticism so as to "read" as a text the social arrangements, collective experiences, idioms, sights, and sounds of living cultures—the whole process of the means by which meanings are socially constructed. In this shift, the ground of the entire debate on culture and society was moved from a literary-moral to an anthropological view of culture.

IDEOLOGY

The development of Cultural Studies through the 1960s and 1970s has been well documented by Hall (1980) and need not be recapitulated here. Of decisive importance, however, has been the emergence within the theory of culture of a nonidealist notion of ideology and a decisive rethinking of the classical Marxist base/superstructure couplet. Though now commonplace in European scholarship, the notion of ideology is only recently entering American parlance, being itself thoroughly ideologized during all the decades of the Cold War that allowed no conceptual space for a "Marxism" that was not also "Soviet." Deeply committed to an idealist conception of the origins of public meanings, particularly the dynamics of mass consciousness and the role played by public forms of communication in establishing widely held meanings, mainstream American academic inquiry, when it could get away from the overwhelming fascination with a narrow "effects" paradigm, asked how the human symbol-using potential orders material reality mythically or in "fantasy themes" or "worldviews." But it neglected to ask how that normative ordering is influenced by the socioeconomic structure of a society, because the symbolist tradition maintained an inherent resistance to discussing the capacity of a "free" (as opposed to a "totalitarian") society to determine mass consciousness.

The notion of ideology, on the other hand, takes the exercise of power as its focal point, particularly the ways in which a certain social order is maintained through the ability of a dominant minority to fashion public meanings that are then "naturalized" throughout the whole of mass consciousness. A systematic orientation of thought, derived from the social and economic conditions of existence and the forms of thought and feeling of a particular group within a culture, becomes ideological as it gains adherence among other social groups and begins to mold their personal convictions into a replica of dominant norms. Since it is built on a narrow social point of view, it is encased within a specific body of unexamined assumptions through which its view of the world is filtered. Ideology in this sense is embedded in general perceptions and explanations of the world, thereby disguising its real roots in the perspective of only one part of society, whose interests it defends and legitimizes. From its empirical base in the experience of a specific social group, it becomes normative for the rest of society, turning what is a fact for one group into an ideal for all, thus legitimizing an existing power structure and reproducing it in a noncoercive way. Actual conflicts of interest are hidden in ideology, which, as Poulantzas (1971) suggests, "reconstitutes on an imaginary level a relatively coherent discourse that serves as the horizon of agents' experience" (p. 207).

The degree to which economic forces "determine" the ideological superstructure has remained controversial down to the present. Two polar positions define the limits of the debate. On the one hand, there is the economistic reduction of ideology to the status of an unilinear emanation from the economic level of society, whereby the superstructure becomes a direct, monolithic reflection of the views of the dominant political forces, manipulated by them to protect their own interests. On the other, there is what Ralph Milliband (1985) dubbed the "new revisionism," which tends to disconnect ideology from its roots in class divisions and deny the existence of any reality that is independent of "discourse." Central to the discussion is the meaning of *determine* in the base-superstructure model and how it may be amplified by cognate terms such as *condition, shape, mold,* or *form* (Parekh, 1982, p. 26) or

Raymond Williams's (1977, p. 84) translation of it as "setting bonds to" or "setting limits to" rather than "causing." Louis Althusser's decisive influence on the debate was the assertion that the ideological superstructure has "relative autonomy" from its base and that it is "over-determined" in the way Freud described the structured, multiple causation of symptoms in psychotic patients.

The theories of Antonio Gramsci, particularly his concept of cultural hegemony, rediscovered some 30 years after his death in a Fascist prison, gave further impetus to the movement of the concept of ideology away from reductionist notions of determinism, and represent a major turning point in European cultural theory. Hegemony, the consensual aspect of political control, is achieved in civil society through those institutions that create and diffuse cognitive and affective structures through which we perceive and interpret social reality: not only the mass media but also family, school, church, political parties, and trade unions.

Contemporary cultural theorists would expand this to include music, television, clothing, architecture, visual design, and the folkways of various subcultures (e.g., Bell, 1985; Chambers, 1986; Ewen & Ewen, 1982; Hebdige, 1979; O'Connor, 1987). Hegemony becomes what Raymond Williams (1977) calls a "saturation of the whole process of living—to such a depth that the pressures and limits of what can ultimately be seen as a specific economic, political and cultural system seem to most of us the pressures of simple experience and common sense" (p. 110).

MEDIA THEORY

Contemporary Cultural Studies owes a considerable debt to Gramsci's recognition that modern industrial societies embody powerful links between political, economic, and cultural activities and the "private" lives of citizens, for example, between the realities of electoral politics, the uses of leisure, the privacy of family life, the cohesion of ethnic, racial, gender, or youth identity and the major consciousness industries that mediate a limited range of meanings.

At the same time, industrial societies, with their structural inequalities and rank differences in power between social groupings, require the consent of the majority to secure the ascendancy of particular groups. The Gramscian argument is that the learning of ideological meanings, in a process of self-identification with the hegemonic forms of the culture, results in the blunting of consciousness through the manufacture of a "common sense" that accepts inequalities as the accidental by-product of the total political system. The suppression of alternative meanings, once carried out mainly through the coercive apparatuses of the state (police, courts, prison, military forces, and so on) is now carried out in the operations of cultural hegemony. With the successful naturalization and universalization of the worldview of a particular social group, critics can then be marginalized as naive, irresponsible, Utopian, or even *ideological,* in the derogatory Napoleonic sense of that term (see Corcoran, 1984).

It must be emphasized that this kind of discussion of the role of the consciousness industries in bringing about a hegemonic social consensus avoids slipping into a conspiratorial view of hegemony because the thrust of contemporary work is to stress that hegemonic maneuvers of the consciousness industries are learned by individuals positioned within the structures of media organizations through their experience of becoming "professionals." They internalize the norms and implicit understandings considered appropriate to particular production roles. Nor does it need proof that one class intentionally pursues its collective ideological interests as a tightly knit group of committed owners or managers through detailed control of cultural production.

Contemporary Cultural Studies is interested in a structural view of how the cultural industries are positioned within the general capitalist economy and how the underlying logic of that position imposes constraints on the range of feasible content and formal options available within the economic imperatives of the market. The emphasis is on political-economic structural analysis rather than on the identity, motivations, and activities of the particular actors involved, since, as Murdock (1982, p. 127) points out, for the purposes of structural analysis, it does not particularly matter who the key owners and controllers are.

As American and European media theory deviated at an accelerating pace over the last 30 years, the latter felt itself under the tug of a centripetal force that induced theoretical connections between such seemingly disparate questions as: Who owns and manages the media of communication? What are the predominant strands of content that are recognizable? and What effects do the media have on audiences? The American tradition by contrast, despite occasional exceptions such as the early work of Melody (1973), maintained its tendency toward fragmentation in theoretical concerns and isolationism in professional identities. Specialists in "ownership," for instance, are generally isolated in a managerialist paradigm and see no connection between economic control and questions of the encoding of messages or audience "effects." The same could be said for specialists in "policy" studies who concentrate on the legal battles fought out within the law by different media interests, large and small, under the watchful eye of the liberal-pluralist state. Questions of content and effect are seen to belong to quite different specialties, clearly visible in university curricula and in professional conferences. Likewise, specialists involved in the quantitative analysis of content or the surveying of audience response generally see no links between (a) economic and political control of consciousness industries and production routines, (b) "content" considered as an active, signifying system, amenable to semiological analysis that constructs meanings consonant with the dominant economic interests supporting it as a profit-making venture, and (c) the complex ways in which audiences engage with those meanings and the feelings they generate.

This segmentation has obvious implications for the question of what will happen as Cultural Studies, built on a commitment to a holistic view of culture (and eschewing the more familiar producer/content/receiver divisions), becomes better known in American universities and academic associations. Will each American specialty relate to and take out of Cultural Studies only what it sees as pertaining to itself and leave the rest, in a kind of pick and choose situation—those interested in management or policy studies, for instance, relating only to the strictly political economic aspects of Cultural Studies? Or will the strength of the integrative force defining Cultural Studies induce American colleagues to dissolve their own self-erected barriers and look across the fences into neighboring paddocks? Will policy or management specialists, for instance, follow Gitlin's (1983) example and consider the light their own work can shed on the kinds of productions that dominate contemporary American media with their impact on American culture in general and ultimately on the thrust of American society, domestically and internationally, in the late twentieth century? Or will the complete holistic project of Cultural Studies be generally rejected because it cannot produce a good "fit" with mainstream media theory?

CODES AND THE SUBJECT

Some aspects of Cultural Studies may be quite unrecognizable to many American academics. Consider the category of "content" and the traditional method of studying it in its fragmentable parts by establishing fixed conceptual categories and then quantitatively determining the presence or absence of the manifest messages. Not only has the European experience been to investigate content semiologically, that is, as a structured whole in which the relationships between elements is probably more important than is the frequency of their occurrence, but it has also underlined the need to analyze codes of expression. One of the major contributions of the British journal *Screen* for many years has been to give continuous attention to examination of the dominant codes of narrative cinema and television, particularly the ideological role of the classic codes of realism. The thrust of the *Screen* argument has been that the forms of realism—intensifying spectator involvement in the imaginary time/space continuum of the drama with all its characters, landscapes, and events, privileging plot linearity, carefully building the credibility of character motivation—have to be critically opened up to scrutiny in order to understand the ideological character of the screen media. These unconscious codes of verisimilitude are so naturalized and exercise such hegemonic control over Western film and television production today that one has to look to other cultures or to the "art cinema" of the West to discover alternative modes of representation, which in turn reveal classical realism to be one mode of representation not *the* mode of representation. From its origins in the bourgeois novel of the eighteenth century, this mode is now becoming an ideal export item for multinational production and distribution concerns and is having a multiplier effect on production practice on a global scale (Hamelink, 1983).

This aspect of content analysis is by now very familiar in the curricula, journals, and conferences of American Film Studies, but as I have pointed out (Corcoran, 1987), the organization of academic labor in American universities means that the insights of film studies are generally kept apart from those of media studies, as had been the case in Britain 20 years ago. The compartmentalization is presently being broken down by journals such as *Jump Cut* and *Social Text* and monographs such as *Regarding Television* (Kaplan, 1983), which discussed the production of the television and film subject by the ideological structures of realism in all its variants. Not only do these forums provide examples of ideological critiques of particular media artifacts, but they also advance ideological theory in general in an American context. When one pursues the strand of Cultural Studies that explores narrative and its codes, the trail leads to a further terrain that may be even more alien for mainstream American academia than semiology has been, because one finds down that path the fusion of two concerns that used to be considered quite distinct: *content* and *effect,* or in semiological terms, *text* and *reader*.

This fusion focuses on one of the most useful and at the same time controversial concepts in contemporary theory, that of the *subject*. This fusion is rooted in the creative confrontation of two intellectual traditions that until recent times seemed to have very little to say to each other: the Marxian and the psychoanalytic. The interface between the two is provided by the tradition of semiology, with its emphasis on analyzing the active processes of signification using a linguistic paradigm. Thus one of the most important strands of Cultural Studies, still in the process of developing, is the attempt to close the theoretical gap between the signifying practices of the text, the subjects induced by contemporary discourse, and the symbolic order of particular social formations in which they both are fashioned. This project is nothing less than the total refusal of the customary compartmentalization of these concerns in mainstream theory, in an attempt to deconstruct what Stam (1983) calls the pleasure-meaning-commodity complex: "Psychoanalytic methods help disengage television's relation to desire, semiotics helps disengage its procedures of meaning and a critical and dialectical Marxism can disengage its status as purveyor and exemplification of commodity fetishism and its place within the competing class discourse" (p. 39).

The vocabulary of "subject" and "pleasure" (and the theoretical baggage these imply) is very strange indeed to mainstream American media theory, within which "effects" were measured by surveys, "content" was conceptualized as a static, manifest phenomenon to be measured quantitatively in discrete categories, and production variables were of interest only to those pursuing questions of "management" or "policy." Some reference to the incorporation of a psychoanalytic perspective in Cultural Studies is therefore in order here, especially as the whole Freudian paradigm has failed to gain a foothold in the face of empiricist psychology in most American universities, not only in communication but also in departments of psychology.

PSYCHOANALYTIC THEORY

The notion of "the subject" gaining ascendancy in Cultural Studies displaces the more familiar notion of the "individual" by giving an important place in human experience to the unconscious and to the determining influence on it of dominant cultural forces. The humanist view of humankind posits a private consciousness that is coherent and autonomous, a stable human essence that is untouched in its freedom by historical or cultural circumstances. These values are called into question, however, by researchers touched by some of the insights of psychoanalysis, in particular the reinterpreting of Freud by Jacques Lacan. Here the notion of "the subject" permeates the view of human reality as a construction that is culturally orchestrated by the signifying activities of the dominant symbolic order, those significations remaining generally unconscious. The writings of Lacan suggest that no aspect of human reality is free from the structuring power of the symbolic order, language itself playing a major role in the construction of subjectivity. The idea of a unitary individual is replaced by the concept of the subject as a set of contradictory "positions," composed of unconscious processes that fix it in a certain relation to both language and visual representation as a means toward knowledge of the world.

Ideology is therefore thought of as "both a practice of representation and the construction of a subject for that representation" (Coward and Ellis, 1977, p. 72). But this subjectivity is discontinous and unstable (quite unlike the notion of "the individual") except when discourse, that is, a signifying system that preexists the individual, provokes its emergence and creates in it the illusion of consistency, an imaginary wholeness. The discontinuous subject has the capacity to occupy multiple and even contradictory sites, within a range of discursive positions, and at these sites specific meanings can be realized even as the subject feels itself to be the coherent source of meaning. Our multifaceted subjective identity is built up out of many different social relations that only partly overlap with one another. Morley (1986, p. 42) for instance, gives the example of a hypothetical white male viewer of the current affairs program "Nationwide," who may be simultaneously a productive worker, a trade union member and shop steward, a supporter of the Social Democratic Party, a consumer, a racist, a home owner, a wife beater, and a

Christian—and goes on to suggest different, even contradictory ways in which that man might "read" different segments of "Nationwide." These readings might be *dominant, oppositional* or *negotiated* in relation to the meanings in the television program that are "structured in dominance" in different ways.

One consequence of this notion of subjectivity is that if individuals and social classes can no longer be thought of as unified subjects whose consciousness exists outside discourse and reflects their underlying economic position, then the notion of classes in the traditional Marxist sense is undermined, and, as we shall see, this realization is being hotly debated today among Marxists in Britain. Another consequence of the notion of subjectivity being outlined here is that it destroys the monolithic conception of "the viewer" that dominated much of the work based on old-style audience surveys with their simplistic notions of message and influence. In its place is a more active conception of the audience and an attention to the social dimensions of reception that criticizes the methodology of external measurement of audience behavior for offering no insight into what the observed behavior means to the people concerned (see Morley, 1986, p. 167). Cultural Studies thus has evolved a respect for ethnomethodology and the paradigm of contemporary anthropology, in the belief that it is only through subjects' own accounts of why they are interested in particular cultural artifacts that we can begin to get any real sense of how meaning is propagated and culture reproduced. It is perhaps significant, in the context of the criticisms of the role of commercial sponsorship on the quantitative thrust of American media research, that Morley's (1986) qualitative study of television viewing within families was sponsored by commercial broadcasting in Britain.

SUBJECT AND SUTURE

The extent to which old distinctions between *content* and *audience* or *effect* are eroded in a radical way in some corners of contemporary Cultural Studies can be seen in the notion of *suture,* an import into British thinking from French film theory. Jean-Pierre Oudart's (1969) outline of how a cinematic subject becomes engaged in the sequences of images in a film is still one of the clearest delineations of this approach.

The first moment of spectator involvement in the screen image is one of sheer joy or ecstasy, what Lacanians call *jouissance.* But the moment of pleasure, free from awareness of frame and screen, is suddenly broken as the limits of the image are perceived. This perception brings an awareness of discontinuity and absence, seen initially in the process of framing (which includes certain portions of the visual field but excludes others) and also in the process of editing (in which shots replace shots in a chain established by an absent Other who is speaking through this chain). This revelation of absence, in the visual field of the camera and in the intervals between shots, initiates the discourse of the film, the active addressing of the spectator and the invitation to respond by psychic involvement through those absences. Characters in the film come to take the place of the absent Other of Lacanian psychoanalysis, recognized by spectators as addressing them, and thus the absence is effaced or filled in with the experience of the film as a continuous whole. This is the essence of the notion of suture—a (psychic) stitching, as in the surgical joining of the lips of a wound. The spectator is sutured into the very structure of filmic signifiers itself. The ceaseless absence or lack posed by a film in its framings and its cuts is sutured into a continuous, flowing experience when spectators insert themselves through fictional characters into the holistic world of the screen in a process that binds them as subjects into the space/time continuum unfolding on the screen. We identify with the camera as narrator through the dynamics of its positionings in which it identifies with different characters within the narrative.

The shot/reverse shot formation was soon identified by those developing a psychoanalytic narrative theory (Oudart, 1969; Dayan, 1974) as a crucial element in the operation of suture, that is, the cinematic set in which a second shot shows the field from which the first shot is assumed to have been taken. Salt (1974) distinguished three variations of this formation that emerged in a certain order in the history of film: the cut from a watcher to his or her point of view, the cut from one long shot of a scene to another more or less oppositely angled long shot, and the cut between just-off-the-eye line angle/reverse angle shots of two people interacting (the set that is, of course, favored in most television studio productions). These sets are closely tied to the 180 degree rule of cinematic and televisual expression, which derives from the realist imperative that the camera deny its own existence by fostering the illusion that the image has an autonomous existence independent of any coercive gaze captured by some kind of technical manipulation of vision. The shot/reverse shot formation locates a fictional spectator in the other 180 degrees of the same circular field, implying that the preceding shot was seen through the gaze of a figure in the narrative. The gaze that directs our look seems to belong to a fictional character rather than to the camera. Thus, as Branigan (1975) points out, suture is achieved through the permutations of the point-of-view shot, whereby we participate in characters' viewpoints and thus experience all the elements of the fictional world contemporaneously with them. The gaze, identified by Mulvey (1975) with the psychoanalytic pleasure of scopophilia, thus lies at the foundation of cinematic suture.

THE QUESTION OF PLEASURE

Since its arrival into the lexicon of critical terms in the 1970s, criticisms of the notion of suture have emerged—criticisms that center on the overly close identification between suture and point-of-view cutting (Rothman, 1976; Salt,

1974; Heath, 1981). Elucidation of these developments must remain outside the scope of this short essay, but it is of crucial importance here to note the whole attempt within Cultural Studies to address the question of pleasure, a question that has had no room for the asking, never mind the answering, in mainstream American theory. The latter has asked very different kinds of questions about the gratification of the individual consumer's "needs" using a very different kind of methodology grounded in a very different theory of the individual-in-society. The notion of pleasure, is, of course, intimately linked to the concerns of the theory of ideology, because it raises the question of how contemporary culture achieves the ideological effect critical scholars claim for it by offering participants what Fredric Jameson (1981) calls "compensatory pleasure," that is, utopian impulses released and managed by cultural texts, in which "substantial incentives are offered for ideological adherence" (p. 291). The question of pleasure asks what is presented in return for submission to the privileged discourse of a particular power structure in society, that is, how individual consciousness takes shape in ideology. In visual media, suture functions to give the viewing subject the illusion of a stable and continuous identity by "interpellating" him or her into familiar discursive positions and thereby articulating the existing symbolic order in ideologically orthodox ways.

The question of pleasure is now getting constant working over, not only in film theory but in relation to television viewing, some of it on the American side of the Atlantic and some of it beginning to counterbalance the emphasis on the "pleasure of viewing" with the other (neglected) Lacanian notion of the "pleasure of hearing," especially in regard to television (e.g., Stam, 1983). Media criticism coming from this direction is concerned not only with textual analysis but with the mode in which a text addresses its spectators in a discursive engagement. Its textual reading might be called psychostructural because of its attempt to take into account formal aspects of the text that serve the role of interpellating viewers in particular ways. Its object is to suggest different ways in which the ideological effect of a text is to place a spectator in a particular subject position in the process of suturing him or her into the text.

This type of psychostructural reading constructs an "ideal" spectator from the text itself. Obviously the danger must be noted (and avoided) of confusing this with a "real" spectator by reverting to a type of hypodermic theorizing that leaves no room between the mode of address of a text and actual audience responses. As Morley (1980) warns, "we must be aware of arguing that the positions of knowledge inscribed in the textual operations are obligatory for all readers" (p. 160). Morley gives the further warning to those using the concept of the subject that the constant intervention of other texts and discourses, which also position the subject, should not be ignored. The subject is the product of discursive practices traversing it throughout its history. Thus a text may be rejected, or renegotiated, by the subject's relation to other texts, institutions, discursive formations, because

> it is clear that the concept of interdiscourse transforms the relation of one text/one subject to that of a multiplicity of texts/subject relations, in which encounters can be understood not in isolation but only in moments of their combination. (p. 166)

This point is amplified in Morley's (1986) more recent criticisms of his own earlier work on the viewing of the television program "Nationwide." Reservations about the theory of the subject articulated by Hall (1980, p. 161) should also be noted at this point, if only because of Hall's enormous influence on the development of Cultural Studies in Britain.

DIVERSITY

North American interest in Cultural Studies can be recognized in the *Journal of Communication's* attention to "Ferment in the Field" (1983); it should also be recognized that description exhibited in several places tends to reduce the great diversity of contemporary approaches to cultural analysis (and resistance to them) to one-dimensional depictions. Perhaps in the context of the polarized framing of "administrative" versus "critical" research and the perceived need to defend and attack opposite positions, this oversimplification is inevitable. Nevertheless, as the "Ferment" gets wider circulation in academia, it is necessary to emphasize the diversity in Cultural Studies as well as its central concerns. Grossberg's (1984) excellent division of the terrain offers a useful model of research that focuses on the culture/society couplet. He delineates 10 different positions, organized into three larger categories, that are worth summarizing very briefly here.

(a) Classical approaches (Grossberg distinguishes three different trends) tend to deemphasize both the text as a set of signifiers and the nature of decoding processes, in favor of focusing on the relationship between the text and the producer, understood as both economic interests behind particular texts and the processes of production themselves. The early work of Dorfman and Mattelart (1975) and Gitlin (1980), for instance, assume rather than investigate the power of the text to fashion everyday consciousness and assume that the text always speaks with one voice. That audiences may negotiate alternative oppositional readings of texts does not enter into the analysis. Much of the research done in the classical mode is political-economic in its concentration on modes of production in the consciousness industries, along with patterns of ownership and systems of distribution.

(b) Hermeneutic approaches (of which Grossberg illuminates four types) pull the domain of experience into the relationship between culture and society and give cultural practices a more active, ideological role in the construction of power relationships. Thus texts are not just reflective of their economic base but are thoroughly ideological in the complex ways in which they produce, transform and shape meaning structures. Using the techniques of literary theory, the critic examines the complex ways in which the text codes and potentially transforms the fabric of everyday lived experience.

(c) Discursive approaches concentrate on the intertextual domain of experience in which the subject is positioned and articulated. They insist that power can not be read off the surface of texts as systems of meaning but must be looked for in the ways in which texts produce meaning by structuring signifiers around the subject. Power must also be sought in how texts are inserted into a network of other texts that both reinforce them and are in turn reinforced by them. In all cases, the notion of the subject is foregrounded, although theories of the subject as diverse as Althusser's and Foucault's are contained in this category. The shortest of shorthand comparisons between these three broad categories is offered by Grossberg in the observation (p. 418) that classical approaches tend to ignore the audience or assume it is passive and view the long-standing Marxist problem of the determination of the superstructure by the base as simply causal. Hermeneutic approaches assume an active audience and view economic determination as a process of defining constraints and exerting pressures. Discursive approaches attempt to insert the audience into the very structures of cultural textuality and see the base/superstructure relationship as a process of "overdetermination."

It should be obvious that the range of approaches to cultural interpretation contains differences not only in theoretical and methodological assumptions but in political implications. As Hanno Hardt (pp. 587-588) notes, Cultural Studies demonstrates a sense of engagement between political practice and theoretical considerations, particularly in the implications for intervention in cultural practice and resistance to the dominant ideological thrust of contemporary culture. It is important for North American academics in this instance to resist monolithic notions about the politics that can come with labels, such as *Marxist*, that are ideological products of decades of Cold War feelings rather than descriptors used with any precision.

It is worth pointing out that within the left in Britain, for instance, there is nothing like unanimity on the questions raised by the various Marxian streams feeding Cultural Studies. The work of people like Stuart Hall and Ernesto Laclau has been dubbed "right wing" and "revisionist" from the standpoint of classical revolutionary Marxism (Ralph Milliband, 1985) because it is perceived as being influenced by Continental Europeans, such as Althusser, Foucault, and Derrida, to the point of denying the existence of any reality that is independent of "discourse." Alex Calinicos (1987), for instance, criticizes the "intellectual surrender" of Stuart Hall to the "new revisionism" of the 1980s, in which Hall is "now confined largely to spouting neoliberal platitudes surrounded by a fog of Gramscian rhetoric" (p. 112). To what is Hall surrendering? The core of the "new revisionism" is seen to lie in the retreat from the traditional hope in the working class as the spearhead of change, a retreat associated in Britain with Eric Hobsbawm and the journal *Marxism Today*.

This retreat is described by Ellen Wood (1986) as being fundamentally "the automisation of ideology and politics from any social basis and more specifically from any class foundation" (pp. 1-2). The central disagreement is again over the nature of the culture/society couplet or the relationship between economic base and ideological superstructure. Are classes coherent, unified groups whose actions and consciousness reflect the economic conditions of their existence, or is there no necessary correspondence between economics and consciousness?

The question has relevance not only for those interested in whether, in its development of the theory of ideology, Cultural Studies has broken with orthodoxy too radically. It is also of interest to media theorists exploring the processes of the formation of consciousness and seeking to accumulate empirical data like Morley's (1980, 1986) on whether, for instance, one can conclude from a person's class, race, or gender how she or he will read a given text.

Clearly, Cultural Studies in all its diversity is well established not only in British academics, but also in the rest of anglophone Europe and Canada. In Ireland, for instance, the National Institute for Higher Education in Dublin and the journal *Cranebag* (until its recent demise) are foci for such work, and in North America, "Ferment in the Field" (Gerbner, 1983) brought together many of those working in the same tradition in the United States and Canada. What of the possibility, raised by Hardt (p. 553) that the potential of radical thought represented in Cultural Studies will be dissipated or co-opted in the accommodation of liberal dissent in the United States? Of obvious relevance to the question of the impact of innovative thinking will be a consideration of the role of academic gatekeepers: journal editorial boards, conference organizers, officers in professional associations, and the survival possibilities of alternatives to the International Communication Association and the Speech Communication Association, such as the Union for Democratic Communications.

Also relevant are academic management structures: tenure and merit review boards, research grant funders, and recruitment and dissertation committees. It remains to be seen, for instance, whether rearguard action will focus exclusively on questions of methodology, as tended to happen in the 1950s (Hardt p. 550), or whether the "Marxism" in Cultural Studies will be seen merely as the old, familiar economic Marxism that has been consistently rejected in American academia (as it was in the Britain of F.R. Leavis), or whether there is sufficient room in American theories of culture for a consideration of the links between the political-economic structures of society and the public meaning systems that coexist with them.

In gazing into the crystal ball to predict how this relatively new intellectual movement will compare with Critical Theory of the 1940s in its impact on mainstream American thought, it is interesting to note Calinicos's (1987, p. 108) observation that one of the centers of the *resistance* to the "new revisionism" of Cultural Studies is North American socialist thinking. It also remains to be seen, therefore, whether American socialist intellectuals, who have not existed in any measurable quantity in departments of communication, which they have tended to shun as excessively industry-driven in their research, will abandon their traditional indifference to questions of culture and see the need for a new kind of critique of contemporary society that transcends the rigid boundaries between economics, anthropology, philosophy, linguistics, psychology, sociology, and political science.

An interesting starting point would be an examination, from within a Cultural Studies rather than an idealist "history-of-ideas" paradigm, of the role of the university in contemporary American culture. This examination could be done by adopting either a political-economic angle, to open out the multifaceted relationships between academia and the hegemonic corporate-military state, or an ethnographic approach, to articulate the lived experience of the subculture of young academics caught in the tenure-promotion-publication nexus, or a discursive perspective, to disentangle the ways in which academics are subjectively positioned as professionals within a powerful ideological apparatus.

REFERENCES

Bell, D. (1985). Contemporary cultural studies in Ireland and the "problem" of Protestant ideology. *Cranebag, 9,* 91-95.

Branigan, E. (1975). Formal permutations of the point-of-view shot. *Screen, 16,* 54-64.

Calinicos, A. (1987). Looking for alternatives to reformism. *International Socialism, 34,* 106-117.

Chambers, I. (1986). *Popular culture: The metropolitan experience.* London, Methuen.

Corcoran, F. (1984). Consciousness: A missing link in the coupling of technology and communication. *Canadian Journal of Communication, 10,* 41-73.

Corcoran, F. (1987). Television as ideological apparatus: The power and the pleasure. In H. Newcomb (Ed.), *Television: The critical view* (pp. 533-552). Oxford: Oxford University Press.

Coward, R., & Ellis, J. (1977). *Language and materialism: Developments in the theory of the subject.* London: Routledge & Kegan Paul.

Dayan, D. (1974). The tutor code in classical cinema. In B. Bichols (Ed.), *Movies and methods* (pp. 438-451). Berkeley: University of California Press.

Dorfman, A., & Mattlelart, A. (1975). *How to read Donald Duck: Imperialist ideology in the Disney comic.* New York: International General.

Ewen, S., & Ewen, E. (1982). *Channels of desire: Mass images and the shaping of American consciousness.* New York: McGraw-Hill.

Gerbner, G. (Ed.). (1983). Ferment in the field. *Journal of Communication, 33.*

Gitlin, T. (1980). *The whole world is watching: Mass media in the making and unmaking of the new left.* Berkeley: University of California Press.

Gitlin, T. (1983). *Inside prime time.* New York: Pantheon.

Grossberg, L. (1984). Strategies in Marxist cultural interpretation. *Critical Studies in Mass Communication, 1,* 392-421.

Hall, S. (1980). *Culture, media, language.* London: Hutchinson.

Hamelink, C. (1983). *Cultural autonomy in global communications.* New York: Longman.

Heath, S. (1981). *Questions of cinema.* Bloomington: Indiana University Press.

Hebdige, D. (1979). *Subculture: The meaning of style.* London: Methuen.

Jameson, F. (1981). The political unconscious. Ithaca, NY: Cornell University Press.
Kaplan, E. (1983). *Regarding television.* Frederick, MD: University Publications of America.
Marx, K., & Engels, F. (1962). *Selected works* (Vol. 1). Moscow: Progress.
Melody, W. (1973). *Children's television: The politics of exploitation.* New York: Longman.
Milliband, R. (1985). The new revisionism in Britain. *New Left Review, 150,* 29-46.
Morley, D. (1980). Subjects, texts, readers. In S. Hall (Ed.), *Culture, media, language.* London: Hutchinson.
Morley, D. (1986). *Family television: Cultural power and domestic leisure.* London: Comedia.
Mulvey, L. (1975). Visual pleasure and narrative cinema. *Screen, 16,* 6-18.
Murdock, G. (1982). Large corporations and the control of the communications industries. In M. Gurevitch, T. Bennet, J. Curran, & J. Woollacott, (Eds.), *Culture, society and the media.* London: Methuen.
O'Connor, B. (1987). *Women and media: Social and cultural influences on women's use of and response to television.* Unpublished doctoral dissertation, University College, Dublin.
Oudart, J-P. (1969). La Suture. *Cahiers du Cinema,* April, pp. 36-39; May, pp. 50-55.
Parekh, B. C. (1982). *Marx's theory of ideology.* Baltimore: Johns Hopkins University Press.
Poulantzas, N. (1971). *Political power and social classes.* London: New Left Books.
Rothman, W. (1976). Against the system of suture. In B. Nichols (Ed.), *Movies and methods* (pp. 452-459). Berkeley: University of California Press.
Salt, B. (1974, Fall). Statistical style analysis in motion pictures. *Film Quarterly,* pp. 13-22.
Stam, R. (1983). Television news and its spectator. In E. A. Kaplan (Ed.), *Regarding television: Critical approaches—An anthology* (pp. 35-49). Frederick, MD: University Publications of America.
Williams, R. (1977). *Marxism and literature.* Oxford: Oxford University Press.
Wood, E. (1986). *The retreat from class: A new "true" socialism.* London: Verso.

Critical Theory and Empirical Critique in Mass Communication Research: Some Methodological Considerations

SLAVKO SPLICHAL
Edvard Kardelj University

THE last decade of the development of communication theory and research is indicated by several attempts to "recreate the past" in the field and, particularly, to (re)examine the relationship between theoretical knowledge about communication and the media, empirical research, and social practice. The centrality of this debate can best be illustrated by a number of dissertations on dominant "paradigms," "traditions" and "schools" in communication studies, particularly those concentrated on the dichotomies between empirical versus theoretical, administrative versus critical, or quantitative versus qualitative research.

However, the large majority of these international debates are (1) extremely *ethnocentric,* overwhelmingly concentrated on the development of the media and communication research in Western societies. Besides, (2) most dichotomizations of the tendencies and strategies in communication research are—if not actually false—at best grave *simplifications* (Slack & Allor, 1983, p. 208) of an almost hundred-year tradition(s) in the field, and (3) they often *obscure historical differences and causes* of different approaches (i.e., that a specific "tradition" is a product of specific cultural and historical conditions and may "produce" different consequences when these conditions are changed). This could be exemplified by the fact that not only may Critical Theory be a "critical impulse" against the ideologized empirical research (as required by Adorno & Horkheimer), but empirical research may be an Empirical Critique (i.e., a "critical impulse") against the ideologized theoretical knowledge. As the former usually applies to developed capitalist

Correspondence and requests for reprints: Slavko Splichal, Faculty of Sociology, Political Science, and Journalism, Edvard Kardelj University, Kardeljeva Ploscad 5, 61000 Ljubljana, Yugoslavia.

Communication Yearbook 12, 618-635

societies, the latter may apply to pre- and postcapitalist societies, where more or less sophisticated empirical research contributed to the abolition of feudal metaphysics and communist dogmatism. Some cases of communication and public opinion research in different historical and social instances demonstrate historical differences of apparently the same "traditions."

In this contribution, I do not mean to add to these debates by analyzing further the differences between the variety of research traditions and their histories, but to concentrate on some important but usually overlooked *methodological* dimensions of (potential) similarity and complementarity among traditions that ought to be radically different. In particular, I would neither sustain the argument of substantive methodological incongruity between Critical Theory and Cultural Studies, and empirical research, nor assume, in contrast to Hardt, that the problem of empirical research remains (or ought to remain) a secondary issue in a critical reexamination of the field, particularly in debates about the relations between critical and other (not to say administrative) "schools." On the contrary, when it comes to diagnosing "what ails the field," communication scholars usually "tend to locate themselves along a continuum that runs from empiricist to theorist," even toward its extremes (Lang & Lang, 1985, p. 49). Smythe and Van Dinh (1983, p. 117) argue that besides the problems chosen and the ideological orientation of the researcher, "the research methods used are commonly thought to be the basis for distinguishing" between administrative and critical research and theory.

Yet there is an important difficulty in the examination of the significance of methodological questions for controversies within communication theory and research. The notion of "empirical research" often pretends not to be socially and historically (and even not theoretically) defined, while the notions of "Critical Theory" and "Cultural Studies" are rather exactly elaborated, at least in the historical perspective, and thus limited to specific authors, ideas, theoretical models, interpretations, and even background assumptions. If there is no doubt about the need and validity of these "limitations" (i.e., as exact as possible conceptualizations of specific theories), there also should be no excuse for the discussions of "empirical research," which consider it as if it were a single compact entity, without its own history (or histories), and independent of specific cultural and historical influences. As Hardt points out in his contribution to this volume, a lack of differentiation among members of the "empirical school" may weaken assertions about the theoretical premises of the "school" as well.

BETWEEN DEAD FACTS AND FICTITIOUS SUBJECTS

Attempting to move beyond the oversimplified characterization of epistemological preferences and methodological options of the "empirical school" as a single paradigm in contrast to different theoretical traditions, Vaillancourt

(1986) correctly asserts the existence of different traditions in both Western and Marxist currents that practice empirical research. Although her differentiation between romanticism, empiricism, and rationalism in Western thought, and philosophical, materialist, structuralist, and Stalinist Marxists is neither exhaustive nor exclusively defined, and her treatment of "currents" or "orientations" can be labeled formalistic (Wenger, 1986, p. 8), Vaillancourt's conceptualization indicates the extreme diversity of research strategies from pure interpretive to completely empirically constrained methodology within both Marxist and non-Marxist traditions. Thus theoretical and empirical traditions in communication science cannot be ordered within only two categories, either. They differ primarily in the dominant questions they are endeavoring to answer, in specific research methods and results that are achieved and explained by the researchers and verified by the users in society, and in semitheoretical assumptions about the nature of society, human individuals, and science itself that are rarely stated explicitly.

However, most attempts to define "just exactly what it means to do critical research oversimplify the differences between critical research approaches and other approaches" (Slack & Allor, 1983, p. 208). One of the mainstreams in communication studies is usually called "empirical" "positivistic" or "administrative," representing a research orientation into specific, measurable, short-term, individual, attitudinal, and behavioral characteristics, particularly into the effects of (mass) communication. The second mainstream is usually referred to as "critical theory" and is linked to the Frankfurt Circle in the period between the two wars. In contrast to the administrative researchers who are concerned neither with the values that "generated" the research problem nor with the social consequences of their research endeavours, for critical scholars, the key questions become the values and political positions of the researcher and the research activity itself. The proposition that absence of an explicit attention to values in the selection of relevant problems for research leads implicitly or explicitly to the support of the social *status quo* and the interests of the ruling classes could be taken as the key "indicator" of the critical orientation.

It is true that a simple dichotomy is insensitive to the variety of critical and empirical approaches. However, most attempts to demystify these oversimplifications concentrate only on the critical extreme (i.e., different critical approaches) and fail to consider the differences within the empirical extreme. Empirical research methods (e.g., experimental designs, surveys, statistical analysis of data) are usually considered almost sufficient evidence of administrative research without any detailed elaboration. Thus it seems that there is no room for Empirical Critique, apart from Critical Theory.

The question of the relationship between Critical Theory and Empirical Critique actually concerns the same questions that the discussion of the relationship between theory and empirical research brought up at the end of the 1950s in Germany ("Positivismusstreit"), when "critical theory renounced any possibility for the positivists to be capable, with their methods, of recognizing reality, and the positivists responded by reproaching the Frankfurters with their incapability of ever achieving reality with their endeavours and theories" (Haug, 1978, p. 644). Contemporary embarrassments and doubts stem from the ranks of both empiricists and theoreticians. The former seem to be becoming more interested in the importance as well as in the truthfulness of the results, and the latter seem to assess, as a criterion of validity, not only the importance but the truthfulness of research findings. Hence, do "traditional" differences between the former and the latter as defined by Merton (1979, p. 153) 30 years ago no longer exist?

Merton's dichotomy between theoreticians and empiricists may seem to be doubtful for both theoretical and epistemological reasons. On the one hand, a number of "empiricists" define "usefulness," "importance," or "effectiveness" as their criterion of "truthfulness" (e.g., the so-called pragmatists), and numerous "theoreticians," in order to prove the "truthfulness" of ideas, rely on the empirical world—social practice. On the other hand, as Horkheimer (1976, p. 43) pointed out, no structural differences exist between the "theoreticians" and "empiricists" in their mode of thinking and notions of theory. There always exists, on one side, theoretical knowledge, and on the other side, the state of things that must be embraced by it. Theoretical explanation is considered the process of subsuming—establishing a link between pure observations or constantizing facts and the conceptual structure of knowledge. Only when the researcher (1) masters the material to the smallest detail, (2) analyzes its different forms of development and (3) tracks out their internal relationships, can she undertake (theoretical) explanation that, by its nature (structure), essentially differs from the research itself (Marx, 1973, p. 27). Indeed, there is no theory that is actually not related to the empirical world, although it may not be created directly on the basis of observed facts. There may exist only a theory that does not want to reflect this connection or wants to be "superior" to it, "more real" than reality itself.

Apart from these "structural identities," different traditions, streams, or "paradigms" in the development of any science (a kind of competition between different streams) are "natural" forms of the process of knowledge growth. As Weber (1986, p. 32-33) emphasized , there is no single, absolutely objective way of explaining and interpreting human activity and social relations, and every scientific thought is bound to remain partial, to grow old and be replaced. Social relations, as the object of research, always in a way also determine the kind and the scope of research, as they not only "give" the object (human practice) to the subject (researcher), but create the subject for the object. As human practice entails theoretical consideration, the latter retroactively acts on its object—social relations, if it is "an actual, positive science, the representation of practical activity, the practical development process of people" and not a "collection of dead facts, as it is in the case of empiricists" or a "fictitious action of fictitious subjects, as in the case of idealists" (Marx & Engels, 1973, p. 27). Hence theory always implies its own relation to practice; according to Habermas (1980, p. 8), theory should reveal the historically created state of the interest, to which it still belongs through the acts of cognition, and, on the other hand, the historical action that theory may actively influence. In this way, theory becomes a catalytic moment of the same social relation that it analyzes. The dependence of the research result on its subject (researcher) may be revealed by considering the degree to which a research work both reflects its own assumptions and distinguishes "the test of truthfulness of a judgment from the test of its vital importance" (Horkheimer, 1976 p. 11). The aptitude for such differentiation Horkheimer (1976) defines with the dialectic function of (critical) theory to

> measure every historical phase, not only in regard to individual isolated data and concepts, but also in regard to its original and complex content. . . . Today a valid philosophy does not exist in the return from concrete economic and social analyses to empty and emptied categories, but on the contrary, in preventing the transformation of economic concepts into empty and emptied details able to conceal reality in all places. (p. 11)

Moreover, Horkheimer (1976, p. 75) even proves that the decisive contextual lines of a theory can be neither transformed nor materialized in action without a "historical overturn," without the rise of a "new society as such."

The question is, however, whether research is sentenced—until such an "overturn" both in theoretical knowledge and social practice—to positivistic identification and classification of facts into as neutral as possible categories, which are "naturally given" and thus functional for the given social relations and defined by them (i.e., to the bare registration of the numerous phenomena, on one side, and the abstract critique of them on the other).

In his critique of the "traditional science," Horkheimer (1976, p. 71) does not express such radical doubts. In his opinion, with the application of processes of "traditional science" to society, "statistics and descriptive sociology originate, which may become important for any kind of purpose, including critical theory." Accordingly, the solution is not in a priori negation of the use, value, and validity of conformist "expert science" or intellectual techniques without a careful examination of their cognitive fertility, (i.e., whether or not something can be rightly or wrongly determined when using a specific theoretical-methodological approach). Rather, one must reveal theoretical background and assumptions as well as cognitive limits of these techniques. There are numerous problems that cannot be approached accordingly, and solved without a previous empirical investigation (though limited to recording of pure facts) of the variety of the concrete development as the basis for the mental reproduction of the material world. Otherwise, theoretical knowledge remains in empty abstractions.

EMPIRICAL RESEARCH AGAINST THE IDEOLOGIZED CONSCIOUSNESS

Within this context, I would list three particular reasons why most critical communication scholars are not likely to accept the thesis of a potential merger between empirical and theoretical research. Their resistance to empirical research is primarily based on what Gouldner (1970, p. 31) denotes as background assumptions rather than on an explicit theory, model, or research logic. *The first reason is "apologetic idealism" of criticism,* that inability to elaborate the phenomena of alienation in the communication sphere with the help of general theory (theories) of society, but only by sophisticated speculations and mingling analysis with interpretation. One of the most important problems of contemporary theoretical (critical) knowledge—perhaps the core of its crisis—lies in the fact that it often overlooks how even the most abstract concepts are the very products of concrete historical conditions; thus they are completely valid only for those conditions and may not be, without further assumptions, generalized. As empirical research procedures and data require theoretical sophistication, theoretical concepts need to be historically contextualized in social practice. "Thus, also in the theoretical method, the assumption of the subject, the society, must always be in the representation" (Marx, 1974, p. 22). Only then can a theory have a historical significance.

As an illustrative example of how the most abstract concepts can be operationalized, we can take Marx's idea that the basic source for revolutionary change in society is the contradiction between the mode of production and the development of productive forces (and not between the means of production and the relations of production that is a famous product of Stalin's revision of Marx's ideas but—incredibly—usually considered Marx's original idea (e.g., Young, 1980). Although Young is misled by Stalin's "theoretical" revisions, it is worth quoting his empirically testable operationalization of Stalin's

> thesis that, as the disjuncture between means of and relations to production [according to Marx, between the development of productive forces and the mode of production] increase, class struggle increases and intensifies. The first variable, disjuncture, is measured by such things as unemployment rates, bankruptcies, and income inequality. The second variable is measured by strikes by workers, higher prices set by owners, political volatility of workers and by speed-up and stretch-out by owners. (p 11)

Yet testing this hypothesis requires both a large amount of appropriate data and appropriate (valid) multivariate statistical methods.

Melody and Mansell (1983) argue that, contrary to the preceding exemplification,

> much critical analysis tends simply to assume that existing institutional structures are the problem and must be changed. But it usually does not provide a clear idea of how these structures should, could, or would be realistically changed to alternative institutional structures that research has shown are better. (p. 110)

For example, "the criticism of global communication structure was developed in a theoretical vacuum, where the thesis of media imperialism was no more than a hypothesis" (Hellman, 1980, p. 8). Empirical testing of such theoretically ill-defined hypotheses might lead to counterevidence and to falsification of hypotheses and the whole theory. Another example might be "a total and blanket rejection by critical scholars of the behaviorist tradition of effects research" as "either inherently uninteresting and/or biased in terms of liberal pluralist assumptions built into it, without a thorough-going critique of such research" (Fejes, 1984, p. 223).

On the other hand, the insight into the development of empirical social research (particularly the collection of interview response data) in pre- and postcapitalist societies undoubtedly falsifies *the thesis of its innate conservative, administrative nature*. On the contrary, these methods were conceived to a great extent (e.g., in the form of "social statistics" of the eighteenth and nineteenth centuries) as a critical impulse—not against the *ideologized science* as Adorno and Horkheimer later defined the role of critical theory versus empiricism, but—*against the ideologized consciousness of the old and afterwards new ruling classes* in the developing capitalist societies. As the beginnings of empirical (opinion) research in the time of progressive bourgeois ideology and the development of new capitalist relations in the developed societies, the empirical recording of the new processes, in itself, contributed to the abolition of feudal metaphysics and thus to the development of a new bourgeois society. Empirical research in socialist countries, almost two centuries later, developed as the direct expression of the democratization of socialist societies. It is unfortunate that the understanding of the development of empirical research has so often been coupled with an antagonism toward quantitative methods, with an aberration that a principal adversity exists between the critical theory and the empirical research. Indeed, the progressive role of empirical research, per se, considerably changed during the development of monopoly capitalism, and *a large part of (mostly empirical) social research in capitalist societies fell under the general law of capitalist production,* as was the case with numerous other human activities, including (mass) communication itself. In such circumstances, the main aim of a research is no longer its scientific relevance, (i.e., its *use value,*) but its *exchange value*. This is why, today, empirical research without *the impulse of* theory would *perpetuate the existing dominant relations in capitalist society,* and it does so to a great extent. In such circumstances, the critical theory, which can and should reveal and (re)create the emancipatory potential of survey research, is of prime importance. A different nature is held by empirical research in the postcapitalist societies, where it acts in the first place as a critical impulse against the ideologized abstract social sciences, against formalism and simplified generalizations, and for investigating differences in interests and social contradictions in the processes of the development of socialism (i.e., actually the same role as it has had against feudalism and for capitalism during the revolutionary social changes almost two centuries ago). Although empirical research (e.g., surveys) in postcapitalist societies retains its manipulative character (Splichal, 1987, p. 259), it neither is "replicative of the alienation implied in the general existence of the commodity form" nor "represents a form of distorted communication associated with a political order," as suggested by Wenger (1986, p. 38). At least, if we consider both—repressive and emancipatory—dimensions, empirical research cannot be simply reduced to administrative research, which is subordinated to commercial and ruling power interests.

It is true, however, that idealism of critical theory is not the only reason that there actually exists a resistance against it. Not rarely, conservative reproaches spring from the true assumption that critical theory prophesies radical social changes that cannot be formulated in the present, other than theoretically, as an interpretation of the actually existing from the standpoint of the possible.

> As it is opposed to the guarantees of a partial world, it itself seems to be partial and unjust. And, primarily, it does not care for any kind of material success. The criticism of dialectic theory does not come from an idea itself. Already in its idealistic form, it has rejected the concept of something that in itself is good and, by itself, opposed to reality. It does not create claims in regard to what is exterior of time, but in regard to what it is already time for. (Horkheimer, 1976, p. 63, 88)

Such a (critical) theory concerns (1) imagination of something not yet existent and (2) a tendency (endeavors) toward abolition or overcoming barriers that do not allow for its practical realization. The historical departure of *critical* theory from theory in general is essentially in that (1) it includes "facts" that do not yet exist, but have an ample possibility of existing; (2) its interests are general but they are not generally acknowledged (accepted) in society; and thus (3) it is less a confirmation and more a critique of social relations. This is why any action congruent with it cannot be productive in existing dominant social relations. Indeed, such a theory is an enemy of both the existing relations and the ideas that contribute to the further existence of the past in the present.

"POSITIVE" AND "CRITICAL" METHOD

Second, there exists misapprehension of the real relationship between the qualitative and the quantitative methods as well as the logic and assumptions of the statistical analysis of data.

The assumption that there exists a methodological difference *in principle* between "positive and critical social science" (Comstock, 1980) overlooks critical points of the latter, particularly the process of transformation of empirically observed facts in theoretical knowledge and, even more importantly, the fact that any empirical fact is *the* fact only from a very specific theoretical perspective (although this perspective may be only implicitly present in empirical research).

The critique of positive science (particularly of empirical research and mathematical-statistical methods of data analysis) should distinguish what is immanent from what is a consequence of a specific (i.e., valid or invalid in regard to the object and aim of the research) use of specific methods. Comstock points out the differences between mainstream science and critical science, but he confuses "epistemologic assumptions of positive science" (i.e., investigative *logic*) and "empirical research of social structures and processes" (i.e., research *procedures and methods).* Consequently, his comparison of two methods is based on the relation of the "steps of the method of critical research" to the *background assumptions* rather than the steps of the positive social science; the latter could be actually denoted as *empiricism,* particularly when omitting the first and the last—theory-related—steps, (i.e., theoretical groundlessness and unreflectedness, frequently even practical uselessness).

Among Comstock's seven "steps in the research methods of positive and critical social sciences," none of the "steps" of the former is simultaneously a "step" of the latter.

By contrasting the "*critical method*" with the "*positive method,*" Comstock suggests that these methods are mutually exclusive. However, he did not answer the essential question: how it is possible, practically, to "identify social groups or movements whose interests are progressive" (first step of critical science) without "previous empirical and theoretical work," observations, surveys, interviews, and other data gathering strategies and techniques, and data analyses (first to sixth steps of positive science). This all the more, as Comstock seems to be of the opinion that this "identification" may be achieved once forever. Although "the critical researcher may fruitfully use empirical findings of past research as well as conduct his or her own empirical studies, . . . these empirical analyses of social structures must be referred to the specific experiences of the study's subjects."

In a way, Comstock's "empirical phase of critical research" could represent a form of "qualitative methods." Although the notion of "qualitative methods" has no precise meaning in any of the social sciences (Van Maanen, 1983, p. 9), it is usually related to "a particular tradition in social science that fundamentally depends on watching people in their own territory and interacting with them in their own language, on their own terms" (Kirk & Miller, 1986, p. 9). However, "qualitative research" does not mean "the absence of counting" or "identifying the presence or absence of something" instead of "measuring the degree to which some feature is present." Indeed, most of the adherents of "qualitative methodology" claim that there is no principal *contradiction* between the quantitative and qualitative approach; qualitative research does not imply a commitment to innumeracy. From this perspective, procedures of the "positive social science" cannot be a priori excluded from the "critical method" as attempted by Comstock.

QUANTITY VERSUS QUALITY IN THEORY AND RESEARCH

The *ungrounded equalization of the administrative research with the quantitative methods* of the empirical research may be considered *the third reason* for the fact that the potential interpenetration of the two historical paradigms is not to be seen by critical theoreticians. An example of this reductionism is Smythe's and Van Dinh's operationalization of the administrative ideology, which they define as "the linking of administrative-type problems and tools, with interpretation of results that supports, or does not seriously disturb, the status quo" (Smythe & Van Dinh, 1983, p. 118). Quite clearly, the definition starts from defining *the problem* and *the aim* of the research as the essential elements of the definition of the administrative ideology. On the contrary, its operationalization goes in a completely different direction:

> Under administrative research the first type of research is for the sake of simplicity called "quantitative." It includes market research. It serves the private corporate interests. Additionally, "Survey research, conducted with rigorous standards for sampling, variance estimates, and control (but not elimination) of biases involved in questionnaire construction and interview and coding techniques, would also qualify as quantitative administrative research." (Smythe & Van Dinh, 1983, p. 118-119)

The abuse of the concept "quantitative research" or logical error is sufficiently evident: it is not the quantitative research but the "market research" (specifying the problem and the aim of research) being a special form of administrative ideology because of the specific aims of research that are subjected to commercial (profit) interests. Reducing the dimensions "theoretical empirical" or even "administrative critical" to the dimension "qualitative-quantitative" places the accent in the wrong place. As the empirical methods are *instrumental* solutions to the problems of gathering, processing, and interpreting information (data), the decision for their application is—if it is to be valid—necessarily dependent on the research problem and aim. The very subject and the aim of research determine whether it is appropriate to choose qualitative or quantitative methods for problem solution. The choice between the two kinds of methods ideally should be based on their respective probabilties of obtaining the evidence being sought (Berger & Kellner, 1981,

p. 46), and no method can be a priori excluded as inappropriate, whether quantitative or qualitative. The research practice is, unfortunately, still far from such an ideal state.

That dichotomies of the "qualitative versus quantitative" and "theoretical versus empirical" do not represent mutually exclusive dimensions, and the theories in the social sciences are no exception, may, perhaps most convincingly, be demonstrated by the example from classical Marxist tradition (Splichal, 1987, p.240). In *The German Ideology,* Marx and Engels prove that "the consciousness develops and forms because of the increase of productivity, the increase of needs and the growth of population that is the basis of both. Along with this develops the division of labour . . . , division of material and mental labour" (Marx & Engels, 1973, p. 31). It is easy to reformulate the preceding sentence into a clear, empirical, testable hypothesis: The *growth* of the population (X) influences the *increase* of needs (Y_1) and the *increase* of productivity (Y_2), as a result of which the consciousness is *developing* (Z_1) and with this the *division* of labor (Z_2). Independent variables (X, Y_1, and Y_2) are—quite obviously—quantitative and can be measured, while the dependent variables (Z_1 and Z_2) are qualitative. This hypothesis is eventually an illustration of Marx's idea of the "qualitative leap" (revolutionary change) as the result of quantitative (evolutionary) changes in the society. Whether or how it is possible to quantify the dependent variables is not essential; the essential question here is whether it is meaningful to quantify them in a valid manner. The scientific productivity of quantitative methods thus depends on the research problem and on the aim of research; a priori preference for qualitative or quantitative methods leads to an unfruitful voluntarism. Of course, the question of the accuracy, reliability, and validity of concrete applications of quantitative methods remains open—as it does for qualitative methods. But the point to be made here is that solutions to these problems depend on the methodological development of the social sciences, on mutual critical impulses between theory, empirical research, and social practice.

As "the most general abstractions occur only with the richest concrete development, where one seems collective to many, collective to all" (Marx, 1974, p. 25), the formulation of these relationships is not only a question of theory, but a question of the empirical evidence. One of the central issues of empirical research is the theoretic ability of a researcher to differentiate between the quantitatively prevailing and the essential characteristics of objects under study. The essential characteristics of society are never determined by the remains of the old in it (although they quantitatively still dominate) but by the elements of the new (i.e., by the direction and aim of the development of society). The new never appears as quantitatively dominant or as an average, but as an "exception" for which only a more thorough and theoretically based research can show that it is actually not just a chance but a rule, a result of historical development. With this, the task of (empirical) research may not be reduced to revealing just new phenomenological forms.

For social research and social practice or policy as well, it is essential to discover the conditions that led to the affirmation of the new and those that prevent or hinder its further development, and to formulate the key relationships between them.

Consequently, research may not be conducted with a self-evident classification of "facts" into already existing conceptual systems, although we are often forced to use simple, "natural" categories when starting a research work. On the other hand, and even if we have fairly well-developed theoretical categories, the process of research must be open-ended: It must allow and make possible the development of categories themselves during research. Gradually, with the progress of research from its "zero" investigating phase, cracks may be revealed in the "natural" categories.

> [These] analytical distinctions, and hence groupings, outweigh the phenomenologically presented categories of the quotidian. In the exposition phase, the structure of the presentation is dictated by the developed analytical categories, with reference to natural world categories principally in exemplification of concrete analytical points being made. (Freiberg, 1980, p. 6)

Quite surely, this process cannot be limited by terminally firmly defined research projects as they are usually conducted in contemporary times, particularly because of financial reasons, and from which, according to Horkheimer (1976), the charlatans receive the greatest benefit:

> A great number of so-called scientific products... are paid for in different ways; a portion of the value produced by truly productive work is spent on them, without this having any influence at all on the productivity of the workers... An activity, which contributes to the existence of society in its given forms does not need to be productivity, i.e., to create values for a certain action. (p. 53)

It is true that "expert-scientific" empiricism represents a form of conservative research because it even consciously avoids considering the dominant social relations in which research itself is embedded or even determined and concentrates only on (measurable) facts, thus reducing theory to generalization of facts and relationships between them. On the other hand, however, if (quantitative) empirical research would remain only a domain of traditional or positive science, would not its results, because of the supposed radical difference between positive and critical science for the latter, always be only an object of critique and never a moment of its own development or "a theoretically grounded program of action which will change social conditions?" Would not, then, critical science be transformed into an abstract human conscience, into a modern kind of Enlightenment without the power to change the world under investigation—as has happened to critical theory? Actually, with such a differentiation of critical science from empirical research, it also turns away from the practical "social conditions," from the practice itself. A productive theory (even if productivity is defined with regard to the possible, not the actually existing) cannot only "count on the existence of knowledge" or "yield investigation to traditional fields."

> Theoretical expositions with little or no applicability as models for the understanding of empirical social reality ignore the transition from the idealist to the materialist dialectical method. Such theoretistic efforts are *at best* suggestive; they contain insights that can be converted by others into research tools. At worst, such unsupported theoretical exposition amounts to little more than a sterile intellectual exercise. (Freiberg, 1980, p. 9.)

Thus it is far from being any kind of productive science as postulated by Horkheimer.

It is not by chance that Critical Theory has practically strayed into a blind alley, precisely because of its perseverance in the transformation of the social whole, the essential change as the main object of the theory and the necessary condition of validation of theory. Owing to its postulate of "being interested in the change, which is necessarily reproduced by the ruling injustice" (Horkheimer, 1976, p. 63-64), which has been practically falsified with the loss of an actual interest of the working class, Critical Theory lost its actual, real subject of the essential change (revolution) as the ferment of the future and, with this, its own foundation (i.e., "that which it is already time for," according to Horkheimer).

CULTURAL STUDIES: NOTHING NEW IN THE DICHOTOMY BETWEEN ADMINISTRATIVE AND CRITICAL TRADITIONS?

Have any of these methodological controversies been resolved by the "newest paradigm" in communication research—the British Cultural Studies tradition and its internationalization? Beyond any doubt, as Hardt argues in his treatise on Critical Theory, Cultural Studies, and American mass communication research, British Cultural Studies constitute a significant contemporary theoretical contribution to the field of mass communication research. Contrary to other European traditions, particularly those in Germany and France (e.g., Marxism and Critical Theory, which were slow in penetrating the United States because of language differences and difficulties), British Cultural Studies were immediately accessible in the original language and challenged predominantly empirical, behavioristic, and scientific American communication research, rejuvenated American cultural/critical tradition(s), but also increased positivist and phenomenological resistance to cultural studies (Carey, 1985, p. 31-37). Certainly, the influence of Cultural Studies in the United States and elsewhere is not caused merely by the absence of language barriers. At least five possible reasons for the spread of Cultural

Studies can be listed: (1) changes in mainstream communication research, (2) changes in receiving societies, (3) a growing internationalization of social events and processes in general and, in particular, of sciences, (4) a growing complexity of the human environment and the world, which needs a more complex, holistic understanding and interpretation, and (5) the uniqueness of concepts used and/or developed within new theory and their greater explanatory power, as compared to older concepts and research traditions.

I believe that there is no need (nor the time) to elaborate in more detail on the first four "reasons" that make Cultural Studies nowadays, particularly in the United States, more popular. The "Ferment in the Field," issue of the *Journal of Communication* (1983)—to take just one example—indicated rather plainly the changing conditions, opportunities and needs of communication research related to the new "information age," "open technologies," "human complexity," "internationalization of the cultural industries," to the neccessity of a "new critical synthesis," "decompartmentalization" and "processual analysis," or the importance of "being critical." The theoretical and epistemological significance or even uniqueness of Cultural Studies, however, deserve some more attention.

In his recent unpublished treatise, presented at the first Colloquium on Communication and Culture in Dubrovnik (1987), Colin Sparks, the editor of *Media, Culture and Society,* which has published major contributions in this field, illuminates some crucial elements of the history of British Cultural Studies. He discussed three major specific features of British Cultural Studies that make this tradition distinct from many others, particularly from what he vaguely calls "Mass Communication tradition," which has been developed within the frameworks of sociology, psychology, political economy, law, and political science. All three differences originate from the pervasive debt of Cultural Studies to *literary criticism.* Indeed, literary criticism as the origin and background of Cultural Studies (in both the biographical and intellectual sense as indicated by Sparks) should be considered a unique characteristic of this tradition: "Consequently a critique of the media in terms derived from a defence of literary values was one of the key elements in the emergence of thinking about the media in Britain" (Sparks, 1987, p. 8).

Thus the first distinctive characteristic of Cultural Studies is its "*evaluative approach to mass media artifacts*" and, consequently, the absence of any endeavor to develop "*analytic instruments* of its own." Rather, Cultural Studies "promiscuously borrowed methods and models from the most diverse of schools" (Sparks, 1987, p. 10)—from the young Marx, the Critical Theory of the Frankfurt School, and from Gramsci to Lévi-Strauss and Lacan. Second, Cultural Studies developed from the very beginning as a "*critical current.*" Although Cultural Studies developed within the Marxian and left-wing (political) tradition (as represented by the *New Left Review),* its critical orientation had "little or nothing to do with formal politics." However, it is not "depoliticized" in the sense usually associated with the mainstream media research in the United States. On the contrary, British Cultural Studies "appealed to the critics of mass communication research with its provocative investigations of contemporary social problems, demonstrating a sense of engagement between political practice and theoretical consideration within the public sphere" (Hardt, 1986, p. 123). The third defining element of Cultural Studies identified by Sparks ought to be "the extent to which it has been a *marginal phenomenon*" up until very recently, in relation to both university education and research funding, and to the media. The first dimension of marginality is trivial, because all new schools or paradigms have been born on the margins of already socially recognized tradition(s) within normal science. Besides, there also exist contrary views on its contribution to the international debate on vital communication issues, considering it influential internationally, particularly through publications. Apart from this controversy, the second dimension of its marginality is rather important: From the very beginning, Cultural Studies' tradition was characterized by its distance from the *media institutions* as their main research object or, as Halloran and Jones (1985, p. 25) maintain, it is "less inclined to have a service, administrative or commercial character." In other words, we are again facing the "old dichotomy" of *administrative versus critical* research, Cultural Studies being located on the "critical side" of the dimension.

However, Cultural Studies tradition departs both from classical administrative research and classical Marxism in its epistemological consideration of causality in social processes—in conceiving the role of structure and superstructure as *interdependent* components of a sociocultural system. In a way, with this reconceptualization of more rigid (although not one-way) relations, as defined by Marx, and its inclination to Weberian interpretive sociology, particularly to his concept of "causal pluralism" that rejects mechanical and unilateral causality, Cultural Studies becomes compatible even with the systems concept in the social sciences. As Bertalanffy (1973, p. 204) points out, the systems model of man as an active personality system "is the common denominator of many otherwise different currents." Both Systems Theory and Cultural Studies contradict the structural-functionalist theory, particularly the linear S-R models, and deny any validity to considering human creative and cultural activities as responses to stimuli, homeostasis or gratification of needs.

> The method of classical science was most appropriate for phenomena that either can be resolved into isolated causal chains or are the statistical outcome of an infinite number of chance processes. . . . The classical modes of thinking, however, fail in the case of interaction of a large but limited number of elements or processes. (Bertalanffy, 1973, p. 34)

Within Cultural Materialism, the crucial question that separates it from other social theories is "to what extent can fundamental changes be propagated and amplified by ideologies and political movements when the modes of production and reproduction stand opposed to them" (Harris, 1979, p. 73). For Cultural Studies,

> complex social formations had to be analysed in terms of the economic, political and ideological institutions and practices through which they were elaborated. Each of these elements had to be accorded a specific weight in determining the outcomes of particular conjectures. (Hall, 1985, p. 83)

Contrary to both critical and positivistic traditional media analyses, Cultural Studies relies upon a systemic concept of wholeness that presupposes the "struggle" between components of the whole, in which the role, significance, or function of any component ultimately results from the interaction of all components, but certain components of the complex social formations affect it substantially and therefore can be denoted as key instances of the system (e.g., of the production and reproduction of the dominant ideologies).

Precisely in this context, I would add one more important, perhaps even essential, characteristic of Cultural Studies in distinguishing it from Critical Theory rather than positivistic tradition, since the major target of the former has often not been society's problems, but administrative (empirical) research (Melody & Mansell, 1983, p. 110). I find very convincing Sparks's (1987) arguments that Cultural Studies is not hostile to empirical research traditions in the field, contrary to the "classical" Critical Theory. However, in Cultural Studies tradition,

> its use of empirical methods has always been eclectic and piratical rather than an integral part of its project. That does not mean a collapse into the worst banalities of the M[ass] C[ommunication] T[radition] number crunchers and model builders. It does, however, mean that the project of critical inquiry has to be reworked from the start as an activity that includes empirical research.

Hall (1985, p. 88) explicitly claims that "*extensive empirical work* is required" (emphasis added) to prove the validity of explanatory terms developed within the new critical paradigm. As certain concepts and models of general systems theory that can be defined in both natural and mathematical languages (e.g., graph theory, hierarchical clustering) are broadly applicable to sociocultural systems, it seems that, in principle, there is no obstacle to empirical validation of some basic theoretical premises of Cultural Studies and thus to make the new critical paradigm not only challenging, but even dominating for both analytical and explanatory reasons.

REFERENCES

Adorno, T. W., & Horkheimer, M. (1980). *Socioloske studije*. Zagreb: Skolska Knjiga. (Original work published 1956)

Berger, P., & Kellner, H. (1981). *Sociology reinterpreted: An essay on method and vocation.* Garden City, NY: Anchor/Doubleday.

Bertalanffy, L. V. (1973). *General system theory.* Harmondsworth: Penguin.

Carey, J. W. (1985). Overcoming resistance to cultural studies. In M. Gurevitch & M. R. Levy (Eds.), *Mass communication yearbook* (Vol. 5). Beverly Hills, CA: Sage.

Cohen, B. (1980). *Developing sociological knowledge: Theory and method.* Englewood Cliffs, NJ: Prentice-Hall.

Comstock, D. E. (1980). A method for critical research: Investigating the world to change it. *Transforming sociology series* (No. 72). Livermore: Red Feather Institute for Advanced Studies in Sociology.

Fejes, F. (1984). Critical mass communication research and media effects: The problem of the disappearing audience. *Media, Culture and Society, 6,* 219-232.

Freiberg, J. W. (1980). Dialectical method. *Transforming sociology series* (No. 57). Livermore: Red Feather Institute for Advanced Studies in Sociology.

Gouldner, A. (1970). *The coming crisis of Western society.* New York: Basic Books.

Habermas, J. (1980). *Teorija i praksa* (Theorie und praxis). Beograd: BIGZ.

Hall, S. (1985). The rediscovery of ideology: Return of the repressed in media studies. In M. Gurevitch et al. (Eds.), *Culture, society and the media.* London and New York: Methuen.

Halloran, J., & Jones, M. (1985). Learning about the media. *Communication and Society,* (Vol. 16). Paris: UNESCO

Hardt, H. (1986). British cultural studies and the return of the critical in American mass communication research: Accommodation or radical change? *Journal of Communication Inquiry, 10*(2), 117-124.

Harris, M. (1979). *Cultural materialism: The struggle for a science of culture.* New York: Random House.

Haug, F. (1978). Dialektische Theorie und empirische Methodik. *Das Argument, 111,* 644-656.

Hellman, H. (1980). *Idealism, aggression, apology, and criticism: The four traditions of research on "international communication."* Paper presented at the 12th Congress of IAMCR, Caracas.

Horkheimer, M. (1976). *Tradicionalna i kriticka teorija/Tradizionalle und kritische Theorie.* Beograd: BIGZ. (Original work published 1936-1937)

Kirk, J., & Miller, M. L. (1986). *Reliability and validity in qualitative research.* London: Sage.

Lang, K., & Lang, G. E. (1985). Method as master, or mastery over method. In M. Gurevitch & M. R. Levy (Eds.), *Mass communication yearbook* (Vol. 5). Beverly Hills, CA: Sage.

Marx, K. (1973). *Das Kapital* (Vol. 1). Berlin: Dietz Verlag.

Marx, K. (1974). *Grundrisse der Kritik der politischen Oekonomie.* Berlin: Dietz Verlag.

Marx, K., & Engels, F. (1973). *Die deutsche Ideologie* (Marx-Engels-Werke, Vol. 3). Berlin: Dietz Verlag.

Melody, W. H., & Mansell, R. E. (1983). The debate over critical vs. administrative research: Circularity or challenge. *Journal of Communication, 33*(3), 103-114.

Merton, R. K. (1979). *O teorijskoi sociologiji* (On theoretical sociology). Zagreb: Naklada CDD.

Slack, J. D., & Allor, M. (1983). The political and epistemological constituents of critical communication research. *Journal of Communication, 33*(3), 208-217.

Smythe, D. W., & Van Dinh, T. (1983). On critical and administrative research: A new critical analysis. *Journal of Communication, 33*(3), 117-127.

Sparks, C. (1987). *British cultural studies.* Paper presented at the first Colloquium on Communication and Culture, Dubrovnik.

Splichal, S. (1987). "Public opinion" and the controversies in communication science. *Media, Culture and Society, 9,* 237-261.

Vaillancourt, P. M. (1986). *Social reality, epistemology, methodology, and research: Marxist assumptions about inquiry.* Paper presented at the XI World Congress of Sociology, New Delhi.

Van Maanen, J. (Ed.). (1983). *Qualitative methodology.* Beverly Hills, London: Sage.

Wenger, M. G. (1986). *Marxism and social research: The mythology of epistemology.* Paper presented at the XI World Congress of Sociology, New Delhi.

Weber, M. (1986). *Methodologija drustvenih nauka* (Gesammelte Aufsatze zur Wissenschaftslehre). Zagreb: Globus. (Original work published 1922)

Williams, R. (1973). *Communications* (3rd ed.). Harmondsworth: Penguin.

Young, T. R. (1980). Cultural Marxism: An introduction. *Transforming sociology series* (No. 77). Livermore: Red Feather Institute for Advanced Studies in Sociology.

SECTION 5

ORGANIZATIONS AND GIFTS

11 One-Way Communication Transfers in Loosely Coupled Systems

LARRY DAVIS BROWNING
University of Texas at Austin

SHEILA C. HENDERSON
St. Edward's University

This chapter integrates the one-way transfer theory of Boulding (1973) and Mauss (1967) with the loosely coupled systems theory of Weick (1976) to advance the thesis that one-way transfers are plausible events under conditions of slack and ambiguity—the prime dimensions of loosely coupled systems. A field research project of in-depth interviews with retirees is reported in narrative form to verify past theory and to search for new theoretical formulations on giving in the organizational setting. The results of the research show that dramatic reports of organizational life are surfaced in the process of searching for one-way transfers. People taking a risk that produces a positive outcome for someone else is a powerful, if traditional, narrative. The surprising finding of the research shows negative gifts (corrections to alter or reshape behavior that are unappreciated at the time but are later valued) are a constant theme in the data.

HISTORICALLY, behavioral science theory has been influenced by an exchange model borrowed from economics, which considers self-interest and an even exchange to be the prime motivator of human behavior (Kau & Rubin, 1979), and therefore assumes that it is a given in social interaction (Homans, 1961; Blau, 1964; Chadwick-Jones, 1976; Burgess & Huston, 1979). However, when we base our interpretations of social systems solely on models of self-interest, we "risk the serious danger of *fostering* such behavior to the exclusion of less self-interested, altruistic acts" (Kaun, 1984, p. 30). For this reason, Kaun (1984) has introduced economists to the concept of "ideology" as an alternative to "self-interest." The influence of the economic metaphor, in which rationality and equivalency are paramount, has channeled the inquiries of communication researchers away

Correspondence and requests for reprints: Larry Davis Browning, Department of Speech Communication, CMA 7.114, University of Texas-Austin, Austin, TX 78712.

Communication Yearbook 12, 638-669

from formulating explanations of phenomena that appear irrational and unstable (Morgan, 1980).

Rather than as randomly occurring aberrations of economic model exchange, these interactions might profitably be considered as different forms of give and take (Polanyi, 1944; Boulding, 1973; Hyde, 1983; Sahlins, 1974; Macneil, 1986), operating according to separate value systems and decision-making strategies. Instead of assuming that logical symmetrical exchange is a given in social systems, we might reasonably posit an "erotic" commerce, opposing *eros* (the principle of attraction, union, and involvement that binds together) to *logos* (reason and logic in general, the principle of differentiation in particular; Hyde, 1983, p. xiv). According to this construct, one-way, rather than two-way, transfers account for a significant part of social interaction. Drawing upon gift theory developed from studies of primitive societies (Mauss, 1967; Boulding, 1973), this chapter builds a noneconomic model for understanding social systems in our information-based society by examining the effects of information abundance (slack) on the conduct of organizational relationships.

One of the problems arising from the dominance of the economic metaphor as a research paradigm is the conceptual ambiguity surrounding what distinguishes one form of exchange from another. At its most concrete or literal, economic or market exchange is a simultaneous two-way transfer of ostensibly "equal" material commodities, although each participant in the exchange is usually assumed to be seeking to maximize his benefits in relation to his costs out of self-interest (Davis, 1973). Yet exchange "is virtually always relational exchange, that is, exchange carried on within relations having significant impact on its goals, conduct, and effect" (Macneil, 1986). In his book, *The Economy of Love and Fear*, Boulding (1973) theorizes that the economic mechanisms that account for one-way transfers (research grants from foundations, for example, or college educations from parents), which comprise from 20 to 50% of all economic transactions, are inherently logical rather than as aberrations from the two-way transfer economic model. Boulding agrees with the sociologists and anthropologists (Polanyi, 1944; Lévi-Strauss, 1964; Mauss, 1967; Ekeh, 1974; Hedican, 1986) and philosophers

AUTHORS' NOTE: An earlier version of this chapter was presented at the Annual meeting of the Speech Communication Association, November 1981, Anaheim, CA. While we consider this a team effort, the author contributions to this chapter merit some details. The original research, conceptual framework, data analysis and write-up were produced primarily by the first author. The manuscript writing of the conceptual section, the second of three waves of library research and the final editing were done primarily by the second author. We would like to thank Jack Whitehead for attending a Kenneth Boulding lecture at the University of Texas and returning with the gift of an oral theory of gifts; Robert Hopper and Jim Gilchrist for comments on earlier drafts of this chapter; Ann Butterfield for arranging the interviews at the church; Charla Ann Baker and Nancy Wilson for help on the literature review; and Jim Bell, Roger Cude, Treva Dayton, Susan Hale, Glen McLaaughlin and Nancy Roth for help in collecting interview data. We would also like to acknowledge Pat and Joe Froehle, Jim Smeeding, and Anne Van Kleek for their human models of one-way transfers.

(Aristotle, *The Poetics,* cited in Taussig, 1980, 1962; Baudrillard, 1981; Miller, 1987) who contend that the economic exchange system is embedded in and reflective of the social exchange system, suggesting that exchange operates on parallel levels—the material and the social—every time some physical commodity changes hands.

But what about situations in which the physical commodity changing hands has little or no utility value beyond serving as a vehicle for the underlying social exchange (e.g., Malinowski's, 1922, conception of ceremonial exchange)? Or, more troublesome still, situations in which the "commodity" is not "physical" at all but communicative, like an arranged introduction or a useful piece of information (Boulding, 1973). As emphasis shifts from the economic to the social, the notions of equivalency, directionality, and logic become slippery. Often it is the social transaction that actually defines the material one. For example, the exchange of Christmas gifts might look like a two-way economic transfer, yet it is actually two simultaneous one-way transfers in which powerful psychological and cultural "messages" are given along with the fruitcake or the pot holder made at camp (Schwartz, 1967; Poe, 1977). When the commodity itself is a "message," like a piece of information, it becomes more difficult to discover whether the exchange is economic or purely social or whether it involves a two-way or one-way transfer. Certainly, we have ample evidence that information in the form of professional expertise or technical secrets is worth money (a salary in the first case and a bribe or payoff in the second) and thus subject to two-way economic exchange on a regular basis. But when someone passes along a recommendation or volunteers his services to his professional association, in most cases, the exchange is obviously a one-way transfer—a communicative grant or gift to which no specific value can be assigned, and thus no *economic* model can be strictly applied.

The concept of *giving,* which is the pedestrian term for one-way transfer, is often lumped with a broad range of altruistic acts and, as a consequence, is not well defined. The terms's usage varies from what 34 apartment dwellers weren't willing to risk to help Kitty Genovese (Latane & Darley, 1970) to what a fisherman does with his spoilable catch exceeding what he needs to feed his family (Mauss, 1967). Motivations in one-way transfers involve a great deal more than simple altruism or benevolence (Krebs, 1970; MacCrimmon & Messick, 1976), ranging from self-interest or egotism (Cook, 1966; Hammond, 1975) to hostility and guilt (Brown, 1959; Schwartz, 1967) to shame (Lynd, 1958) to status anxiety (Schwartz, 1967) to security, power, and control (Korn & McCorkle, 1954; Whyte, 1964; Levi-Strauss, 1964). The German word for *gift* is also the term for *poison* (Bailey, 1971), which suggests the potential for a gift to be both attractive and suspect at the same time. Boulding (1973) accounts for the dark side of one-way transfers by suggesting that in addition to the *gift,* which is a pure expression of benevolence, there is the *tribute,* which is a grant made out of fear. He acknowledges that few transfers clearly rest at one end of the spectrum or the other; most grants are mixes of good will and threat. To add more context to the understanding of the motivation for and the circulation of gifts, consider the following two examples.

Example one. In his book, *The Devil and Commodity Fetishism in South America* (1980), Michael Taussig tells the story of a culture both registering and fending off "the historical forces of encroaching capitalism" (Sass, 1986). He describes the experience of peasants in a precapital society in which work carries spiritual properties and is weighted according to use-value (comparable to the pride and honor of "earning your living by the sweat of your brow" in American culture), as they become proletariat in a commodity-based society in which exchange-value dominates. As long as the peasants cultivate their own land according to their own customs, they partake in and contribute to the spirit of use-value. However, as they become landless wage earners, either on sugarcane plantations or in tin mines, they are thought to "enter into secret contracts with the devil in order to increase their production and hence their wage" (p. 13). As luck would have it, these contracts with the devil produce baneful consequences: The land they purchase with their wages becomes barren; their livestock dies; the maker of the contract, invariably a man, dies prematurely and in pain (Taussig, 1980, p. 13). As long as their contribution is autonomous, it has spiritual validity; when the same effort is exchanged, its substance is lost.

Example two. This comes from Hyde's (1983) description of an Indian gift: When the puritans first landed in Massachusetts, they discovered a thing so curious about the Indian's feelings for property that they felt called upon to give it a name. In 1764, when Thomas Hutchison wrote his history of the colony, the term was already an old saying: "An Indian gift," he told his readers, "is a proverbial expression signifying a present for which an equivalent return is expected." We still use this, of course, and in an even broader sense, calling that friend an Indian giver who is so uncivilized as to ask us to return a gift he or she has given (p. 3).

Hyde (1983) goes on to invite us to imagine a scene: An Englishmen comes to an Indian lodge and is offered a smoke from a ceremonial pipe that is traditionally circulated among neighboring tribes. After sharing the tobacco, the Englishman is offered the pipe when he leaves. He is ecstatic about his new gift and can already imagine sending it back to the British Museum. He is later visited by another neighboring tribe and is surprised when his translator tells him that if he wishes to show his good will, he should offer them a smoke and give them the pipe.

> In consternation the Englishman invents a phrase to describe these people with such a limited sense of private property. The opposite of "Indian giver" would be something like "white man keeper" (or maybe "capitalist"), that is, a person whose instinct is to remove property from circulation, to put it in a warehouse or museum (or, more to the point for capitalism, to lay it aside to be used for production). (Hyde, 1983, p. 4)

The Indian giver understood the same principle that Mauss (1967) found among Indian tribes of the Pacific northwest and the southern Pacific—the obligation to give, receive, and circulate. In his book, *Muddling Toward Frugality* (1978), Warren Johnson posits a future world affected by electronic information to look more like communities of the turn of the century than like the urban centers of the 1980s. This chapter uses theory on the abundance of raw materials in the past (Mauss, 1967) to consider the abundance of information in modern communities (Sowell, 1980).

GIFTS IN LOOSELY COUPLED SYSTEMS

The thesis of this chapter is that one-way transfers in organizations occur under conditions of abundance and ambiguity, traits that are characteristic of loosely coupled systems. As mechanisms for the redistribution of resources, one-way transfers operate according to a logic broader than efficiency (Najjar, 1978; Bolnick, 1975), which, as Bourgeois (1981) points out, is another characteristic of loosely coupled systems. The slack resources in loosely coupled systems allow them to achieve high levels of autonomy and effectiveness with disregard for the constraints of efficiency. When systems are loosely coupled, subunits have ample or redundant resources in the form of time, personnel, finances, and discretion over decision making and exist in larger systems that are uncertain as to means-ends connections, the flow of influence, coordination processes, feedback and evaluation procedures, and causes of outcomes. In loosely coupled systems, the interactions between subsystems do not occur in predictable, stimulus-response ways; instead, interactions are *dampened* by subunits that absorb them, or are *eventually* (and possibly *suddenly*) passed on by subunits that reach a threshold level with them, or are *symbolically* made by subunits that are unable to make explicit connections between intentions and actions (Weick, 1980; Salancik, 1975). Possessing resources beyond mere adequacy or even comfort, but *not* possessing control mechanisms to monitor resource use or outcomes from that use, puts a system in the position in which one-way transfers are both likely and logical: "A gift is a thing we cannot get by our own efforts. We cannot buy it; we cannot acquire it through an act of will" (Hyde, 1983, p. 1).

In the cornerstone conceptual piece on loosely coupled systems, Weick (1976) directly addresses the qualities exhibited by loosely coupled systems. They can be organized under the dual headings of slack and ambiguity. These 15 qualities are cross-coded in Table 11.1.

The combination of slack resources and the inability to predict or control outcomes in loosely coupled systems means that organizational subunits are able to retain self-control and persistence but are unable to control others (Glassman, 1973; Ouchi, 1978). Subunits cannot be sure that exchanges will occur; other subunits may withhold resources or attention even though they

TABLE 11.1
Qualities that described loosely-coupled systems

Slack	Ambiguity
(1) slack times—when there is an excessive amount of resources relative to demands	
	(2) occasions when any one of several means will produce the same ends
	(3) richly connected networks in which influence is slow to spread and/or weak
	(4) a relative lack of coordination, slow coordination, or coordination that is dampened as it moves through the system
(5) a relative absence of regulations	(5) a relative absence of regulations
(6) planned unresponsiveness	
(7) actual causal independence	
	(8) poor observational capabilities on the part of the viewers
(9) infrequent inspection of activities within the system	(9) infrequent inspection of activities within the system
	(10) decentralization
(11) delegation of discretion	(11) delegation of discretion
	(12) theory-based absence of linkages
	(13) an observation that an organization's structure is not coterminous with its activity
	(14) those occasions when no matter what you do things always come out the same
	(15) few prerequisites—unrestricted entry

SOURCE: Weick (1976, p. 5).

are formally expected to participate (Cohen, March, & Olsen, 1972). Neither can subunits be certain of the value their contribution will be assigned, nor know how much will be received back in relation to what is given (Pettigrew, 1973). If, however, the subsystems are effective and self-sustaining, their perspective on the environment may not be directed toward equitable exchanges with other subunits, but instead, may be focused on how to ensure that their resources will be the ones applied to organizational problems (Benson, 1975). Such a perspective upends the traditional assumption that organizations are problem-solving systems that respond to uncertainties in their environments by planning, organizing, controlling, and evaluating outcomes (Taylor, 1923; Koontz & O'Donnell, 1964). Instead, organizations appear to be "garbage cans"—collections of choices looking for problems; issues and feelings looking for decision situations in which they might be aired; solutions looking for issues to which they might be the answer; and decision makers looking for work (Cohen & March, 1974, p. 81).

ONE-WAY TRANSFERS OF COMMUNICATION

Transfers of communication in loosely coupled systems meets the requirements of requisite variety (Weick, 1979). If a loose or garbage can system is characterized by uncertainty, one-way transfers within the system must be equally varied. Variety must be matched with variety. The net effect of the compounding of looseness and communication gifts provides loose systems with the basics for survival—creativity, commitment, and momentum. Glassman (1973) calls commitment persistence; Peters (1987) calls creativity the acceptance of failure; and Weick (1979) and Peters and Waterman (1982) call momentum action bias. The argument for one-way transfers in loosely coupled systems as an enabling condition for these three dimensions will be developed by detailing the ambiguous and abundant qualities of communication and linking them to creativity, commitment, and momentum in organizations.

The Ambiguity of Communication Gifts

Communication gifts have six paradoxical qualities that heighten their ambiguity and distinguish them from transfers of other types. Communication is (1) *abundant*—it's going on all the time (Mauss, 1967), (2) *ephemeral*—it passes quickly and is hard to capture: "The spirit of a gift is kept alive by its constant donation" (Hyde, 1983, p. xiv), (3) *intangible*—it eludes precise identification and definition (Hyde, 1983), (4) *reusable* and *replenishable*—it doesn't get "used up" and can be given away and kept at the same time (Sowell, 1980), (5) inherently *value-free*—what is priceless in one situation might be worthless in another: "You cannot put a price on it" (Hyde, 1983, p. 60), and (6) *time-bound*—its timing is the greater part of its significance (Sowell, 1980). Communication grants in a "garbage can" system would be given generously (because they are abundant, reusable, and replenishable) and made sense of retrospectively (because they are ephemeral, intangible, value-free, and time-bound).

Timeliness is particularly significant when grants are communicative because timing makes the value of the gift ambiguous. Because they are ephemeral commodities, depending upon the total situational context in which the donor and recipient find themselves, the value of communicative grants depends as much upon the need of the recipient as on the resource abundance of the donor. In a "garbage can" situation, the convergence of donor, recipient, need (i.e., problem), and resource (i.e., solution) is in many ways random and unpredictable. Therefore, the exact value of any communicative gift remains ambiguous prior to the gift-giving. The value often remains somewhat ambiguous afterward as well, since the feedback loops tend to be long and tenuous (Weick, 1976, 1980). Any single communicative act potentially is less related to the immediately prior and subsequent acts than to an act occurring between the participants weeks or even years before. People remember gifts for a long time. Patterns that appear weak or fuzzy within a narrow time frame have high resolution when viewed through a longer perspective. By assuming a developmental, "macro" perspective of one-way transfers, we discover a rationality and stability in previously disturbing "anomalous" phenomena (Kadushin, undated; Granovetter, 1973; Ekeh, 1974).

As timing is an ambiguous dimension in determining a gift's value, it is also a crucial element in determining whether or not a transfer is a gift at all. If one expects (and receives) an immediate return for his effort, then the event more closely fits the definition of a two-way transfer or economic exchange. Although the argument was made earlier that the exchange of Christmas gifts could not be considered a form of two-way transfer, its ritualization places it at the pole closest to exchange on the continuum of gifting, while at the other pole are transfers anonymously and spontaneously given (Arrow, 1975), like those dispensed for several seasons during the 1950s on the television show "The Millionaire." If one has no expectations for a return in kind, expressing a "don't worry about it" attitude, then the interaction exemplifies gifting. While the donor may or may not receive a grant in return at some future time, the span of time that elapses prior to return serves an important social integration function: so long as the recipient is in the donor's "debt," so to speak, he or she is more likely to behave in a peaceful and loyal fashion (Gouldner, 1960; Malinowski, 1922).

One-way transfers operate independently of direct, immediate exchange or feedback that lengthens their loop and increases their ambiguity. This operation has both good and bad effects; good because such independence gives the donor more choice over the selection or creation of what she or he has to give or say; bad because it operates without regulation. If the presentation is unappreciated or has a negative effect upon the recipient, the donor might never know to alter his or her behavior. Boulding (1973) captures the no-feedback-no-standards-of-success principle in "Edsel's Law":

> When the Ford motor company produced the Edsel automobile, it soon discovered the demand was not adequate to justify its production. There was very rapid feedback, and as a result the mistake was corrected and the Edsel withdrawn. In contrast, if the Ford Foundation produced an "Edsel" in the form of grants for purposes that were not particularly socially useful or did not produce the intended results, the Foundation might never know. (p. 24)

The lack of knowledge of immediate results (or even the desire thereof) helps to explain why gifts or one-way transfers in organizations are usually connected to positions, subunits, or organizations that are "privileged" (Glidewell, 1973, p. 4) and buffered from demands of short-term success, but are expected to emphasize ideology and internal standards as guides for evaluation (Selznick, 1957; Ouchi, 1978).

The Abundance of Communication Gifts

The reusability and replenishability of communication as a resource importantly affects its use as a granting commodity. When a donor has a replenishable supply of a resource, the applicability of the costs-benefits model is altered because his ability to absorb costs will give him more decision-making freedom (Prattis, 1973). The strategic function of slack is that it allows for a distinction between different forms of risk-taking decisions. When the outcomes of a particular choice (such as making a grant) are unclear, the consequences of taking that action are a matter of probability and the decision is called "risky" (Ellsberg, 1961; Yates & Zukowski, 1976). Deutsch (1960) distinguishes between two types of decisions that could be considered risky—gambling and trusting: "In the present terminology, one gambles when one has much to gain or little to lose and one trusts when one has much to lose or little gain" (p. 124). Because slack reduces constraints, it allows subunits to make decisions having uncertain outcomes with less concern for the efficiency of gambling or trusting in any particular situation. Under conditions of uncertainty, decisions are often made serially and are greatly affected by situational factors, such as the order in which the decisions are made and even momentary impulses (Bolnick, 1975). Thus if the *benefit* ratio of a grant or one-way transfer is high relative to costs (no matter how high costs might be), then the donor is likely to be more willing to give resources (Boulding, 1973) and, importantly, is less likely to monitor the outcomes of his or her giving to see if returns are paid on the grant-investment. This tendency is dramatically increased when the situation is a "garbage can," in which the value of decisions or the outcomes of giving can be discovered only later and usually only by paying close attention. A problem with Boulding's (1973) work is that it is dominated by the phenomenon of scarcity, which means that if "A" gets a grant, some unfortunate "B" will not. However, communication as an intangible and infinitely renewable resource does not have the same limitations as material goods. The three forms of communicative grants—providing information, providing linkages, and providing emotional support—can be one-way transfers with high potential benefit that can be distributed to unlimited numbers of "A's" and "B's" (Browning & Johnson, 1984).

High-level positions in organizations provide members with abundant resources. Certainly, one of the reasons high-level positions are prized is the broader span of resources at one's disposal as well as the greater freedom of action in dealing with those resources (Thompson, 1967). Boulding (1973) suggests that authority is established not solely by the possession of resources but also by the dispensing of them:

> The ability to make internal transfers is one of the principal marks of status in a hierarchy. The higher a person stands in the hierarchy (the more he is a "boss and less he is bossed) the more internal grants he has the power to control. (p. 3)

Resource allocation is a political process that is the basis for stratifying social systems (Salancick & Pfeffer, 1977; Prattis, 1973); grants are an important part of the "political economy" (Boulding, 1973)—the process by which roles are created and things get done. But the "political economy" has always been assumed to operate according to the exigencies of scarcity, wherein power accumulation is designed to assure unequal access to scarce resources (Velzen, 1973; Cyert & March, 1963; Moch & Pondy, 1977). Information has traditionally been understood to circulate asymmetrically (Ramos, 1976), making it a resource that is differentially distributed at some levels and subject to careful control (Prattis, 1973). The more information an organizational member possesses, the higher his structural-functional position is presumed to be. The assumption is that organizational members at higher positions in the hierarchy will jealously hoard their limited information resources, denying others access in order to reinforce their positions (Prattis, 1973; Ramos, 1976) and accrue power (Velzen, 1973).

Grants, or one-way transfers on an interpersonal level tend to take place at higher strata in organizations, in which role and task definitions are less prescribed and work flows less predictable than at the more bureaucratically structured, lower strata (Weick, 1979; Pfeffer, 1981). At lower organizational levels, information travels along work flow networks (Brass, 1981) and tends to be narrowly confined to the specifics of the well-defined task to be accomplished. Decisions are typically made using particularistic criteria (Salancick & Pfeffer, 1977), with an emphasis on maximization of short-term, and often parochial, goals (Prattis, 1973). In states of uncertainty, people in bureaucratic positions will tend to adopt "rational" economic exchange patterns to minimize their social costs, out of self-protection (Deal & Kennedy, 1982; Davis, 1973).

The combined effect of slack and ambiguity is to foster creativity, commitment, and momentum.

CREATIVITY

The donor in one-way transfers has more personal control over the shape and form of his or her input, increasing the potential for creativity. Slack resources and restricted or ambiguous feedback allow a donor to experiment, to find or create environments in which the criteria for input evaluation are loose and flexible. For example:

> Hoffer remembers with pleasure the day he drew the worst worker on the docks, a fellow so clumsy and inept that the others took pains to avoid working with him. "We went to work," Hoffer recalls, "and started to build our load. On the docks it's very simple—you build your side of the load and your partner builds his side, half and half. But that day I noticed something funny. My partner was always across the aisle, giving foreign aid to somebody else. He wasn't doing his

> share of the work on our load, but he was helping others with theirs. There was no reason to think that he disliked me. But I remember how that day I got started on a beautiful train of thought. I started to think why it was that this fellow, who couldn't do his own duty, was so eager to do things above and beyond his duty. And the way I explained it was that if you are clumsy in doing your duty, you will never be ridiculous in helping others—nobody will laugh at you. The man was trying to drift into a situation where his clumsiness would not be conspicuous, would not be blamed. (Tomkins, 1968, pp. 31-32)

At the organizational level, this creative license permits organizations to experiment with new strategies to compete more boldly in their environment (Bourgeois, 1981) and even independently to redefine those environments (Benson, 1975).

One-way transfers are also voluntary, and while informal voluntary relationships are less dependable (by definition, one can't be assured continuation of a voluntary relationship), participation in them provides members greater freedom and less obligation than do relationships that have clear definitions for what each party expects from the other. Greater freedom means more options, which meets a central requirement for successful human (White, 1949) and organizational adaptation (Pondy & Mitroff, 1979; Ashby, 1960). As much research on altruism suggests (Krebs, 1970), a key component of the willingness to provide help is the giver's perception that the assistance is not expected or demanded.

COMMITMENT

The effect of voluntary participation and the power to withdraw is a mighty one (Hirschman, 1970, Emerson, 1962). *Not* withdrawing—maintaining a commitment despite less-than-satisfying immediate outcomes—is an even mightier option available to donors in granting relationships. Najjar (1978) points out that

> one-way transfers often reflect an inner normative stance or sense of commitment on the part of the donor and are usually intended to promote social and political ends that are often held as value preferences and cannot be demonstrated or refuted on allocative grounds alone. (pp. 502-503)

The concept of commitment is also reflected in Gouldner's (1960) discussion of the persistence and stability found in granting relationships.

Buchanan's (1975) game theory matrix of the Samaritan's dilemma demonstrates the power of the commitment option. The Samaritan's dilemma presumes two roles: potential Samaritan and potential parasite. In the negotiation game, the parasite predicts that the Samaritan will maximize short-term utilities in ways that allow the parasite to benefit, assuming that the cost of immediate rejection of his demands is too high for the Samaritan to bear. Because the Samaritan has slack, he or she will not be willing to capitulate in the short-term; awareness that he or she will gain genuine advantages by locking into a strategic behavior pattern in advance of any observed response on the part of the parasite, along with a willingness to accept the prospect of short-term injury as a result of such strategic rigidity, determines the outcomes of the game. The one-way transfer of action and a conscious inattention to immediate feedback from the action bolster the Samaritan's original decision, despite the fact that the immediate attractive solution would be to acquiesce to the parasite's demands (Buchanan, p. 77). Real world examples of this action include prisoners going on hunger strikes, terrorists kidnapping diplomats and the North Korean capture of the Pueblo (Buchanan, p. 79; Prattis, 1973). An unfortunate potential outcome of commitment is the "sacrifice trap" (Boulding, 1973), in which the identity of the donor becomes so tightly bound up in the one-way transfers or grants he or she can become trapped in a disadvantageous pattern of giving indefinitely.

Although some modern observers suggest that the affiliative, integrative social ties gluing modern social structure together have almost completely dissolved under the pressures caused by exclusive subscription to an economic market "mentality" (Hardin, 1968; Slater, 1971), others suggest there are "paraeconomies" (Ramos, 1976), that is, nonmarket-centered social systems, existing at both formal and informal levels, which rely heavily upon grants or one-way transfers to exist (Najjar, 1978). It is the *para*economic, social transfers that account for the "counterrational" (Browning, 1982) aspects of formally "rational" systems and that, rather than representing "breakdowns" of rational models, may actually prevent them from falling apart. "Gifts are made to create social solidarity" (Macneil, 1986, p. 573). Weick (1976) suggests that the connotations of tacitness and impermanence arising from loose coupling are also potentially crucial "gluing" devices holding organizations together (p. 3).

The idea of one-way transfers to foster commitment may be foreign to organization theory, but it is familiar in theories of community (Najjar 1978; Ramos, 1976). A community may be the essential example of a loosely coupled system: a collection of actors, with unclear and varying status and power, who lead their lives in the same space, having the collective goal of survival or continuation and sharing values or ideals about fair play, success, ambition, and special care for favorites. In these terms, loosely coupled organizations and the upper regions of most other types of organizations are communitylike in their norms for give and take. In a mobile society (such as an organization characterized by changing membership), serial or generalized reciprocity is a way of maintaining continuity and a sense of community.

MOMENTUM

Social exchange, unlike economic exchange, is by its very nature not only incapable of balance (because of the fluidity of the "commodities" exchanged, such as status, recognition, support, and so on) but actually *strives* for disequilibrium. The stretch for disequilibrium, like the runner stretching for the tape, creates momentum. When social exchange is institutionalized in roles and rituals (Schwartz, 1967), the expectations or anticipations that arise generate what Simmel (1950) called "inertia," in the form of gratitude (or grudge, as Schwartz, 1967, points out). The inertia created by the giving of grants or one-way transfers produces an integrative social indebtedness that keeps society both stable (Simmel, 1950) and evolving (Mauss, 1967; Boulding, 1973; Ekeh, 1974). Gouldner (1960) suggests that the requirement for rough, rather than exact, equivalency in repayment of a gift is a mechanism for generating uncertainty over time as to who is in debt to whom. According to Schwartz (1967), violating the rule of approximate reciprocity—"returning a gift in near, but not exact, value of that received" (p. 6)—by striving for too close an equivalency of return, drains the relationship of its personalness and sentiment, reducing it to pseudoeconomic exchange. The more one-way transfers look and act like economic exchange, the greater the likelihood of exploitation and gifts becoming precursors to demands (Bohanan, 1955, p. 60). Further, Gouldner (1960) points out that the most important use of what he calls hemeomorphic reciprocity (exact return of that which was received) is in the negative norm for return of an injury—"an eye for an eye." Keeping a state of "balance" by immediately returning a gift is a way of maintaining independence (Poe, 1977), which is as "unfriendly" as is seeking balance by gift equivalency. Gouldner (1960) quotes Seneca to make this point: "A person who wants to repay a gift too quickly with a gift in return is an unwilling debtor and an ungrateful person" (p. 75, footnote). Any presentation is made into a gift simply by the lack of explicit return by the recipient. In this way, the recipient, even more than the donor, defines the transaction and reduces equivocality. If he perceives the interaction as a grant, he defines the nature of it by the timing and content of his reciprocation.

Marcel Mauss (1967) adds to the argument for momentum by describing the three underlying tenets of gift giving: the obligations to give, to receive, and to reciprocate. Although Boulding (1973) suggests that these obligations highlight the difficulty of distinguishing grants or gifts from exchanges, Mauss's discussion of reciprocity emphasizes the mediated nature of repayment in gifting. His perspective (as well as those of Malinowski, 1922, and Gouldner, 1960) implies a nonimmediate equity—serial and generalized reciprocity that transforms repayment from *individual* obligation to *community* activity. Ekeh (1974) elaborates on this idea by distinguishing between the various combinations of numbers of actors and directionality of reciprocation. When the relationship is between isolated actors in dyads (exclusive restricted exchange) or between dyads that are implicated in a network with other dyads (inclusive restricted exchange), investigating the balance or rewards or outcomes is manageable. However, when multiple parties are recipients of an action taken by a single individual (group focused, generalized exchange), it is more difficult to determine the balance of rewards. The same is true for the gift from many to one (individual focused generalized exchange). Confusion activates momentum. Examples of the latter two situations might be in leading a troop of Boy Scouts—the gift is to the parents—and a barn raising.

The *first* gift is powerful for momentum because it is unique both temporally and symbolically. Adler (1981) calls this the "fresh impulse" or "primitive force" (p. 57). As Simmel (1950) points out, the first gift is the only one that can be considered to arise out of completely "pure" motives (he talks of pure benevolence, but Boulding would also include pure threat). All subsequent grants are subject to the intrusion of a sense of obligation or ingratiation, and thus lack the spontaneity of the first. However, this is more likely the case when partners engage in direct reciprocity; it is only in a partnership that "second" or "third" gifts can exist logically. With serial (Mauss, 1967; Gouldner, 1960) or circular (Malinowski, 1922) reciprocity, although the sense of obligation continues, it is indirect or generalized, felt as a sense of *social* obligation that is not person-specific. This circumstance suggests that when engaging in serial reciprocity, donors are enjoying an autonomous, "duty-free" role that is unavailable to them otherwise.

Moving from gift to exchange alters momentum by creating reciprocal trading. While the forms of social exchange—its rules and rituals—are predictable, its substance is not (Schwartz, 1967). An important attribute of the norm of reciprocity is that its requirements can change significantly from situation to situation (Gouldner, 1960). Indeed, according to Simmel's (1950) concept of "sociability" or Goffman's (1961) "rule of irrelevance," the content of a social interaction should be unimportant and have no consequence for future interaction beyond the merely symbolic. In common parlance, "it is the thought that counts." Irrelevance is an inexorable producer of slack resources, because it immeasurably broadens the range of acceptability of a grant or gift. When it doesn't matter what one gives, only that it is given, and when the meaning or value of the gift can usually be discovered only retrospectively anyway (as is the case with communicative grants), then social indebtedness arises from the acts of giving and receiving themselves. Not only will paying too much attention to the content of a grant put a strain on the social bonds it represents (Schwartz, 1967), but it can be an after-the-fact signal that the bonds have already been broken. For example:

> When life in the group runs smoothly, the obligations binding members are not explicitly recognized. . . . It is only when the relationship breaks down that the underlying obligations are brought to light. While Alec and Frank were friends I

> never heard either one of them discuss the services he was performing for the other, but when they had a falling out. . . each man complained to Doc that the other was not acting as he should in view of the services that had been done for him. (William F. Whyte, *Street Corner Society*, quoted in Gouldner, 1960, p. 176.)

IN-DEPTH INTERVIEWS ON ONE-WAY TRANSFERS

Our approach to data collection about the conditions, expressions, and outcomes of one-way transfers was to follow Weick's (1981) suggestion to build a case by "affirmation rather than falsification" (pp. 24-25), linking theory to common sense as a reminder of what we "know but forget" when we subscribe too thoroughly to a single paradigm (Weick, 1981, pp. 33-34). Rather than taking a critical perspective, these were interviews of appreciation (Vickers, 1965). Brockreide (1974) argues that appreciation risks failing as critical research because it avoids reporting its reason for its like or dislike. We make this research trade-off (Weick, 1979) for the possibility of surfacing new understandings of communication exchanges between people. A set of informal pilot interviews completed while constructing the conceptual section of this chapter showed us that the economic exchange model did not account for all reports of resource interchanges in organizations. Because Boulding (1973) acknowledges that gifts may be a small but important part of resource exchange, we were less interested in the frequency of gifts than in their impact when they did occur, even if in isolated circumstances. To increase the likelihood of interviewees having an integrative rather than competitive perspective toward gifts, we selected individuals in late adulthood who had held positions of leadership in their careers and who would be more able to reflect "on one's life and its meaning" (Schott, 1986, p. 661). Interviewees were retirees selected from a chapter of the Service Corps of Retired Executives (SCORE) and from an Austin, Texas church.

The method was to begin the interviews by clarifying what we meant by one-way transfers and then to seek out sensitizing examples (Bacharach & Lawler, 1980) through in-depth questions. Snow, Zurcher, and Sjoberg (1982) call this "interview by comment" and suggest that this strategy is particularly applicable for surfacing a respondent's meaning for a term or topic. Our goal was to strike a balance between focusing the interviews on the topic of giving and allowing enough freedom to assure the interviewees' comments and interpretations were their own. The interviewers used follow-up probes to elicit specific examples and summarizing techniques to control for dross (Webb, Campbell, Schwartz, & Sechrest, 1966). The interviews ranged in length from 30 minutes to an hour and 15 minutes, with an average length of approximately 45 minutes. The tape recorded interviews were transcribed to manuscript for theme analysis.

The data are presented in narrative form (Anderson, 1987) to take advantage of the relation between life story and giving communication gifts. Of the 15 interviews completed, we have selected four to showcase because they provide interesting examples (Davis, 1971) and yet represent the content of the other 11 interviews. Names have been changed. The interview narratives are a mix of researcher interpretations and direct quotes.

To take advantage of the opportunity to discover theory as well as verify theory in case studies (Glaser, 1978; Glaser & Strauss, 1967), we generated a chart of 48 sentence statements from the literature review to sharpen the comparison to the cases (seen in Table 11.2). The points in the cases where the theory section is affirmed are identified by a parenthetical number that corresponds with the number of the statement in Table 11.2. After each case has been described from the interview data, it will be analyzed in comparison to the items in Table 11.2 to show the places where theory has been verified and where new findings have been discovered. In the conclusion we will compare verified and discovered findings from the cases.

The Commodities Broker

This interview began with a quick bridge of commonality. One of the authors had played high-school basketball against the team from this man's hometown (20 years before and 400 miles away from where the interview took place), when the interviewee's team had a player who was a fondly remembered regional star. This moment of familiarity and recognition meant this interview would be a charged exchange and would require a guidance system to give it direction rather than a means to get it off the ground.

Early stereotypical cues in this interview made the interviewer doubt that this man would have many examples of gifts. He was bald-headed and cigar-chomping, and one of his first examples of his early career successes was the business opportunities he had pursued when buying farm land from dust-bowl refugees in the 1930s for a few cents on the dollar in order to acquire the oil leases on their windblown farms. The image of the interviewee arriving to purchase a farmer's land as the farmer loaded his family onto the truck to head West did not establish a foundation for discovering one way-transfers in loosely coupled systems. But as the interview progressed, the man moved very quickly to his example of when he had helped another person, in fact an entire population of people. Following is the first half-page of transcript from his interview:

ER: What I'm looking for is personal experiences of businessmen who had times in their career where there wasn't a direct connection, but someone who helped them out and gave them some kind of unrepayable gift. A benefactor who helped you out or gave you information, helped you through.

EE: Subject to where they were not to benefit themselves? Well, I can think of a lot of them where . . . there would be *some* ulterior motive on the part of those who

TABLE 11.2

Dimensions of One-Way Transfers in Loosely-Coupled Systems
(1) Exchange is a given in social interaction.
(2) Two-way transfers account for a signficant part of social interaction.
(3) Participants in exchange seek to maximize benefits in relation to costs.
(4) The social transaction often defines the material one.
(5) When the commodity is a message, it is difficult to distinguish between economic and social exchange.
(6) Information (expertise or secrets) is worth money.
(7) Motivations in one-way transfers involve more than altruism or benevolence.
(8) The gift has potential to be simultaneously attractive and suspect.
(9) Most gifts are mixes of goodwill and threat.
(10) A spiritual gift is autonomous; when the same effort is exchanged, its substance is lost.
(11) The capitalist is a person whose instinct is to remove property from circulation.
(12) Gifts occur under conditions of abundance and ambiguity.
(13) Gifts operate according to a logic broader than efficiency.
(14) LCS have abundant resources—time, personnel, finances, and decision discretion.
(15) LCS are uncertain as to means-ends connections, the flow of influence and coordination processes.
(16) In LCS, interactions between subsystems do not occur in predictable, stimulus-response ways.
(17) Possessing resources without control and monitoring mechanisms increases one-way transfers.
(18) A gift is a thing we cannot acquire through our own efforts.
(19) Organizations are a collection of choices looking for problems.
(20) Communication gifts are abundant and constant.
(21) Communication gifts are ephemeral.
(22) Communication gifts are intangible.
(23) Communication gifts are reusable and replenishable.
(24) Communication gifts are inherently value free.
(25) Communication gifts are time bound.
(26) In garbage-can situations, the convergence of the donor, recipient, need, and resource are unpredictable.
(27) Value of gifts is uncertain when feedback loops are long and tenuous.
(28) People remember gifts for a long time.
(29) If one expects (and receives) an immediate return for his or her effort, the event more closely fits the definition of economic exchange.
(30) As long as the recipient is in the donor's debt, he or she is more likely to behave in a peaceful and loyal fashion.
(31) One-way transfers operate independent of direct, immediate feedback.
(32) When the donor has a replenishable supply of a resource, the applicability of the cost-benefits ratio is altered.
(33) If the benefit ratio of a grant is high, the donor is more likely to give resources.
(34) Information, linkages, and emotional support can be distributed to unlimited numbers of individuals.
(35) High level positions in organizations provide members with abundant resources.
(36) Grants are an important part of the political economy—the way roles are created and things get done.
(37) Control over the shape and form of a gift increases the potential for creativity.

(continued)

Table 11.1 Continued

(38) One-way transfers involve less obligation than do exchanges with clear definitions of expectations.
(39) A key component of the willingness to give a gift is the giver's perception that the assistance is not expected or demanded.
(40) One-way transfers reflect an inner normative stance or sense of commitment on the part of the donor.
(41) Gifts create social solidarity.
(42) The inertia created by giving keeps society evolving.
(43) The requirement for rough, rather than exact, equivalency generates uncertainty as to who is in debt to whom.
(44) Immediately returning a gift is a way of maintaining independence.
(45) Serial and generalized reciprocity transforms repayment from individual obligation to community activity.
(46) The *first* gift is powerful for momentum.
(47) Moving from gift to exchange alters momentum.
(48) Too much attention to the content of a gift signals that social bonds may already be broken.

went out of their way to give them some help alright (1, 2), *but* they also derived benefit from it when it did work. I don't know if that's what you. . . .

ER: How long did it take for the benefit to come in?

EE: Oh, in a couple of years (27, 29).

ER: Was there any guarantee on their part?

EE: No. Well it was kind of like a risk *venture*? (22, 24) Well, I'll just give you kind of a thumbnail picture. This was an endeavor I embarked on in 1939 (28). It was a wholesale shipping, marketing service. We started with three products, but shortly we reduced it to *one*. With the object of being the biggest and the best that there was. This was the marketing of watermelons for farm organizations in three states. Some of 'em were co-ops in a pure sense, some were just an association, a few guys would get together and set up a program.

The farm commodities marketing operator went on with great animation to tell his story of how he traveled to four large metropolitan areas, talking to dealers and learning their complaints about the *ills* of the product when they received it, and then how he went back to the growers and gave them instruction on how to produce watermelons that matched the preferences expressed by the wholesale purchasers (6, 34). Because watermelons were so heavy to ship, even by rail, the cost of spoiled or wasted product reduced the amount paid to the grower. The goal was to ship uniform fruit that eliminated the cost of waste at the receiving end. The broker reported that the growers increased their payoff by four to one over their previous experience with selling watermelons. The buyers provided the information on product requirements, the grower produced the product, and the interviewee

> started and operated the whole program from A to Z, and took a percentage or a service charge (33), set up a cash operation based on all the markets in the nation, not all of 'em—all the *big*, about 24 in all (32).

In this role, his self-perception of a gift was an act that is often derided and hated—the middleman, the broker (Sowell, 1980). But his gift to everyone was information (6): to the buyers—"I know farmers who will deliver watermelons to you that are uniform, and high quality"; to the farmers—information on how to change their practices:

> The old way of doing it was: just go out in the field and gather what you got, and throw it in the car, and send it off. We had to start with the land it was grown on. And we set up an educational program, to *indoctrinate* all the growers and the farmers, so that everybody does everything he does in exactly the same way for the same purpose, so these dealers, receivers on the other end, were very helpful in providing the necessary information that we might go back and know what to do, or figure out what to do (36). Never before had there been a common variety where a dealer up in Detroit would order ten car loads of watermelons—and get the same product. I've often said to many people, I wouldn't have taken the risk now knowing what I know, but I was just too dumb to know any better (26, 31, 36).

In the single opportunity of talking to the interviewee, it was impossible to determine how much of a milestone this project was to him, but the story rang true as a major life experience.

> EE: I came back and was running my dad's old country department store—and I was about six blocks on the west side of town—and between my house and town, up the street there was what was called "Chisler's row." That's where the peddlers all gathered in and the farmers would bring their stuff and sit along there on the side of the street, an empty block there, trees, and that's where the trading went on. And these old boys who came in from Kansas, Nebraska, sometimes Iowa, Colorado, Denver. They'd come in there and sit all day and they'd get their heads together and they'd say: "now we don't buy anything until sundown, you see they gotta go home then, and they've got to get rid of it and we'll get it cheap."
>
> So I'd go by everyday, three or four times a day, and especially at night, and I'd be walking by, and I'd see them sell those watermelons for two cents a piece or three cents a piece, sometimes give them away, cause they had to get home—[the interviewee is emotional and speaks a word unintelligibly] their trucks and chores. And this bothered me; there ought to be a better way to do that [sigh, holding back tears]— than that and if we could find a better way we could create a *cash* market for a product that we could grow without end there (4, 7, 15, 19, 20, 25, 34, 39).

This narrative exemplifies the costs of moving from a value-based to a commodity-based culture, from the South American peasant example that began this chapter. But instead of paying costs to the devil like the peasants, the watermelon farmers in dust-blown Oklahoma reaped the benefits of having a commodities broker or exchange agent to transform the value of their product by moving it to another location. Rather than having a just price, based on objective costs incurred by the producer as Marxist use-value might hold, "a given physical object has a value that varies greatly according to the location of that object in time and space, and according to the risks associated with it" (Sowell, 1980, p. 67). The middleman changes the location of things in space and time, and as a result is changing the value of things by relocating them (34).

The final theoretical tie within this narrative is the connection to efficient gifts mentioned by Boulding (1973). People make one-way transfers when it is not costly for them to do so. The broker describes the ease with which he transformed the lives of the farmers he helped. The payoffs for him were high. He created win-win opportunities for himself and others. Given his position in the general store in his community (35), he had central information to perceive what was possible and the economic slack to create a solution that few others would have had the chance to give.

The Reluctant Lawyer

As in the first interview reported, the lawyer's initial contribution did not suggest he had examples of one-way transfers. "In the law business, time is about all you can give" (1, 2). Because a lawyer is a wage earner and an hourly worker, and his time is his "inventory," it is not surprising that he had some caution about identifying an ideology of benevolence as his own.

> ER: My purpose is to look at the kinds of experiences you might have had where somebody gave something to someone else without wanting anything in return. This may be a means of support, information, or a connection. Can you think of some experiences you might have had?
>
> EE: In business you usually don't find people giving anything. There is an old cliche in the legal business: The advice you get is what you pay for. Its worth what you pay for it. If you get it for nothing you don't get anything (1, 2).
>
> In most instances, no one is willing to give you anything. Through hard work you develop the facts of a case you want to present to the court. You document that so that it's not a question of anyone giving you anything. It's: "judge, here it is."

But as he progressed in the interview he began to qualify his beginning "you don't find people giving anything" stance. First, he made a claim for protecting one's own and one's favored. When people in your organization have a problem "you are going to help them out in any way that you can. You will support them in any way that you can. How far that goes depends on the circumstances and the persons involved (34)." This claim suggests selective giving to those in close proximity and special attention to the favored. He also identified instances of giving to those who were beginning in business.

EE: I have helped a lot of people. People starting out in business that really couldn't afford the work. I encouraged them in development until they reached a time when they could afford services (43). Some became my best clients (7). Some go somewhere else as soon as they can afford to go somewhere else. Fifty percent of it will go bad on you as far as time, effort, and goodwill (17). The other half will pay off.

While he seemed acutely conscious of the possible long-term payoff rather than immediate return (27, 29), he was equally conscious of Boulding's (1973) ratio of "efficient gifts." For him the efficiency threshold is 50/50; which seems generous for a person whose time is money (33). In addition to efficient gifts, the lawyer helped people in dire straits. He reported about a client in trouble with the Internal Revenue Service for not paying taxes over a five-year period. He no longer had a business or a job; his wife's job was their sole source of income. They did not own a home or car, because the government would claim it. The government had levied the wife's income, and there was, therefore, no money to pay an attorney with.

EE: I've tried to help them. I've made arrangements for installment payments. The government has agreed to remove the levy from the salary on the basis that perhaps the wife could get a raise. As a result, a friend of theirs who is also in tax trouble wants to come in today. I have to draw the line somewhere. I can't stand unlimited hours of helping those who got themselves in a jam because they didn't recognize their own responsibilities in paying their taxes. There was an attorney here in town, down on his luck and became an alcoholic. I used to handle all his tax work for him and not charge him a thing. I still help his wife.

The lawyer's interview is important because it establishes a context for giving in a help-giving profession. He espouses little gift ideology; he makes no claims for the goodness of humans or the likelihood of norms for giving. Yet his behavior shows him to help people in emergencies and to risk being asked for more help from even more distant strangers as a result. This example points to the importance of considering the help-giving professions as special categories of one-way transfers. Therapists, doctors, lawyers, and accountants, because their principal product is assistance or support, may paradoxically have less orientation toward models of one-way transfers than this research method would identify. Because the people with whom they are in contact are seeking help, they have little chance to behave voluntarily, a key dimension in the theory of one-way transfers developed in this chapter (38).

EE: You don't have time anymore. My biggest criticism of society today is people don't have time for family, friends, etc. Keep your head down and stay on the job. If you have to do it, you expect everyone else to do it too. If you expect everyone else to do it, you're not speaking in terms of giving them anything.

The lawyer ends with a statement of tight, not loose, coupling. The person is restricted by his time and expects that others are similarly.

The Mail Train to Texarkana

Buddy reviewed his career, beginning as an undercover agent for the Texas Liquor Control Board before the sale of alcohol was legal in Texas. During his seven years with the Board, he moved from undercover work into management. With the onset of World War II, he entered the Navy. After the war, Buddy took a job as a postal railway clerk and worked his way up to Chief Officer in the Dallas Service Branch. He had many compelling images of gifts over his career, but the strongest one came from a description of the mail train to Texarkana, Texas.

During Buddy's tenure as a postal railway clerk, he worked on a four- to six-man crew sorting third-class mail according to destination (including packages and newspapers) during the 14-hour train trip between San Antonio and Texarkana, Texas. During the interview, he described a demerit system for "misthrowing" the mail. Certain employees were responsible for "checking" clerks and reporting sorting errors. The possible negative effects of this type of watchdog relationship were transformed into a positive sense of community by the manner in which the negative reports were handled.

> EE: But your reporting employee, like at the end of the run, you would meet each other. Like you would meet in Texarkana, and this group, they were checking me, is what they called it. We would talk there in the hotel, and they would sit down and explain to me what I was doing wrong. And then we would do the same thing ourselves. Now that's a very minor deal, but it was a total "giving" thing (41).

In their section on conflict in organizations, March and Simon (1958) build on interdependence and the timing of acts as a central issue in the negotiation of differences in organizations. When subunits (like crews) overlap in responsibility and manage a shift change from one group to the next, the likelihood for conflict is increased. These conditions are familiar in organizational conflict: "The last shift did not fill out the paperwork properly, which accounts for the administrative errors that are causing problems organization-wide." Or, in another firm, "They did not clean the vat after their last batch, which explains why large amounts of the product are tainted." And in a final familiar example, "They are leaving the back door unlocked, which accounts for the theft and loss rate of missing goods." Conflicts with this structure are not easy to resolve, because once they are passed from one shift to the next, the norm is set for acting in the same way toward the next shift. Because no shift wants to be taken advantage of, no one is willing to resolve the problem and pass on to the next shift careful paperwork, clean vats, and secure doors. Buddy's example shows in a simple way how the gift of helping the next crew set a tone for the workplace that transcended the normal structure of the conflict. According to Buddy, one-way transfers or support gifts were a norm among the postal railway workers during his employment.

> EE: And for instance, the clerk in charge on railway mail was not required at any time to [help] if I was having difficulty in completing my workload. I mean they would be caught up with their work (14) and come up and help me, or anyone else that was having difficulty. And we in turn, who had no responsibility to the letter carriers, [would help] if they were running behind with their registered mail (42), and letters hadn't been distributed before we would be reaching the next town. [The work group was] a family. [We were always] helping one another (36, 45).

One can interpret the extra time on the train as slack time, which created conditions for the gift (12). This giving is outstanding when one considers the stereotype of seniority in uncomplicated settings: wasting time while goading the overworked newcomer (42). Louis's (1980) prescription for socializing newcomers is a match for this case. Rather than testing them in a sink-or-swim environment as an initiation rite, she suggests helping them out.

Over the years of his career, Buddy had the opportunity to extend the "family" feeling directly in specific one-way transfers of support and advice.

> EE: I had a case where a person was drinking too much, and having problems, and I talked to him several times. . . . And the amazing thing about that, a couple of years later (28), I'd been long gone, and I got a letter from him thanking me for working with him and the advice that I had given him (5, 34).
>
> He was a young man. He said that if it hadn't been for talking to me, that he didn't know [what would have happened to him]. Well, that makes you feel real good (7).

The correction of errors on the mail train set up a theme that ran through Buddy's examples of gifts over his career. His examples focused on developing trustworthy relationships that included a component of correction or handling "bad news." And in addition, he knew he would be listened to:

> EE: There's such things as listening and not hearing, but there's also people who listen and then consider. I might have been wrong about what I was talking about, but it was considered. And in the relationships I had, after they'd considered, and they thought I was wrong, they'd come back and say "Look, this is really just not going to work."

Buddy's interview was a study in serial transfers in which at times he was the recipient of gifts from others and at subsequent times he was the donor. In all the cases, he described the effects of the gifts as norm-setting actions in his personal organizational history. The gifts tended to focus on a type of communication that acknowledges errors, accepts when a plan or design is not working (6), and assumes that people get out of relationships what they put into them. Buddy's early experience set a tone for how he was to interact over a series of decades.

One of the planning tenets for loosely coupled systems is the importance of personnel selection. Because there are so few control devices, having people who match with system conditions becomes imperative (Weick, 1987). Under conditions of slack and ambiguity, people who persist (Glassman, 1973) with a set of norms or beliefs are more likely to achieve Buchanan's Samaritan's outcome (1975). Buddy reported experiences that can be coded as a norm for one-way transfers. Yet his view remained balanced. Buddy closed his interview by responding to the interviewer query about whether "you never get something for nothing."

> EE: I think that's wrong. Any time that you can get constructive criticism—now remember, I said 'constructive criticism'—you're getting something for nothing. You're not paying for it.

He then added that there are a number of things that people get for free.

> EE: You get respect for nothing, is one thing. If you are a dedicated employee, conscientious, a loyal employee, you're gonna get recognition. That comes about as a result of your own particular make-up. It might be interpreted that you're giving something to get the respect from that person, but . . .
>
> If yourself is the type person that I'm talking about. I think it helps to like people. But I think people pretty well give what they receive (1).

The Desk Jockey Lightens the Load

Gary had retired after 20 years in the Air Force (first as a pilot and later on in project management) and was a student in an MBA program at the time of his interview. The interviewer's anecdotal experience with Gary gave little evidence of anything other than a utilitarian or Machiavellian approach to life. In one class, he had disposed of Carl Rogers in a sentence: "People aren't inherently good; they're bad. And that's why we need religion to keep us in line."

Because of his familiarity with Gary's outlook, the interviewer was concerned that the interview would produce few examples of altruistic behavior. However, Gary responded quickly and directly to the initial question.

> ER: When you look back over your career, can you think of specific examples where people in your organization have given somebody something altruistically, not expecting an immediate payback for what they've given?

EE: Yes. I think the examples come under the general heading of being a mentor, providing advice and assistance. In my case, I had an example of that where the commander of an organization I was in had to, because of the rating system used in the Air Force at that time, had to select one of nine people.
ER: Promising young fellows.
EE: Promising young fellows—at least that was the description—that were being cultivated for promotional material for the rank of Colonel. And I was fortunate enough to be so identified. I would say that there was no thought that the individuals involved felt they would benefit from that. It was an action taken, in their minds, to maintain the quality of the Air Force management structure. In my case, I was very grateful. (Laughter)
ER: When they were selecting you, did they give you any tips or hints—or did they simply have the nine people lined up and one day they announced that it was you?
EE: The commander used profile folders and chose me. After that, yes, there were a lot of tips. For example—I'll give you a specific—at that stage I had just attempted to grow a mustache. And it was suggested to me that I shave it off to have my picture taken for the promotion folder that would go forward to the promotion board (6, 33).

Gary went on to explain how this exchange had occurred:

EE: Basically he called me in and said, "As you know, you've been sponsored for candidacy, and it will improve your posture with the promotion board if you shave off your mustache."
ER: Straight.
EE: Straight, yeah. And I said, "Thank you very much." (Laughter) And then when I reflected on it—my first reactions, as I said, were kind of frustration and anger—not at him but at the system. I respected him very much. I thought he was trying to give me a good steer (41).

Gary reports that this commander continued to offer insider tips until his retirement.

EE: Incidentally, I've seen him since then, and he's still the same kind of person. There appears to be no other motivation than he wants to help (12). In fact, he's working for a contractor in Dallas, and when I saw him several months ago, he said that if I wanted to call on him, he thought that I might be able to help with some technical writing, I might be able to work it into my program.

Later on in his career, Gary worked with a man who had family problems, particularly with his 15-year-old daughter who was using drugs. The co-worker talked to Gary about the emotional blowups they had. Gary listened, but did not try to counsel him, except to give him sympathy and an opportunity to talk it out (34):

EE: Probably because of the rapport that we had, he came and told me one day that she had run away. At that point, having had kids myself, I was very concerned and could see that he was stressed (7).

At that time, Gary was monitoring research and development projects for the Air Force and was responsible for manpower management and hiring—trying to fill vacant positions (26).

EE: I took over the manpower part of his activity and one part of his R & D projects. Because the research and development organization was a lot looser than the Air Force line organizations, their supervisor supported the shift in responsibilities, as long as everything was covered (14, 26).

The way we left it was, "Doug, we'll keep on doing this as long as necessary," knowing that he would not abuse it (20). The deal was that when he could resume the activities he would come in and say, "I'm ready. I can handle it." He came in, as I recall, and said things are better at home, they've turned the corner, and he thought he could handle everything now (24). So I very happily turned everything back over to him. (Laughter)

ER: Was it a noticeable increase in workload? Did you have to really . . .

EE: No, I can't claim any great sacrifice on my part (38, 12, 14,).

ER: Well, that's a good story.

EE: But the realization was there that he would do the same thing (41, 43).

ER: Yes, I wanted to ask you that. I mean, obviously it was a good deal, but I wonder what it meant to him. Did he ever give any indication later that he . . .

EE: He said that he appreciated it, and nobody ever pressed him that I know of (43, 31). Last time I saw him he indicated that everything was okay at home.

ER: It could have meant a whole lot.

EE: If you're talking altruistic, maybe I don't qualify there (7), because I felt good when he said everything was still all right. Because I felt I'd contributed to that in some small way (13, 32). I felt good. The good feeling, I guess, is the payoff (7). I will say that this guy, Doug, I'd classify him as a good friend. Whereas at the time that this occurred, we were working associates (41). So maybe it wasn't that altruistic after all, because—no, I shouldn't say that. I did not do it to get his friendship. It resulted from that.

Gary contrasted the situation in research and development with his experience as a pilot, pointing out the lack of slack in the line organization.

EE: There was a far greater urgency there. There wasn't much latitude for error or personal feelings. For example, you have what they call lines to fly—you have so many planes to launch—and if you don't launch them, then somebody's got to provide an explanation why. And that's embarrassing. There's more of a production mentality. Maybe I was caught up in it when I was younger, earlier in the Air Force, but I don't remember anything that I would even attempt to qualify as altruistic behavior. It was quite the opposite. It was really kind of murderous (12).

In March and Olsen's (1974) description of garbage-can decision processes, they describe four relatively independent "streams" within an organization: problems, solutions, participants, and choice opportunities (p. 26). Their description of problems is relevant here.

> Problems are the concern of people inside and outside the organization. They arise over issues of lifestyle; family; frustrations of work; careers, group relations within the organization; distribution of status, jobs, and money; ideology; or current crises of mankind as interpreted by the mass media or the nextdoor neighbor. All require attention. Problems are, however, distinct from choices; and they may not be resolved when choices are made.

This case focuses on a problem in the family of an organizational participant. Drug and alcohol use among teenagers worries parents and floods into the workplace. The gift in this case is a combination of oversight (March & Olsen, 1976) and "let it pass" (Garfinkel, 1967) with uncertainty absorption (March & Simon, 1958), which means a leader absorbs or "sits on" information that is relevant and could be damaging legally if surfaced. Because organizational rules for family problems cannot cover all circumstances and would be problematic to administer if they did, these issues are handled outside the rational system and are circumstances of one-way transfers. The bonding they potentially create is a good example of the glue in loosely coupled systems (Weick, 1976) that, rather than being disintegrated, actually hold organizations together.

CONCLUSION

The most compelling themes of the data were the examples of drama and character embedded in the interviews on communication gifts. If organizations are organized around emotional issues (Weick, 1979) and personal dynamics that compete for individual attention (Cohen, March, & Olsen 1972), the search for gifts surface a side of organizational communication traditionally unexposed in our research. The dignity of a recovering teenager supported by the father's workplace, the recovered agricultural production of farmers after a drought (the Oklahoma farm town now claims to be the watermelon capital of the world!), the correct movement of mail on a rumbling train in an organization stereotyped for its bureaucracy, show the dramatic interpretation of relationships and give them an interest and vitality that would not be possible with exchange theory alone. The character development could easily take another turn. Following Boulding's (1973) assumption of one-way transfers (gifts or tributes) in a world equally capable of good and bad, one could design an interview schedule to draw out examples of the one-way system of tributes or times when people were emotionally taxed, badgered, or robbed in nonexchange ways, and produce valid narratives of the workplace.

The cases also showed dramatic narratives of organizations because of the unplanned intersection of people, resources, information, and support that resulted in things getting done. Loose coupling is a theory of dimensions intersected by time—not logic (Weick, 1976). Garbage cans are co-occurring streams of solutions, people, problems, and opportunities. Asking for reports of gifts is asking for times when gift-giving is the opportunity chosen. Opportunity and success makes a good story—especially when preceded by risk and sacrifice.

There are items in Table 11.2 that received insignificant verification. These cases did not verify mixed gifts for which it was hard to determine whether a gift was given (9), possibly because gifts based upon mixed motives are usually delivered with subtlety and finesse. They are like a double bind, which make them more difficult to remember and surface. The listing of dynamic communication qualities (20, 21, 22, 23, 24) may also be too fine-grained in loose systems to be highly visible in interviewee recall; while they were represented, they were not a major or outstanding part of the coding completed on the cases from Table 11.2 and they did not provide much explanation for the cases.

Another discovery theme that had little theoretical stance in the literature on one-way transfers (possibly because it is parental), was the communication of negative information as a gift. Bailey (1971) said that gifts may be poison; a theme of the findings here is that poison may be a gift. "Negative gifts" (poison) refer to messages that are not easy to hear and are corrections that address a personal topic, even those as trivial as shaving off one's mustache. The negative gifts have a not-ness in common that disciplines or directs the recipient to change his or her behavior. The interpretations over time are classically parental, with the person at the time reluctantly accepting the correction and later thanking, often in person, the individual for setting straight a course of action that transformed their lives.

The change from negative to positive interpretation made by these people—from "threat" to "benevolence" (Boulding, 1973) as the underlying thrust of the negative gifts—and the time lapse in which the transformations occurred, are interesting issues in each example. Tracy, Van Dusen, and Robinson (1987) find that "well-given criticism offers the added bonus of making both interactants feel that their relationship is stronger" (p. 46). If a person is constrained by being pulled from in front of a moving car, the appreciation for the rough handling is immediately obvious and the discontent over the action is brief. This response contrasts with constraints or admonitions that take years to be appreciated. This difference raises a number of questions about how the transformation from threat to benevolence takes place: What is the lag time like? How long does it take? What events intervene to change the interpretation? Do negative events change the preceding negative grants into positive ones? Albert Ellis (Ellis & Grieger, 1977) discusses the topic of self-constraint as "long-term hedonism," in which a person suffers or is denied immediate payoffs for future outcomes. This intrapsychic concept could be usefully translated into long-term benevolence when looking at interpersonal rather than self-directed negatives.

Mauss (1967) and Boulding (1973) have both suggested that positive, benevolent gifts or grants are societally integrative, while negative, threatening gifts or grants are societally disintegrative. Our data incline us to believe that it is instead the ambiguous combination of these two—the dynamic tension created by the inevitable mix of benevolence and threat—that is integrative in the final analysis.

REFERENCES

Adler, P. (1981). *Momentum: A theory of social action.* Beverly Hills, CA: Sage.

Arrow, K. J. (1975). Gifts and exchanges. In E. S. Phelps (Ed.), *Altruism, morality and economic theory* (pp. 13-28). New York: Russell Sage.

Ashby, W. R. (1960). *Design for a brain.* London: Chapman & Hall.

Astley, W. G. (1978). *Sources of power in organizational life.* Unpublished doctoral dissertation, University of Washington, Seattle.

Bacharach, S. B., & Lawler, E. J. (1980). *Power and politics in organizations.* San Francisco: Jossey-Bass.

Bailey, F. G. (1971). *Gifts and poison.* New York: Shocken.

Baudrillard, J. (1981). *For a critique of the political economy of the sign* (C. Levin, Trans.). St. Louis, MO: Telos.

Benson, J. K. (1975). The interorganizational network as a political economy. *Administrative Science Quarterly, 20,* 229-250.

Blau, P. M. (1964). *Exchange and power in social life.* New York: John Wiley.

Bohanan, P. (1955). Some principles of exchange and investment among the Tiu. *American Anthropologist, 57,* 60-70.

Bolnick, B. (1975). Toward a behavioral theory of philanthropic activity. In E. S. Phelps (Ed.), *Altruism, morality and economic theory* (pp. 197-223). New York: Russell Sage.

Boulding, K. E. (1973). *The economy of love and fear.* Menlo Park, CA: Wadsworth.

Bourgeois, L. J., III. (1981). On the measurement of organizational slack. *Academy of Management Review, 6,* 29-39.

Brass, D. J. (1981). Structural relationships, job characteristics and worker satisfaction and performance. *Administrative Science Quarterly, 26,* 331-348.

Brockreide, W. (1974). Rhetorical criticism as argument. *Quarterly Journal of Speech, 60,* 165-174.

Brown, N. (1959). *Life against death.* New York: Random House.

Browning, L. D. (1982). The ethics of intervention: A communication consultant's apology. *Journal of Applied Communication Research, 10,* 101-116.

Browning, L. D., & Johnson, B. (1984). Communicating outside the chain: Developing and using personal communities. In J. L. Whitehead (Ed.), *Readings for business and professional communication.* Lexington MA: Ginn.

Buchanan, J. (1975). The Samaritan's dilemma. In E. S. Phelps, (Ed.), *Altruism, morality and economic theory.* New York: Russell Sage.

Burgess R. L., & Huston, T. L. (Eds.). (1979). *Social exchange in developing relationships.* New York: Academic Press.

Chadwick-Jones, J. K. (1976). *Social exchange theory: Its structure and influence in social psychology.* New York: Academic Press.

Cohen, M. D., March, J. G., & Olsen, J. P. (1972). A garbage can model of organizational choice. *Administrative Science Quarterly, 17,* 1-18.
Cohen, M. P., & March, J. G. (1974). *Leadership and ambiguity.* New York: McGraw-Hill.
Cook, S. (1966). The obsolete "anti-market" mentality: A critique of the substantive approach to economic anthropology. *American Anthropologist, 68,* 323-345.
Cyert, R. M., & March, J. G. (1963). *A behavioral theory of the firm.* Englewood Cliffs, NJ: Prentice-Hall.
Davis, J. (1973). Forms and norms: The economy of social relationships. *Man, 8,* 159-176.
Davis, M. S. (1971). That's interesting: Towards a phenomenology of sociology and a sociology of phenomenology. *Philosophy of Social Science, 1,* 309-344.
Deal, T. E., & Kennedy, A. A. (1982). *Corporate cultures: The rites and rituals of corporate life.* Reading, MA: Addison Wesley.
Deutsch, M. (1960). The effect of motivational orientation upon trust and suspicion. *Human Relations, 13,* 123-139.
Ekeh, P. H. (1974). *Social exchange theory: The two traditions.* London: Heinemann.
Ellis, A., & Grieger, R. (Eds.). (1977). *Handbook of rational emotive therapy.* New York: Springer.
Ellsberg, D. (1961). Risk, ambiguity, and the savage axioms. *Quarterly Journal of Economics, 75,* 643-669.
Emerson, R. M. (1962). Power-dependence relations. *American Sociological Review, 27,* 31-40.
Garfinkel, H. (1967). *Studies in ethnomethodology.* Englewood Cliffs, NJ: Prentice-Hall.
Glaser, B. (1978). *Theoretical sensitivity.* Mill Valley, CA: Sociology Press.
Glaser, B., & Strauss, A. (1967). *The discovery of grounded theory: Strategies for qualitative research.* Chicago: Aldine.
Glassman, R. B. (1973). Persistence and loose coupling in living systems. *Behavioral Science, 18,* 83-98.
Glidewell, J. C. (1973). *A social psychology of laboratory training.* Unpublished manuscript, University of Chicago.
Goffman, E. (1961). *Encounters: 2 studies in the sociology of interaction.* Indianapolis: Bobbs-Merrill.
Gouldner, A. W. (1960). The norm of reciprocity: A preliminary statement. *American Sociological Review, 25,* 161-176.
Granovetter, M. S. (1973). The strength of weak ties. *American Journal of Sociology, 78,* 1360-1380.
Hammond, P. (1975). Charity: Altruism or cooperative egoism? In E. S. Phelps (Ed.), *Altruism, morality and economic theory.* (pp. 115-131). New York: Russell Sage.
Hardin, G. (1968). The tragedy of the commons. *Science* (Vol. 162). 1243-1248.
Hedican, E. J. (1986). Some issues in the anthropology of transaction and exchange. *Canadian Review of Sociology and Anthropology, 23,* 97-117.
Hirschman, A. O. (1970). *Exit, voice and loyalty.* Cambridge, MA: Harvard University Press.
Homans, G. C. (1961). *Social behavior: Its elementary forms.* New York: Harcourt, Brace & World.
Hyde, L. (1983). *The gift: Imagination and the erotic life of property.* New York: Random House.
Johnson, W. A. (1978). *Muddling toward frugality.* San Francisco: Sierra Club.
Kadushin, C. (Undated). *On the problem of formalizing emergent networks among innovators in education.* Unpublished manuscript, Columbia University, New York.
Kau, J. B., & Rubin, P. H. (1979). Self-interest, ideology, and logrolling in Congressional voting. *Journal of Law and Economics, 22,* 355-385.
Kaun, D. E. (1984). The economists' theory of ideology: Competing views. *Economic and Industrial Democracy, 5,* 29-50.
Koontz, H., & O'Donnell, C. (1964). *Principles of management: An analysis of managerial functions* (3rd ed.). New York: McGraw-Hill.

Korn, R., & McCorkle, L. (1954). Resocialization within walls. *Annals of the American Academy of Political and Social Science, CCXCIII*, 90-107.
Krebs, P. L. (1970). Altruism: An examination of the concept and a review of the literature. *Pychological Bulletin, 73*, 258-302.
Latane, B., & Darley, J. (1970). *The unresponsive bystander: Why doesn't he help?* New York: Appleton-Century-Crofts.
Lévi-Strauss, C. (1964). The principle of reciprocity. In L. A. Coser & B. Rosenberg (Eds.), *Sociological theory: A book of readings* (pp. 76-95). New York: Macmillan.
Louis, M. (1980). Surprise and sense making: What new comers experience in entering unfamiliar organizational settings. *Administrative Science Quarterly, 25*, 226-249.
Lynd, H. M. (1958). *On shame and the search for identity*. New York: Harcourt Brace.
MacCrimmon, K. R., & Messick, D. M. (1976). A framework for social motives. *Behavioral Science, 21*, 86-100.
Macneil, I. R., (1986). Exchange revisited: Individual utility and social solidarity. *Ethics, 96*, 567-593.
Malinowski, B. (1922). *Argonauts of the Western Pacific*. New York: Dutton.
March, J. G., & Simon, H. A. (1958). *Organizations*. New York: John Wiley.
March, J. G., & Olsen J. P. (1976). *Ambiguity and choice in organizations*. Bergen, Norway: Universitesforlaget.
Mauss, M. (1967). *The Gift*. New York: Norton.
McWhinney, W. (1973). Phenomenarchy: A suggestion for social redesign. *Journal of Applied Behavioral Science, 9*, 163-180.
Miller, D. J. (1987, May). *From symbol to sign: The process of ideological labor in Jean Baudrillard's "For a critique of the political economy of sign."* Paper presented at the International Communication Association Conference, Montreal, Canada.
Moch, M. K., & Pondy, L. R. (1977). The structure of chaos: Organized anarchy as a response to ambiguity (review of March & Olsen's *Ambiguity and Choice*). *Administrative Science Quarterly, 12*, 296-320.
Morgan, G. (1980). Paradigms, metaphors, and puzzle solving in organization theory. *Administrative Science Quarterly, 25*, 605-622.
Najjar, G. K. (1978). Social systems delimitation and allocative mechanisms: Perspectives on budgeting for development. *Administration and Society, 9*, 495-577.
Ouchi, W. G. (1978). Coupled vs. uncoupled control in organizational hierarchies. *Environments and Organizations*. San Francisco: Jossey-Bass.
Pearce, J. L., & Peters, R. H. (1985). A contradictory norms view of employer-employee exchange. *Journal of Management, 11*, 19-30.
Peters, T. (1987). *Thriving on chaos*. New York: Knopf.
Peters, T., & Waterman, R. (1982). *In search of excellence: Lessons from America's best run companies*. New York: Harper & Row.
Pettigrew, A. (1973). *The politics of organizational decision-making*. London: Tavistock.
Pfeffer, J. (1981). The ambiguity of leadership. *Academy of Management Review, 6*,27-37.
Poe, D. B., Jr. (1977). The giving of gifts: Anthropological data and social psychological theory. *Cornell Journal of Social Relations, 12*, 47-63.
Polanyi, K. (1944). *The great transformation*. New York: Rinehart.
Pondy, L. R., & Mitroff, I. I. (1979). Beyond the open systems models of organizations. *Research in Organizational Behavior, 1*, 3-39.
Prattis, J. I. (1973). Strategising man. *Man, 8*, 46-58.
Ramos, A. G., (1976). Theory of social systems delimitation. *Administration & Society, 8*, 249-272.
Salancik, G. R. (1975). *Notes on loose coupling: Linking intentions to action*. Unpublished manuscript, University of Illinois, Champaign-Urbana.
Salancick, G. R., & Pfeffer, J. (1977). Who gets power and how they hold on to it: A strategic-contingency model of power. *Organizational Dynamics, 5*, 3-21.

Sahlins, M. (1974). *Stone age economics*. London: Tavistock.

Sass, L. A. (1986, May). Anthropology's native problems: Revisionism in the field. *Harpers* (Vol. 273), pp. 49-57.

Schott, R. L. (1986). The psychological development of adults: Implications for public administration. *Public Management Forum*, 657-667.

Schwartz, B. (1967). The social psychology of the gift. *American Journal of Sociology, 73*, 1-11.

Selznick, P. (1957). *Leadership in administration*. Evanston, IL: Row, Peterson.

Simmel, J. (1950). *The sociology of Georg Simmel* (K. H. Wolff, Trans. and Ed.). Glencoe, NY: Free Press.

Slater, P. (1971). *The pursuit of loneliness: American culture at the breaking point*. Boston: Beacon.

Snow, D. A., Zurcher, L. A., & Sjoberg, G. (1982). Interviewing by comment: An adjunct to the direct question. *Qualitative Sociology, 5*, 385-411.

Sowell, T. (1980). *Knowledge and decisions*. New York: Basic Books.

Taussig, M. T. (1980). *The devil and commodity fetishism in South America*. Chapel Hill: University of North Carolina Press.

Taylor, F. W. (1923). *The principles of scientific management*. New York: Harper & Row.

Thompson, J. D. (1967). *Organizations in action*. New York: McGraw-Hill.

Tomkins, C. (1968). *Eric Hoffer: An American odyssey*. New York: Dutton.

Tracy. K., Van Dusen, D., & Robinson, S. (1987). "Good" and "bad" criticism: A descriptive analysis. *Journal of Communication, 37*, 46-59.

Velzen. T. V. (1973). Robinson Crusoe and Friday: Strength and weakness of the big man paradigm. *Man, 8*, 592-612.

Vickers, G. (1965). Appreciation. In *The art of judgment* (pp. 36-74). New York: Basic Books.

Webb, E. J. (1966). In D. T. Campbell, R. D. Schwartz, & L. Sechrest (Eds.), *Unobtrusive measures: Nonreactive research in the social sciences*. Chicago: Rand McNally.

Weick, K. E. (1981, July). *Organizational communication: Toward research agenda*. Paper presented as keynote address at the SCA-ICA Joint-Sponsored Summer Conference on Interpretive Approaches to the Study of Organizational Communication, Alta, Utah.

Weick, K. E. (1980, April). *Loosely coupled system*. Paper presented at the annual convention of the American Educational Research Association, Boston.

Weick, K. E. (1976). Educational organizations as loosely coupled systems. *Administrative Science Quarterly, 21*, 1-21.

Weick, K. E. (1979). *The social psychology of organizing*. Reading MA: Addison Wesley.

Weick, K. E. (1987). *Notes on loose coupling*. Unpublished paper, University of Michigan, Ann Arbor.

White, L. (1949). *The science of culture: A study of man and civilization*. New York: Farrar, Straus.

Whyte, W. F. (1964). *Street corner society*. Chicago: University of Chicago Press.

Yates, J. F., & Zukowski, L. G. (1976). Characterization of ambiguity in decision making. *Behavioral Science, 21*, 19-25.

Social Indicators of One-Way Transfers in Organizations

KENNETH E. BOULDING
University of Colorado

BROWNING and Henderson's chapter is an important contribution not only to grants economics but also to the general study of one-way transfers. It also makes an important contribution to the theory of loosely coupled systems, a phenomenon of great importance in social and organizational life, but very much neglected by the social scientists and especially by economists. The chapter also contains an excellent survey of a burgeoning literature that is seldom brought together by social scientists. The anecdotal reports on surveys at the end, while very interesting, cannot claim to be more than a hint at what should be an important but much neglected empirical field. Social indicators in the area of one-way transfers on a mass scale are virtually nonexistent. Our ignorance in this field is a serious handicap and may be very costly. We do not really understand why some societies, like Lebanon, Northern Ireland, Mozambique, Haiti, Madagascar, and so on—the list is a long one—fall into internal violence and disintegration, while other societies that may be just as heterogeneous seem to hold together and prosper. The study of communication is an important clue to this problem and the extent to which a society is loosely or tightly coupled, especially in its component parts, may be a very important clue as to why societies do, or do not, fall apart.

What seems to be emerging here is an important part of a general theory of integrative systems. I have argued that there are three major interactive systems in society that provide sources of power: One is the threat system. Another is the system of production and exchange, which is mainly the economic system. The third is the integrative system, which deals with such

Correspondence and requests for reprints: Kenneth E. Boulding, Campus Box 484, University of Colorado, Boulder, CO 80309.

Communication Yearbook 12, 670-674

matters as respect, legitimacy, community, friendship, affection, love, and of course their opposites, across a broad scale of human relationships and interactions. I have argued, indeed, that in the long run the integrative system is the most dominant of the three systems. Thus without some form of legitimacy, threat is very ineffective—compare the mugger with the tax collector—and without legitimacy and some sort of community acceptance, exchange is extremely difficult. And complex communities are impossible without trust and a widespread sense of "belongingness."

The dynamics of the integrative system, however, are extremely complex and, at times, very puzzling. The three systems rarely, if ever, exist in a pure form. There is nearly always some mixture of threats, production or exchange, and integrative relationships, although in different aspects of society these have very different proportions. On the whole, political and especially military structures tend to specialize in threat, although this has to be legitimated and has to be financed to be successful. Economic structures rest mainly on production and exchange, though there is an underlying threat system in property rights and regulation and there has to be an integrative aspect in trust and respect and even courtesy. Institutions like the family, the church, and the club, have a strong integrative component, although these too are not immune to threat and, again, have to be financed.

I became interested in grants economics and was instrumental, along with Janos Horvath and Martin Pfaff, in forming the Association for the Study of the Grants Economy (1967), feeling that one-way transfers of economic goods had been much neglected by economists and were a very important component of all economic systems. This concern came in part out of a search for some kind of measure of integrative structures, and it occurred to me that a grants matrix, that is, who gives what to whom, would be, at least, some kind of indicator as to where integrative structures lie. It soon occurred to me, however, that there were two sources of grants. One could be described as "love," at least in some degree, and the other as "fear" (which is mainly why I pay my income tax), so that the grants matrix is a very imperfect measure of the integrative system, although it is highly relevant to it.

Browning and Henderson now go beyond the grants economy, which deals mainly with commodities, and expand the grants concept to information and communication. The difference between grants of goods and grants of information is very significant. We can see this difference if we look at a transaction from an accounting point of view. An economic grant represents a transfer of net worth, whereas an exchange is merely a rearrangement of assets among owners. When I buy a car, the car dealer has one less car on his balance sheet, I have one more car on mine, he has $10,000 or so more on the money sector of his balance sheet, I have $10,000 less if I paid cash. If I buy the car with a loan, the situation is even more complex. My cash may not go down so much, but my debts go up. It is a convention of cost accounting that exchange is always of equal values. This convention raises an interesting question, incidentally, as to where profits come from. From a cost accounting point of view, exchange is just a rearrangement of assets among owners. There is no immediate change in anybody's net worth until some kind of revaluation takes place, which is where profits come from. If I am a car producer and produce a car at a cost of, say, $8,000, it means that in producing the car I have diminished my other assets of cash, depreciation of machinery, the using up of raw materials, and so on, to the tune of $8,000 and I now have a car that cost accountants value at $8,000. If then I sell it for $10,000, of course, my net worth goes up $2,000, which is profit, and the total value of all assets, including mine, has risen.

If in an economic transaction, however, I give somebody $10,000 cash or a car worth $10,000 and what I get is a nice smile, on which the accountant does not put a value, my net worth goes down by $10,000 and the recipient's net worth goes up by $10,000. This is where "scarcity" comes in, as Browning and Henderson note. Economists, indeed, are rather obsessed by scarcity, because we deal with goods and things, not for the most part with information. When information is transferred, however, from A to B, B gets it and A doesn't lose it. Information has this extraordinary capacity of being cloned. This notion, of course, goes right back to DNA and the origins of life.

When a cell divides, the genetic information that was previously only in one cell is now in two. When an egg is fertilized and a child is born, the parents still have the genetic information in their bodies that the child has, though the child has a different combination, having gotten roughly half of its genes from each parent. When I tell somebody a story, the person I tell it to now knows it, and I still know it. This telling is what has been called the "memes" of society, and the parallel with genes is quite strong. It is quite right, therefore, to say that information itself is not scarce and is not a limiting factor, because of its capacity for self-reproduction.

What is scarce is the communicative act. If 30% of human beings are illiterate, it is not because reading and writing are scarce, but because teachers are scarce. When I teach a good class, I do not lose the knowledge that the class learns. In fact, it is a rare class in which I do not add something to my own knowledge in the very act of trying to teach it. It is a good question, therefore, to ask: Why I am paid for teaching? The answer, I think, is that the communication process requires effort, energy, and time, which are scarce. Much as I love teaching—and I do a certain amount of it for free—I would probably not teach full-time or even half-time unless I was paid. The same goes for the man who likes to fish on weekends. He would not become a full-time fisherman unless he was paid. This is the good old principle of increasing marginal disutility, of any particular form of using time, with an increase in the proportion of time so used. Scarcity in economics arises from the fact that each of us has only 24 hours a day to spend. There is no possible way of making this 25. Economics, therefore, does raise its ugly head even in the expansive field of information and communication.

Economists have been surprisingly slow to recognize that something like a learning process is the key not only to biological evolution, but also to economic development. Mutation and selection are essentially a learning process by which the genes "increase in their skill," from the earliest viruses up to humans. Economic development, likewise, is primarily a learning process, as Adam Smith recognized very clearly, by which not only skills are acquired through the division of labor but also the "know-what" that is developed by science in scholarly activity and is translated into know-how that produces chemicals, electricity, and hybrid corn. Economic development is primarily an increase in human productivity per hour, achieved by learning, which in turn is achieved by communication and the "cloning" of know-what and know-how.

The role of loosely versus tightly coupled social structures in the learning process is a very interesting problem that has not received the attention that it deserves. A society in which the learning process is very tightly coupled and organized is not going to change very much. Paleolithic human culture was a good example; it remained virtually unchanged as far as we can judge from the meager records, with each generation reproducing the knowledge and skills of the parents for an extraordinary number of generations, in spite of the fact that genetically paleolithic humans were much the same as we are. This reproduction without expansion may have been a result of their societies being very small and tightly coupled in the family and the kin group, along with a short expectation of individual life, so that there really was no time to expand human knowledge. All the resources of scarce communication had to be used to reproduce the knowledge of the parents in the minds of the children, with nothing left over for innovation. It was only with the coming of agriculture, indeed, that we seem to have started a cumulative learning process. With the development of larger societies and storable food it was possible to have specialized teachers, sages, and even inventors.

Even among quite complex societies, however, there is a difference between those which are open to change and those which are not. Islam, from about 1300 AD on, is an example of a society too well-organized; China may have been similar, so that science was not able to originate in it as an independent subculture, but in more disorganized Europe, with the separation of church and state between the pope and the king or emperor, and a great variety of small states, science was able to develop as a mutation and then survive as a culture.

One of the things that is apt to be overlooked by organization theorists with tidy minds is the tremendous importance of redundancy in the evolutionary process, whether it be in biology or in social systems. I have sometimes called this the "squirrel's law," for squirrels are a very good example of it. They seem to spend most of their time fooling around and having fun. An efficient species that spends all its time gathering food and propagating will expand to the outer limits of its niche without much flexibility. Then when conditions change it will be wiped out. In evolution, the race is to the adaptable, not to the well adapted, in the long run. I am pretty sure that there are relationships—pretty hard to specify—between adaptability and loose coupling. The enormous evolutionary impact of the invention of sex, for instance, introduced the potentiality for enormous change. While an amoeba can reproduce only itself, except under very rare circumstances, sexual species can produce an enormous variety of individuals because of the loose coupling of the sexes, although it is also quite easy for sexual selection to lead to extinction.

A very interesting question is the relation of loose coupling to vulnerability. A very tightly coupled organization is likely to corrupt the information that goes to the top of the hierarchy, as each level of the hierarchy passes on only the information it thinks will please its superiors. President Johnson, for instance, was carefully shielded by his staff from accurate knowledge of what was going on in Vietnam. Only the good news got through. A loosely coupled structure, however, with a lot of informal relationships—chit-chat on the golf course and that sort of thing—is less likely to have this kind of corruption of information and, hence, is more likely to be adaptable and to survive. Obviously there are limits to this process. Most of us have known organizations that have been so loosely coupled that they simply fell apart. There is clearly some optimum degree of looseness or tightness in the organizational structure. Just where this optimum is, is often very hard to judge. What is very clear is that a passion for efficiency may be very dangerous. Mutations tend to appear in the cracks of the system and in the eddies and are often eliminated in the mainstream.

Browning and Henderson are to be congratulated for opening up a very interesting line of thought. It is to be hoped that this will penetrate the more conventional social sciences, each of which tends to be trapped in a spurious search for efficiency, and this tends to lead up a number of elegant blind alleys. A little craziness does nobody and no organization any harm.

One-Way Transfers and Organizational Cohesion

KARL E. WEICK
J. DOUGLAS ORTON
University of Michigan

All contacts among men rest on schema of giving and returning the equivalent.

—Georg Simmel (1950, p. 387)

The argument that an understanding of grants, gifts, kindness, support, and altruism—all themes of "eros"—should be developed just as fully in organizational theory as are themes of "logos" is a distinct contribution of the Browning and Henderson chapter. Their effort to uncover "kinder" organizations is not just a sentimental exercise, but is a closer look at some possible affective and communicative consequences of newer characterizations of organizational form. Organizational forms that cohere despite their anarchic qualities, programmed actions, excess resources, ambiguity, proclivity toward redesign, high turnover, and unshared goals, are both a puzzle and an everyday occurrence. The puzzle is not solved by appealing to formalization, mechanistic procedures, routinization, plans, or goals, as sources of coherence, because these are altered and redefined by the informal organization. More binding sources of cohesion must be sought in more basic human and social tendencies. Browning and Henderson suggest that communication grants and gratitude for their unsolicited transfer are where we should start to look for the mechanisms by which an anarchy remains organized.

In studying this proposal, we discovered just how pervasive reciprocity is in organizations, how difficult it is to make gifts and grants when reciprocity is pervasive, how important ambiguity, action generation, and central exchanges may be as additional prods to one-way transfers and how relatively unimportant the concept of a loosely coupled system is to the basic argument. In the following, we describe the reasoning by which we arrived at each of these conclusions.

Correspondence and requests for reprints: Karl E. Weick, University of Michigan, Ann Arbor, MI 48109.

Communication Yearbook 12, 675-687

ONE-WAY TRANSFERS AND RECIPROCITY NORMS

One-way transfers occur as figures against the virtually universal ground of exchange, equity, and the norm of reciprocity.

> Both exchange theory and equity theory take it as established that in all societies at all times it is and has been considered right (normative) that people should benefit those who benefit them. Indeed the rule seems universally to take the stronger form: for a benefit received, an *equivalent* benefit ought eventually be returned. (Brown, 1986, p. 47)

Pressure for swift, equivalent return should be especially high in organizations in which trust (definable in this context as the length of time over which nonequivalence can be tolerated) is rare and the relationships are time-limited, nondisclosing, and circumscribed, all of which encourage explicit, completed exchanges rather than implicit, dangling obligations.

Although Browning and Henderson try to convey a world of grants and nonexchange, their assertion and stories betray the reciprocities that lie behind them. It is difficult for them to maintain the figure of one-way transfers against the ground of economic exchanges. For example, we are told that one-way transfers "might profitably be considered different forms of give and take" (p. 639) "that one-way transfers ideally operate independent of direct, immediate exchange of feedback" (p. 645) (unless they routinely operate independent of exchange they aren't one way), that one-way transfers may be made "in order to appear superior (and thus accrue power)" (p. 647), and that subsystems will make grants "to ensure their resources will be the ones applied to organizational problems" (p. 643) (in return for a grant of resources the subsystem gains influence, power, and uncertainty reduction).

When Browning and Henderson explicitly ask people to tell them about occasions when people received "an unrepayable gift," when "somebody gave something to someone else without wanting anything in return," or when "people in your organization have given somebody something altruistically—not expecting an immediate payback for what they've given," respondents invoke the language of exchange rather than the language of grants. The railway mail clerk says "people pretty well give what they receive" (p. 661), 50% of the people in whom the lawyer invests time, effort, and goodwill repay "by becoming some of my best clients" (p. 658), and the commodity broker whose gift is to create an exchange system also "took a percentage or service charge" (p. 655) from this gift.

The point is that apparent outcroppings of altruism, help, and grants that look like only half an exchange often turn out to be a complete exchange in which help is exchanged for esteem, influence, or approval. The evidence for this lies in the fact that when esteem, influence, and approval are withheld, grants and help often dry up.

So, having seen how hard it is to break free of exchange—and further illustrations will be developed throughout this commentary—and how quickly a one-way transfer can dissolve into a two-way transfer, we conclude that exchange is a more fundamental property of relationships in organizations than we had realized. Furthermore, we begin to sense that it may take an unusual set of conditions to produce one-way transfers. And we find ourselves with growing interest in the question of just what those conditions might be.

ONE-WAY TRANSFERS AS COMPLEX GIFTS

Browning and Henderson's interest in gifting is understandable because of their feeling that gifts increase social solidarity (p. 649) and that gifts create "integrative social indebtedness" (p. 651). It is assumed that when people feel indebted, they behave peacefully and loyally, which promotes solidarity. This plausible scenario runs into difficulty, however, when it is imposed on a background of reciprocity and exchange.

Gifting is often equated with giving but, as we saw earlier, giving per se is an incomplete transaction that invites the more complete transaction of give and take. Simmel (1950) was keenly aware that mere giving is open-ended:

> For, giving is by no means only a simple effect that one individual has upon another: It is precisely what is required of all sociological functions, namely interaction. By either accepting or rejecting the gift, the receiver has a highly specific effect upon the giver. The manner of his acceptance, gratefully or ungratefully, having expected the gift or being surprised by it, being satisfied or dissatisfied, elevated or humiliated—all this keenly acts back upon the giver, although it can, of course, not be expressed in definite concepts and measures. Every act of giving is, thus, an interaction between giver and receiver. (p. 389)

Several complications of gifting are implied in this quotation, at least six of which are relevant to Browning and Henderson: Gifts create a social exchange, the first gift can't be repaid, gratitude mediates gift effects, gifts obligate, gifts demote, and gifts puzzle.

Social Exchange and Gifts

The processes that Browning and Henderson describe sound less like a contrast between exchange and nonexchange and more like a contrast between economic exchange and social exchange. The difference between these two has been described by Brown (1986). An economic exchange is enforceable by law, a matter of calculated costs and benefit; there is an explicit definition of equivalence; and the terms are discussable. In contrast, a social exchange is never enforceable at law; costs and benefits are more difficult to calculate; equivalence is subjective rather than objective; and the terms are not discussable.

The difference between these two forms of exchange becomes apparent when friends find themselves faced with the awkward situation of "splitting the check" at a restaurant.

> To do so is to suggest an unwillingness to take turns, an inability to sustain trust and enter upon real friendship. We have similar feelings even when we do split the check. To insist on *exactly* equal shares is either gauche or a joke: "I owe you twenty dollars *and seven cents*." To return hospitality at once and in almost identical form is again too economic a procedure. Did I have dinner at your house last night with six guests, two wines, and five courses. Very well, you must have six, two, and five with me tonight. It is not done. (Brown, 1986, p. 54)

Social exchange is most likely to replace economic exchange when interaction is face-to-face and when the commodity being offered is difficult to value and equivalence is hard to establish. Communication grants, which are described as ephemeral, intangible, reusable, value-free, time-sensitive, and abundant, clearly do not have the clear valuation found in commodities associated with economic exchange, nor does one feel free to haggle over the terms of such communication grants. Thus the world that is portrayed by Browning and Henderson may be more a world of social exchange than economic exchange, even though both unfold in organizations. Furthermore, communication grants may have their effects in organizations because they are an effective means to turn economic exchanges into social exchanges.

It is possible, however, for gifts to turn a social exchange into an economic exchange. This possibility is described by Homans (1974) in his discussion of "doing favors." He notes that resentment often occurs when a double repayment is exacted for favors. If Person asks for a favor, and Other does the favor, Person usually responds with approval, admiration, and an acknowledgment of Other's superiority. If Other then asks Person to do a favor in return, this request implies that Person is an equal rather than a subordinate, which also implies that the earlier approval and deference were gained under false pretenses. To avoid these consequences, when Other is asked to do a favor, he or she should do the favor out of pure kindness and lay no claim to a counter favor (Homans, 1974, pp. 221-222).

First Gifts

Browning and Henderson are aware that first gifts have a quality of uniqueness (p. 651), but we feel that they underestimate how influential this unique quality may be in the development of relationships in organizations. If gifts promote cohesion, this result is more likely for early gifts than later gifts. The presence or absence of solidarity lies in beginnings. This situation is evident in Simmel's (1950) description of the first gift:

> Once we have received something good from another person. We no longer can make up for it completely, no matter how much our return gift or service may objectively or legally surpass his own. The reason is that his gift, because it was first, has a voluntary character which no return gift can have. For, to return the benefit we are obliged ethically; we operate under a coercion which, though neither social nor legal nor moral, is still a coercion. The first gift is given in full spontaneity; it has a freedom without any duty. (p. 392)

Systems with short memories, high turnover, multiple projects, and rapidly shifting tasks should have lots of "beginnings," more occasions for first gifts, and a more dense web of obligation and indebtedness. As change increases, so too should solidarity because there are more opportunities to make binding first gifts.

Gratitude

A topic of interest to Browning and Henderson, given this background, may be "gratitude" as glue. Simmel (1950) suggests that "gratitude actually consists, not in the return of a gift, but in the consciousness that it cannot be returned" (p. 392), which suggests that gratitude is the source of an "atmosphere of obligation" (p. 395). Notice that gratitude maintains its claim even after a return gift has been made because freedom is always missing from the return gift. Relationships live on in the form of gratitude, and this continuance seems to be what we sense when we listen to the mail clerk and the clean-shaven military officer handpicked for promotion. The point is not to ask about help, which could be either a spontaneous gesture or a partial repayment for something that happened earlier, but to ask grateful action which lingers around good turns received in the past.

At first glance, gratitude may seem as foreign to organizations as altruism. Browning and Henderson taken the important step of suggesting that there are several reasons to expect altruism, help, and grants in "heartless" organizations. What we have added is the suggestion that people may be more willing to discuss this aspect of organizations if the inquiry is framed in terms of the more familiar feeling of gratitude than in terms of the less familiar cognition of an "unrepayable gift"

Thus we suspect that Browning and Henderson are not interested in gifts of all kinds, but more in first gifts and the conditions in organizations that affect their frequency, visibility, and capability for binding others.

Obligations Imposed by Gifts

So far we have maintained a neutral tone when we said that gifts obligate. Obligation has a dark side, however, and this side is why we doubt that gifts are as strong a source of solidarity as the authors do. Browning and Henderson note that "any presentation is made into a gift simply by the lack of explicit return by the recipient" (p. 645).

The problem with that assertion is that people feel compelled to reciprocate even if they can't. Help that cannot be reciprocated is the problem of underdeveloped countries, people on welfare, and so on. The loss of control recipients often experience when gifts and claims are forced on them and which they must repay with more costly reciprocations of compliance, loss of stature, loss of esteem, heightened deference, or other subjective equivalents, explains why resentment and withdrawal are often the unexpected responses to gifts. This sequence is dramatically evident in the statement that "foreign aid is a psychological substitute for war" (Brown, 1986, p. 64). "Donations" of foreign aid often mask an expectation of reciprocal exchange when, in return for surplus commodities, a nation obtains military bases, political influence, or protection of investments.

Because of the dark side of indebtedness, we might expect less of the peacefulness and loyalty in response to gifts than Browning and Henderson expect (p. 654), and more responses, such as derogation of gifts, transformation of a social exchange into an economic exchange so that repayment can be made swiftly and exactly, efforts to recall prior favors that preceded the gift and therefore make it a repayment rather than an obligation, and termination of relationships in order to break the imperatives of reciprocity and exchange. Furthermore, we would expect all of these to occur before the last resort to the humiliation of a loss of status.

Status and Gifts

If a recipient accepts a gift and fails to make a return,

> he [*sic*] then confesses himself, not only to the giver but to any other beholder, to be neither the giver's enemy [he would refuse the gift] nor his friend [he would make a fair return] but his social inferior. He may even, in becoming the giver's inferior, become his subordinate too; the only way he can work off his debt may be to accept the orders of his creditor. Since status is a relative matter, the same act that brings one man down in the world brings another up, and some givers may use the norm of reciprocity to enhance their own status. (Homans, 1974, p. 218)

If we think of gifts as occasions when status may get realigned, some assertions in Browning and Henderson take on a different meaning. The observation that gifts are usually connected to positions which are privileged (p. 645) may also mean that gifts are a powerful means to preserve privilege by demonstrating superiority. The use of unrepayable grants to raise status may be a key aspect of "organizational politics." Gifts that cannot be reciprocated lower the status of those who have some status to lose. If one has no status to lose, then it is easier to accept gifts that cannot be repaid. In the stories told to Browning and Henderson, we see this dynamic operating when an alcoholic attorney down on his luck and a family that is captive of the IRS, accept the gift of an attorney's expertise which they cannot repay either objectively or subjectively.

Is Communication a Gift?

Aside from all of these complications for one-way transfer associated with the activity of gifting, there are questions raised by the unusual nature of the gifts themselves. Browning and Henderson proposed that one-way communication grants give information, provide linkage, or give emotional support. The problem is that it is not always clear that communication is a gift, from the standpoint of either the giver or the recipient.

From the giver's side, if communication is intangible and ephemeral it may not have enough substance to be something that can be given and something that moves from a donor to a recipient. Futhermore, if communication is abundant, reusable, and renewable, then it costs very little for the donor to provide, should not require much repayment from the recipient, and, therefore, should have only a small, transient effect on cohesion.

From the recipient's side, it would seem difficult to assign value to communication: Communication can interrupt ongoing activities and produce overload; what looks like help to the donor may be irrelevant to the recipient ("I am from the government and I have come to help you"). If the donor thinks a message offered as a gift represents a big investment and entitles the donor to a large repayment but the recipient feels that talk is cheap as well as disruptive because it interrupts and overloads, then cohesion is unlikely to result from views that are this far apart. Because organizations sometimes encourage people to inflate the worth of their contributions, the misunderstandings and fragmentation we have just described should be fairly common.

Summary

In summary, one-way transfers may be a mechanism of social cohesion, but only under special conditions. Giving is an incomplete transaction that sets in motion a variety of social processes. Gifts may be a force for cohesion if they are spontaneous (first gift), if they evoke feelings of gratitude, if they can be approximately, but not fully, reciprocated, and if they occur when someone already feels inferior to the giver or the question of relative status has not arisen or when the gift has been asked for by the receiver (costs have already been incurred by the receiver in the act of requesting and there is no residue for resentment).

Gifts may be a force toward fragmentation if they are repayments, impossible to reciprocate, forced upon the recipient, or take place between status equals and pose a status threat.

The only way to strip gifts of their overlay of reciprocity is to follow the "Millionaire's" recipe (p. 645): make gifts spontaneously and anonymously.

SOURCES OF ONE-WAY TRANSFERS

In our efforts to learn more about one-way transfer and the conditions under which it will occur and produce cohesion, we initially probed more deeply into the qualities of gifting. We now enlarge our search for conditions favoring one-way transfers by looking first at the proposal by Browning and Henderson that one-way transfers are encouraged by slack and ambiguity, and second by suggesting that one-way transfers may be associated with action generators and central exchanges.

Slack

Slack may be the occasion for one-way transfers as in the examples in which mail sorters had time on their hands, Gary helped Doug at no great sacrifice (p. 663), the commodity broker had both excess watermelons and time to visit metropolitan markets, and the lawyer initially had time on his hands because he had few steady clients (p. 658). These examples of "resources beyond mere adequacy" (p. 641) suggest that slack, when it occurs, may encourage one-way transfers. The frequency with which slack occurs would seem to be decreasing in organizations, which suggests to us that it may be relatively less common as a source of one-way transfers than is true for ambiguity. The decrease in slack can be attributed to several factors. Individuals typically expand their work to fill the time allotted to it, cost consciousness leads to zealous pruning, staff positions are now seen as more dispensable than they had been, time management encourages people to fill whatever idle moments they find, lean and mean organizational cultures gain their identity precisely from the fact that they have no resources beyond mere adequacy, downsizing has gained new stature as a responsible means to cope with competition, and small size is valued over large, which means that usually fewer people do more activities with less time left over. Furthermore, if slack does exist and if its existence is common knowledge, then any transfers that result from it should be seen as cost-free donations that need no repayment and incur no obligations.

Ambiguity

Ambiguity is more common than is slack in loosely coupled systems because a defining property of such systems is indeterminacy. "Loose coupling exists if A affects B (1) suddenly (rather than continuously), (2) occasionally (rather than constantly), (3) negligibly (rather than significantly), (4) indirectly (rather than directly), and (5) eventually (rather than immediately)" (Weick, 1982, p. 380). As indeterminacy and ambiguity increase, one-way transfers may also increase because they could be an effective means to reduce ambiguity. The clue to this possibility lies in the earlier discussion of foreign aid as a device for building obligation and dependency. Indebted people should be more predictable than should nonindebted people, assuming they have some interest in maintaining status. One-way transfers may stabilize the behavior of recipients. Recipients remain more attentive and responsive to donors, compliance and deference may increase, and recipients think twice before they resist. All of these responses reduce ambiguity in the social environment of donors.

One-way transfers, even if they do not immediately obligate, do represent sense-making experiments that may reduce ambiguity. They are not trial and error, but simply trials. It is the discovery of "error" that is the first step toward making sense of what one faces. One-way transfers can be viewed as pure trials in search of outcomes, including error. Any outcome represents a potential contingency between action and reaction, and any contingency is a potential regularity that can be a welcome replacement for ambiguity.

Thus a large family of organizational theories that describe proactive behavior, retrospective sense making, justification, experimentation, and nonroutine problem solving all share the idea that action is underrationalized in its early stages and that the reasons for its occurrence are built up and become clearer as the behavior unfolds and outcomes become attached to it. Action undertaken for insufficient reasons looks much like a one-way transfer, because it has not been preceded by an elaborate calculation of profit or undertaken to achieve clear-cut, guaranteed gains. Instead, gains, if they even occur, are post hoc discoveries rather than a priori certainties. One-way transfers are powerful sense-making devices, not just because they strengthen alliances, but because they make things happen. And when things happen in a contingent manner, order is discovered and ambiguity decreases.

Thus it seems to us that ambiguity may be the more important of the two antecedents of one-way transfer proposed by Browning and Henderson.

Action Generation

While we have emphasized that one-way transfers represent action that is instrumental to the reduction of ambiguity, one-way transfers can also be understood in terms of pure action. The clue to this possibility is the assertion by Browning and Henderson that one-way transfers may be common in garbage can organizations (p. 644). An organization in which people, solutions, choices, and problems flow in separate streams and converge fortuitously, may have frequent one-way transfers, not because those independent streams contain slack and ambiguity, but because they represent action as a programmed output (Starbuck, 1983). Any system that is programmed to produce action will make things available to people, whether they request them or not. And the value of these provisions will be determined by what is being considered at the moment of their arrival. Thus, while we agree with Browning and Henderson that one-way transfers should be common in an organized anarchy (a hypothesis that has yet to be tested), we disagree that this is because anarchies are loosely coupled or have an abundance of slack and ambiguity. Instead, we feel that anarchies have many one-way transfers because they are programmed to generate action independent of demand, stimulation, or specific requests.

The juxtaposition of one-way transfers, organized anarchies, and systems of action generation, suggests a fascinating set of questions, the most basic of which is: What happens to the norm of reciprocity in a system that is programmed to ignore it? Are all gifts in an organized anarchy first gifts? Do people punctuate streams of noncontingent activities into contingent exchanges? Is the level of trust in an organized anarchy chronically high because equivalent repayment is so difficult to calculate and so slow in coming? The questions are endless, but the focus is constant. The theme remains, what happens to one-way transfers when they are imposed on a background of exchange? The variation suggested by Browning and Henderson's inclusion of organized anarchies is that organizations that are action generators produce one-way transfers with such frequency that they may alter the background condition of reciprocity and exchange that we have assumed up to this point. If the background condition is not altered, then phenomena associated with exchange—phenomena such as indebtedness, subjective equivalents, gratitude, status threats, trust, obligation, and repayment—should unfold in a different way than is associated with systems in which conventional exchange is easier.

Central Exchange

One-way transfers may increase under conditions of slack, ambiguity, and action generation, but they may also increase when people presume that there is a "central exchange." People may make one-way transfers on the assumption that

> a benefit withdrawn calls for a benefit deposited. With whom the deposit is made could be a matter of indifference; the point is to maintain a balance in the centrally kept accounts. Whether one believes there is Someone actually keeping those accounts seems to be a question of religion, but many act as if they were even though they do not say they believe it. (Brown, 1986, p. 57)

Browning and Henderson's opening example of peasants whose work initially carried spiritual qualities and was weighted according to use values, and the later examples of barn raising, boy scout leading, and community activity, all suggest that one-way transfers may involve less concern for repayment by a specific, proximate recipient, and more concern with the books kept by a more inclusive, more distant body.

It may well be that the people Browning and Henderson study are in an exchange relationship with some other entity than their immediate interaction partner. That possibility need not be read mystically. Consider the example of a barn raising. When 20 farmers help one farmer build a barn, that may look like 20 farmers making one-way resource transfers to one farmer, as the one farmer is not expected to repay the 20. But the one farmer is expected to repay the community by future involvement in its activities and 20 farmers who make deposits can expect repayment from the community at some future time, should they need it.

The point is that face-to-face one-way transfers may be sustained by the promise of reciprocation from some other entity that keeps score. To find the source of one-way transfers is to look beyond slack, ambiguity, and action for beliefs about balances kept in central accounts. One-way transfers at one level of analysis, may be exchanges at another level of analysis.

ONE-WAY TRANSFERS AND LOOSELY COUPLED SYSTEMS

The basic model used by Browning and Henderson is that loosely coupled systems create slack and ambiguity, which then encourages one-way transfers. Their proposals seem to be just as robust and more economical if loose coupling is dropped as a driving variable. The people whom Browning and Henderson interviewed were not asked about loosely coupled systems and apparently felt no need to invoke them. While commodity markets; professions, such as law; and public sector organizations, such as the post office and military, have all been mentioned in discussions of loose coupling, they have not been uniquely tied to one-way transfers, communication, or slack and ambiguity. Thus these four variables can be discussed by themselves without the further problem of arguing that slack and ambiguity are the primary causal forces associated with a loosely coupled system or that organized anarchies are the prototypic loosely coupled system.

If loosely coupled systems were to be given more prominence in the Browning and Henderson argument, the number of complications would increase. If we argue that "loosely coupled elements are responsive but that each element also preserves its own identity and some evidence of its physical and logical separateness" (Weick, 1976, p. 3), then we are faced with the paradox that elements are simultaneously coupled and uncoupled. Elements are both responsive and separate, and autonomous and interdependent. One-way transfers have the potential to preserve this paradoxical quality because they too are simultaneously coupled (Person transfers resources to Other) and uncoupled (Other does not transfer resources back to Person). So one-way transfers are not encouraged by a separate, loosely coupled system, they are instead the very form of the system itself.

Futhermore, loosely coupled systems are usually discussed in association with hierarchies, a convention that dates back to Simon's (1962) important essay on the "architecture of complexity." The specific assertion is that subsystems are tightly coupled within and loosely coupled with other subsystems. This assertion suggests that one-way transfers should be an intergroup phenomenon and two-way transfers should be an intragroup phenomenon. This speculation, however, becomes complicated because we usually expect that social exchange dominates within a group, and economic exchange (e.g., transfer pricing) dominates between groups. Thus it may be that when we look closer, social exchange and one-way transfers play a bigger role in intergroup networks and ties than we have though up to now and that intragroup relations are more pure exchange and more economic than we may have seen before. Or, a closer look may suggest that the rule of thumb, tight within and loose between, has limited accuracy when placed alongside the more pervasive paradox that all systems are mixtures of tight and loose coupling. Or, when we look at the frequency of coupling, we may find that many loose couplings and one-way transfers within a subsystem approximate the tightly coupled system we expect to find.

The overriding question is: What does happen to exchange in loosely coupled systems? Because indeterminacy is higher in such systems it should be harder to be explicit about exchanges, harder to find exact equivalents for gifts, and harder to enforce repayment, all of which should encourage social exchange, one-way transfers, gratitude, and indebtedness. And yet, a loosely coupled system also has separate entities with distinct identities, formal relations that are more explicit and discussable, and more inclination to move toward impersonal economic exchange than toward more personal social exchange. Just as the loosely coupled system itself is paradoxical, the exchanges that it fosters may be an odd mixture of the personal and the impersonal. And one-way transfers may be a unique window on these odd mixtures.

Norms of reciprocity can certainly span and constrain the diversity and separateness of a loosely coupled system, so the mere fact of looseness does not cancel the influence of reciprocity. And yet looseness also makes it more difficult to agree on the value of transfers, there are fewer occasions to monitor repayment, and the very fact of separateness may weaken the claims of exchange. Nevertheless, there are dependencies among the actors in loosely coupled systems; coalitions do form among separate actors; and people and groups do remember favors given and favors received.

Perhaps reciprocity in a loosely coupled system is no different from that in a tightly coupled one. It is to Browning and Henderson's credit that they have alerted us to look more closely at this issue with more precision. But their argument that one-way transfers may be common in organizations, and that these transfers are made in the form of communication, and that the imprecision of repayment for these transfers is a source of cohesion among members, is sufficient stimulus to inquiry that the more troublesome question of the role of loosely coupled systems in all of this, need not be added.

REFERENCES

Brown, R. (1986). *Social psychology: The second edition.* New York: Free Press.

Homans, G. C. (1974). *Social behavior: Its elementary forms* (rev. ed.). New York: Harcourt Brace Jovanovich.

Simmel, G. (1950). *The sociology of Georg Simmel.* Glencoe, NY: Free Press.

Simon, H. A. (1962). The architecture of complexity. *Proceedings of the American Philosophical Society, 106*, 467-482.

Starbuck, W. H. (1983). Organizations as action generators. *American Sociological Review, 48*, 91-102.

Weick, K. E. (1976). Educational organizations as loosely coupled systems. *Administrative Science Quarterly, 21*, 1-19.

Weick, K. E. (1982). Management of organizational change among loosely coupled elements. In P. Goodman (Ed.), *Change in organizations* (pp. 375-408). San Francisco: Jossey-Bass.

INDEX

Anti-Semitism, 83-92
and ideology, 83
and language, 83
and scapegoating, 85-86
and social class, 84
and spontaneous speech, 89-92
function of, 84-85
in newspaper stories, 86-89

Communication technology design, 498-530, 533-535, 547-555
action science methodology, 504-509; example of 506-508; versus hypothetico-deductive science, 504-505
and adaptable systems, examples of, 523-528
and bureaucratic decision making, 501-502
and conversation, 517-519
and designers' assumptions concerning human communication, 498-499, 529
and designers' assumptions concerning technology, 499, 501, 509
and designers' assumptions concerning users, 499-501, 509, 518-523, 529; and system functionality, 522-523; and user knowledge, 519-520; versus users' perspectives, 518-519
and evaluative research, 502-503, 509
and expanding user choice, 539-540
and functional equivalence with older systems, 533, 538, 540-541
and information exchange, 548, 550-552
and interactive media, 547
and level of program structure, 549-550
and novelty, 538-541, 543
and Taylorism, 510, 514
and the computer news project, 539-541
and the information society, 510
and the role of users, 533, 542-543
and user adapted systems, 551-553
and user convenience, 538-541
and user reflexivity, 533, 543-544
and user self-monitoring, 536-537
contextual instability of, 534
cybernetic model of, 500, 509-511, 513; organizational applications, 511-512
designer-user relationship, 501
definitions of, 501
distracting features of, 534-535
homeostatic model of, 510-511, 513; organizational applications, 512-513
importance to communication researchers, 499-500
influence of social context on, 500, 514-518, 528; and employee participation, 514-516; and organizational decision making, 516-517; and technological innovation, 517, 519
problems associated with technical sophistication, 534, 537-538
psychosocial context of application, 536-537, 543, 547-553
"socially open" approach to, 499, 509, 529, 533, 542, 544, 547, 549, 553-555
sociotechnical analysis of, 508
user redefinition of, 535

Computer-Mediated Communication Systems, 436-470, 477-488, 490-494
and communication researchers, 490
and computers, 481
and "conversation," 438
and differentiating constructs, 482-483
and educational applications of microcomputers, 494-496
and information processing, 485
and information richness, 481-482
and information society, 455
and integrating research efforts, 477
and interpersonal communication, 481-482, 488
and perspectives on information, 462-467; as commodity, 463-464; as interpretive activity, 465-466
and program evaluation, 490-493
and technology, 478
and types of functions, 484
channel based, 487
classification schemes of, 481-488
definitions of, 437-438, 478
differentiation within, 480-481
forms of, 439
four dimension model of research concerning, 440-462, 469-470, 478; *stakeholders*, 440-448, 479, 491, 493; differences among, 442, 444; and evaluation, 442; critique of, 443; and systems rationalism, 444; and segmented institutionalism, 444; types, 444-448; *goals*,

440, 448-452, 479; formative research, 448, 491; summative research, 448-452, 491; *domains*, 441, 453-455, 480; categories of, 453-454; *tools*, 441, 455-462, 480; research design, 457-458; generalizability, 457-458; control/randomization, 458-459; types of data, 459; analytic methods, 460-462
functioned based, 484-487
functions of, 437-438
media systems versus media systems research, 479-480
proliferation of, 480
relationship to other media, 439-440
relationship among dimensions, 467-469; across dimensions, 467-468; constraints across dimensions, 468-469; within dimensions, 467-469
research methods appropriate to, 493-496; case studies, 496; structured interviews, 494-496; surveys, 493-495; quantitative/qualitative, 493
variety of approaches to study of, 436
Conversation (see also Discourse), 31-32, 60-74
and job interviews, 35
and minority groups, 33-34
between doctors and patients, 35-37
between parents and children, 32
between men and women, 32-33
in the classroom, 37
in the courts, 37-39
practices of, 60-74; logics of status, 68-69; and time and space, 70-74; and turn-taking, 65-66, 70-73
Conversational coherence, 95-123, 130-143, 146-155
and causality, 132, 135-138
and cognitive information processing, 97, 100, 106, 109-112, 114-115, 120-121
and cohesive devices, 102, 105, 117
and comprehension process, 106-108, 112, 120, 135-138, 147-148, 151, 154
and connectedness, 95
and conversational cues, 117-122, 153
and expectancies, 134, 138-139
and meaning, 130, 133-135, 149-150, 152
and memory, 123
and perception, 134
and probability, 132
and relationship to knowledge structures, 133, 138-139, 147, 152-155
and relevance, 98-100, 105, 118, 151-152
and structural correctness, 104-105, 118
and textual attributes, 147
as element of subjective experience, 146-147
as evaluative judgment, 96, 101, 106-108, 115-116, 120, 122-123, 131, 133-135, 146-147, 150
as independent variable, 140
assumptions concerning, 96-97
definition of, 95, 131
locus of, 96, 116
micro and macroscopic, 131
necessary conditions for achieving, 100, 102, 104, 108
relationship to knowledge structures, 109-122
sufficient conditions for achieving, 101-102, 105, 108-109
textual and psychological attributes of, 141-142
Critical mass communication research, 559-595, 613-633
American pragmatic tradition, 559-567, 585, 591, 593; and social reform, 563-565; and technological innovation, 561; and the American press, 563-564; the formation of democratic community in, 560-562, 566; the reconciliation of morality and science in, 560, 567; versus European approaches, 562, 567
British cultural studies tradition, 559, 586-595, 630-633; American adaptations of, 588-592, 595, 630-631; and empirical investigation, 623-633; and politics, 631; and the administrative/critical dichotomy, 623; and the empirical tradition, 590; as evaluative approach, 631; discourse in, 587; emphasis on active audiences, 587-588; influence of literary theory on, 631; Marxist influence on, 586, 588, 591-592; role of ideological analysis in 586-588, 590-592; role of intellectual in, 592
critical theory tradition, 571-573, 576-585, 594-595; emphasis on history and culture, 582; emphasis on social power, 578, 581; Habermas' emancipatory project, 582-585, 594; influence of Frankfurt School theorists on, 571-573; relationship to Marxism, 576, 578, 580-581
empirical/theoretical synthesis, 619, 623-624; methodological similarities between approaches, 619; resistance to, 623-624
empirical/social scientific tradition, 567-576, 579-580, 594, 618-625, 628-629;

and administrative research, 571, 575; and capitalist development, 624; and conservatism, 624, 629; and efficiency, 570; and individualism, 570; and Marxism, 623, 628; and the Frankfurt School, 622, 630; and the process of phenomenological description, 629; and the rise of structural/functional sociology, 567-568; approach to political power advocated, 570, 572-574; as critique, 618, 620; diversity within, 619-620; encounters with the critical tradition, 571-576, 579-580, 594; media effects research, 570, 572; models of communication, 568-569; relation to critical theory, 620-621, 625, 630; socioeconomic context surrounding, 568; versus theoretical emphasis, 621-622, 624, 628;
methodological issues in, 619, 625-628; quantitative versus qualitative research, 626-628; and administrative research, 627
traditions of, 618, 620
Cultural Studies, 601-616
and ideology, 603-605, 612, 614-615; and materialism, 604, 614-615; and base superstructure debates, 604-605, 615
and hegemony, 605, 607-608; role of media in, 605-606; structural analysis of, 606
and Marxism, 602-604, 614
and the ideological environment surrounding media institutions, 602
and the role of American academics, 601, 603, 606-608, 615-616
categories of, 613-614
disciplinary diversity in, 601, 616
semilogical perspective on, 607-612; and spectator pleasure, 608, 611-612; role of discursive codes, 607-608; role of Marxism and psychoanalysis in 608-612; role of the subject in, 608-612
Culture and Communication, 383-410, 417-425, 427-434
and conditions for cultural development, 421-422, 424
and cultural content, 420-421
and cultural identity, 389, 393, 431
and cultural knowledge, 428-429
and cultural logic, 384
and epistemology, 392
and grass-roots social movements, 409, 433
and ideology, 390-391, 393, 408-409, 417
and institutions, 424-425
and media imperialism, 432
and modernity, 427, 434
and persona analysis, 420
and power, 388-389, 393, 408-409, 417, 420, 425, 431, 433
and problems of a universalized subject, 420
and structuralism, 428-430
and structure, 390
and Third World modernization, 385-388; relativity of, 385-386, and one world, many cultures view concerning, 386-387; cultural identification, 387-388
and Westernization, 383-384, 400-408
as process, 424-425
culture as perspective on society, 389
cultural identity, critique of, 418-421; clarity, 418; usefulness, 418; individualistic bias, 418-419; types of identity, 419
definitions of, 391, 393, 431-432
dynamism of, 393
emic/etic approaches to, 391-392
forces of resistance to cultural development, 422-424
influence of contemporary literary theory on, 428-430; and textual interpretation, 428; and textual production, 428-429 relevant concepts of, 433-434
internal/external factors effecting, 384, 404
macro/micro levels of 384, 417
materialism/idealism dichotomy, 408
media imperialism approach to, 400-408; alternatives to, 405; criticism of, 403-405; in nonThird World countries, 406-407, 432, 433; language, 402; modes of influence, 401-402; practices of media organizations, 402; role of audience in, 403; technology, 402
modes of communication, 417, 425
research agenda in, 408-409
synthesized perspective on, 417
theoretical diversity in, 427-428
Western versus Eastern approaches to, 394-430; direct/indirect communication, 399; individual/collectivity, 396-397; in terms of language, 395-396; power, 395; social relations, 397-398;

Dialectics of friendship, 157-185, 190-200, 203-212
Aristotelian view, 205-210
ambiguity in, 170, 190-192

and continuity/discontinuity, 191
and cultural forms, 192, 195-199
and empirical discourse, 203-205, 211-212
and encapsulation, 162, 184
and eros, 207, 208
and gender, 178-180, 183-185, 193, 197
and hermeneutics, 203-212
and institutionalization, 165-166, 169, 182-183, 192, 199, 203-204
and intimacy, 166, 180, 183, 194-195
and marriage, 180-181, 193
and morality, 205-207, 209-210
and moral/tactical meanings, 168
and praxis, 210-211
and public spaces, 198-199
and reflexive time, 190-191
and relatedness, 192
and same-sex relationship, 178-181
and self-concept, 174-176, 180-181, 185
and selfishness/altruism, 173-174
and self-monitoring, 183
and social contexts, 191
and social research, 190, 199-200
and sociohistoric norms, 167, 169
and symbol systems, 190-191
and the economy of rewards, 173-174
and the philosophy process of naming, 204-205
and work, 181-183, 185, 193
and young adulthood, 178, 180-182, 185, 193
basic elements of, 158-164; contradiction, 157, 159-160, 164, 192; motion, 157, 160, 164, 192; praxis, 157, 163-164, 185, 192; totality, 157-158, 164
contextual dialectics, 157, 164-169, 177-178, 184; public/private, 157, 165-167, 185, 192; real/ideal, 157, 167-169, 192
historical transformation in, 191, 193-199; ecology of friendship, 191, 196-198; strangers to friends, 191, 193-196
interactional dialectics of, 157, 169-178, 184; effect/instrumentality, 157, 170-174, 178, 192, 199; expressiveness/protectiveness, 158, 170, 176-177, 180; independence/dependence, 157, 170-171, 192, 199; judgment/acceptance, 157-158, 170, 174-176, 179
transendence and transformation, 161, 184
Discourse, 18-50, 60-64 (see also Conversation)
and common sense, 72
and conversational formats, 66-67
and conversation, 31-39
and cultural Marxism, 61
and ideological reproduction, 25-26
and ideology, 23-27, 60-74
and personal power, 61, 63
and power, 19, 26-31, 49-50, 59-62, 69-70, 73
and practice, 61
and social interaction, 27
and structural Marxism, 61
and text, 41-42, 60
and the utterance, 65, 67, 70
genres of, 28-29
levels of, 28
mediated, 42-49
organizational, 39-40
political, 40-41
production of, 21-22
social approach to, 18
social power 19-29, 42, 49-50, 61, 63; access to, 22; and discourse, 49-50; and symbolic elites, 22-23, 25-26; dimensions of, 28-29; properties of 19-21; structures of, 28-29, 42; versus personal power, 19, 61, 63
Western news media, 42-46; and advertising, 47; and labor, 47; and other minorities, 47; and portrayals of Third World countries, 43-45; and power, 42-47; effects of, 45

Ideology, 23-27, 62-68, 72
and class consciousness, 63
and cognition, 63
and consciousness, 62, 65
and conversational practice, 63, 65-68, 72
and discourse, 24-25
and language, 62
and news media, 25-26, 42
and subjectivity, 63-64
and the State, 63, 73-74
as false consciousness, 23-24
as social cognition, 24
Classical Marxist, 24
function of, 62
reproduction of, 25-26, 43
Intercultural Communication, 278-303
acculturation process studies, 287-288
and cultural adoption, 292, 301-302
and cultural sense-making, 312, 322
and diffusion of information studies, 288
and nationalism 297
and power, 297-298
and racial and ethic issues, 280
and scholarly cooperation, 281-283, 303

and soujourn studies, 287
and the individual, 284, 295
and the media, 297-299
and the perception of difference, 283-286
and "third culture" model, 292-298, 300-302, 311-312; interactional roots of, 294
and uncertainty reduction, 286
conceptual diversity in, 310-311; attributionists, 311; conceptualizers, 311; cultural discounters, 311; cultural particularists, 311; ethicists, 311; resolutionists, 311; specifiers, 311
culture versus its artifacts, 289
diversity within, 279-280, 282-283, 303
evaluation of, 280
history of, 279-283
homogeneity/heterogeneity pardox of, 283-286
in organizations and families, 295-296
in post war period, 281
internal challenges to, 278
methodological issues in, 280, 282, 291, 302
perspectives on culture, 288-293
possibilities for merging perspectives, issues in, 311-313; role of environment, 312; role of history, 313; role of ideology, 313; role of language, 313; role of motivation, 313; role of part/observer, 312
relationship to interpersonal communication, 284
technological model of, 289-290, 292-293, 299, 301
Western influence in, 290-292, 297, 299-301
Interpersonal relationship development, 315-348, 355-368, 371-380
and context, 378, 380
and perceptions of cultural difference, 334-335, 337, 339, 348
and perceptions of cultural similarity, 333-334, 337-338, 348
and relational "universals," 321
and research context, 347
as dialectical process, 375-375, 379
cross-cultural variation in, 321-333, 360-368, 371, 373, 377-380; and individualism/ collectivisim, 322-325, 328; and masculinity/feminity, 323, 325-326, 328; and ongoing relationships, 363, 367; and power, 323-324; and uncertainty avoidance, 322, 324, 328; and Western ideology of intimacy, 379-380; in high versus low context cultures, 332, 329-333, 340-341, 377-378; in ingroup/outgroup relations, 324-325, 327-329, 333, 340; in initial interactions, 360, 363, 366
predicted outcome value theory approach to, 356-368; and intimacy, 364-365; and liking, 367; and reciprocity, 365; and relational development, 358-359, 367; and similarity, 366-367; and verbal communication, 361; major tenets of, 356; role of uncertainty reduction in, 357-358, 361-363, 365-367
social penetration approach to, 316-317, 325-329, 334-338, 345, 355, 371, 374, 377-378; and culture, 378; and dyadic reciprocity, 377; and gender, 318; communicative dimensions of, 317-318, 335-337; importance of self-disclosure to, 317; in Korea, 328-329; in United States versus Japan, 325-327; linear assumptions of, 374; stages of 317, 338
uncertainty reduction approach to, 315-316, 318-321, 329-333, 337, 348, 355-356, 362-368, 371-379; and ambiguity, 346; and attributional confidence, 330-333, 337, 340-341; and behavioral predictability, 319; and cognitive predictability, 319; and culture, 379; and dispositional factors, 373-374; and ethnolinguistic identity theory, 339-340, 343-344, 348; and initial interactions, 316, 374; and intergroup anxiety, 341-343, 346; and interpersonal/intergroup salience, 343-344, 347; and intimacy, 364; and relational instability, 374, 379; and self-consciousness, 320-321; and self-disclosure, 330, 337, 340-341; and self-monitoring, 320; and situational factors, 374; and uncertainty increases, 345, 376; and understanding, 319; as dialectical process, 345; intercultural elements of, 342-343; in United States versus Japan, 330-333, 340; linear assumptions of, 374, 377; major tenets of 319-320, 341; motivational bases for, 372-373

Organizational Communication, 638-666, 670-686
and communication exchange, 671-672
and communication "gifts," 640-647, 665-666; abundance of, 646; and feedback, 645; and resource allocation, 647; para-

doxes of, 644-645; threat versus benevolence, 665-666; timing of, 644-645
and economic exchange, 640, 670-672
and evolutionary processes, 673-674
and integrative systems, 670-671
and loosely-coupled systems, 640-666, 670, 673-674, 682-686; action in, 683-684; role of ambiguity in, 682-683, 685; role of exchange in, 686; role of slack in, 682, 685; vulnerability in, 674
and one-way transfers, 640-666, 670, 676-686; and creativity, 647; and economic versus social exchange, 677-678; and emotions, 652-653; and first gifts, 678; and gratitude, 679; and obligation, 679-680; and organizational committment, 648-649; and organizational momentum, 650-651; and status, 680; and the ephemeral nature of communication, 681; and variety, 644; as complex exchanges, 677; difficulty in identifying, 676-677; dimensions of, 654-655; examples of, 641; interview methods for studying, 652-653; motivations for, 640; narrative dimensions of, 653, 664-665; role of ambiguity in 642-643, 645; role of slack in, 642-643, 646, 649
and reciprocity, 675-677, 681, 684-686
and scarcity, 672
and threat systems, 670
economic models of, 638-640
rational models of, 643, 649
role of emotions in, 675
role of grants economics in, 670-671
role of self-interest in, 638-639

Power, 76-92
and dialectic of individual and collective discourse, 79-80, 86, 92; and ideology, 83
and language, 81-91
and multi-level analysis of, 79
and powerlessness, 82
and prejudice, 83-92
and the non-English speaking world, 77
definitions of, 78
effects on those subjected to, 77
ethnopsychoanalytical approach to, 79-82
interdisciplinary approach to, 76
internal perspective on, 76
irrationality of, 76, 81
multidimensionality of, 77-78, 92
relational character of, 77

Second-guessing theory, 213-242, 249-262, 266-274
and attributional claims, 215
and cognitive-behavioral factors, 255
and context, 232-233, 255
and deception, 213-214, 239
and duration of information processing, 255-256
and evaluating ability, 259
and extracting bias cues, 225-230, 232-233, 238-239, 258
and general suspiciousness, 257
and information gathering, 215, 220, 235-237, 241-242
and internal/external truth standards, 232
and Machiavellianism, 257
and message salience, 215
and mindlessness, 272
and nontransactional episodes, 269
and organizations, 240-242
and perceptions of message bias, 213-214, 219-220, 223, 231-233, 239-240, 249, 253-254, 256-261, 271-274
and personality, 259
and rationalistic assumptions, 268-270, 272-274
and receiver knowledge, 215, 230
and relationship to communication theory, 216-219, 240, 242, 267; connecting communication and cognition, 218-219; emphasizing indirect episodes, 217; emphasizing nontransactional episodes, 218, 242; expanding the role of the receiver, 216-217, 240
and selective application of, 257-260
and self-monitoring, 224
and social strategic considerations, 235-237
and task conditions, 228-229, 235
and the need for accurate information, 223-226, 229, 231, 234-235, 240, 249, 252-253, 257
and the role of the hearer, 254-255, 268-269
and uncertainty reduction, 223, 228, 255
antecedents and consequences of, 256
as a skill, 222, 226, 271
attitudes toward source, 259-260
connections of communication and cognition, 269, 271
definition of, 214
four-stage model of, 219-238; preconditions for, 222-226; reinterpretation assessment phase, 220-221; reinterpretation phase, 220, 230-237; social tactic choice

phase, 220, 222, 237-238; theoretical linkages between variables, 226-230; vigilance phase, 220, 222, 230, 234, 238
historical relation to allied disciplines, 266-267
illustrations of, 214-215
perspectives on active message gathering, 250-256; attributional analysis of opinion change, 253-254; cognitive response approach, 251; knowledge bias, 253-254; need for cognition, 253; personal relevance, 252; reporting bias 253-254; the elaboration likelihood model, 251-253
undirectional biases of, 269

ABOUT THE EDITOR

JAMES A. ANDERSON (Ph.D., University of Iowa, 1965) is Professor of Communication at the University of Utah. His scholarly writing concerns the relationship between theory and method in science, an area he most recently explored in *Communication Research: Issues and Methods* (1987). His research interests focus on the communication structure and practices of social action routines, political campaigns, media literacy, and family ethnographics.

ABOUT THE AUTHORS

STEPHEN R. ACKER (Ph.D., University of Utah, 1981) is Associate Professor of Communication at Ohio State University. His principal research interests are in the design and implementation of new communication technologies and the processes of visual communication.

NOBLEZA C. ASUNCION-LANDE (Ph.D., Michigan State University, 1960) is Professor of Communication Studies at the University of Kansas. Her expertise and theoretical interests include intercultural communication, cross-cultural conflict, communication in multinational organizations, development communication, and communication policy. She is coauthor of *The United States and Japan in the Western Pacific* (1981), editor of *Ethical Perspectives and Critical Issues in Intercultural Communication* (1980), and coeditor of *Building Bridges Across Cultures—Perspectives on Intercultural Communication Theory and Practice* (1981).

KENNETH E. BOULDING (M.A., Oxford, 1939) was born in Liverpool, England, in 1910, and educated at Oxford and the University of Chicago (Commonwealth Fellow, 1932-1934). He is Distinguished Professor of Economics, Emeritus, at the University of Colorado, Boulder, as well as a Research Associate and a Project Director in the Program of Research on Political and Economic Change at the university's Institute of Behavioral Science. His major interests are economic theory, grants economics, conflict and peace studies, evolutionary theory, general systems, and the study of human knowledge and learning.

JAMES J. BRADAC (Ph.D., Northwestern University, 1970) is Professor of Communication Studies at the University of California, Santa Barbara. He is the author of many publications in the area of language and communication. He is the coauthor, with Charles Berger, of *Language and Social Knowledge* (1982, published by Edward Arnold). He is currently working on a chapter on language attitudes and impression formation for the forthcoming *Handbook of Language and Social Psychology,* edited by Howard Giles and W. Peter Robinson (John Wiley). His major interests are in language and communication, interpersonal communication, and language and power.

LARRY DAVIS BROWNING (Ph.D., Ohio State University, 1973) is Associate Professor of Organizational Communication at the University of Texas at Austin. His M.A. and B.A. are from the University of Oklahoma. His research interests, in addition to one-way transfers in loosely coupled systems, include qualitative and ethnographic methodology, the communication surrounding organizational accidents, the symbolic use of information, and the relationship between narrative and argumentative rationality in organizations.

FRED L. CASMIR (Ph.D., Ohio State University, 1961) is Chairman of the Graduate Committee, Communication Division, Seaver College/Pepperdine University, and Director of the International Affairs Sequence. His major interests include international negotiation processes and the impact of mass media on cultures and societies.

FARRELL CORCORAN (Ph.D., University of Oregon, 1978) is Head of the School of Communications and Dean of the Faculty of Communications and Human Studies at the National Institute for Higher Education in Dublin, Ireland. He has published analyses of the rhetoric of the Cold War and contributions to the theory of ideology.

ERIC S. FREDIN (Ph.D., University of Michigan, 1980) is Assistant Professor in the School of Journalism at Ohio State University. His main research interests are design of new technology systems and cognitive aspects of political communication.

DIANA GAGNON (Ph.D., Harvard University, 1986) is a Research Associate and Lecturer at the Massachusetts Institute of Technology Media Laboratory. She is also serving as Study Director for the Media Laboratory's new Audience Research Facility, where she is conducting research on the design and influence of the next generation of consumer media technologies. Her current research focuses on prototype development and testing of interactive-entertainment television, future fiber optic services, and electronic publishing. Her research has spanned a variety of topics including the social and psychological effects of new media, video game addiction, video games and spatial skills, human factors of media design, and learning through interactive versus observational media.

MAUDIE L. GRAHAM is currently completing her Ph.D. at the University of Illinois, Urbana-Champaign. She is an Assistant Professor of Communication at the University of Wisconsin, Milwaukee. Her research interests include the regulation of social interaction, discourse processing, social cognition, and interpersonal communication.

WILLIAM B. GUDYKUNST (Ph.D., University of Minnesota, 1977) is Professor of Communication at Arizona State University. His major interest is in developing a theory that explains interpersonal and intergroup communication and incorporates cultural variability. An initial statement of such a theory appears in *Theory in Intercultural Communication* (Sage, 1988), a volume he coedited with Young Yun Kim. A more complete formulation of the theory will be presented in "Strangeness and Similarity: A Theory of Interpersonal and Intergroup Communication" (*Multilingual Matters,* in progress). He recently completed *Cultural and Interpersonal Communication* (with coauthors Stella Ting-Toomey and Elizabeth Chua), which has been published by Sage in 1988. He currently is coediting, with Molefi Asante, the *Handbook of Intercultural and Development Communication* (Sage, in press).

CEES J. HAMELINK, Ph.D., is Professor of Communication at the University of Amsterdam and member of the faculty of the Institute of Social Studies at The Hague, Netherlands. His publications include 10 books on different aspects of international communication. He is convenor of training courses in communication policy and planning in the African and Asian region, and Vice President of the International Association for Mass Communication Research.

HANNO HARDT (Ph.D., Southern Illinois University, 1967) is John F. Murray Professor of Journalism and Mass Communication at the University of Iowa. His interdisciplinary work is rooted in a cultural/historical tradition of communication studies and has focused most recently on contributions toward an intellectual history of communication and media studies in the United States.

LEONARD C. HAWES (Ph.D., University of Minnesota, 1970) is Professor of Communication at the University of Utah. His research interests include organizational theory and practice in the postindustrial age.

CARRIE HEETER (Ph.D., Michigan State University, 1985) is Director of the Communication Technology Laboratory at Michigan State University where she earned a B.A. in communication in 1982. The Comm Tech Lab is a multidisciplinary association of faculty and students studying new communication technologies. Her research interests include mediated communication systems, the human interface, interactivity and applications, and the impact of new communication technologies. Her recent work has examined the choice process with cable television, uses of videotex for information retrieval, and, currently, the emergence of computers as a new medium for communication.

SHEILA C. HENDERSON (M.A., University of Texas at Austin, 1982) is on the faculty of St. Edward's University in Austin. Her research interests lie in the nonrational aspects of organizations, with particular emphasis on socially constructed reality. She is a professional writer and editor, specializing in management topics. She also provides communication training and consultation.

DEAN E. HEWES (Ph.D., Florida State University, 1974) is Professor of Speech Communication at the University of Minnesota. His research interests include cognitive approaches to communication, small group communication, message campaigns, rumors and gossip, and methods for studying social interaction processes.

SALLY JACKSON (Ph.D, University of Illinois, 1980) is Associate Professor of Communication at the University of Oklahoma. Her research interests are in the areas of interpersonal argumentation and discourse analysis. She has been published in *Human Communciation Research, Communication Monographs, Quarterly Journal of Speech,* and *Journal of Child Language,* and serves on the editorial boards of numerous journals. She is currently studying processes of argumentation in mediation programs for the resolution of disputes.

SCOTT JACOBS (Ph.D., University of Illinois, 1982) is Associate Professor of Communication at the University of Oklahoma. He has also taught at the University of Nebraska and at Michigan State University. His scholarly interests include communication theory, discourse analysis, and argumentation theory. He is currently working on research in the nature of rules and discourse and is studying processes of argumentation in third party mediation of disputes.

JEROME JOHNSTON (Ph.D., University of Michigan, 1971) is Associate Research Scientist at the Institute for Social Research, Adjunct Associate Professor in the School of Education at the University of Michigan, and Senior Researcher at the National Center for Research in Postsecondary Teaching and Learning. He has been conducting studies of media since 1975. He began studying the potential of prosocial television (*Positive Images: Breaking Stereotypes with Children's Television,* Sage), and later did a major review of the educational potential of all electronic media (*Electronic Learning: From Audiotape to Videodisc,* Lawrence Erlbaum). In the 1980s he became concerned with the rapid evolution of the new information technologies, and the problems this presented for researchers (*Evaluating the New Information Technologies,* Jossey-Bass). Recently, he has been studying the evolving use of computers in higher education, using the video case study as his preferred methodology (*The Electronic Classroom in Higher Education,* NCRIPTAL). He thinks the medium of electronic text and graphics (computers) presents unique challenges to educators because of the subtle differences between print and electronic media (*Electronic Information: Literacy Skills for a Computer Age,* NCRIPTAL).

KATHY KELLERMANN (Ph.D., Northwestern University, 1983) is currently on the faculty of Michigan State University. Her research interests include interaction analysis focusing on the relationship between thought and talk.

DAVID R. MAINES (Ph.D., University of Missouri, 1973) is Associate Professor in the Department of Sociology at Pennsylvania State University. His areas of interest include interpersonal relations, gender and the life course, and social organization. He has recently coedited, with Carl J. Couch, *Communication and Social Structure* and is at work on *Time and Social Process.*

GERALD R. MILLER (Ph.D., University of Iowa, 1961) is Professor and Chair, Department of Communication, Michigan State University. The author of numerous articles and books in areas such as interpersonal communication, persuasion, and legal communication, he is a past editor of *Human Communication Research* and *Speech Monographs.* He is a past President of ICA, and is a Fellow of ICA and of the American Psychological Association.

J. DOUGLAS ORTON (M.A., Brigham Young University, 1985) is a doctoral student who has done graduate work in organization studies at Brigham Young University, the University of Texas at Austin, and the University of Michigan. He has studied contradictory innovation strategies within computer companies, satire as organizational communication, loose coupling, and organizational downsizing.

SYED A. RAHIM (Ph.D., Michigan State University, 1968) has worked for the planning commission in Bangladesh, and is currently a research associate at the Institute of Culture and Communications, East-West Center, Honolulu. His current research interest is the cultural construction of knowledge and communication in development.

WILLIAM K. RAWLINS (Ph.D., Temple University, 1981) is Associate Professor of Communication at Purdue University. His ongoing research concerns the communicative achievement and management of friendship across the life course. He is also interested in the reflexive quality of social inquiry and the necessity of linking its processes and products to broader contexts to appraise their significance.

RONALD E. RICE (Ph.D., Stanford University, 1982) received his B.A. in English literature from Columbia University and his M.S. in communication research from Stanford University. In between, he worked for a publishing firm in New York, was a faculty member of an international school in Rome, and was a communication analyst and data processing manager of a statewide bank in Virginia. He has published in the fields of telecommunications policy, organizational communication systems, network analysis, the diffusion of innovations, and popular music. He is coeditor or coauthor of *Public Communication Campaigns* (Sage, 1981), *The New Media: Communication, Research, and Technology* (Sage, 1984), *Managing Organizational Innovation* (Columbia University, 1987), and *Research Methods for the Study of New Media* (Free Press, 1988). He is Assistant Professor at the Annenberg School of Communications, University of Southern California.

MICHAEL E. ROLOFF (Ph.D., Michigan State University, 1975) is Professor of Communication Studies at Northwestern University. His research interests include social exchange within intimate relationships, persuasion, interpersonal conflict resolution, and bargaining and negotiation. He wrote *Interpersonal Communication: The Social Exchange Approach*, and coedited *Persuasion: New Directions in Theory and Research* and *Interpersonal Processes: New Directions in Communication Research*, both with Gerald R. Miller, and *Social Cognition and Communication*, with Charles R. Berger.

ALLEN SCULT (Ph.D., University of Wisconsin, 1975) is Professor and Chair of the Department of Speech Communication at Drake University. His recent scholarship has focused on hermeneutics and scholarly conversation and the rhetorical analysis of Biblical texts. The two interests came together when he collaborated with Michael McGee and J. Kenneth Kuntz on a recently published essay, "Genesis and Power: An Analysis of the Biblical Story of Creation" (*Quarterly Journal of Speech*, Vol. 72, May 1986, pp. 113-131).

JAN SERVAES (Ph.D., Leuven University, Belgium) is working on international communications at the Department of Mass Communication, Catholic University of Nijmegen, The Netherlands. In 1987-1988 he was in the United States as a Fulbright Scholar. He has taught at the Catholic University of Leuven, Belgium, and Thammasat University, Thailand. He is the author of six books in Dutch and two in English, and has written numerous articles for international journals.

CARRA SLEIGHT is a Ph.D. candidate at Michigan State University. Her primary interest focuses on the impact of cognition on communication in a variety of settings. Her current research concerns the effect of deception attributions on relational communication.

SLAVKO SPLICHAL (Ph.D., University of Ljubljana, 1979) is Professor and Head of the Department of Journalism and Centre for Social Communication Research at the Faculty of Sociology, Political Science and Journalism in Ljubljana, Yugoslavia, where he teaches communication theory and methodology. He is the president of the Yugoslav section of Mass Communication and Public Opinion Research, and a member of the International Council of the International Association for Mass Communication Research and of several editorial boards of journals in Yugoslavia and elsewhere. He has published a number of books and articles on communication theories, public opinion, political propaganda, advertising, media policy, and methods for communication research in Slovene, Serbo-Croat, English, Polish, French, and Spanish.

WILLIAM J. STAROSTA (Ph.D., Indiana University, 1973) is Graduate Professor of Communication at Howard University, and editor of the *Howard Journal of Communications*, which focuses on analyses of communication and culture. He has conducted sponsored field research in India or Sri Lanka three times. Reports on his research on rhetoric and social change in rural Third World campaigns and on related matters of persuasion and culture/ethnicity have appeared in a variety of journals and collections over a 20-year period.

MICHAEL SUNNAFRANK (Ph.D., Michigan State University, 1979) is Associate Professor of Speech Communication at Texas A&M University. His research interests are in the areas of interpersonal communication, social cognition, and the dynamics of personal relationships.

STELLA TING-TOOMEY (Ph.D., University of Washington, 1981) is Associate Professor at Arizona State University. Her research focuses on cross-cultural conflict styles in interpersonal relationships. Her most recent books include *Culture and Interpersonal Communication*, with William Gudykunst and Elizabeth Chua, and *Communication, Culture, and Organization Processes*, coedited with William Gudykunst and Lea Stewart.

TEUN A. VAN DIJK (Ph.D., University of Amsterdam, 1972) is Professor of Discourse Studies at the University of Amsterdam. After earlier work in literary theory, text grammar, and the cognitive psychology of text processing, his more recent research focuses on social, psychological, and critical aspects of discourse, with special interest in the reproduction of racism in various types of discourse, and in the structures and functions of news in the press. On these topics he has published many books, most in English, of which the most recent are *Strategies of Discourse Comprehension* (1983, with Walter Kintsch), *Prejudice in Discourse* (1984), *Handbook of Discourse Analysis* (1985, 4 Vols.), *Communicating Racism* (1987), *News as Discourse* (1988) and *News Analysis* (1988). He is cofounder and present editor of *TEXT*.

KARL E. WEICK (Ph.D., Ohio State University, 1962) is Rensis Likert Collegiate Professor of Organizational Behavior and Psychology at the University of Michigan. Since graduating from Ohio State, he has been associated with faculties at Purdue University, the University of Minnesota, Cornell University, and the University of Texas. He has also held short-term faculty appointments at the University of Utrecht in the Netherlands, Wabash College, Carnegie-Mellon University, Stanford University, and Seattle University. In addition to his work as editor of *Administrative Science Quarterly*, he is on the editorial boards of *Contemporary Psychology, Small Group Behavior, Organizational Behavior Teaching Review, The Journal for the Theory of Social Behavior*, and *Accounting, Organizations and Society*. He studies and writes about such topics as how people make sense of confusing events, the effects of stress on thinking and imagination, techniques for observing complicated events, self-fulfilling prophecies, the consequences of indeterminacy in social systems, the craft of applying social science, substitutes for rationality, determinants of effective managerial performance, high reliability organizations, and the management of professionals.

RUTH WODAK (Ph.D., University of Vienna, 1974) was born in 1950 in London. She is Professor of Studies in Slavic Languages, Eastern European History, and Linguistics at the University of Vienna. Since 1983 she has been full Professor for Applied Linguistics at the University of Vienna. Her research interests include socio- and psycholinguistics and discourse analysis (class and sex-specific language behavior, language minorities, mass communication, therapeutic discourse, legal discourse, doctor-patient discourse, and language and ideology). She has published nine books and more than 80 articles in these fields.

NOTES

For Product Safety Concerns and Information please contact our EU
representative GPSR@taylorandfrancis.com
Taylor & Francis Verlag GmbH, Kaufingerstraße 24, 80331 München, Germany

www.ingramcontent.com/pod-product-compliance
Ingram Content Group UK Ltd.
Pitfield, Milton Keynes, MK11 3LW, UK
UKHW022208190926
475702UK00003B/265
* 9 7 8 0 4 1 5 8 7 3 2 0 8 *